Preschool and School-Age Language Disorders

First Edition

Betsy Partin Vinson, M.Med.Sc., CCC/SLP

Clinical Associate Professor
University of Florida

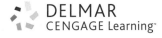

DELMAR
CENGAGE Learning

Australia • Brazil • Japan • Korea • Mexico • Singapore • Spain • United Kingdom • United States

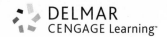

DELMAR
CENGAGE Learning™

Preschool and School-Age Language Disorders, First Edition
Betsy Partin Vinson, M.Med.Sc., CCC/SLP

Vice President, Editorial: Dave Garza

Director of Learning Solutions: Matthew Kane

Senior Acquisitions Editor: Sherry Dickinson

Managing Editor: Marah Bellegarde

Product Manager: Laura J. Wood

Editorial Assistant: Anthony R. Souza

Vice President, Marketing: Jennifer Baker

Marketing Director: Wendy E. Mapstone

Associate Marketing Manager: Jonathan Sheehan

Content Project Management: PreMediaGlobal

Production Director: Carolyn Miller

Senior Art Director: David Arsenault

Compositor: PreMediaGlobal

For product information and technology assistance, contact us at
Cengage Learning Customer & Sales Support, 1-800-354-9706

For permission to use material from this text or product, submit all requests online at **www.cengage.com/permissions.**
Further permissions questions can be e-mailed to
permissionrequest@cengage.com

Library of Congress Control Number: 2011922485

ISBN-13: 978-1-4354-9312-4

ISBN-10: 1-4354-9312-5

Delmar
5 Maxwell Drive
Clifton Park, NY 12065-2919
USA

Cengage Learning is a leading provider of customized learning solutions with office locations around the globe, including Singapore, the United Kingdom, Australia, Mexico, Brazil, and Japan. Locate your local office at:
international.cengage.com/region

Cengage Learning products are represented in Canada by Nelson Education, Ltd.

To learn more about Delmar, visit **www.cengage.com/delmar**

Purchase any of our products at your local college store or at our preferred online store **www.cengagebrain.com**

Printed in the United States of America
1 2 3 4 5 6 7 15 14 13 12 11

Dedication

This book is dedicated to my father, Clyde Partin, Sr.,
who passed away June 16, 2009.

He taught me to love the game of baseball, to work hard, to do my best,
and most importantly to believe in myself. He was a role model for and an
inspiration to our family, to his students at Emory University, where he taught for
over 50 years, and to all who knew him. He taught me that, as Ralph Waldo
Emerson said, "The secret to education is to respect the pupil."

He continues to be loved and is sorely missed.

Contents

CHAPTER 9   **Language-Based Learning Disabilities in the School-Age Population   387**

CHAPTER 10   **Spelling and Reading Disorders   441**

Preface

Preschool and School-Age Language Disorders is an introductory undergraduate textbook designed to create a basic understanding of language disorders in children. It is hoped that this understanding will serve as the foundation for a continuing curiosity about communication disorders. A wide variety of pediatric communication differences, delays, and disorders are presented from the perspectives of causes and defining characteristics, in a format that facilitates the student's understanding of these aspects of communication disorders. Differences related to multicultural aspects of language and communication are incorporated into the text, as well as delays and disorders related to developmental language deficits, language-learning disabilities, reading disorders, attention deficit disorders, and traumatic brain injuries.

The primary objective of this book is to provide the undergraduate student with an overview of pediatric language differences, delays, and disorders. Basic knowledge of language development and neuroanatomy is assumed, as topics related to these areas of the communication sciences are addressed throughout the book. High school students who are considering entering the profession of speech-language pathology may also find that this book provides an overview of the types of childhood language deficits with which our profession works. I hope that by studying this book, the student will gain the desire to explore and integrate continuing study of language disorders from three perspectives: the researcher's, the clinician's, and the academician's.

Organization of the Text

Chapter 1 focuses on delays, disorders, and differences and the classification of language deficits in children. This includes providing a framework for analyzing pediatric language disorders based on the features of language—semantics, syntax, phonology, morphology, and pragmatics. Included in this chapter is information about the impact of poverty on the development of language. The content of Chapter 2 includes syndromes that have language delays and disorders as part of their characteristics, as well as a section addressing the effects of alcohol, illegal drugs, and nicotine on the developing fetus. Chapter 3 is dedicated to a discussion of language delays and disorders seen in children on the autism spectrum. Chapter 4 focuses on factors in preschool language development and deficits that could impact future academic and social abilities and on how to "set the stage" for good outcomes when young children enter school. Chapters 5 and 6 provide an overview of the assessment and treatment of language disorders in preschool-aged children.

Chapter 7 focuses on the federal legislation and case laws that affect delivery of speech-language pathology services in the public schools.

Implications of the legislation for speech-language pathologists and educational audiologists are provided.

Chapters 8 through 14 are dedicated to the school-aged child and adolescent. Because so many school districts rely on the labeling of disorders to determine a child's eligibility for services, these chapters are based on an etiological perspective. Chapter 8 covers language development in the school years and the impact of language deficits on school performance. Chapter 9 provides definitions of language-based learning disabilities and addresses curricular issues that may be affected by the presence of a language-based learning disability. Chapter 10 encompasses the effects of language deficits on reading and spelling, as well as their potential effect on school performance. Chapter 11 looks at the impact of attention deficit disorder (with or without hyperactivity) on language skills and academic performance. Although ADHD is not a language disorder, the impact it can have on language and learning is an area of increasing study in our field. In addition, there is high co-morbidity of ADHD with language-based learning disabilities, which is another reason I believe it warrants attention in a book about language disorders. Chapter 12 addresses traumatic brain injury, an area that affects all ages. I included this chapter because the highest incidence of brain injury is in the adolescent population. Chapters 13 and 14 address assessment and treatment considerations in the school-aged population.

Appendices A and B provide reading lists the reader can use to increase his or her knowledge of preschool (Appendix A) and school-age (Appendix B) language delays and disorders. Appendix C lists additional readings on cultural influences on speech and language development. Appendix D lists memoirs, biographies, and autobiographies of individuals with communication disorders. It is a list of books about the impact of lifelong language delays and disorders such as cognitive impairments, autism spectrum disorders, and learning disabilities on children and adults. Even though this book focuses on preschool and school-aged children, I believe it is important to read about adults living with these disorders, so I included adult-focused books as well. It is my hope that the students (and professionals) who interact with persons who have communication disorders will read these books to learn more about the *personal* impact having a communication disorder can have on day-to-day life. Finally, Appendix E is the key to the answers for the review questions at the end of each chapter.

Features of the Book

Marginal notes highlight the vocabulary introduced in each chapter. The Think About It questions encourage students to think "outside the box" and apply their knowledge to real-life situations. Think About Its pose questions, some theoretical, some philosophical, some ethical, and some involving personal reflection about various issues and situations we face as speech-language pathologists and audiologists working with children who have communication deficits.

Illustrative case studies appear at the end of each chapter. Learning objectives are presented at the beginning of each chapter, and review questions at the end of each chapter. Illustrations and tables expand upon and clarify information in the text. Appendices provide a wide range of resources related to language deficits in each of the age categories of the book.

Author Acknowledgements

This book does not pretend to be a scientific approach to the study of language delays, disorders, and differences. It is clinically based on my experiences, research, and literature reviews over the last 34 years as a speech-language pathologist. I am indebted to those who have taught me so much about language deficits throughout my educational and professional career. This includes my professors at Emory University, my colleagues over the years, the students I have taught, and the many children and families I have had the opportunity to serve. I am also grateful to those who have taught me life skills, including patience and perseverance. These people include my parents—my late father, Clyde, to whom this book is dedicated, and Betty Partin, my mother. My husband, Tim, and my three children, Elizabeth, Jennifer, and Will, have been a source of support and encouragement, particularly Elizabeth who was a tremendous help in tracking down references. I would also like to acknowledge Laura Wood, Biswa Jyoti Sur, Daniel Nighting, and all those I do not know whom she has enlisted for their support and guidance in this project. I would also like to acknowledge and thank three of my graduate students, Liz Duda, Kristen Lewandowski, and Liz Mazzochi, for their contribution of the case study in the autism chapter. Thanks are also extended to the anonymous reviewers who had many helpful hints along the way. All these individuals had a vision; I hope that I have been able to fulfill that vision and that you, the undergraduate student, will benefit from this book.

Betsy Partin Vinson, M.Med.Sc., CCC/SLP
Clinical Associate Professor
University of Florida

REVIEWERS

S. Jay Kuder, Ed.D
Professor and Chair
Rowan University
Glassboro, NJ

Paula R. McGuire, Ph.D., CCC/SLP
Clinic Director
Northwestern University
Evanston, IL

Martha L. Smith, Ph.D, CCC/SLP
Clinical Professor
East Carolina University
Greenville, NC

Marianna Walker, Ph.D., CCC/SLP
Associate Professor
East Carolina University
Greenville, NC

Chapter 1

Delays, Disorders, and Differences

1

LEARNING OBJECTIVES

After completion of this chapter, the reader will be able to:

1. Explain the differences between a language delay, a language disorder, and a language difference.

2. Differentiate between linguistic competence and linguistic performance.

3. Discuss the role of cognition in the development and organization of language.

4. Describe the role of the listener in the development and interpretation of a child's language.

5. Discuss the impact of socio-economic status and the mother's level of education on a child's language development.

6. Explain the theoretical basis for the Bloom and Lahey model of language disorders.

7. Discuss the impact of cultural influences on storytelling.

INTRODUCTION

Language delay. The acquisition of normal language competencies at a slower rate than would be expected given the child's chronological age and the level of functioning.

Language disorder. A disruption in the learning of language skills and behaviors. It typically includes language behaviors that would not be considered part of normally developing linguistic skills.

When discussing disturbances of language functioning in preschool children, it is necessary to distinguish among a language delay, a language disorder, and a language difference. Briefly, a language delay can be defined as the acquisition of normal language competencies at a slower rate than would be expected given the child's chronological age and level of functioning. For example, a child who does not speak his first word until 24 months (instead of 10–12 months) or combine words until 36 months (instead of by 24 months) would have a delay.

As defined by the American Speech-Language-Hearing Association (ASHA), a language disorder is "impaired comprehension and/or use of spoken, written, and/or other symbol systems. The disorder may involve (1) the form of language (phonology, morphology, syntax); (2) the content of language (semantics); and/or (3) the function of language in communication (pragmatics) in any combination" (ASHA, 1993). A child who has a language disorder uses language behaviors that would not be considered part of normally developing linguistic skills. An example of this is found in the case study at the end of this chapter. When a delay extends into the early elementary school–age years, it may appear as a language disorder. This is further discussed in Chapter 6. However, a language disorder may be diagnosed during any point in life, depending on a variety of etiological factors.

As discussed by Bloom and Lahey (1978), this aberration of development differs from normal development in terms of the actual behaviors demonstrated by the child, the sequence in which aspects of language are learned, and the rate at which they are learned. The breakdown of the definition of language disorders into the components of language is a major topic in this first chapter.

Finally, language difference is the term applied to language behaviors and skills that are not in concert with those of a person's primary speech community or native language. ASHA defines language difference as "a variation of a symbol system used by a group of individuals that reflects and is determined by shared regional, social, or cultural/ethnic factors. A regional, social, or cultural/ethnic variation of a symbol system should not be considered a disorder of speech or language" (ASHA, 1993). Language differences exist owing to unfamiliarity with a language or to cultural variations of the person's native language. Individuals who speak English as a second language may experience instances in which lack of familiarity with English impairs a communicative exchange. In such instances the language is considered different, but not disordered or delayed.

Another semantic dichotomy that a clinician must understand is the difference between linguistic competence and linguistic performance as it relates to delays, disorders, and differences (Bloom & Lahey, 1978). Both of these aspects of language must be considered in terms of the person's native language as well as any cultural setting in which he or she may be. Linguistic competence refers to the language user's underlying knowledge about the system of rules of the language he or she is using to communicate in any given setting. It is the understanding a person has of the operating principles needed to use language in a functional manner, whether it is the person's native language or not. Linguistic performance, on the other hand, refers to the utilization of the child's or adult's linguistic knowledge in daily communication. Whether an individual (of any age) is described as having a language delay, a language disorder, or a language difference, the assessment of language skills must address his or her linguistic competence, what he knows about communicating, and linguistic performance, how he communicates.

Language difference. Language behaviors and skills that are not in concert with those of the person's primary speech community or native language.

Linguistic competence. The language user's underlying knowledge about the system of rules of the language he or she is using to communicate.

Linguistic performance. The utilization of the person's linguistic knowledge in daily communication.

WHO IS AT RISK?

There are numerous factors that can place a child at risk for developing a language delay or a disorder. Some of these are intrinsic factors (i.e., biological or "within" the child), and some are extrinsic (i.e., environmental). In the ASHA position statement on *Learning Disabilities and the Preschool Child*, at-risk indicators "refer(s) to biological, genetic, and perinatal events as well as adventitious diseases or trauma that are known to be associated with adverse developmental

TABLE 1–1 Factors that put a child at risk for developmental delay

1. Serious concerns expressed by a parent, primary caregiver, or professional regarding the child's development, parenting style, or parent–child interaction.
2. Parent or primary caregiver with chronic or acute mental illness, developmental disability, or mental retardation.
3. Parent or primary caregiver with drug or alcohol dependence.
4. Parent or primary caregiver with a developmental history of loss and/or abuse.
5. Family medical or genetic history characteristics.
6. Parent or primary caregiver with severe or chronic illness.
7. Acute family crisis.
8. Chronically disturbed family interaction.
9. Parent-child or caregiver-child separation.
10. Adolescent mother.
11. Parent has four or more preschool-age children.
12. The presence of one or more of the following: parental education less than ninth grade; neither parent is employed; single parent.
13. Physical or social isolation and/or lack of adequate social support.
14. Lack of stable residence, homelessness, or dangerous living conditions.
15. Family inadequate health care or no health insurance.
16. Limited prenatal care.
17. Maternal prenatal substance abuse or use.
18. Severe prenatal complications.
19. Severe perinatal complications.
20. Asphyxia.
21. Very low birth weight (<1,500 g).
22. Small for gestational age (<10th percentile).
23. Excessive irritability, crying, and tremulousness on the part of the infant.
24. Atypical or recurrent accidents on the part of the child.
25. Chronic otitis media.

Source: Communication intervention: Birth to three, by L. M. Rossetti, pp. 5–6. Copyright 1996 by Delmar, Cengage Learning.

outcomes" (ASHA, 1987). Many factors, ranging from syndromes to the education level of the mother, can be risk factors. Table 1–1 lists several factors that place a child at risk for developmental delay.

An indicator that a child may be at risk is the late development of speech and language. Reviewing the research literature, Plante and Beeson

(2004) define late talkers as "young children (between approximately 16 and 30 months) whose language skills fall below 90 percent of their age peers. These children are slow to acquire their first fifty words and slow to combine words into phrases" (p. 177). Some, but not all, children do eventually reach the language and speech levels of their age peers. But, frequently, late talkers have none of the risk factors cited earlier in this section, yet they experience language deficits as they mature. Numerous studies and reports have shown that children with preschool language delays often present learning disabilities, autism spectrum disorders, or attention deficit disorders when they reach school age (Hagberg, Miniscalco, & Gillberg, 2010; ASHA, 2009; NEILS, 2007; NJCLD, 2007; Snowling, Bishop, & Stothard, 2006; Woods & Wetherby, 2003; Snowling, Adams, Bishop, & Stothard, 2001; Bishop & Edmundson, 1987; ASHA, 1987).

The National Early Intervention Longitudinal Study (NEILS, 2007) was sponsored by the Office of Special Education Programs (OSEP) of the U.S. Department of Education to analyze the birth–3 intervention programs established in accordance with Part C of the Individuals with Disabilities Education Act (see Chapter 7). The study focused on four questions:

1. Who are the children and families served through Part C?

2. What early intervention services do participating children and families receive?

3. What outcomes do participating children and families experience?

4. How do outcomes relate to variations in child and family characteristics and services received? (p. 1).

The study gathered outcome data on "developmental accomplishments in the domains of functional mobility; independence in feeding, dressing, and toileting; expressive and receptive communication; and object and social play" (p. 2). Speech and communication problems were the most prevalent reasons for referral for early intervention (41 percent). Other reasons were pre- and perinatal problems (19 percent), motor delays (17 percent), and overall delay (12 percent). The study also noted that "children with developmental delays related to language and communication" are rarely identified before 12–18 months, and 75 percent of the children entering early intervention after the age of 24 months had some variant of a speech or communication problem (p. 2–3).

Another factor that can impact the development of speech and language is socio-economic status. Many children who are raised in impoverished conditions frequently do not have the wide variety of experiences needed to develop a versatile and comprehensive language. Infants of teenage mothers are often at risk for language problems due to socio-economic deprivation. Often the adolescent mothers themselves are from single-parent homes (NEILS, 2007). Statistics from the Children's Defense Fund indicate that 25 percent of today's adolescents are living in a single-parent home. "Black adolescents are twice as likely as white adolescents to live with one parent and four times

TABLE 1–2   Risk factors exacerbated by persistent poverty (Polakow, 1993)

Teen-age pregnancy
Premature birth
Poor health
Inadequate nutrition
Lack of housing
Instability in family relationships
Later school failure

Delmar/Cengage Learning.

as likely to live not with a parent at all but with some other relative" (Polakow, 1993, p. 76). Table 1–2 lists risk factors exacerbated by persistent poverty.

It is important to note that 27 percent of the children enrolled in the early intervention programs established by Part C were from families with household incomes of less than $15,000 per year (21 percent of the general population of families with 3-year-old children have a comparable level of income; see Table 1–3). It is stated in the study that "poverty is one of the strongest predictors of poor developmental outcomes in children, and its co-occurrence with a delay or disability before age 3 suggests these children are especially in need of effective interventions" (p. 2–4).

Tied in with poverty is the education level of the mother. This factor is considered to have predictive value with regard to children's language abilities, particularly in relation to reading. This is discussed further in Chapter 10. However, the highest population of children in the Part C early intervention programs was children of mothers with a GED or high school

TABLE 1–3   Household income of children enrolled in Part C early intervention programs

Income Level	% in EI Population	% in General Population*
$15,000 or less	27	21
$15,001–$25,000	16	16
$25,001–$50,000	29	31
$50,001–$75,000	16	16
Over $75,000	13	16

*General population data from National Household Education Survey (1999) for children up to 3 years of age.

Source: Data compiled from *Early Intervention for Infants and Toddlers with Disabilities and Their Families: Participants, Services, and Outcomes,* January 2007, pp. 2–7.

TABLE 1–4 Education level of mothers of children enrolled in Part C early intervention programs

Education Level	% in Education Level Population	% in General Population*
Less than a high school degree	16	17
GED or high school degree	32	27
Some college	28	28
Bachelor's degree or higher	24	27

*General population data from National Household Education Survey (1999) for children up to 3 years of age.

Source: Data compiled from *Early Intervention for Infants and Toddlers with Disabilities and Their Families: Participants, Services, and Outcomes,* January 2007, pp. 2–7.

degree. A breakdown of the population based on the mother's education level is shown in Table 1–4.

While it is difficult to predict which children will continue to have language problems as they get older, some factors under consideration as having predictive power are limited vocabulary, poor use of gestures to augment communication, lack of conventional gestures, poor comprehension skills, social and communication impairments, lack of joint attention, and lack of symbolic play (NEILS, 2007; Woods & Wetherby, 2003; Thal, Bates, Goodman, & Jahn-Samilo, 1997; Thal & Tobias, 1992). That is why it is so important that parents and other caregivers take advantage of opportunities in everyday life to develop and expand a child's language. An example of this is depicted in Figure 1–1. Early intervention is also critical in preventing the development of persistent speech, language, communication, and learning deficits. In an updated study of children served in Part C early intervention programs, Hebbeler (2010) provided statistics with regard to the percentage of children enrolled in the programs with a primary diagnosis of hearing impairment or speech or communication problems (see Table 1–5).

The percentage of children receiving speech-language pathology services in the early intervention programs was 53 percent, second only to the general category of "service coordinator," which was at 63 percent. The next highest percentage of service was held by physical therapy and occupational therapy, with both of these together providing services to 38 percent of the children. The average length of service for children who only had speech or communication problems was 9.7 months. This may be low (it was the lowest length of service of all the programs) because many of these children were not identified until after 24 months of age.

As discussed in Chapter 7, a primary goal of the provision of federally funded early intervention programs is to decrease the number of students who need special education services when they enter school. However, according

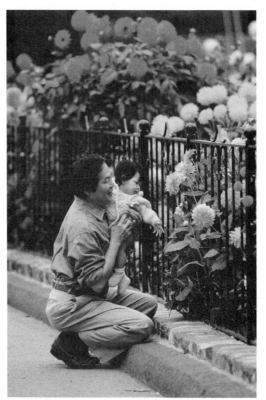

FIGURE 1–1 A variety of opportunities are needed to facilitate language development. A trip to a garden provides opportunities to stimulate the senses as well as to expand a child's language by exposing him or her to a variety of colors, smells, and textures. (*Delmar/Cengage Learning.*)

TABLE 1–5 Percentage of children enrolled in Part C early intervention programs with Hearing Impairment or speech/communication problems as primary diagnosis

Age When First Enrolled	Hearing Impairment	Speech/ Communication
0 to less than 12 months	2%	5%
12 to less than 24 months	2.3%	48.5%
24 to 36 months	1.5%	75.4%

Source: Data compiled from *Characteristics of children served in Part C.* PowerPoint presentation by Kathy Hebbeler, 2010.

to the 2007 report of the NEILS project, 63 percent of the children who received the Part C early intervention services until they were 36 months old still needed special education services in the public schools.

> **think about it**
>
> In what ways would you expect the education level of the mother in the household to impact her child's language development?

LANGUAGE DEVELOPMENT

Robert Owens (1984) delineated five principles that must be considered when describing the development of language and communication in infants:

1. Development is predictable.

2. Developmental milestones are attained at about the same age in most children.

3. Developmental opportunity is needed.

4. Children go through developmental changes or periods.

5. Individuals differ greatly. (Rossetti, 1986, p. 18)

While it is not the intent of this book to provide a treatise on language development, a brief review of philosophies dedicated to explaining the growth of language in a child is offered. The reader is referred to the reference list at the end of this chapter for in-depth resources addressing the broad scope of language development and to further study the components of each of the theories mentioned in this section.

McLaughlin (1998) describes two approaches to the study of language development. One is to describe the sequence of language acquisition based on normative development. The other approach addresses the question of how language develops, looking at the underlying processes and mechanisms. McLaughlin refers to various "-isms" when exploring the question of how language develops. One of these "-isms" is nativism. Those who are proponents of this school of thought believe that when a child is born, he or she has the capacity to learn all the language aspects, and that the knowledge of language comes to fruition as the child matures biologically. This viewpoint closely ties in with the "nature" side of the "nature versus nurture" philosophy of child development. McLaughlin cites Parker and Riley (1994) in saying that language development is inherent in a child's genetic makeup or nature. The concept of nativism is often associated with mentalism, which also holds that "knowledge primarily derives from inborn mental processes" (McLaughlin, 1998, p. 129). Those who ascribe to the nativism theory

Nativism. The idea that the capacity to develop language is innate, with language knowledge coming to fruition as the child matures biologically.

Mentalism. Often associated with nativism, the mentalism philosophy posits that one's knowledge is derived from innate mental processes.

believe that the structure of language is independent of the use of language (Hulit & Howard, 2002).

Nativism is on the opposite side of theories of language development from the empirical perspective, which holds that children are genetically equipped to learn, but the individual is not born with the knowledge he or she gains over the life span. Empiricism and behaviorism embrace the nurture side of the argument with regard to what constitutes the process of developing language (McLaughlin, 2006). Behaviorists and empiricists tend to believe that children are relatively passive in their language acquisition, and that "their emerging language is determined not by self-discovery or creative experimentation but by the selective reinforcements received from their speech and language models" (Hulit & Howard, 2002). Arguments can be made for the role of nature and the role of nurture in a child's development of language. McLaughlin (2006) points out that most researchers favor a compromise between nature and nurturing. This compromise is referred to as interactionism. Proponents of interactionism ask, "What is the nature of the interaction between children's genetic makeup and their experiences that results in language learning?" (McLaughlin, 2006, p. 129).

Piaget put forth a model based on the interaction between cognition and language called the cognitive theory. Piaget believed that nurture, not nature, played the primary role in the development of language. He paid particular attention to the ages of birth to 2 years, a period of tremendous development of cognition and, coincidentally, speech and language. Hulit and Howard (2002) summarize this relationship as follows:

> It should be noted that all theorists accept that a relationship exists between cognitive development and language development. What separates cognitive theorists from others is their belief that language does not hold an absolutely unique position in overall development. They believe that language itself is not innate, even though the cognitive precursors for language are innate. (p. 33)

Cognitive theorists also believe that language is a result of cognitive development and organization. It is not genetically preordained, nor is it structured around learning principles. Rather, these theorists believe that language is rooted in environmental opportunities and cognitive processes, and that language is one ability, among others, that is developed for the manipulation and representation of concepts the child has learned (Hulit & Howard, 2002).

Other researchers and practitioners look at language development in terms of the features of language (form, content, and use). Noam Chomsky strongly believed that the capacity to learn language is innate and developed a theory that he called transformational generative grammar (TGG). TGG refers to Chomsky's belief that there are rules, or transformations, that govern how syntactic components of our language are combined. TGG is based on

Empiricism. The belief that a child's language is not innate but develops as a result of experiences.

Behaviorism. Like empiricism, the belief that a child's language is not innate but develops when verbalizations are positively reinforced.

Transformational generative grammar (TGG). A theory of rules, or transformations, that govern how syntactic components of our speech are combined to express language.

linguistic universals and the language acquisition device. Linguistic universals are the shared principles that underlie the variety of languages and form the foundation for a relatively universal structure of language. For example, all languages have a basic subject/predicate structure of language, and a method for negation. In keeping with the belief that there are certain universals in language, Chomsky's theory holds that language structure is an innate capacity specific to human beings (McLaughlin, 2006; Gleason, 2005).

Chomsky also proposed the concept of a language acquisition device (LAD) that serves as the neurological foundation for language development. The LAD is not a specific structure in the brain; rather it is a means of looking at the neurological network responsible for language development in children, even in the absence of input from adults in the child's world. Chomsky (1965) further maintained that the LAD is unique to humans. The LAD was reconceptualized as universal grammar (UG) in Chomsky's later works (Steinberg, 1993). Universal grammar is based on the belief that there are general rules and categories of grammar common to all languages (Gleason, 2005).

Chomsky's propositions are grouped together as the psycholinguistic theory. The psycholinguistic theory, which explains the relationship between language form and cognitive processing, helps us to understand the syntactic component of language. Chomsky, the leading proponent of the psycholinguistic theory, described language from an innate, rule-governed, psychological perspective and argued that universal linguistic rules of grammar underlie language acquisition. A child's knowledge of linguistic rules allows him or her to understand and generate language.

A more recent theory of grammar proposed by Chomsky (1982) is known as government and binding theory (GB). The components of GB are represented in Figure 1–2, and below is a brief definition of each component. Chomsky maintained that grammatical theories must be universal (apply to all languages) and recognize that all children learn grammar without being "taught."

The components depicted in Figure 1–2 can be defined as follows:

- D-structure: the relationship between units of grammar

- S-structure: how words are organized in a sentence

- Phonetic forms: sounds of a language

- Logical forms: bring semantics into the picture

- Phrase structure rules: rules governing the placement of clauses within a sentence

- Lexicon: the syntactic, morphological, and phonological aspects of each word

- Lexical category: nouns and verbs

- Functional category: syntax (grammar) (Gleason, 2005; Chomsky, 1982).

Linguistic universals. The shared principles that underlie the variety of languages and form the foundation for a relatively universal structure of language.

Language acquisition device (LAD). The LAD is not a specific structure, but rather a conglomeration of innate capacities of language that governs the input and output of language form.

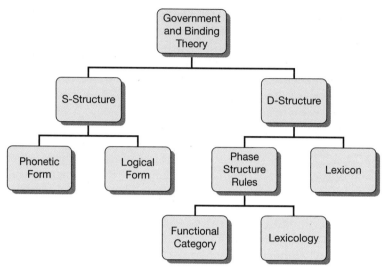

FIGURE 1–2 Depiction of Chomsky's government and binding theory. (*Source:* Gleason, 2005; Chomsky, 1982.)

While Chomsky studied language and its development in terms of its structure, Fillmore (1968), Chafe (1970), and others sought to explain language development in terms of the content, or semantics, of language. One notion espoused by Fillmore is that of case grammar. Fillmore believed that the semantic deep structure of a sentence is formed prior to the syntactic representation of the sentence. He looked at language in terms of the basic relationships in a sentence. In Fillmore's model of case grammar, there is an effort to study the influence that semantics has on the structure of language. According to Fillmore, the relationship between nouns and verbs is determined by universal semantic concepts at a level beneath the deep structure (Hulit & Howard, 2002).

Fillmore further believed that there are two components to sentences. The first component is modality, which has to do with sentence characteristics such as negation, interrogation, and verb tense. The second component is proposition, which examines the relationship between nouns and verbs within a sentence. Fillmore maintained, "the relationship between the noun and verb in a given sentence determines the meaning underlying that sentence" (Hulit & Howard, 2002, p. 30). When contrasting Chomsky's and Fillmore's theories, it is important to note the role of cognition. In Chomsky's transformational generative grammar, cognition and interaction with the environment had no role in the development of language; rather, language required linguistic input only. In Fillmore's case grammar, language is based largely on the child's understanding of his experiences, with the revelation of cognition relying on language. This belief, cognitive determinism, is a driving force behind the model of language development

Modality. According to Fillmore, one of two components of sentences, which looks at the influence of semantics on grammar, particularly as applied to verb tense, the question form, and negation.

Proposition. According to Fillmore, the second component of a sentence, which regulates the relationship between nouns and verbs.

proposed by Bloom that is explained in further detail later in this chapter. Cognitive determinism denotes the belief that a child's knowledge of the world is expressed through his or her language, and that meaning precedes form (McLaughlin, 2006; Bloom & Lahey, 1978).

The connectionist theory of language development has received much attention in recent years. The proponents of this theory believe that language is innate, but, unlike previous theorists, do not believe there is a specific gene that is responsible for the development of grammar. Rather, they say, language development occurs in a neural network composed of "nodes" that store input from the environment. Also, linguistic input is stored in long-term memory, with the input heard more frequently being more likely to be stored there (Rumelhart & McClelland, 1986; Elman et al., 1996; Pinker, 1999; Lizardi, 2000). A third belief of connectionist theorists (as described by Lizardi, 2000) is that "language production is a solution to the problem of transferring multidimensional representations into a linear (monodimensional) string of words" (p. 7). As Pinker (1999) writes, "learning is impossible without innately organized circuitry to do the learning" (p. 210). Thus, connectionists maintain that language develops as the result of interaction between nature and nurture.

The first researchers to propose the connectionist theory were Rumelhart and McClelland (1986) when they set out to explain how children learn the past tense. They maintained that language is organized in a neural network of nodes, and that learning occurs when the nodes interconnect in a new way. The ability to develop unlimited interconnections is what allows us to continue to learn. Children can learn language without having to figure out all the rules; indeed, they do not even have to know that there are rules governing language.

Finally, a model of language development based on pragmatics, or use, of language was presented by Searle and is referred to as sociolinguistics. The concept of sociolinguistics is addressed in more detail in the section "Language Differences" in this chapter. In the theory of speech acts, the "social, emotional, and legal ramifications" (McLaughlin, 1998) of words are studied. As explained by the speech acts theory, the speaker's intent, or use, is focused on more than the speaker's word choices. Searle went on to delineate three types of intent: ordering, requesting, and asserting (Plante & Beeson, 2004). Speech acts are analyzed in terms of forces and components. The forces are propositional force, which is the literal meaning of a sentence, and the illocutionary force, which is the intention of the speech act. The three primary components of speech acts are words and propositions (otherwise known as the locutionary component of language), the intent (the illocutionary component), and the perlocutionary component, which is the listener's interpretation of the speech act (McLaughlin, 2006). The pragmatic theorists were the first to acknowledge the role that the listener plays in the development and interpretation of language.

Cognitive determinism. The belief that cognition relies on language for a child to understand his or her experiences; the child's knowledge of the world is expressed through his or her language, with meaning preceding form.

Sociolinguistics. The study of social and cultural influences on language structures.

Speech acts. In a communicative exchange, expressions verbalized by the speaker such as receiving information, giving information, or acknowledging an individual (greeting and departing words).

Propositional force. The literal meaning of a sentence.

Illocutionary force. The intention of a speech act.

think about it
Do you believe that nature or nurture has the greater impact on language development? Justify your choice.

LANGUAGE DELAYS

Some children develop language as described earlier, but later than one would consider to be within normal limits. Language behaviors related to delays can be characterized in five different ways. A wide range of normal development of language is exhibited across a wide demographic spectrum, and the speech-language pathologist needs to analyze this knowledge through application of the principles outlined by Owens. Without this knowledge as the foundation for studying language abnormalities, he or she cannot possibly understand the complexities inherent in the diagnosis and treatment of language delays, disorders, and differences. The first three categories of language delays represent degrees of difference in delays. The last two categories of language delays represent deviations from normal schedules and sequences that are rarely seen.

The first and most prevalent characterization of children's abnormal language is language delay (Shames, Wiig, & Secord, 1994). As stated in the introduction to this chapter, a child is considered to be language delayed if he or she exhibits normal language behaviors, but the language skills fall below those expected based on his or her chronological age and level of cognitive or intellectual functioning. In other words, everything he or she does typically would be observed in a normally developing child, and the behaviors are typically in the normal sequence of acquisition. However, the child with a language delay acquires these skills at a slower rate than would be expected given his or her age and other abilities. This delay can refer to the onset of usage of the language skill, the rate of progression through the acquisition process, the sequence in which the language skills are learned, or all of these (Bloom & Lahey, 1978).

A second type of delay occurs when a child exhibits a language delay with a plateau (Shames, Wiig, & Secord, 1994). Children in this category follow a normal sequence of acquisition of language skills but never acquire all of the skills expected for children of their age. That is to say, the child progresses up to a point but then levels off. If the acquisition of the language skills of such a child were charted, the child's learning curve would flatten out or plateau. For example, a child who develops language normally until 24 months of age but then fails to progress would be characterized as having plateaued at 24 months. He or she may have small bursts of improvement followed by another plateau or may remain at the 24-month level. It is also possible that, once the child starts to improve, improvement may continue until he or she has caught up with age-level peers. This kind of plateau could be the result of a physical illness, a trauma, or a psychological insult of some kind. However, not all plateaus are due to a developmental deficit or insult. Sometimes a plateau is indicative of progress in another area of development. For example, a child who is delayed in both speech and language skills and motor development may plateau in his or her speech and language development during periods of growth in motor skills. These types of plateaus occur because the immature central nervous system is unable to handle the simultaneous growth in two systems.

A third category of language abnormalities based on normal sequence and schedules describes children who exhibit significant language delay (Shames, Wiig, & Secord, 1994). Again, the child acquires linguistic features in the normal sequence, but tremendous discrepancies occur between the ages the features are acquired and the age at which they are integrated. Linguistic features that frequently coincide with increasing length and complexity of utterances may be delayed in acquisition. For example, a child whose language is categorized in this manner may acquire his or her first words around 28 months of age but may not combine words until he or she is 4 to 5 years of age.

Less frequently seen language abnormalities based on developmental schedules and sequences are the use of normal error patterns with unusual frequency or the use of unique language or phonological features that have never been documented as a normal part of acquisition (Shames, Wiig, & Secord, 1994). Both of these types of language patterns are seen relatively infrequently. An example of normal error patterns with unusual frequency would be the reversal of the position of two sounds in a word, a linguistic behavior known as metathesis. It is not uncommon for a child to mispronounce the word "animal" as "aminal," but with a good model he or she typically corrects the pronunciation in a relatively short period of time. If the child continues to do this reversal consistently for all similar combinations, with unusual frequency, or in many different combinations, it could indicate a language disorder. In the case described previously, the child would not make the correction and would continue to call animals "aminals."

> **Metathesis.** The reversal of the position of two sounds in a word (e.g., "aks" for "ask").

An example of the use of a unique language or phonological feature that has never been documented as a normal part of acquisition is documented in an unpublished thesis at the University of Florida (Schaffer, Dyson, & Vinson, 1989). The child, Edward, was born approximately 3 weeks early after a high-risk pregnancy. Developmental milestones were at the low end of the normal limits, but his speech attempts were essentially unintelligible. Edward had a speech pattern of using the phoneme /h/ for all consonants (See the case study at the end of this chapter). Clearly, Edward's pattern of speech was not a normal pattern of acquisition with regard to sequence or schedule.

think about it

Why is it important for a speech-language pathologist or audiologist to have in-depth knowledge of speech and language development?

LANGUAGE DISORDERS

Semantics. The knowledge and ideas a person has about the objects and events in the world that make up the content of language.

When analyzing linguistic competence, the clinician must look at the child's knowledge of language in terms of content, form, and use. The content domain includes semantics, meaning the knowledge and ideas children have about the objects and events in their world. The form domain consists of specific structures of language, including phonology, morphology, and syntax. Pragmatics, the broadest of the language domains, reflects the different uses, or functions, of language that the child communicates through language.

The following discussion of language deficits attributed to the features of language is based primarily on the work of Bloom and Lahey (1978). These two researchers define a language disorder as "a broad term to describe certain behaviors, or the lack of certain other behaviors, in a child that are different from the behaviors that might be expected considering the child's chronological age" (Bloom & Lahey, 1978, p. 290), and their study of language disorders is based on the following premises:

1. Objects have distinctive properties, including causality, action, time, location, possession, and object permanence.

2. It is necessary to have an understanding of object categories, object knowledge, object relations, and event relations.

3. There are two aspects of language use: language functions (interaction, regulation, control) and linguistic selection (choosing words to fulfill a function based on intent, perceptions of the listener, information sharing, and the situation).

In the Bloom and Lahey model of language development, all features of language are intertwined, so a deficit in one may be accompanied by, or result in, a deficit in another. These investigators also have developed models that represent the different types of language disorders related to the features of language. These models form the basis of the subsequent discussion in this section.

Children may have difficulty formulating ideas or conceptualizing information about the world (content); they may have difficulty learning a code to represent their knowledge (form); or they may learn a code that does not conform with that of their speech community or learn the conventional code but be unable to use it (use). In Figure 1–3, normal language is section D.

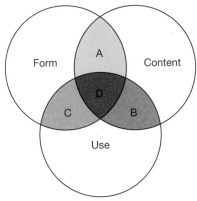

FIGURE 1–3 Bloom and Lahey's model of normal language. Complete development of the components and the interactions are denoted by the solid lines. (*Source:* Lahey, LANGUAGE DISORDERS AND LANGUAGE DEVELOPMENT, Figure 2-1 "The Interaction of Content/Form/Use in Language" p. 22, 1988. Reproduced by permission of Pearson Education, Inc.)

If the description of a child's language fell in area D, but later than expected, the child would exhibit a delay. Disordered language consists of a disruption within one or more of the three components or in the interaction among and between the components.

The Semantic Domain: Deficits in Content

Description of the Semantic Domain

Early semantic rules appear to be universal. Regardless of their native language, children learn that basic rules exist governing meaning and relationships between meaning units, and other rules exist that dictate the relationship of language form to objects and events, and to words and word combinations. We also know that children combine words cross-culturally in similar ways to express basic meaning. For example, children typically use agent + action, action + state, and attribute + object to govern their early word combinations, regardless of their native language.

According to Bloom and Lahey (1978), word meaning is made up of semantic features that characterize and define the word and selection restrictions that prohibit certain word combinations (redundancy). Using this definition of word meaning, synonyms are words with identical semantic features and antonyms are words with opposite semantic features. When faced with a word that has multiple meanings, the listener must rely on selection restrictions, linguistic context, and nonlinguistic context. For example, if I saw a football player showing off, I might say, "He is a real hot dog!" Using your knowledge of semantic features and selection restrictions, you would be able to understand that this is a metaphor, and that the football player is not actually a hot dog. However, if a child has semantic deficits, he or she may envision an actual hot dog without understanding that I meant the player was being pompously demonstrative.

Language is a fundamental way of representing experience. Therefore, experiences are needed for language development and enhancement. Conceptual development occurs when a child has the ability to organize cognitively many different experiences and to reorganize these concepts as more information is learned. When children are developing their semantic repertoires, it is not uncommon for them to identify several objects by one descriptor or name, based on other experiences with objects or events that have the same semantic features. A child who has been exposed primarily to dogs most likely will go through a stage in which he or she identifies all animals with four legs as dogs. However, as the child learns more about the animals and develops the restrictions that guide word selection in any given experience, he or she will begin to label animals by their correct names using conventional semantic categories. A child who was shown a Christmas tree in an office referred to it as a "hot flower." The mother explained that the child identified all trees and plants as flowers and used the word "hot" for all lights; hence, the "hot flower" in the lobby.

Another consideration in describing the concept of semantics is that a word may have two types of meaning. The first type is denotative meaning, which is the literal definition of a word as found in a dictionary. In contrast, connotative meaning is the meaning of a word based on emotional and/ or associative factors. Nicolosi, Harryman, and Kresheck (1996) provide an example of connotative meaning in the use of the word "pig." "Pig" can be literally, or denotatively, defined as a large, domesticated farm animal from which pork is derived. The connotative meaning of "pig" may refer to a sloppy individual or an unsavory character. Thus, the connotative meaning depends on an interpretation by the communication partners.

Children who have weaknesses in conceptual development (i.e., the development of ideas about the world, which make up the content of language) fall into the category of those with semantic deficits. A pure semantic deficit is rare because conceptual knowledge is necessary to develop form and use. Some research indicates that children who are blind may, early in their language development, have language disorders that are restricted to the semantic category (Bloom & Lahey, 1978). However, they usually outgrow their deficits when they learn to compensate for the sensory deficit. Children who have hydrocephalus also demonstrate semantic deficits in many cases. Children whose language could be illustrated using the drawing in Figure 1–4 would have more advanced form and use interactions than content interactions.

These children may speak in grammatically correct sentences but have little to say. The term "cocktail party speech," which is common in individuals with hydrocephaly, is an apt descriptor of content-specific disorders. Most interactions at cocktail parties consist of forms and uses that are appropriate for social interaction but are weak on content. Typically, a child with a

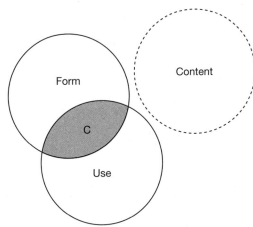

FIGURE 1–4   Bloom and Lahey's model of content disorders. Complete development of the components and the interactions are denoted by the solid lines; dashed lines represent incomplete development of the component, the interactions, or both. (*Source:* Lahey, LANGUAGE DISORDERS AND LANGUAGE DEVELOPMENT, Figure 2–2 "Disruption of Content" p. 24, 1988. Reproduced by permission of Pearson Education, Inc.)

semantic deficit may give commands and ask many questions. He or she may be extremely social and may even be described as verbally aggressive. Some children in this category may be echolalic, which means the child repeats, or echoes, what he or she hears spoken by others (Bloom & Lahey, 1978).

Disorders of Content

Clinically, children who have semantic deficits are slow in acquiring their first words and in subsequent vocabulary development. These children have difficulty in acquiring temporal and spatial relationships. Another clinical red flag that can be indicative of a semantic deficit or disorder is difficulty in grasping synonyms and antonyms (Lahey, 1988).

 How does a child develop knowledge of the world?

The Form Domain: Phonology, Syntax, and Morphology

Defining the Form Domain

Children who have form deficits may use gestures or early forms of communication, such as crying and cooing, because they have difficulty learning and using the conventional codes. Figure 1–5 shows a partial overlay of content and use with the separation of form. This is a graphic representation of how

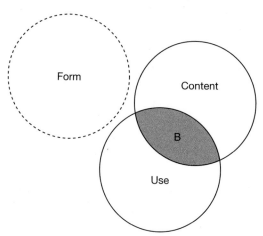

FIGURE 1–5 Bloom and Lahey's model of form disorders. (*Source:* Lahey, LANGUAGE DISORDERS AND LANGUAGE DEVELOPMENT, Figure 2–3 "Disruption of Form" p. 25, 1988. Reproduced by permission of Pearson Education, Inc.)

knowledge and ideas about the world's objects and events, and the abilities to communicate these ideas, may be intact, while the child's knowledge of the linguistic system for representing and communicating these ideas is impaired. Children who have difficulties acquiring word endings (such as *-ed, -ing, -er,* and *-est*) fall into this category, which Bloom and Lahey have designated as a disruption between form and content.

Phonology Deficits The form of the structures puts the knowledge children have about their world into words, phrases, and sentences. This aspect of language connects sounds with the conventional system of symbols. The first form component we will discuss is phonology. Phonological rules govern the distribution and sequencing or organization of phonemes (sounds) within a language. Children who have phonological deficits have difficulty establishing correct correspondences between the adult's and the child's linguistic forms. This may be evidenced in consistent misuse of specific phonemes despite being able to correctly articulate the sound. For example, the child may be able to say /s/, but when shown a saw will identify it as a "taw." Some children with phonological deficits may have more pervasive speech-motor difficulties, and the role the speech-motor deficits play in the phonological deficit needs to be clarified before a phonological approach is used as the basis for remediation.

Phonology. The distribution and sequencing or organization of phonemes within a language.

Syntax Deficits Syntax refers to the appropriate, rule-based ordering of words in connected discourse. Rules exist that govern word order, sentence organization, and the definition of relationships between words, word types (questions, passive voice, etc.), and word classes (nouns and verbs).

Syntax. Appropriate, rule-based ordering of words in connected discourse.

Clinically, syntactic deficits may manifest as depressed utterance length, the use of telegraphic speech, frequent word reversals, and problems with the auxiliary verb system. Around 18–20 months, children who are developing in a typical manner begin to combine words into two-word utterances with astounding accuracy with regard to syntax. For example, they may use verb–noun combinations such as "see kitty," adjective–noun combinations such as "dirty shoe," adverb–noun combinations like "more milk," or pronoun–verb combinations such as "I go." Children continue to progress, sometimes making errors such as omitting the subject of a sentence, as when saying, "Want cookie" instead of "I want (a) cookie" (Bernstein & Levey, 2009, p. 42). Over the next 2 years, through the emergence of noun phrases, verb phrases, adjectives, negations, and questions, form continues to develop and, by age 4.0 years, most children have adult-like syntax (Bernstein & Levey, 2009).

Morphology Deficits Morphemes are the smallest units of meaning that make up the grammar, or morphology, of language. They are the rules that modify meaning at the word level. Morphological deficits are demonstrated clinically as problems with prefixes, suffixes, verb tense, plurality, and word usage. Morphemes can be free or bound. Free morphemes can stand alone and have meaning (single words), while bound morphemes must be attached to words in order to have meaning. An example of a bound morpheme is the prefix -un. By itself, that prefix has no meaning; however, it gains meaning when attached to a word as in "undone." Thus, bound morphemes change the meaning of a word. Bound morphemes also may change the syntactic category of a word, as when -ly is added to an adjective and changes the word into an adverb (e.g., "glad" is an adjective that becomes an adverb when -ly is added) (Plante and Beeson, 2004).

> **Morphology.** Units of meaning that make up the grammar of language by modifying meaning at the word level.

In 1975, Brown studied the language development of three American English-speaking children, paying particular attention to their morphological endings and use of function words. Brown summed up the children's language by dividing it into six stages, matching a corresponding mean length of utterance (MLU) and approximate chronological age with each stage. These stages are summed up in Table 1–6. Furthermore, Brown described 14 obligatory morphemes. By "obligatory," Brown means that the use of these morphemes is required in order to develop adult-like forms of language.

Bernstein and Levey summed up these obligatory morphemes as found in Table 1–7.

think about it
How does a child's exposure to books affect his or her development of syntax and morphology?

TABLE 1–6 Brown's stages of language development

Stages	Characterized by	Features	Examples
Stage I MLU: 1.0–2.0 Age: 12–26 mos.	First words: semantic roles expressed in simple sentences	Single word utterances combining semantic roles	Naming significant objects, persons, and events in their daily experiences (*cup, spoon, Mommy, Daddy*, etc.). Agent + Action, Action + Object, Action + Location, Entity + Location, Entity + Attribute, Demonstrative + Attribute
Stage II MLU: 2.0–2.5 Age: 27–30 mos.	Modulation of meaning	Emerging of grammatical morphemes	Present progressive (*-ing*), prepositions (*in, on*), plural (*-s*), irregular past (e.g., *ran, ate*), possessive (*-s*), articles (*a, the*), regular past (*-ed*), third person regular, third person irregular, auxiliary and copula verbs (*is, are, was, were*)
Stage III MLU: 2.5–3.0 Age: 31–34 mos.	Development of sentence form	Noun phrase elaboration and auxiliary development	Noun phrases elaborated in subject and object positions (*Big boy running fast, Billy ate my cookie*); auxiliary verbs allowing more mature interrogatives and negatives
Stage IV MLU: 3.0–3.75 Age: 35–40 mos.	Emergence of complex sentences	Embedding sentence elements	Object noun phrase complements (*I know you are my friend*); bedded wh- questions (*I know who is hiding*); relative clauses (*I helped boy who is nice*)
Stage V MLU: 3.75–4.50 Age: 41–46 mos.	Emergence of compound sentences	Conjoining sentences	Conjoining two simple sentences (*I have a book and you have a toy*)

Source: Adapted from *A First Language: The Early Stages* by R. Brown, 1973. Cambridge, MA: Harvard University Press.

The Pragmatic Domain: Deficits in the Functional Use of Language

Defining Pragmatics

> **Pragmatics.** The social use and functions of language for communication.

Pragmatics refers to the social use of language. A person must have pragmatic competence in order to analyze and understand contexts in which language is used and the functions for which it is used. Language is used in a variety of ways for a variety of purposes, but a child with a pragmatic deficit will not be able to use language in context appropriately (see Table 1–8).

At a very early age, a child develops the ability to choose alternative structures to influence the listener and create change. Prior to the development of language, the child's communicative signals are expressed through

TABLE 1–7   Order of emergence of 14 grammatical morphemes*

Grammatical Morphemes	Examples	Age of Mastery (months)
1. Present progressive verb ending -ing	Mommy push*ing* Johnny throw*ing*.	19–28
2. Preposition *in*	Put *in* box.	27–30
3. Preposition *on*	Put *on* table.	27–30
4. Plurals (regular)(-s)	Eat cookies. More blocks.	24–33
5. Past irregular verbs (*came, fell, broke, went*)	He *went* outside. Johnny *broke* it.	25–46
6. Possessive noun ('s)	Jimmy's car. Mommy's coat.	26–40
7. Uncontractible copula (*be* as the main verb; *am, is, are, were, was*)	He *was* bad. They *are* good.	27–39
8. Articles (*a, the*)	Billy throw *the* ball. Give me *a* big hug.	28–46
9. Past regular (-ed)	He jump*ed*. She push*ed* me.	26–48
10. Third person singular regular	He cooks. Johnny goes.	26–46
11. Third person singular irregular	He *has* books. She *does* work.	28–50
12. Uncontractible auxiliary (*be* verbs preceding another verb: *am, is, are, was, were*)	The boys *are eating*. The baby *is crying*.	29–48
13. Contractible copula	I'*m* good. She'*s* nice.	29–49
14. Contractible auxiliary	I'*m* eating. She'*s* jumping. They'*re* playing.	30–50

*Used correctly 90 percent of time in obligatory contexts.

Source: From "Language Development: A Review" by Bernstein, D. K., & Levey, S. In *Language and Communication Disorders in Children* by D. K Bernstein and E. Tiegerman-Morris, pp. 28–100, copyright 2009. Allyn & Bacon.

cooing, crying, jargon, and echolalia as he or she attempts to establish and maintain contact with other people in his or her environment. As children mature, they learn why people speak and begin to use conventional language forms and content to effectively communicate their intentions.

Jargon. Correctly articulated utterances with appropriate prosody; typical of children aged 10–14 months; decreases as words emerge.

TABLE 1–8   Uses of language

Social	Greeting
Learning	Giving information
	Requesting information
Control	Turn-taking
	Initiating
	Maintaining
	Giving feedback

Source: Delmar/Cengage Learning.

Metalinguistic skills. Skills that form the basis for effective ability to think about language, thus allowing the interpretation of language.

In the early school years, children begin to develop metalinguistic skills, which form the foundation for effective pragmatic skills. Embedded in metalinguistic skills are the knowledge and interpretation of rules of language. For example, the child learns that a word is a word, it is made up of sounds, it can be defined, and it can be spoken and written.

Children who have pragmatic deficits learn the system to code ideas but have difficulty putting it into use.

Disorders of Use

The child with a disorder of use often talks about something that is out of context with the conversation or topic at hand. Some authors have described the interaction pattern as intrapersonal communication because the child rambles repetitively or tangentially with little regard for the listener (see Figure 1–6) (Bloom & Lahey, 1978).

Pragmatic deficits may appear as difficulty in maintaining a topic or as lack of communication despite relatively normal use of speech sounds, morphology, and syntax. Often the child with a pragmatic deficit has poor communication fluency, poor conversational skills, and poor nonverbal social skills.

think about it   Why is it important for preschoolers to have playmates?

Deficits in the Interaction Among the Components of Language

Occasionally, a child has some development of each component of language but incompletely developed or distorted interactions among the components (see Figure 1–7). That is, he or she has failed to integrate form, content, and use completely during the acquisition of language.

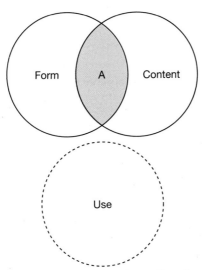

FIGURE 1-6   Bloom and Lahey's model of use disorders. (*Source:* Lahey, LANGUAGE DISORDERS AND LANGUAGE DEVELOPMENT, Figure 2–4 "Disruption in the Use of Language" p. 28, 1988. Reproduced by permission of Pearson Education, Inc.)

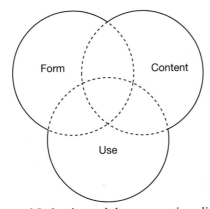

FIGURE 1-7   Bloom and Lahey's model representing disordered interactions between the components of language. (*Source:* Lahey, LANGUAGE DISORDERS AND LANGUAGE DEVELOPMENT, Figure 2–5 "Distorted Interactions of Content/Form/Use" p. 32, 1988. Reproduced by permission of Pearson Education, Inc.)

According to Bloom and Lahey, the child uses forms to communicate ideas, but the forms he or she uses may be inappropriate to the content and meaning intended to be conveyed. Typically, this child uses very little meaningful speech; in fact, it may be limited to stereotypic speech. On occasion, the child may use what appear to be appropriate utterances; but, most likely, these are complete utterances that the child has learned to use in response to certain situations or ideas, even though he or she may not know the semantic-syntactic relations that are represented within the sentences (Bloom & Lahey, 1978).

Stereotypic speech. The unintentional use of a real or invented word or phrase that has little meaning.

With regard to differential diagnosis, unlike children who have a form deficit, these children might produce sophisticated examples of the conventional language structures. They differ from children with semantic deficits because they may have complex ideas about the world, but they do not have the ability to appropriately code the ideas they have. Finally, they differ from children with more isolated pragmatic disorders because they do use forms for personal interaction. When a child has distorted interactions among form, content, and use, messages are well formed and used for specific purposes in the situation; however, there is a mismatch between the content of a message and its use and between the content and its form, even though some element of the content is related to the message or the situation in which it occurs.

Lack of Interaction Among the Components

Even more rare is the child who has incomplete development of each component of language and no interaction among the components (see Figure 1–8). Children in this category use stereotypic speech utterances that have little or no relation to the situation at hand. No apparent function is evident for speech, other than possibly to maintain some form of communication contact. The child may recite TV or radio commercials or repeat utterances heard previously that are, in some idiosyncratic way, associated with the present context. It is important to note that, in this example as well as in all of the disorders based on features of language, isolated instances are not a basis for determining the existence of a problem. The use of commercial jingles

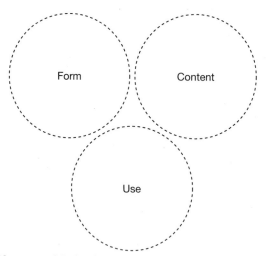

FIGURE 1–8 Bloom and Lahey's model of distorted interactions and incomplete development of the components. (*Source:* Lahey, LANGUAGE DISORDERS AND LANGUAGE DEVELOPMENT, Figure 2–6 "Separation of Content, Form and Use" p. 33, 1988. Reproduced by permission of Pearson Education, Inc.)

and idiosyncratic utterances must be prevalent in the child's communicative exchanges. A few years ago, one of my son's friends came to the door and inquired as to whether or not my son could go to the movie with the friend's family. My husband asked where the movie was playing, and the child responded, "At theaters everywhere!" This child could not be labeled as having a lack of interaction of his form, use, and content based on this one utterance. However, if this statement were made randomly, frequently, and without any relation to the existing context, and if it were the standard mode of communication, there would be reason for concern.

LANGUAGE DIFFERENCES

A speech community is a group of people who routinely and frequently use a shared language to interact with each other (Fasold, 1990). A communication difference exists when communication behaviors meet the norms of the primary speech community but do not meet the norms of standard English (Shames, Wiig, & Secord, 1994). This difference can exist whether the person in question is a child from a different country or simply a different neighborhood in the same city. The slight variations that occur in a language are systematic, patterned, and rule-governed and constitute a dialect. Dialects often develop along lines of geographic separation or social difference (Fasold, 1990). Dialects may be distinguished from each other by word choices and/or variations in how a sound or word is pronounced.

Speech community. A group of people who routinely and frequently use a shared language to interact with each other.

Dialect. Systematic, patterned, rule-governed variations in a language.

Regardless of the degree of variation, all dialects are considered to be linguistically valid and legitimate. They develop as a result of the mixing of a variety of languages of different cultural groups. When the minority language mixes with the language of the native speakers, dialects emerge. Frequently, the distribution of political and economic power plays a role in determining which language becomes the dominant one, with the language of those in power becoming the primary language and the application of the cultural differences developing the dialect. Thus, regional dialects and cultures emerge based on geographical boundaries, social and legal boundaries, and political and economic power.

Coleman and McCabe-Smith (2000) define culture as "the shared beliefs, values, traditions, assumptions, and lifestyles of a group of people" (p. 5). The study of culture can be based on an ethnography of the communication or on sociolinguistics.

Ethnography is the study of language use for communicative purposes, considering social and cultural factors. It tends to be descriptive in nature.

Sociolinguistics is the study of social and cultural influences on language structures. Sociolinguists study the communicative interactions of people in social situations. The field of sociolinguistics is relatively new in the social sciences. It developed at the end of the first Head Start program in 1965 when psycholinguists and anthropologists met in an attempt to explain why

Culture. The philosophies, ideas, arts, and customs of a group of people that are passed from one generation to the next.

Ethnography. The study of language use for communicative purposes, considering social and cultural factors.

some children had problems in school and others did not (Nelson, 1993). Together, the professionals in these two sciences initially approached the topic from a psycholinguistic viewpoint. That is to say, they looked at the "interrelationships between the structures and processes underlying the ability to speak and understand language" (Nelson, 1993, p. 26). Eventually, the sociolinguistic viewpoint developed. Instead of looking for psycholinguistic problems within children, they came to the conclusion that they needed to look at language differences between the homes and schools of children who succeeded and of those who did not succeed in school (Nelson, 1993).

Ethnographic and sociolinguistic researchers have studied several factors that influence language acquisition, language behavior, and communication and discourse rules. Together, these social scientists identified seven areas of concentration that need to be considered when studying the issue of dialectal variations in individuals (see Table 1–9).

The first domain of study is race and ethnicity, based on cultural attitudes and values, not on biology and genetics. Samovar and Porter (1994) summed up the issue as follows:

> Language is the primary vehicle by which a culture transmits its beliefs, values, norms, and world views. Language gives people a means of connecting and interacting with other members of their culture and a means of thinking. Language thus serves as a mechanism for communication and as a guide to social reality (pp. 16–17).

The second domain is based on the study of social class, education, and occupation. To address these issues, it is necessary to evaluate the effects of the home environment, child-rearing practices, family interaction patterns, travel, and experiences. It would be expected that children who have stable homes with consistent parenting do better in school than those who do not. However, it is critical that children not be labeled as deficient in their

TABLE 1–9 Seven areas of concentration that need to be considered when studying the issue of dialectal variations in individuals

---

Race and ethnicity

Social class, education, and occupation

Region

Situation or context

Peer group association and identification

First language community or culture

Gender

Source: Compiled from *Human Communication Disorders: An Introduction* (4th ed.), by G. H. Shames, E. H. Wiig, and W. A. Secord, 1994, pp. 143–144. New York: Macmillan Publishing Company.

cognition or language because of personal biases related to a specific social group or speech community. Some children have the opportunity to travel and learn about regional dialects firsthand, whereas others have few opportunities to go beyond their hometowns and neighborhoods. An enriched environment is one in which children are exposed to a variety of experiences, and these experiences do not need to be of epic proportions. Taking a child to a grocery store and letting the child feel and smell fresh produce is a wonderful experience that dovetails with events that occur in the daily lives of families.

Regional issues constitute the third domain that needs to be addressed when studying language. As stated earlier, many dialects emerge as a result of geographic boundaries. In the lower 48 states, at least 10 regional dialects are recognized (Nist, 1966). These dialects consist of phonological features, word choices, idioms, and characteristic patterns in syntax, prosody, and pragmatics. Speech-language pathologists need to analyze their own dialects to see if they could impact the intervention process.

The social context of a situation often influences a person's choice of a language or dialect. With regard to situation or context, peer group associations, and the first language community, it is sometimes necessary to speak a more standard dialect; at other times the native dialect emerges. The ability of an individual to switch dialects or languages depending on the situation is called code-switching. Teenagers may speak in one dialect when they are with their peer group and in another dialect when they are with their families. Frequently, these dialectal variations are semantic in nature. For example, a teenager came home from school and announced that she had a boyfriend and that they were going steady. The mother assumed that this meant they were dating only each other (based on the definition of "going steady" when she was in school), only to find out that "going steady" meant you held hands in the halls at school.

The effects of gender are a topic of much interest to those who study the sociolinguistic aspects of language. However, this aspect of dialectal variations does not play a role in most patients seen by the speech-language pathologist. Nonetheless, an astute speech-language pathologist needs to study the gender-related and/or age-related issues of clients who are from a different culture. For example, one culture does not allow a woman to establish eye contact with a male and permits a child to speak only when spoken to first. Another culture may focus on loudness, with women being very soft-spoken in comparison to the men in their environment. It is important to understand the effects of gender in different cultures in order to effectively plan diagnostic and therapeutic services.

A major impact on language use comes from the cultural influences of storytelling. In some cultures, stories are primarily topic-centered narratives, whereas in others topic-associated narratives take precedence. In addition, an oral storytelling tradition, as opposed to a written storytelling tradition, is a cultural factor that affects language development and language use. Storytelling facilitates the development of critical cognitive functions, such

Topic-centered narrative. A tightly structured discourse on a single topic or a series of closely related topics and events.

as conceptualization, social interaction, and problem-solving skills. A topic-centered narrative is characterized by a tightly structured discourse on a single topic or a series of closely related topics and events. Such narratives tend to have a temporal organization or a thematic focus that prevails throughout the story. Frequent exposure to storybooks helps a child to understand topic-centered narratives, which can eventually influence the development of cognitive and language foundations. Most storybooks assume that the reader has little information about the subject. Typically, storybooks have an orientation section that sets up the story and introduces the characters, an elaboration that develops the story, and a resolution that completes the story.

Topic-associated narrative. A series of narratives linked to a topic with no particular theme or point to the narrative.

In contrast, topic-associated narratives are more traditional in countries where stories are told orally but are usually not written down. A topic-associated narrative consists of a series of narratives linked to a topic, with no particular theme or point to the narrative. Rather, the stories are a source of entertainment, with the details frequently altered as the stories are passed through the oral tradition. The listener must make the shifts and links in the story on the basis of presumed knowledge about the topic, which typically has no temporal or focal connections between the segments of the story. Often the temporal aspects and segmental shifts are provided by pitch and tempo changes instead of by words. Topic-associated narratives usually are more common among children of working-class parents whose families may not have money available for many storybooks (Payne & Taylor, 2006).

think about it

How can a school-based speech-language pathologist facilitate the integration of a child from a foreign culture into a primarily English-speaking classroom?

SUMMARY

As clinicians, we need to determine what the individual knows about language and how adept he or she is at using knowledge in a functional manner. In other words, the question guiding the assessment of language must be based on the concept of functional application of the person's knowledge of his or her language. Can this individual integrate the rules that govern language use and language knowledge in a manner that allows him or her to be understood in interactions with others?

Throughout this book, the term "language disorder" is used as a diagnostic entity to refer to any disruption in the learning of language in the absence of primary intellectual, sensory, or emotional deficits (Bloom & Lahey, 1978). The term "language delay" is used as a description of qualitative differences from normal with regard to the time of onset, rate of development, actual behavior learned, or sequence in which the behavior was learned. By taking this view of language delays and disorders, we are forced to describe what the child can do without difficulty, what the child can do with some degree of difficulty, or what the child cannot do. This enables us to have a better understanding of possible disruptions in the child's language development and to design more appropriate plans of intervention.

CASE STUDY

History

Edward is a 5-year-6-month-old child who presents in the clinic with problematic speech intelligibility. He was born at 37 weeks gestation by C-section following a high-risk pregnancy. Edward's mother started premature labor at 13 weeks gestation and remained on bed rest for the remainder of the pregnancy. She received terbutaline and morphine to slow down contractions throughout the pregnancy. Edward has two older sisters who both attend public school and are doing well. Both of Edward's parents have masters' degrees. His father is a biologist and his mother is a teacher. Edward started kindergarten in August at the same public school where his sisters are enrolled. His teachers report that he is very social, well behaved, and has adapted well to the school setting. He gets along well with his peers. They note that he has befriended a classmate who has physical disabilities and is in a wheelchair. He does have difficulty with fine motor tasks and shows little interest in coloring and puzzles. He does those tasks when asked to, but never chooses tasks requiring fine motor coordination during free time.His mother expressed interest in pursuing private therapy to improve her son's speech. He had received therapy for about 6 months, but it was discontinued when the family moved to this city 4 months ago. The reports from his previous therapist were lost in the move, but Edward's mother reported minimal improvement.

Evaluation

In the preassessment interview, Edward's mother described his unique sound acquisition pattern. When Edward began talking around 15 months of age, he used the sound /h/ in place of all consonants and also had some vowel distortion. When he learned a new sound, such as /p/, he would drop the /h/ and use /p/ in place of all consonants. When he figured out where to appropriately use a /p/, he would revert to using the /h/ for all consonants other than /p/. This pattern continued until Edward had acquired most of the consonants. Vowel distortion remained a consistent problem.

Edward's speech was evaluated using the Assessment of Phonological Processes–Revised (APP-R) and a spontaneous language sample. On the APP-R, Edward had a phonological deviancy score of 33. Based on Edward's performance, the clinician concluded that Edward had a moderate phonological disorder that consisted of fronting (cat → tat), liquid gliding (red → wed; lock → wock), consonant deletion, and vowel distortions. In spontaneous speech he was approximately 40 percent unintelligible. His intelligibility is compromised not

(continues)

CASE STUDY *(continued)*

only by his phonological patterns, but also by a rapid rate of speech that borders on cluttering. Edward tested within normal limits on a hearing screening.

On language testing using the Test of Language Development–P:3, Edward scored in the 91st percentile with a composite score (quotient) of 120. The word articulation subtest was the only subtest that was problematic. Edward has an excellent command of sound-symbol correspondence, and he reads at a first-grade level. It should be noted that when Edward reads aloud, he has an accelerated rate just as he does in spontaneous speech. Content and use of language are intact.

Summary

Edward is a bright young man who presents with phonological difficulties that interfere with his intelligibility. A review of his speech and language development reveals that Edward had an unusual pattern of sound acquisition that impacted the ability of others to understand him. At the single-word level, Edward has fronting, liquid gliding, and consonant deletion. He also has distortion of the vowels. Edward has no difficulties with semantics and pragmatics, and phonology is the only aspect of form that is affected.

	Strengths	Weaknesses
Communicative	Oral decoding and segmentation abilities Hearing WNL Pragmatics Semantics	Phonological processes that interfere with intelligibility, including fronting, liquid gliding, and consonant deletion Rapid rate of speaking that interferes with intelligibility
Noncommunicative	Good home environment Enrolled in a well-respected public school Positive personality	Mild frustration when he cannot make himself understood Poor eye-hand coordination Weak fine motor skills

Recommendations

It is recommended that Edward receive phonological therapy using the cycles approach two times a week. Following 10 weeks of therapy, it is suggested that he be reevaluated to determine if he needs additional therapy.

Mrs. L will contact the previous therapist to get copies of her reports. Edward will also be referred to an occupational therapist for evaluation of his fine motor skills and eye-hand coordination problems.

> **think about it**
> Is Edward's speech a delay, a disorder, or a difference, or can this even be determined based on the information provided? Do you think there is any relationship between his fine motor difficulties and his speech difficulties?

REVIEW QUESTIONS

1. Cross-cultural studies suggest that
    a. Early semantic rules are universal.
    b. Early phonological rules are not universal.
    c. There are no similarities in grammar across cultures.
    d. Early semantic rules are not universal.

2. Sociolinguistics is defined as the study of
    a. Social institutions.
    b. Language assimilation.
    c. Causes of language disorders.
    d. Social and cultural influences on language structure.

3. Which of the following "-isms" (McLaughlin) support the nature philosophy of language development?
    a. Empiricism and behaviorism
    b. Interactionism and nativism
    c. Mentalism and nativism
    d. Mentalism and behaviorism

4. Which of the following set of "red flags" is most typical of a disruption of content or semantics?
    a. Slow acquisition of first words, slow in understanding temporal and spatial relationships, lack of understanding of antonyms and synonyms
    b. Slow acquisition of first words, delayed understanding of category words, difficulty maintaining a topic
    c. Slow acquisition of first words, slow in understanding temporal and spatial relationships, normal communication
    d. Slow acquisition of first words, slow in temporal and spatial relationships, frequent word reversals

5. Use of "cocktail party speech" could be indicative of which of the following?

   a. Disruption in interactions between content and form

   b. Incomplete development of content

   c. Disruption in interactions between use and content

   d. Incomplete development of use

6. A child who has knowledge and ideas about events and objects, can communicate ideas, but often uses gestures because he has difficulty learning conventional codes for expressive language has a disruption in

   a. Form

   b. Content

   c. Use

7. Plante and Beeson define late talkers as children between the ages of 16 and 30 months whose language skills fall below 80 percent of their age peers.

   a. True

   b. False

8. Topic-centered narratives are traditional in countries where stories are told orally but usually not written down.

   a. True

   b. False

9. Students who exhibit a language difference are considered to be language disordered.

   a. True

   b. False

10. Use of limited functions of language is indicative of a pragmatic disorder.

    a. True

    b. False

REFERENCES

American Speech-Language-Hearing Association. (1993). *Definitions of communication disorders and variations* [relevant paper]. Available from www.asha.org/policy. Retrieved May 15, 2010.

American Speech-Language-Hearing Association. (1987). *Learning disabilities and the preschool child* [position statement]. Available from www.asha.org/policy.

Bernstein, D. K., & Levey, S. (2009). Language development: A review. In D. K. Bernstein and E. Tiegerman-Morris (eds.), *Language and communication disorders in children* (pp. 28–100). Boston: Allyn & Bacon.

Bishop, D. V. M., & Edmundson, A. (1987). Specific language impairment as a maturational lag: Evidence from longitudinal data on language and motor development. *Developmental Medicine and Child Neurology, 29*, pp. 442–459.

Bloom, L., & Lahey, M. (1978). *Language development and language disorders.* New York: John Wiley and Sons.

Chafe, W. (1970). *Meaning and the structure of language.* Chicago: University of Chicago Press.

Chomsky, N. (1965). *Aspects of a theory of syntax.* Cambridge, MA: MIT Press.

Chomsky, N. (1982). *Some concepts and consequences of the theory of government and binding.* Cambridge, MA: The MIT Press.

Coleman, T. J., & McCabe-Smith, L. (2000). Key terms and concepts. In T. J. Coleman (ed.), *Clinical management of communication disorders in culturally diverse children* (pp. 3–12). Boston: Allyn & Bacon.

Elman, J. L., Bates, E. A., Johnson, M. H., Karmiloff-Smith, A., Parisi, D., & Plunkett, K. (1996). *Rethinking innateness: A connectionist perspective on development.* Cambridge, MA: The MIT Press.

Fasold, R. (1990). *The sociolinguistics of language.* London: Basil Blackwell.

Fillmore, C. (1968). The case for case. In E. Bach and R. Harmas (eds.), *Universals in linguistic theory.* New York: Holt, Rinehart & Winston.

Gleason, J. B. (2005). *The development of language* (6th ed.). Boston: Allyn & Bacon.

Hagberg, B. S., Miniscalco, C., Gillberg, C. (2010). Clinic attendees with autism or attention deficit/hyperactivity disorder: Cognitive profile at school age and its relationship to preschool indicators. *Research in Developmental Disabilities: A Multi-disciplinary Journal, 31*(1), pp. 1–8.

Hebbeler, K. (2010). *Characteristics of children in Part C.* NECTAC Webinar Series on Early Identification and Part C Eligibility. Powerpoint presentation.

Hulit, L. M., & Howard, M. R. (2002). *Born to talk: An introduction to speech and language development.* Boston: Allyn and Bacon.

Lahey, M. (1988). *Language disorders and language development.* New York: Macmillan Publishing Company.

Lizardi, L. O. (2000). A connectionist approach to language acquisition. ERIC #ED39434.

McLaughlin, S. (1998). *Introduction to language development.* Clifton Park, NY: Delmar, Cengage Learning.

McLaughlin, S. (2006). *Introduction to language development* (2nd ed.). Clifton Park, NY: Delmar Cengage Learning.

National Early Intervention Longitudinal Study (NEILS). (2007, January). *Early intervention for infants and toddlers with disabilities and their families: Participants, services, and outcomes.*

National Joint Committee on Learning Disabilities (NJCLD). (2007, October). *Learning disabilities and young children: Identification and intervention* [technical report]. Available from www.asha.org/policy.

Nelson, N. W. (1993). *Childhood language disorders in context: Infancy through adolescence.* New York: Merrill.

Nicolosi, L., Harryman, E., & Kresheck, J. (1996). *Terminology of communication disorders* (4th ed.). Baltimore, MD: Williams & Wilkins.

Nist, J. (1966). *A structural history of English.* New York: St. Martin's Press.

Owens, R. E. (1984). *Language development: An introduction.* Columbus, OH: Charles E. Merrill.

Parker, F., & Riley, K. (1994). *Linguistics for non-linguists: A primer with exercises* (2nd ed.). Boston: Allyn and Bacon.

Payne, K. T., & Taylor, I. L. (2006). Multicultural differences in human communication and disorders. In N. Anderson and G. H. Shames, *Human communication disorders: An introduction* (7th ed.). Boston: Pearson Education, Inc.

Pinker, S. (1999). *Words and rules: The ingredients of language.* New York: Basic Books.

Plante, E., & Beeson, P. M. (2004). *Communication and communication disorders: A clinical introduction* (2nd ed.). Boston: Allyn and Bacon.

Polakow, V. (1993). *Lives on the edge: Single mothers and their children in the other America.* Chicago: University of Chicago Press.

Rossetti, L. M. (1986). *High risk infants: Identification, assessment, and intervention.* Boston: College-Hill Press.

Rossetti, L. M. (1996). *Communication intervention: Birth to three.* Clifton Park, NY: Delmar Cengage Learning.

Rumelhart, D. E., & McClelland, J. L. (1986). On learning past tenses of English verbs. In J. L. McClelland, D. E. Rumelhart, & The PDP Research Group, *Parallel distributed processing: Explorations in the microstructure of cognition. Vol. 1: Foundations.* Cambridge, MA: The MIT Press.

Samovar, L. A., & Porter, R. E. (1994). *Intercultural communication: A reader* (7th ed.). Belmont, CA: Wadsworth Publishing Company.

Schaffer, S., Dyson, A., & Vinson, B. (1989). *Phonological development: A case study.* Unpublished master's thesis. Gainesville, FL: University of Florida.

Shames, G. H., Wiig, E. H., & Secord, W. A. (1994). *Human communication disorders: An introduction* (4th ed.) New York: Macmillan College Publishing Company.

Snowling, M. J., Adams, C., Bishop, D. V. M., & Stothard, S. E. (2001). Educational attainments of school leavers with a preschool history of speech-language impairment. *International Journal of Language and Communication Disorders, 36,* pp. 173–183.

Snowling, M. J., Bishop, D. V., & Stothard, S. E. (2006, August). Psychosocial outcomes at 15 years of children with a preschool history of speech-language impairment. *Journal of Child Psychology and Psychiatry and Allied Discipline, 47,* pp. 759–765.

Steinberg, D. D. (1993). *An introduction to psycholinguistics.* New York, NY: Longman.

Thal, D. J., Bates, E., Goodman, J., & Jahn-Samilo, J. (1997). Continuity of language abilities: An exploratory study of late- and early-talking toddlers. *Developmental Neuropsychology, 13,* 239–274.

Thal, D. J., & Tobias, S. (1992). Communicative gestures in children with delayed onset of oral expressive vocabulary. *Journal of Speech and Hearing Research, 35,* 1281–1289.

Woods, J. J., & Wetherby, A. M. (2003, July). Early identification of and intervention for infants and toddlers who are at risk for autism spectrum disorder. *Language, Speech, Hearing Services in the Schools, 34,* pp. 180–193.

Chapter 2

Syndromes, Developmental Disabilities, and Motor and Sensory Impairments that Affect Language and Speech

LEARNING OBJECTIVES

After completion of this chapter, the reader will be able to:

1. Identify the primary characteristics of a variety of disorders associated with pediatric language deficits.

2. Differentiate between a sequence and a syndrome.

3. Differentiate between the descriptive terms *genetic, chromosomal,* and *hereditary.*

4. Describe the effects of hearing loss on a child's development of form, content, and use of language, then discuss the impact of cochlear implantation on language and speech.

5. Discuss the impact of prematurity on cognition and language development.

6. Discuss the effects of alcohol, nicotine, and other drugs on speech, language, and cognitive development.

INTRODUCTION

As defined by the American Speech-Language-Hearing Association (1993), a language disorder is

> impaired comprehension and/or use of spoken, written and/or other symbol systems. The disorder may involve (1) the form of language (phonology, morphology, and syntax), (2) the content of language (semantics), and/or (3) the function of language in communication (pragmatics) in any combination (p. 1).

Although it certainly is preferable to address a language disorder in terms of the language abilities and disabilities that the child demonstrates within his or her linguistic system, it often becomes a legal and financial necessity to officially "label" a child's disorder with a diagnostic descriptor on the basis of etiological considerations. Funding for special education and related services in the public schools often hinges on the diagnostic label that has been used to classify the disorder with regard to the child's abilities and disabilities. Eligibility for Medicaid and other reimbursement programs also requires the application of a diagnostic label. Therefore, whether the clinician philosophically supports or opposes the concept of labeling, it is a necessity in many settings. Together, the professional and the family must consider the benefits and drawbacks of labeling a child's disorder and act accordingly.

Actually, it is not the act of labeling that is the major problem; rather, it is the *assumption* of the presence or absence of specific skills and traits that often accompanies a label that is problematic. In instances such as this, even though it is the condition that is labeled, the clinician should not forget that it is the *child* who is being assessed and treated, not the disorder. If the child's speech and language patterns do not interfere with the message being understood, the problem may not be labeled a communication disorder. However, if interference occurs with the message being received by the listener, it is most likely that some professional, such as a teacher or speech-language pathologist, may label the problem a communication disorder. For purposes of discussion, the remainder of this chapter addresses the language aspects of a communication disorder. Also, information presented in this chapter includes the gamut of speech and language impairments often associated with specific syndromes and disorders. However, not all children exhibit every characteristic, and children often demonstrate characteristics not normally associated with a particular diagnosis. Some children have more than one disorder, and that, too, affects which behaviors and skills a child demonstrates.

GENETIC AND CHROMOSOMAL SYNDROMES

Frequently, the terms *genetic* and *chromosomal* are used as if they are synonymous. Genetic disorders refer to those that are carried on genes. Genetic disorders may be acquired, as when a gene undergoes a mutation, or they may be inherited. Chromosomal disorders refer to deviations of the genes that are located on the chromosomes, and they also may be inherited or acquired. A chromosomal disorder is defined as "a disorder of the number or structure of the chromosomes as they are distinctively arranged for a particular individual" (Johnson, 1996, p. 80).

Two other terms that are frequently misapplied are *sequence* and *syndrome*. According to Shprintzen (1997), a sequence is "a disorder where many of the anomalies are actually secondary disorders, caused by a single anomaly which sets off a chain reaction of changes in the developing embryo that result in other anomalies" (p. 75). Robin sequence is discussed in the next section. A syndrome is defined as "the presence of multiple anomalies in the same individual with all of those anomalies having a single cause" (Shprintzen, 1997, p. 53). It is possible for a child to have a syndrome and a sequence, such as having the Stickler syndrome in the Robin sequence. Down syndrome, fragile X syndrome, and velo-cardio-facial syndrome are discussed in this chapter.

Down Syndrome (Trisomy 21)

Down syndrome is a chromosomal disorder that is caused by the presence of three copies of chromosome 21 rather than the usual two; this disorder also is labeled trisomy 21. The most prevalent of the chromosomal anomalies,

Genetic. Specific characteristics or traits passed from one generation to the next.

Chromosomal disorder. A disorder in the structure or number of chromosomes or both.

Sequence. A disorder in which many of the anomalies are actually secondary disorders caused by a single anomaly, which sets off a chain reaction of changes in the developing embryo that result in other anomalies.

Syndrome. The presence of multiple anomalies in the same individual, with all of those anomalies having a single cause.

Down syndrome, occurs once in approximately every 600 to 800 live births (Nyhan, 1983). Historically, children with Down syndrome were assumed to have moderate to severe mental retardation. However, more recent evidence does not support that assumption, and the range of mental deficits in children with Down syndrome is documented as mild to severe. The more contemporary findings may, in part, reflect the greater availability of early intervention and increased understanding of the importance of structuring a rich and redundant language environment to facilitate the development of nonlinguistic and linguistic language and communication in children with Down syndrome.

Down syndrome is recognizable by its common features, which are generally well known. The children typically have a round face with abnormal development (dysplasia) of the tissues of the midface area and a prominent jaw (prognathism). The oral cavity is relatively small, which limits movement of the tongue and affects speech intelligibility. Also, these children tend to be mouth breathers with a habitually open mouth. The mouth breathing is also due to the fact that the nasopharyngeal area is underdeveloped. Due to hypotonia, the tongue is typically carried forward in the oral cavity and may protrude. Teeth are late to develop and are frequently incompletely developed or missing. Submucous clefts are fairly common in individuals with Down syndrome, and the hard palate may be high and narrow and may also be a cleft (Jung, 1989; Shprintzen, 1997). (See Figure 2–1.)

Dysplasia. Underdevelopment of tissue.

Prognathism. Abnormal facial construction in which the upper and/or lower jaws project forward.

Hypotonia. Abnormally low muscle tone; sometimes referred to as athetosis.

Although the degree of disability varies quite a bit, all babies with Down syndrome show a developmental delay with regard to their motor, speech, and language development. Children with Down syndrome typically demonstrate slow motor development, intellectual disabilities, limited lexicon, memory problems, and speech problems (Berk, 2004). After reviewing several studies, Stoel-Gammon (1981) concluded that there was little difference in terms of the quality and quantity of vocalizations in babies with Down syndrome up to age 12 months. However, as they reach the age of 1 year, the delay begins to become evident as many children with Down syndrome do not begin to use words until 24–36 months of age, with some beginning verbalization as late as age 7–8 years (Stoel-Gammon, 1981).

Accardo (2008) stated that, as a general rule, children with Down syndrome achieve developmental milestones at about twice the age that typically developing children develop the milestones. For example, children with Down syndrome typically sit at 11 months, creep at 17 months, walk unsupported at 26 months, and utter their first word at 18 months (note: this is earlier than Stoel-Gammon found).

Speech and Language Skills in Children with Down Syndrome

Articulatory errors tend to be inconsistent when compared to typical children and children with other forms of intellectual disability. The vocal quality is characterized as being lower pitched than normal, breathy, and husky

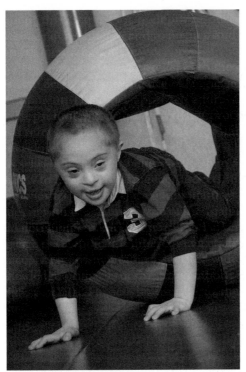

FIGURE 2–1   Children with Down syndrome are often happy and playful. Note the facial features discussed in the text. (*Delmar/Cengage Learning*)

(Jung, 1989). Stuttering is fairly common, along with prosody and phrasing problems (Shprintzen, 2000).

In Italy, Caselli and colleagues (1998) conducted a study to investigate the development of language and communication in children who had Down syndrome. They studied 40 children between the ages of 10 and 49 months who had Down syndrome and 40 typically developing children aged 8 to 17 months in order "to examine the relations among verbal comprehension, verbal production, and gesture production in the very early stages of development" (p. 1125). Specifically, Caselli and colleagues wanted to determine if a dissociation between comprehension and production exists, and if so, whether it affects speech only or speech and gestures. The Italian version of the MacArthur Communicative Development Inventory (CDI) (Fenson et al., 1993) was administered to each child, and they found that the children with Down syndrome were severely delayed in reaching the developmental milestones compared to the typically developing children. Although differences in semantics and syntax between typically developing children and children with Down syndrome appear to be minimal in the early stages, the differences become more pronounced as the children get older. This is true particularly in relation to phonology and morphosyntactic abilities, with lexicon often being spared. The older children with Down syndrome typically use simple sentences with words such as articles, pronouns, and prepositions being omitted (Fowler, 1990; Chapman, 1995; Rondal, 1993; Fabbretti, Pizzuto, Vicari, & Volterra, 1997). The results of the Caselli study concluded that "a dissociation emerged in children with DS between verbal comprehension and production, in favor of comprehension, whereas synchronous development was found in vocal lexical comprehension and gestural production" (Caselli et al., 1998, p. 1132). The dissociation between comprehension and production is similar in typically developing children and children with Down syndrome when the children are matched based on lexical comprehension, but children with Down syndrome use more gestures, especially when comprehension of the lexicon exceeds 100 words.

In general, the communication skills of children with Down syndrome fall below what would be expected based on cognitive ability, although these children are typically very social. Receptive language typically is more intact than expressive language, and the language abilities frequently plateau around the 3-year-old developmental level. Auditory and short-term memory are also impacted (Pore & Reed, 1999; Shprintzen, 2000). Children with Down syndrome may be more delayed than they appear in the first 2 years of life due to the fact that they are known to be highly social, which can mask their cognitive skill deficits up to 24 months of age. However, at 24 months, the delays compared to their neurotypical peers become more evident (Roizen, 2002).

As previously mentioned, children with Down syndrome have intelligence quotients that range from mildly impaired to profoundly handicapped. Regardless of the level of functioning, as the child with Down syndrome advances in age, the gaps between his or her language skills and those of his or her peers at the same mental age widen. This is particularly true in the areas of morphology and syntax. Chapman and colleagues (1998) found that children with Down syndrome tend to omit morphemes and grammatical function words more than their mental-age peers. Thus, it makes sense that therapy with children who have intellectual disabilities, and particularly those with Down syndrome, should have syntax and morphology as major foci of therapy. Chapman and colleagues stated that adolescents with Down syndrome can improve these areas of expressive language, thereby increasing the length and complexity of their sentences. Kumin, Councill, and Goodman (1998) conducted a study to determine when children with Down syndrome start talking about events in the past and in the future, as well as when they use *–ed* and *–ing* word endings. Their findings are summarized in Tables 2–1 and 2–2.

Typical mean length of utterance in children with Down syndrome is 1.5 words at 4 years of age, 3.5 words at 6 years of age, and 5+ words at 15 years (Kumin, 2003). In the early years, their lexicon consists primarily of

TABLE 2–1   When children with Down syndrome use *–ed* to form the past tense

Age	Never	Sometimes	Often
2	100%	—	—
3	93%	7%	—
4	78%	19%	3%
5	77%	18%	5%

Source: From *Early communication skills for children with Down syndrome,* by L. Kumin, p. 111. © 2003 by Woodbine House. Reprinted with permission.

TABLE 2–2   When children with Down syndrome use *–ing*

Age	Never	Sometimes	Often
2	96.3%	3.7%	—
3	73%	13%	13%
4	61%	27%	12%
5	52%	36%	22%

Source: From *Early communication skills for children with Down syndrome,* by L. Kumin, p. 111. © 2003 by Woodbine House. Reprinted with permission.

concrete, referential words that denote objects or things experienced by the child. Grammatical classification words such as *or* and *however* are typically not used until age 5 at the earliest, and use of words with grammatical meanings usually does not develop until approximately age 6 (Kumin, Councill, & Goodman, 1998). It should be noted that when children with Down syndrome are compared to their chronological-age peers, they have a smaller vocabulary. But, when compared to mental-age peers, they may have a larger vocabulary. This may be explained in part by the fact that when compared to mental-age peers the child with Down syndrome is most likely older chronologically and has had more life experiences (Rondal, 1978; Miller, 1988; Kumin, 2003). This is important clinically in that these children need to be taught to organize their vocabulary into concepts, thus forming a basic organization to their language that enables them to generalize their vocabulary.

Children with Down syndrome usually have language deficits that are greater than would be predicted when looking at their nonverbal cognitive skills (Chapman, 1995). Using a test of nonverbal intelligence, Buckley (1993, 1995a) tested 12 teenagers who had Down syndrome. The mean age of the teenagers was 14:11. On the Ravens Progressive Matrices Test (Raven, 1995), which tests nonverbal reasoning skills, they scored a mean age of 7:0. On a picture vocabulary comprehension test the mean age for the group was 5:6, and on a grammar comprehension test the average score was 5:0 years.

Reading Skills in Children with Down Syndrome

Reading levels in children with Down syndrome frequently exceed their language and cognitive levels. Several studies have been done to evaluate reading skills in children with Down syndrome. Buckley (1995b) did a study in which a group of cognitively matched children with Down syndrome was divided into two subgroups. One subgroup was taught to read, and the other was not. When the study concluded, Buckley found that the language and memory skills of those children who were taught to read were more advanced than those in the nonreader group. In addition, the speech, language, and educational achievements by the readers were more advanced by the time the children reached age 10 to 11. These findings support the importance of introducing a literacy component into the educational and therapeutic plans for students who have Down syndrome.

In another study on reading ability in children with Down syndrome, Kay-Raining Bird, Cleave, and McConnell (2000) followed 12 children with Down syndrome over a 4.5-year period, looking at the impact of three literacy skills (language, cognition, and phonological awareness) on reading acquisition. The purpose of the study was to determine the roles of word recognition and decoding abilities in the reading of children with Down syndrome. Two predictors of literacy development in the Down syndrome population are cognitive ability (Sloper et al., 1990) and expressive-receptive language skills (Carr, 1995). Children who have better cognitive and language skills typically do better in the academic setting.

Sloper and colleagues (1990) studied 123 children with Down syndrome aged 6 to 14 years. They investigated child, parental/family, and school variables and their effects on academic achievement. Their findings were that mental age was the most predictive variable. Other predictors included "older ages, mainstream placements, female gender, and fathers' feelings of control over the outcomes of their children" (Kay-Raining Bird, Cleave, & McConnell, 2000, p. 320). Carr (1995) did a longitudinal study in which she followed 54 children with Down syndrome. When the individuals were 11 and 21 years of age, she assessed their language, cognition, and academic achievement. She assessed reading using the Neale Analysis of Reading Ability (Neale, 1958), and found that two-fifths of her sample could be scored, even though some additional subjects had letter recognition skills. Carr's findings supported the findings of Sloper and colleagues in that IQ is a significant predictor of reading success, and that there are

"significant correlations between reading and both vocabulary comprehension and production skills" (Kay-Raining Bird, Cleave, & McConnell,
2000, p. 320).

In a study by Fowler, Doherty, and Boynton (1995), 33 young adults with
Down syndrome were divided into four subgroups based on their reading
performance. The assessment consisted of three subtexts of the Woodcock
Reading Mastery Test-Revised: Word Identification, Word Attack, and
Passage Comprehension (Woodcock, 1987), and the Auditory Analysis Test
(AAT) (Rosner & Simon, 1971). Kay-Raining Bird and colleagues summa-
rized Fowler's findings as follows:

- As measured by the Word Attack subtest, decoding skills lagged behind
  word identification abilities except in the most skilled readers.

- The poorest performances were on the Passage Comprehension subtest.

- Even taking out the variable of cognitive status, the children's performance on the AAT was generally poor; however, the performance was
  variable across participants and was significantly correlated with their
  performance on the Word Attack and the Word Identification reading.

- Those individuals who scored beyond the first-grade level on Word
  Attack skills on the WRMT-R also scored at least a 10 on phonological
  awareness on the AAT.

- Based on this, phonological awareness is a necessary component of
  decoding, but alone is not sufficient for decoding ability to develop.

- Other measures correlating significantly with reading ability in the
  subjects with Down syndrome (again, after cognition was partialled out)
  were word retrieval, auditory memory, and visual memory.

Other studies have supported these findings and shed additional light on
the role of phonological awareness in reading, both in normally developing
populations and Down syndrome populations (Kay-Raining Bird & McConnell,
1994; Kay-Raining Bird et al., 1998).

The implications of these studies for therapy with children with Down
syndrome are that it appears that it may be beneficial to incorporate preliteracy and literacy skills commensurate with their cognitive age into the
therapeutic curriculum of children with Down syndrome.

Motor Development in Down Syndrome

Another factor to consider in looking at language development and use in
preschool children with Down syndrome is that their motor development
is delayed, and they are hypotonic and hyporeflexive owing to immature
development of the central nervous system (Sparks, 1984). Hypotonia refers
to abnormally low muscle tone, which leads to a characteristic description
of Down syndrome babies as "floppy." Hyporeflexia refers to an abnormally

low response when the reflexes are stimulated. Therefore, babies with Down syndrome may not do as much environmental exploration as a normal baby would. This decreased exploration of the environment impacts the child's ability to have experiences that help in language development.

Hearing Impairment in Down Syndrome

Another factor is the frequent occurrence of hearing impairment in children with Down syndrome. Small auricles and congenital malformations of the Eustachian tube and of the nasopharynx typically are present. It is not uncommon for children with Down syndrome to suffer from impacted wax (Jung, 1989). Conductive hearing loss coupled with frequent middle ear infections also can affect language development. Pueschel (1987) reported that over 75 percent of children with Down syndrome suffer from a hearing loss, with the majority of these individuals having mild to moderate losses in the 15- to 40-dB range. These losses may be conductive, sensorineural, or mixed, although the conductive hearing loss is the most common.

Conductive hearing loss. A breakdown in the ability of the middle ear to receive acoustic signals from the environment and then to transmit the acoustical information to the inner ear.

Generally speaking, the individual with Down syndrome has the following major systems affected: central nervous system, craniofacial system, cardiac system, gastrointestinal system, hematologic system, limbs, and ocular systems (Shprintzen, 2000). The occurrence of cancer is higher in individuals with Down syndrome, and they frequently have congenital heart and respiratory disorders. Obesity, blood disorders (particularly leukemia), and immune deficiencies are common. All of this has the potential to reduce life expectancy to 30 to 40 years (Shprintzen, 1997; Pore & Reed, 1999; Shprintzen, 2000).

In addition to all of the above, one must take into consideration social and behavioral issues. Individuals with Down syndrome are typified as being very social, happy, and affectionate. Actually, their social and behavioral characteristics are more in line with those of the general population when compared based on age.

Co-Morbidity of Down Syndrome with Other Disorders

There is a low prevalence of co-morbidity of autism and Down syndrome, but it does occur. Co-morbidity with autism is seen more often in children with fragile X syndrome, tuberous sclerosis, and Prader-Willi syndrome (Accardo, 2008).

There is a higher prevalence of ADHD in the population of children with Down syndrome than in the population of neurotypical children, but it is lower in the Down syndrome population than in groups of children with other intellectual disabilities. One study found that ADHD was reported in 56 percent of boys with Down syndrome and 42 percent of girls with Down syndrome. Yet another study found that 31 percent of preschoolers with Down syndrome had signs of ADHD (Lipkin, 2008).

Issues for Adolescents with Down Syndrome

Various studies have identified problems frequently seen in adolescents with Down syndrome. Accardo (2008) summarized the research and found that the following issues are reported relatively frequently in the literature:

- Behavioral problems, including acting out and aggressive behaviors

- Obesity (due to slower metabolism combined with puberty)

- Problems with sexuality (children with intellectual disabilities have difficulty understanding the physical, social, and emotional changes associated with puberty)

- Poor self-management skills

- Increased hearing and vision problems

- Dermatological manifestations (folliculitis related to hygiene problems and obesity, atopic dermatitis, seborrheic dermatitis, and fungal infections)

- Periodontal disease and other dental problems

- Cardiac concerns (often present from birth)

- Psychiatric disorders (see Table 2–3).

TABLE 2–3   Behavioral and psychiatric disorders exhibited by children with Down syndrome

Behavior	Percentage
Aggressive behavior	7%
Attention deficit disorder with hyperactivity	6%
Oppositional disorder	5%
Stereotypic behaviors	3%
Elimination difficulties	2%
Phobias	2%
Autism	1%
Eating disorders	1%
Self-injurious behaviors	1%
Tourette syndrome	0.4%
Pervasive developmental disorders	7%

Source: From Down Syndrome, by N. J. Roizen in *Children with disabilities* (5th ed.), M. Batshaw (ed.). Paul H. Brookes, 2002.

Another confounding factor that occurs when the child with Down syndrome approaches adulthood is the early occurrence of senility and Alzheimer's disease (Shprintzen, 1997). In fact, 15–20 percent of individuals with Down syndrome over the age of 40 years develop Alzheimer's disease (Roizen, 2002). Both conditions (Down syndrome and Alzheimer's disease) show the accumulation of beta-amyloid plaques, along with presynaptic cholinergic deficits resulting from the plaques (Accardo, 2008).

> **think about it**
>
> You are a pediatric speech-language pathologist in a large urban hospital. Mr. and Mrs. Jackson, college-educated professionals, are the new parents of a baby boy who has Down syndrome. They did not know the diagnosis prior to his birth. How would you approach your first meeting with them and their 2-day old baby?

Fragile X Syndrome

The second most common genetic syndrome is fragile X syndrome, caused by "a fragile site on the long arm of the X chromosome" (Pore & Reed, 1999, p. 80). It is also referred to as Martin-Bell syndrome (Shprintzen, 1997). Fragile X syndrome is the most common genetic precipitant of mild to moderate cognitive impairments. In addition, it is linked to 2–3 percent of all cases of autism (Berk, 2004).

Figure 2–2 is a drawing depicting the facial characteristics of a boy with fragile X syndrome. An easily missed abnormality that is believed to account for one-third to one-half of all X-linked cases of mental handicaps (Sparks, 1984), physical symptoms of fragile X syndrome often do not become apparent until the child reaches later childhood and puberty.

Articulation delays are common, as are language problems. Typically, children with this syndrome demonstrate deficits in auditory reception, visual and grammatic closure, and auditory sequential memory (Sparks, 1984).

Disorders in speech and language range in degree from very mild to very severe, and the speech and language deficits often are the first sign that something is wrong with the child (Johnson, 1996). The diagnosis of fragile X syndrome hinges on the presence of cognitive deficits of unknown cause, autism, or four or more of the following characteristics: mental retardation, perseveration in speech, hyperactivity, short attention span, negative reaction to physical contact, hand flapping, hand biting, poor eye contact, hyperextensive finger joints, large and prominent ears, large testicles, simian crease, and family history of mental retardation (Johnson, 1996). Also associated with fragile X syndrome is a prominent forehead and chin and flat feet. The syndrome is more prevalent in males than in females, with incidence figures of 1 in 1000 male births and 1 in 2,000 female births (Pore & Reed, 1999).

Grammatic closure. The ability to determine the missing elements in a sentence.

Auditory sequential memory. The ability to remember sounds, words, phrases, and sentences in a specified sequence.

Recent delineation of fragile X syndrome represents a significant advance in our understanding of mental retardation. It is second only to Down syndrome as a genetic cause of mental retardation (Turner et al., 1986). Persons with fragile X syndrome are said to have distinctive personalities, with shyness and friendliness being common attributes. The clinical phenotype includes (see list):

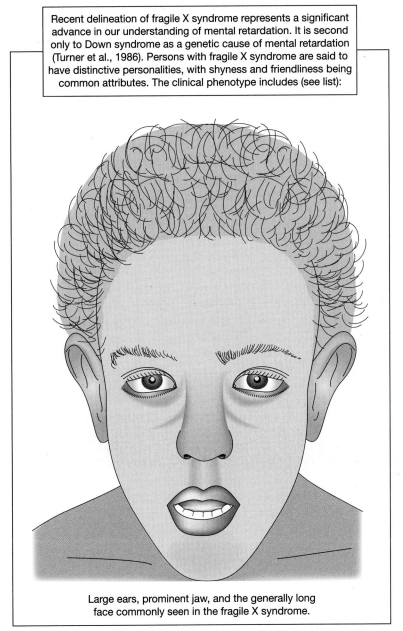

Large ears, prominent jaw, and the generally long face commonly seen in the fragile X syndrome.

FIGURE 2–2   Characteristics of children with fragile X syndrome. (*Source: Based on Genetic Syndromes in Communication Disorders. Austin, TX: Pro-Ed, 1988.*)

Speech and Language Characteristics of Children with Fragile X Syndrome

Although the language symptoms can range from mild to severe, there is not a direct relationship between the severity of the retardation and the degree of the language impairment. Children with fragile X syndrome exhibit intellectual impairment, along with a variety of speech, language, and learning deficits such as poor eye contact, hyperactivity, social deficits that mimic autism, social withdrawal, and a limited attention span (Roberts et al., 2002). According to Percy (2007, p. 132), "fragile X is the most common inherited intellectual disability." When comparisons are made between male children with fragile X syndrome and male children with Down syndrome who have the same cognitive levels, those with fragile X syndrome have more depressed language skills. The development of expressive language skills frequently lags significantly behind the development of receptive language skills. Boys with fragile X syndrome demonstrate much individual variability in their language skills, with marked delays in overall receptive and expressive communication and language development (Roberts, Mirrett, & Burchinal, 2001). Some children with fragile X syndrome may show a strength in their lexicon but have poor abstract reasoning skills; others may have poor development of their lexicon. A poor short-term memory and the presence of an auditory processing disorder are also characteristic.

In an effort to further study the communication and symbolic behaviors of boys with fragile X syndrome, Roberts and colleagues (2002) studied the language of 22 males diagnosed with fragile X syndrome. The boys ranged in chronological age from 21 to 77 months and developmentally were younger than 28 months. Each boy was tested using the Reynell Developmental Language Scales and the Communication and Symbolic Behavior Scales. All of the boys demonstrated significant delays, and there was substantial individual variability. Generally speaking, the testing indicated that the boys had weaknesses in the use of gestures, reciprocity, and symbolic play skills. The boys had specific weaknesses in "the use of repair strategies, conventional gestures (i.e., pushing away), distal gestures (pointing at a distance), and complex action schemes" (pp. 300–301). Strengths were found in vocal and verbal communication, specifically in using a wide variety of words, sounds, and word combinations. On repeat assessment after one year had passed, "children who (initially) scored higher in communicative functions, vocalizations, verbalizations, and reciprocity scored higher in verbal comprehension. Children with higher scores in verbal communication also scored higher in expressive language development" (p. 295).

Girls with fragile X syndrome typically are less impaired than boys with fragile X syndrome. Approximately 50 percent of girls with fragile X syndrome exhibit typical cognitive functioning but may show signs of a non–language based learning disability. Males and females have strengths in reading, verbal memory, and simultaneous processing (learning information in totality as opposed to in parts) (Meyer & Batshaw, 2002).

Their findings of Roberts and colleagues (2002) relative to the types of gestures that were found to be weak in boys with fragile X syndrome is somewhat supported by the conclusions drawn by Flenthrope & Brady (2010), who studied the "relationship between gesture types and later expressive language use in natural communication situations" (p. 139). They did not find a significant relationship between the use of prelinguistic gestures and later language outcomes in young children with fragile X syndrome who also exhibited several symptoms of autism. Although initially surprised by their results relative to other studies, they concluded that the type of gestures used, as opposed to the variety of gestures used, could be more predictive of language outcomes, specifically word production. For example, enhanced natural gestures (Calculator, 2002), social gestures, conventional gestures, and pointing are more advanced gestures than contact gestures and reaching as a requesting gesture.

Speech is usually delayed, and the more severely affected children may be nonverbal. Articulation errors, stuttering, and cluttering are frequent symptoms, and these individuals typically have a hoarse and breathy quality of voice. A high-arched palate and/or cleft palate and feeding problems are also common (Pore & Reed, 1999; Shprintzen, 1997). Boys with fragile X syndrome do not use as many gestures to support their verbal attempts at communication. Rather, they use more jargon, and they tend to have more echolalia and perseveration than their counterparts with Down syndrome. In fact, their communicative behaviors are more typical of children with autism (Wolf-Schein et al., 1987). However, unlike children with autism, some children with fragile X tend to be very social, with a good sense of humor. Nonetheless, approximately 25 percent of children with fragile X syndrome have enough characteristics that overlap with those seen in children with autism that they meet the criteria for a secondary diagnosis of autism spectrum disorder (Meyer, 2007).

Cognitive deficits are more common in males than females, with the females having mild to severe learning disabilities and males having moderate to severe mental retardation (Pore & Reed, 1999).

Cognitive and language deficits can hinder the academic and social growth of children with fragile X syndrome. As in children with autism, many of these characteristics are typical of those seen in individuals with attention deficit disorder with hyperactivity. Specifically, a boy with fragile X syndrome may be hyperactive, have a short attention span, be impulsive, and have poor interactive skills (Paul, 2001). Boys may also exhibit some signs of autism such as repetitive hand flapping, lack of eye contact, hypersensitivities, and tactile defensiveness, which means that they usually have a negative reaction to being touched. They also frequently have fine motor control deficits (Spiridigliozzi et al., 2001).

With regard to cognitive skills, Paul (2001) writes that the individuals with fragile X syndrome do better on tasks that require "simultaneous processing" than on those that require "sequential processing." For example,

Echolalia. The unintentional repetition of words spoken by others.

Perseveration. Unintentional repetitive movements or vocalizations.

Tactile defensiveness. A pronounced dislike of being touched, usually accompanied by a negative emotional reaction.

identifying the missing part of an object when shown an incomplete picture of that object is an easier task than reproducing a series of words in the same order as presented. Strengths that can foster academic progress include good long-term memory and visual memory. Individuals with fragile X syndrom are good at repetition and verbal imitation, skills that can also contribute to academic success when provided with a good model (Spiridigliozzi et al., 2001).

However, children with fragile X syndrome also have several weaknesses that can hinder academic, social, and vocational growth. Spiridigliozzi and colleagues (2001) found that calculation, abstract reasoning, and problem solving are problematic for children with fragile X syndrome. Initiating and completing tasks are also problematic, but they do respond to prompts to help in these areas. They also found that IQ in this population declines over time because their rate of development slows down as they get older (when compared to normally developing peers). Because of the decline as the boys get older, efficient and effective early intervention is critical.

The extent to which these children have speech and language deficits is tied, to some degree, to the level of intellectual disability that is present. Thus, one could expect to see some of the same behaviors and characteristics that are described in the section on cognitive handicaps. In addition, children with fragile X syndrome demonstrate delays in expressive language. Receptive language and semantics are relatively unaffected when compared to the level of expressive language. These children use numerous phonological processes for an extended amount of time when compared to their age-level peers. Their speech is also characterized by a rapid rate and reduced intelligibility, particularly as sentences increase in length (Scharfenaker, 1990). In addition, they demonstrate word-finding difficulties (which impacts their abilities to answer direct questions), have delayed syntax, and exhibit pragmatic deficits including lack of clarifying gestures, poor turn taking, and poor maintenance of a topic (Schopmeyer & Lowe, 1992).

Other Characteristics of Children with Fragile X Syndrome

According to Pore and Reed (1999), approximately 63 percent of boys who have fragile X syndrome also have otitis media. Seizures are seen in approximately one-fifth of the afflicted individuals. It is not unusual to see attention deficit disorders with hyperactivity (ADHD). Motor development is typically delayed, partially due to possible hypotonia, and sensory integration skills are also deficient (Pore & Reed, 1999). Another characteristic found in individuals with fragile X syndrome (and coincidentally, also in Down syndrome) is late-onset psychosis (Shprintzen, 1997). Behavioral patterns of children with fragile X syndrome are delineated in Table 2–4.

TABLE 2–4 Behavioral patterns in fully affected males with fragile X syndrome

Behavior	Percentage
Hand flapping	85%
Lack of eye contact	90%
Tactile defensiveness	76%
Hyperactivity	73%
Inattention	95%
Aggression	25%
Anxiety	64%

Source: Data compiled from Fragile X Syndrome, by G. A. Meyer & M. L. Batshaw in *Children with Disabilities* (5th ed.), M. Batshaw (ed.). Paul H. Brookes, 2002.

Robin Sequence/Stickler Syndrome

Historically, Robin sequence has been called Pierre Robin syndrome. Based on the definition previously discussed, it should be called Pierre Robin sequence or Robin sequence. Affected babies have a very small jaw and a U-shaped cleft palate. Both of these characteristics compromise the upper airway system. These children are obligatory mouth breathers, which interferes with feeding and the more natural nasal breathing. This is an example of a sequence in which the child's tongue cannot be positioned anteriorly due to the small jaw. Thus, the pharynx (breathing space) does not expand because when the child's mouth is closed, the tongue falls back into the oropharynx. This in turn causes an obstruction to the upper airway, and the child cannot breathe nasally. This condition is called glossoptosis, which is secondary to the inherited genetic trait of micrognathia (very small jaw) (Shprintzen, 1997).

Stickler syndrome is the most common cause of the Robin sequence. In fact, one-third of the patients diagnosed with Robin sequence are also diagnosed as having Stickler syndrome. Stickler syndrome shares the characteristics of Robin sequence in addition to skeletal anomalies such as a clubfoot and eye problems. Stickler syndrome is "a common genetic form of connective tissue dysplasia and perhaps the second most common syndrome associated with cleft palate in the absence of cleft lip" (Shprintzen, 1997, p. 84). Figure 2–3 depicts a girl with characteristic facial features of Stickler syndrome. Figure 2–4 shows the mandibular hypoplasia and cleft palate associated with Stickler syndrome.

Robin sequence is typically classified as either the Robin deformation sequence or the Robin malformation sequence. In the Robin deformation sequence, the causes of the abnormality are extrinsic to the fetus. That is to

Glossoptosis. Displacement of the tongue into a downward position.

Micrognathia. A very small lower jaw that is frequently paired with a recessed chin.

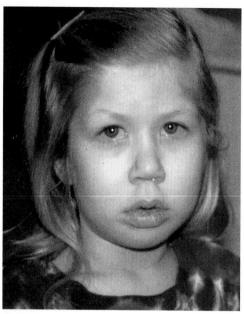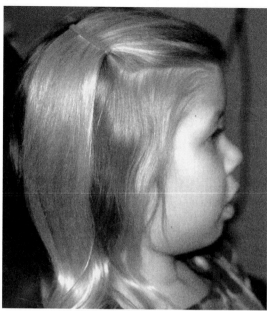

FIGURE 2–3 A girl with characteristic facial features of Stickler syndrome. (*Source:* From Kummer, Ann W. *Cleft Palate & Craniofacial Anomalies: Effects on Speech and Resonance,* 2nd ed. © 2008 Delmar, Cengage Learning.)

say, the anomalies are caused by positional deformities that are not likely to be repeated in subsequent pregnancies. The child may inherit a familial trait such as a small jaw, which is exacerbated by compression problems that would occur if the mother's uterus and/or pelvis were too small, resulting in compression of the baby. In Robin malformation sequence, the cause(s) of the problems are intrinsic to the baby. The baby could have a malformation such as a small mandible that could result in the tongue's abnormal positioning, resulting in poor palatal growth (Shprintzen, 1997).

Speech and Language Characteristics of Stickler Syndrome/Robin Sequence

Speech and language problems can result from the cleft palate and hearing loss exhibited by many individuals with Robin sequence and Stickler syndrome. As mentioned previously, the child with Robin sequence has a cleft palate and possible a cleft lip, and the speech is hypernasal. Hyponasality is sometimes seen when the nasal cavity is extremely small. The posterior location of the tongue may contribute to feeding and breathing problems that result in failure to thrive, dysphagia, and apnea.

The child typically has dentition abnormalities that could contribute to poor articulation. Lingual protrusion distortions and backing are common. The child may develop abnormal compensatory articulation patterns. Intellectual disabilities, possibly due to a lack of oxygen to the brain and upper airway obstruction, sometimes occurs (Jung, 1989; Pore & Reed, 1999; Shprintzen, 2000).

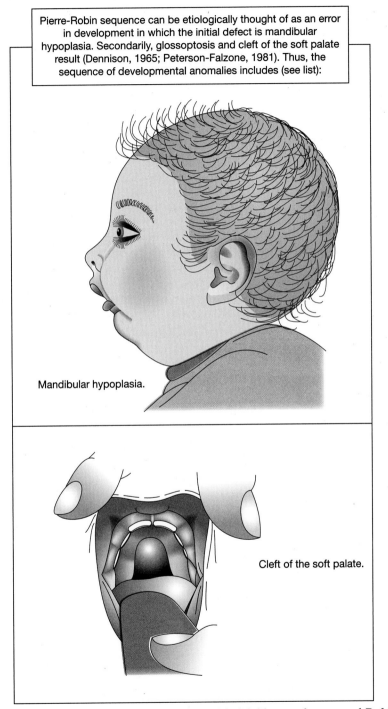

Pierre-Robin sequence can be etiologically thought of as an error in development in which the initial defect is mandibular hypoplasia. Secondarily, glossoptosis and cleft of the soft palate result (Dennison, 1965; Peterson-Falzone, 1981). Thus, the sequence of developmental anomalies includes (see list):

Mandibular hypoplasia.

Cleft of the soft palate.

FIGURE 2–4   Characteristics of children with Stickler syndrome and Robin sequence.   (*Source: Based on Genetic Syndromes in Communication Disorders.* Austin, TX: Pro-Ed, 1988.)

Other Characteristics of Stickler Syndrome/Robin Sequence

Approximately 15 percent of patients with Stickler syndrome exhibit a sensorineural hearing loss that typically affects the high frequencies. In those with cleft palate, chronic middle-ear effusion may lead to a conductive loss. The child with Robin sequence often has anomalies of the middle and external ears. These anomalies include low-set ears, an abnormally angled external auditory meatus, deformed outer ears, and structural defects of the middle ear ossicles (Jung, 1989; Shprintzen, 2000). Eye problems include retinal detachment, occasional cataracts, myopia, and vitroretinal degeneration. Thus, is it essential the child diagnosed with Robin sequence and/or Stickler syndrome receive frequent eye examinations (Pore & Reed, 1999; Shprintzen, 2000).

Velo-Cardio-Facial Syndrome (VCFS)

Velo-cardio-facial syndrome was first documented in 1978 and has received additional attention in recent research. Shprintzen (2000) reports that it "is probably the second most common multiple anomaly syndrome in humans with an estimated population prevalence of 1:2,000 people and a birth incidence that is higher because some babies do not survive the neonatal period" (p. 411). It affects multiple systems: the central nervous system, the craniofacial system, the digestive system, the genitourinary system, the immune system, the limbs, the mental system, the metabolic system, the renal system, the respiratory system, and the skeletal system. Drawings depicting characteristics of an ear and hand in a child with VCFS can be found in Figure 2–5; Figures 2–6 and 2–7 depict children with VCFS.

Speech and Language Characteristics of Children with VCFS

Typically, there is severe velopharyngeal insufficiency in individuals with VCFS, and cleft palate is common. These individuals have severe articulatory impairment that is usually characterized by a preponderance of glottal stop substitutions. Unlike other children with cleft palate, children with VCFS usually do not develop other abnormal substitutions, pharyngeal

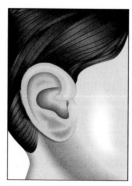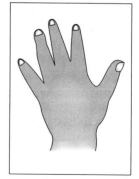

FIGURE 2–5   Characteristics of children with velo-cardio-facial syndrome (VCFS). (*Delmar/Cengage Learning*)

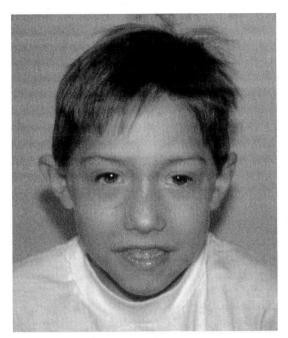

FIGURE 2–6   A boy with velo-cardio-facial syndrome.   (*Source:* From Kummer, Ann W. *Cleft Palate & Craniofacial Anomalies: Effects on Speech and Resonance,* 2nd ed. © 2008 Delmar, Cengage Learning.)

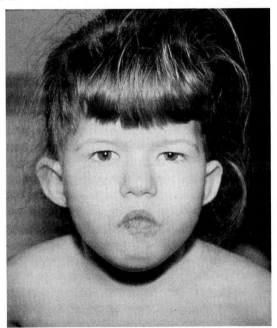

FIGURE 2–7   A girl with velo-cardio-facial syndrome.   (*Source:* From Kummer, Ann W. *Cleft Palate & Craniofacial Anomalies: Effects on Speech and Resonance,* 2nd ed. © 2008 Delmar, Cengage Learning.)

stops, pharyngeal fricatives, or middorsal stops. The voice is high pitched, hoarse, and breathy, and is typically highly hypernasal (Shprintzen, 1997; Shprintzen, 2000). Riski (1999) identifies VCFS as the most common cause of clefting associated with syndrome manifestation. However, with extensive speech therapy and surgical reconstruction of the velopharyngeal valve, the individual with VCFS can achieve normal-sounding speech.

Children with VCFS typically demonstrate a mild language delay but catch up with their typically developing peers between 36 to 48 months of age. They frequently have learning disabilities and difficulty with abstract thinking. ADHD may be evident, and occasionally mild intellectual disabilities is noted. Deficits in auditory memory and processing have also been documented (Shprintzen, 1997; Shprintzen, 2000).

Learning disabilities are characteristic in children with VCFS, a genetic syndrome. In fact, 99 percent of individuals with VCFS experience learning disabilities. Golding-Kushner, Weller, and Shprintzen (1985) found that, regardless of age, children with VCFS had perceptual motor weaknesses. Intellectual functioning and language skills were essentially normal by the time the child turned age 6. However, as they grew older, the children with VCFS demonstrated poor abstract reasoning skills when compared to typically developing children, partially due to the fact that they remained at a relatively concrete level of cognitive functioning. Thus, the academic, language, and psychological skills were negatively impacted. This impact is expected given that as the child advances in school, there are increased linguistic and cognitive demands. Complicating the speech, language, and academic problems is the fact that children who have VCFS characteristically have recurrent bouts of fluid accumulation and infection, also known as **otitis media with effusion** (Faires, Topping, & Cranford, 1993; Gravel & Wallace, 1996).

As children with VCFS get older, the ability to form appropriate social interactions may be negatively affected by stress. Papolos and colleagues (1996) have documented that approximately 70 percent of the cases they assessed presented with some form of bipolar affective disorder such as dysthymia and psychotic manic depression (Shprintzen, 1997). In addition, a study by Goldberg and colleagues (1993) found a wide variety of psychiatric disorders, including attention deficit disorder with hyperactivity, generalized anxiety disorder, obsessive compulsive disorder, severe personality disorder, and paranoid disorder. All these factors vary in terms of their occurrence, but nearly all children with VCFS have "some degree of cognitive impairment and social communication deficits" (Carneol, Marks, & Weik, 1999, p. 28). These impairments may be relatively subtle, and the lack of proper diagnosis may prevent the child from receiving appropriate services in the public schools.

Other Characteristics of Children with VCFS

Individuals who are diagnosed with VCFS often have hearing loss. Although the loss may be sensorineural (15% of the VCFS population), a conductive loss is more common, with the conductive loss occurring secondary to middle-ear effusion. The external canals are usually narrow, and the helix is overfolded. Ears may be small and/or cup-shaped, with attached auricular lobules. The hearing loss is usually mild to moderate and unilateral. The individual may demonstrate an exaggerated startle response (Shprintzen, 2000).

The craniofacial system is characterized by upper-airway obstruction during infancy, an anterior laryngeal web, a large pharyngeal passageway, absent or small adenoids, asymmetrical movement of the pharyngeal walls, and a unilateral vocal cord paresis. The infant may have difficulty feeding, leading to the baby's failing to thrive. Gastroesophageal reflux, nasal vomiting and regurgitation, and constipation are problematic (Shprintzen, 2000).

Behavioral problems in individuals with VCFS are common. During infancy, these babies may be irritable and have poor bonding (although frequent illnesses and hospitalizations may contribute to this).

Williams Syndrome

Initially described by J. C. P. Williams and colleagues in 1961, Williams syndrome (a genetic disorder) was identified based on a distinctive set of cardiovascular anomalies. "In 1978, the multisystem nature of the syndrome was recognized to include specific heart defects (which occur in approximately 80% of cases), developmental disabilities, and unusual facial features" (Percy et al., 2007). Children with Williams syndrome typically exhibit mild to severe intellectual disabilities. They are frequently classified as extroverts due to a friendly personality and extreme talkativeness (hyperverbalism).

The facial features are characterized by the following:

- Broad forehead
- Medial eyebrow flare
- Depressed nasal bridge
- Star-like pattern in the iris
- Wide-spaced teeth
- Full lips (Percy et al., 2007, p. 259t)
- "'Elfin' faces (full lips and cheeks, fullness of area around the eyes)" (Scacheri, 2002, p. 772)

Often, these children are mildly microcephalic and have low birth weight and delayed growth. Difficulties with feeding persist, resulting in failure to thrive during infancy, digestive disorders, and constipation. Middle-ear infections are also common (Percy et al., 2007).

Microcephaly. Head size smaller than age- and gender-appropriate size.

Individuals with Williams syndrome typically are highly social and extroverted. With regard to vocal quality, their voices are usually hoarse. Ogliodontia (absence of one or more teeth) is often present (Acs, Ng, Helpin, & Rosenberg, 2002). They have various physical ailments such as

Hypercalcemia. Abnormally elevated calcium levels in the blood.

congenital heart defects, hypercalcemia, kidney anomalies, contractures of the joints (particularly in the legs), and hypertension (Percy et al., 2007; Scacheri, 2002).

Children with Williams syndrome are sometimes mistakenly diagnosed as having fetal alcohol syndrome or fetal alcohol spectrum disorder due to similarities in their physical features and neurodevelopmental characteristics (Nulman, Ickowicz, Koren, & Knittel-Keren, 2007).

According to Percy and colleagues (2007), Williams syndrome is also characterized by a descriptive, characteristic behavioral pattern. Specifically, the following are typical:

- Developmental delays occur; cognitive abilities range from severe disability to average ability.

- Auditory sensitivity is present.

- There is increased risk of anxiety disorders and ADHD.

- Despite lower overall mental age and visuospatial functioning, higher-level language behaviors are evident. For example, individuals with Williams syndrome often display "cocktail party speech."

- Emotional and behavior difficulties can include irritability, poor concentration, temper tantrums, overactivity, eating difficulties, poor peer relationships, and sleep disturbances.

- Individuals may display inappropriate attention-seeking behavior.

- Affected children show lack of social constraints (e.g., friendliness toward adults, including strangers). (p. 259t)

- Individuals may also demonstrate unusual musical skills.

As mentioned previously, individuals with Williams syndrome are often hypersocial. Nonetheless, they do demonstrate pragmatic deficits; many of these deficits are seen in individuals on the autism spectrum although they are not as pervasive or intense in children with Williams syndrome. They have problems with turn taking, language structure, and topic maintenance. They do not provide sufficient information to facilitate their conversation partner's participation in an exchange, and they tend to rely overly on the leads and contributions of their communication partners (Philofsky, Fidler, & Hepburn, 2007). Philofsky and colleagues summarized pragmatic behaviors of individuals with Williams syndrome as follows:

- Difficulty understanding communicative nonverbal gestures

- A lack of use of communicative nonverbal gestures

- Overtalkativeness

- Difficulties with conversational reciprocity

- Perseverations with language
- Difficulties with topic coherence
- Use of tangential language
- Difficulties interpreting abstract language
- Difficulties with friendships
- Restricted and repetitive interests

Given these characteristics in the language of children with Williams syndrome, speech-language therapy should focus on pragmatic behaviors, including use of social skills in a variety of settings.

Noonan Syndrome

Noonan syndrome is named after Dr. Jacqueline Noonan, a pediatric cardiologist who, along with Dorothy Ehmke, a pediatrician, described a child with a defining set of symptoms. However, she was not the first to describe it. In 1883, Koblinsky noted "a boy with webbing of the neck, incomplete folding of the ears, and a low posterior hairline" (Percy et al., 2007, p. 245). It affects one in every 1,000–2,500 births, and due to highly variable presentations, it is not always identified early. Noonan syndrome is the most common genetic syndrome associated with congenital heart disease. Ninety-five percent of individuals with this syndrome have vision problems.

The principle feature is congenital heart malformation, with 50 percent of the cases being valvular pulmonary stenosis. Ten percent have atrial septal defects, and a small percentage have ventricular septal effects. A heart murmur and/or cardiomyopathy are also common. Short stature, learning disabilities, chest indentations (with the breastbone prominent or depressed), webbing of the neck, and impaired blood clotting are typical. Scoliosis is commonly accompanied by scapular winging. Frequently the affected individuals are hypotonic.

Ears and eyes also have a characteristic appearance; 95 percent have hypertelorism. Other common eye abnormalities include ptosis (drooping) of the eyelids, epicanthal folds, proptosis, strabismus, and nystagmus. Over 90 percent have low-set and backward-rotated ears. More than 90 percent also have a thickened helix. Sensorineural hearing loss is common (Scacheri, 2002), as is chronic otitis media.

Decreased appetite and digestive problems frequently lead to failure to thrive during infancy. The patients often have swallowing difficulties and may have frequent or forceful vomiting. With regard to the oral cavity, more than 90 percent of individuals with Noonan syndrome have a deeply grooved philtrum. Micrognathia (small jaw) is common, as is hypsistaphylia. Dental problems are common. All of these factors combined with poor tongue control lead to disordered articulation.

Epicanthal folds. A fold of skin, sometimes crescent-shaped, on the inner and sometimes outer corners of the eyes.

Proptosis. Bulging of the eyes.

Strabismus. The deviation of the eye(s) from center when looking forward.

Nystagmus. Uncontrollable rapid eye movements.

Hypsistaphylia. A high, narrow palate.

Developmentally, children with Noonan syndrome have a general delay of motor milestones, demonstrating poor motor coordination and general clumsiness. Full-scale IQ scores average around 86 (range of 48–130) (Percy et al., 2007). Approximately 25–33 percent have intellectual disabilities, usually mild. Almost all have learning disabilities. The author's experience includes a child with Noonan syndrome who had profound mental deficits. As many as 50 percent of individuals with Noonan syndrome have a high-frequency sensorineural hearing loss. As one would expect, speech and language delays are consistently present in these children. Percy et al. (2007) report that many individuals with Noonan syndrome have autistic features.

Angelman Syndrome

Although Angelman syndrome was first described in 1965, it was not noted until 1987 that about 80 percent of children with Angelman syndrome have a small piece of chromosome 15 missing (chromosome 15q partial deletion) (Brown & Percy, 2007). Angelman syndrome is a classic example of genetic imprinting in that it is usually caused by deletion of genes on the maternally inherited chromosome 15. Other causes include uniparental disomy, translocation, or single-gene mutation in the region of chromosome 15. Individuals with the UBE3A gene mutation are usually the least affected, while those with the larger deletions of genes on chromosome 15 are thought to be the most affected (Towbin, Mauk, & Batshaw, 2002). Angelman syndrome is a "sister syndrome" of Prader-Willi syndrome. Both are caused by deletion of genes on chromosome 15 (Percy, 2007). The prevalence is not generally known, although a Danish study showed 1 in 10,000 births and a study in Sweden showed 1 in 20,000 based on an eight year study of approximately 45,000 births (www.news-medical.net/health/What-is-Angelman-Syndrome.aspx).

Diagnosis of Angelman syndrome is frequently based on a history of delayed motor milestones, later delay in general development (especially of speech), unusual movements, characteristic facial appearance (in some cases), history of epilepsy and abnormal EEG tracing, a happy disposition with frequent laughter and/or smiling, and the deletion on chromosome 15. Usually diagnosed between the ages of 3 and 7 years, Angelman syndrome is a neurogenic disorder additionally characterized by intellectual and developmental delay, sleep disturbance, seizures and EEG abnormalities (seen in 90 percent of cases), and jerky movements (especially arm and hand flapping). Some describe the gait as being "puppet-like" because the individuals have uplifted, flexed arms when walking and use a stiff, wide-based stance. Motor delays are typical. These individuals have a happy disposition and laugh frequently.

Craniofacial effects include dental spacing, tongue protrusion, and a persistent open-mouth posture. There is relative prognathia secondary to a long mandibular body and maxillary deficiency. Typically, individuals with Angleman syndrome have microcephaly and brachycephaly, as well as a flat occiput. They have deep-set eyes. Facial features become more prominent as

Brachycephaly. Head shape characterized by tallness of the head and flatness of the back of the head.

the child gets older. Some, especially if they have chromosome 15 deletion, have fairer complexions than the rest of their family members.

One hundred percent of children with Angelman syndrome have severe to profound developmental delay that is evident by 6–12 months of age (Percy et al., 2007; Scacheri, 2002). Neurological markers include cortical atrophy, a thin corpus collosum, cerebellar hyperplasia, unilateral hypoplasia of the temporal lobe, and decreased myelination. Progressive ataxia, hyperactive reflexes, and hypotonia in infancy are typical.

Developmental milestones are delayed. These children may fall on the autism spectrum although, as previously mentioned, many show a happy, sociable personality (Percy, 2007). Receptive and expressive language delays are characteristic. There is minimal receptive language development, and the hallmark feature is lack of development of expressive language. About 33 percent develop no speech; many never exceed 5–10 words. Lack of speech is partially due to the level of language functioning, but may also be due to oral motor difficulties. However, children with Angelman syndrome do not use signs as a rule. Some may learn a few signs, but most rely on simple gestures for their communication. They also prefer gestures to signs and other forms of augmentative and alternative communication (AAC) (Alvares & Downing, 1998; Jolleff & Ryan, 1993; Penner, Johnson, Faircloth, Irish, & Wlliams, 1993).

Calculator (2002) studied the use of enhanced natural gestures (ENGs) in interactions between parents and their child with Angelman syndrome. Calculator defined ENGs as "intentional behaviors that are present in a child's motor repertoire or can be easily taught based on a child's extant motor skills" (p. 340). In Calculator's study, the parents were the primary providers of intervention, and the child's home was the site of intervention. ENGs require instruction but are enhanced versions of movements associated with an object or activity that already are being done by the child. Calculator provides an illustration of a natural gesture by describing a child lifting a cup to her mouth using both hands. This action is a natural gesture (NG) because it involves contact with an object. If the child were to use this same gesture without touching the cup, she would be using an enhanced natural gesture. Calculator further describes the differences between ENGs and NGs:

- ENGs are always assumed to be intentional.

- ENGs are readily understood by others in context

- ENGs may involve modifying a natural gesture to make it more comprehensible to others.

- ENGs are limited to distal gestures that do not rely on actual physical contact with the referent or interactant. (p. 343)

Results (based on parent interview) indicated that the use of ENGs as a communication system was effective, reasonable, and easy to teach others. Compared to other systems previously implemented, parents believed

TABLE 2–5   Additional characteristics of Angelman syndrome

Feeding problems in infancy (poor sucking and poor weight gain) in 75%

Frequent drooling, protruding tongue

Tongue thrusting; sucking and swallowing disorders

Prominent mandible

Excessive chewing and mouthing behaviors

Delay in sitting and walking

Poor attention span and hyperactivity

Unusual movements (find tremor, hand-flapping, jerking movements)

Frequent inappropriate laughter

Poor sleeping pattern

Strabismus in 40%

Scoliosis in 10%

Increased sensitivity to heat

Attraction to or fascination with water

Sources: Hyman & Towbin, 2007; Percy, M, (2007); Percy, M., et al. (2007); Scacheri, C. (2002); Towbin, Mauk, & Batshaw (2002); Shprintzen, R. J. (2000); Alvares & Downing (1998); Shprintzen, R. J. (1997); http://www.dmoz.org/Health/Conditions_and_Diseases/Neurological Disorders, http://www.ncbi.nim.nih.gov/bookshelf, http://www.angelman.org/; http://www .news-medical.net/health/What-is-Angelman-Syndrome.aspx.

that the use of ENGs would result in "permanent improvements in their children's communication success at home" (p. 354).

Learning disabilities are seen, but intellectual disabilities in the severe range are more common. General health is good as a rule. A list of additional key features can be found in Table 2–5.

As adults, the persistence of the affectionate nature can pose social and pragmatic issues. They have increased medical complications including the development of joint contractures, curvature of the spine, esophageal reflux, and seizures. Other characteristics of adults are listed in Table 2–6.

An informational agency and websites are listed in Table 2–7. Parents, friends, and caretakers may find these resources to be helpful in learning about Angelman syndrome, and in providing support.

Prader-Willi Syndrome

Prader-Willi syndrome is a chromosomal disorder that occurs in approximately 1 in 25,000 births. Physical characteristics of this syndrome include short stature, almond-shaped eyes, small hands and feet, morbid obesity, and delayed puberty with hypogonadism and cryptorchidism. Hyperphagia, viscuous (thick) saliva, and hypotonia—particularly in the neck muscles— are also symptomatic. Individuals with Prader-Willi syndrome are often

Hypogonadism. Underdevelopment and decreased function of sex organs.

Cryptorchidism. Undescended testicles.

Hyperphagia. Compulsive eating for an extended period of time.

TABLE 2–6 Characteristics of adults with Angelman syndrome

Less hyperactive than when they were younger

Better concentration span than when they were younger

Decreased sleep problems as they get older

Remain dependent on others, but acquire some activities of daily living

Puberty and menstruation begin around normal time

Dressing skills variable (avoid use of buttons and zippers)

Most can eat with a knife and fork

May be able to do simple household chores

Source: http:// www.news-medical.net/health/What-is-Angelman-Syndrome.aspx.

TABLE 2–7 Resources for information about Angelman syndrome

Angelman Syndrome Support Education and Research Trust (ASSERT)

P. O. Box 13694

Musselburgh

EH21 6XZ

Telephone: 01268 415940

E-Mail: assert@angelmanuk.org

www.dmoz.org/Health/Conditions_and_Diseases/Neurological Disorders

www.ncbi.nim.nih.gov/bookshelf

Angelman Syndrome Foundation, Inc.

www.angelman.org/

Special Needs Reads

http://specialneedsreads.com

Delmar/Cengage learning

classified as failing to thrive in infancy, and cognitive deficits are characteristic. The involvement of speech-language pathologists in the management of patients with Prader-Willi syndrome usually centers on the cognitive disabilities (Batshaw, 2002). Typically, the cognitive deficits are in the mild to moderate range or may be learning disabilities (www.ghr.nlm.nih.gov/condition=praderwillisyndrome). In addition, according to the National Institutes on Health, affected individuals have temper tantrums, behavior problems, and stubbornness (www.ghr.nlm.nih.gov/condition=praderwillisyndrome). Sleep disorders are common.

Obsessive-compulsive disorder and self-injurious behaviors are also associated with Prader-Willi syndrome (Reber, 2002). Sometimes, males with fragile X syndrome have truncal obesity, small genitals, and short, broad hands and feet. These boys are frequently referred to as having a "Prader-Willi-like phenotype," but despite some common characteristics, this obesity variant of the fragile X phenotype is not the same disorder as Prader-Willi syndrome (Mazzocco & Holden, 2007).

As mentioned earlier, a hallmark characteristic of Prader-Willi syndrome is hyperphagia. This syndrome affects the hypothalamus, which results in the abnormal eating behaviors. Individuals with Prader-Willi syndrome have a "constant feeling of hunger that can lead to obsessive eating and morbid obesity" (Percy, Brown, & Lewkis, 2007, p. 320). The compulsive eating behaviors typically develop in childhood (see the National Institutes of Health page on Prader-Willi syndrome, www.ghr.nlm.nih.gov/condition=praderwillisyndrome). Along with the eating disorder, these individuals are at increased risk for cardiovascular disease and Type II diabetes (Bigby, 2007). Obesity becomes an issue during the preschool years.

Speech and Language Characteristics of Children with Prader-Willi Syndrome

Lewis, Freebairn, Heeger, and Cassidy (2002) evaluated the speech and language skills of 27 boys and 28 girls between 6 and 42 months of age who had been diagnosed with Prader-Willi syndrome. They used standardized tests as well as an analysis of speech samples. They found a great deal of variability in the speech and language characteristics; some remained nonverbal, while others approximated normal speech and language skills as adults. Based on their findings, Lewis and colleagues made the assertion that oral motor impairments and poor articulation skills can be considered as hallmark symptoms of Prader-Willi syndrome. It is possible that the oral motor difficulties are due in part to hypotonia and have an impact on the difficulties these children have in developing intelligible speech. Other factors that may impact articulation include a narrow overjet, a narrow palatal arch, micrognathia, xerostomia (dry mouth due to insufficient production of saliva), and dental decay (p. 286). In Lewis and colleagues' study, 85 percent of the subjects had mild to severe articulation impairments, with the preschoolers all having articulation deficits in the moderate to severe range that consisted of vowel errors, imprecise articulation, sound distortions, and difficulty sequencing syllables (p. 292). However, 21 percent of the school-age children and 31 percent of the adolescents and adults had normal articulation.

Hypotonia leads to reduced velopharyngeal movement, which affects nasality. Lewis and colleagues (2002) found that 75 percent of their subjects were hypernasal and 14 percent were hyponasal (hyponasality had not been reported previously). Endocrine dysfunction and the use of growth hormones in the medical management of children with Prader-Willi syndrome contribute to altered pitch and vocal quality. Compared to children of the same age and gender, 20 percent of Lewis and colleagues' subjects had high pitch and 24 percent had low pitch. Pitch was within normal range

Micrognathia. A small jaw, typically referring to the mandible.

Xerostomia. Persistent dry mouth secondary to poor saliva production that can be due to extrinsic factors such as medications or intrinsic factors such as Sjogren's disease.

for 44 percent of the preschoolers, 75 percent of the school-age children, and 54 percent of the adolescents and adults.

In regard to language abilities, Lewis and colleagues found that expressive language is more impaired than receptive language. Pragmatics are also affected by a variety of factors including the effects of compulsive behaviors and temper tantrums, as well as language-based difficulties such as "problems with maintaining a topic, judging appropriate proximity to the conversational partner, and turn taking" (p. 287). Other language-related deficits are found in lexical comprehension and expression, and may be due to difficulties with auditory short-term memory and auditory and verbal processing abilities. Relative strengths were found in vocabulary, decoding, reading comprehension, and visuospatial skills.

Lewis and colleagues (2002) studied narrative skills as well, which had not been researched previously. They found that their subjects had "substantial deficits" (p. 291) in narrative retelling tasks and difficulties comprehending narratives. Although the children's narrative skills improved as they got older, the skills never reached normal.

A major contribution by Lewis and colleagues (2002) is the breakdown of speech and language characteristics of children with Prader-Willi syndrome by age:

- 6–24 months: "weak cry, early feeding difficulties, hypotonia and delayed onset of speech/language"

- 18–24 months: a few single words emerge, but no two-word combinations

- 2–5 years: "first words appear and the child acquires vocabulary, two-word combinations, and some syntax"; poor oral-motor skills, mostly unintelligible speech with "many sound errors"

- 5–12 years: residual articulation errors; decreased intelligibility in connected speech; delayed receptive and expressive language; hypo- or hypernasality; difficulties with pitch and vocal quality; poor narrative skills; behavior problems impact social interactions

- 12 years–adult: persistence of articulation errors; persistence of receptive and expressive language deficits, persistence of narrative deficits, "poor conversational skills," and abnormal pitch and vocal quality (p. 293)

Prader-Willi syndrome shares some symptoms and behaviors associated with autism spectrum disorder (ASD) or pervasive developmental disorders (PDD), and therefore may "mask" as one of these disorders. In fact, some surveys show that disorders such as Prader-Willi syndrome, fragile X syndrome, tuberous sclerosis, and Angelman syndrome account for as many as 15–25 percent of all ASD cases. However, these disorders are genetic disorders, not ASDs (Percy, 2007).

Information Source for Prader-Willi Syndrome

The Prader-Willi Syndrome Association is a national clearinghouse for information about Prader-Willi syndrome. They provide information to anyone interested in learning about this disorder. Their website is www.pwsusa.org and their e-mail address is national@pwsusa.org (Rose, 2002).

CHARGE Association

CHARGE is an acronym for

- Coloboma (a defect in the iris or retina)
- Heart defect
- Atresia choanae, or "congenital blockage of the nasal passages" (Scacheri, 2002, p. 753)
- Retarded growth and development
- Genital hypoplasia
- Ear anomalies/deafness

Association. A pattern of malformations occurring at an unusual rate with no known etiology.

Etiology. Causative factors that lead to a delay or disorder.

Association refers to a "pattern of malformations that occur at a rate that is inconsistent with chance alone. This represents a nonrandom association of structural defects, the origin of which is not known. Associations are descriptions of patterns of defects that may, with time and better understanding, become syndromes" (Montgomery, 2008, p. 313). Associations are one category of multiple anomaly disorders (the other two categories are syndromes and sequences). They have a recurrent pattern, but there is no known specific etiology. They do not "domino" as do symptoms found in sequences (Shprintzen, 1997).

Facial features of CHARGE association include a square-shaped face with a prominent forehead. Other facial features include arched eyebrows, occasional ptosis, and large ears. There is a prominent nasal bridge and area between the nostrils. Typically the individual has a flat midface with facial asymmetry and a small mouth. Over 50 percent have anomalies of the outer ear, and middle ear anomalies with accompanying conductive hearing loss are common. Furthermore, sensorineural hearing loss and balance problems plague 90 percent of individuals who have CHARGE association. Effects on the central nervous system include brain malformations and cognitive impairment.

Moebius Syndrome

Moebius syndrome is a rare neurological disorder, present at birth, that affects primarily the sixth and seventh cranial nerves. Other cranial nerves may be affected, usually the third, fourth, fifth, ninth, tenth, and twelfth

(Scacheri, 2002). Individuals with this disorder are unable to move their face: that is, they cannot smile, frown, suck, grimace, or blink their eyes. The articulators have limitations in their speed of movement and in their strength and range of movement (Jung, 1989). Other speech and oral-motor symptoms include the following:

- Drooling

- High palate

- Short or deformed tongue

- Limited movement of tongue

- Submucous cleft palate

- Dental problems

- Articulation and speech disorders

- Swallowing and choking disorders (Jung, 1989; Shprintzen, 2000)

Affected individuals may have skeletal involvement causing hand and foot anomalies, and motor problems due to upper body weakness are common. Approximately 30 percent are on the autism spectrum. Other disorders include sleep disorders, sensory integration dysfunction, vision problems, and respiratory problems. Vision problems include an inability to move eyes laterally, strabismus, and eye sensitivity due to an inability to squint and blink.

Speech therapy includes feeding modifications such as a Haberman or Pigeon feeder, assistance with articulation, and addressing oral-motor control skills to help with feeding. Children with Moebius syndrome may need feeding tubes to maintain nutrition. Furthermore, plastic reconstructive surgery can be done in which there are nerve and muscle transfers to the corners of the mouth to provide the ability to smile. Other surgical procedures to repair limb and jaw deformities, fixing of strabismus, and various forms of facial surgery can be done.

Physical therapy focuses on gross motor skills and coordination, and occupational therapy can be done, frequently focusing on sensory integration therapy.

de Lange Syndrome

de Lange syndrome is known variously as Cornelia de Lange syndrome, Brachman de Lange syndrome, CdLS, Amsterdam syndrome, and typus degenerativus amsteiodamensis. de Lange syndrome is a syndrome of multiple congenital anomalies characterized by a distinctive facial appearance, prenatal and postnantal growth deficiency, feeding difficulties, psychomotor delay, behavioral problems, and associated malformations that mainly involve the upper extremities. Cornelia de Lange, a Dutch pediatrician, first described it as a distinct syndrome in 1933, though Brachmann had described a child with similar features in 1916 (Percy et al., 2007). Diagnosing classic cases of de Lange syndrome is usually straightforward, but diagnosing mild cases may be challenging, even for an experienced clinician.

There are several intrauterine growth issues; 68 percent of individuals with de Lange syndrome have intrauterine growth retardation, with an average birth weight of 4 pounds 12 ounces for boys and 4 pounds 10 ounces for girls. In most cases, growth occurs at rates lower than those on normal growth curves throughout life. Height velocity is equal to the reference range, but pubertal growth is slow. Weight velocity is lower than the reference range until late adolescence. Average head circumference remains less than the second percentile. Failure to thrive can be directly attributed to respiratory and feeding difficulties in the newborn period and throughout infancy. Associated findings include gastroesophageal reflux (30–60%) which affects many children in that it causes irreversible esophageal scarring by the time intervention is attempted. Three percent have pyloric stenosis. Other common findings are a congenital diaphragmatic hernia and malrotation or duplication of the bowel with obstruction (www.emedicine.com/PED/topic482.htm).

Individuals with de Lange syndrome have psychomotor delay. Causes of this have been found post-mortem to include cerebral dysgenesis, with a decreased number of neurons, neuronal heterotopias, and focal gyral folding abnormalities.

Principal clinical characteristics include the following:

- Delay in growth and development
- Hirsutism (excessive growth of hair)
- Bluish, mottled skin
- Structural anomalies in limbs
- Missing or joining phalanges
- Dental problems
- Vermian hypoplasia
- Feeding difficulties
- Psychomotor delay
- Behavioral problems
- Sensorineural hearing loss (90%)
- Self-injurious behaviors

- Gastroesophageal reflux (Shprintzen, 1997; Scacheri, 2002; Percy et al., 2007; Robb & Reber, 2007; Lefler, 2008; www.revolutionhealth.com/ articles/cornelia-de-lange-syndrome/nord30?msc=ehdlp_cornelia-delange-syndrome; www.cdlsusa.org/CdLS%20Diagnostic%20 Criteria%202007%20_3_.pdf)

Distinctive facial characteristics include:

- Short, upturned nose with anteverted nares (88%)

- Depressed nasal bridge (83%)

- Thin, downturned lips (94%)

- Long philtrum

- Low set ears

- Possible cleft palate

- Dentition problems such as eruption difficulties

- Confluent eyebrows that meet at midline (synophyrs) (99%)

- Long, curly eyelashes (99%)

- Low anterior and posterior hairline (92%)

- Underdeveloped orbital arches (100%)

- High, arched palate (sometimes cleft) (86%)

- Late eruption of widely spaced teeth (86%)

- Micrognathia (84%) (Shprintzen, 1997; Scacheri, 2002; Acs, Ng, Helpin, Rosenberg, & Canion, 2007; Percy et al., 2007; Lefler, 2008; www.revolutionhealth.com/articles/cornelia-de-lange-syndrome/ nord30?msc=ehdlp_cornelia-delange-syndrome; www.cdlsusa.org/ CdLS%20Diagnostic%20Criteria%202007%20_3_.pdf; www.emedicine. com/PED/topic482.htm)

Other dental problems include misalignment, delayed teething, microdontia (small teeth), dental erosion due to gastric reflux, and periodontal disease. About 50 percent have ophthalmologic manifestations including the following:

- Myopia (Nearsightedness) (58%)

- Ptosis (drooping of eyelids) (44%)

- Blepharitis (inflammation of eyelids) (25%)

- Epiphora (excessive secretions of the lacrimal glands producing an overflow of tears) (22%)

- Microcornea (small cornea) (21%)

- Strabismus (16%)

- Nystagmus (14%)

- Astigmatism (unequal curvature of the eyes' refractive surfaces, i.e., cornea, creating a visual problem)

- Optic atrophy

- Coloboma of the optic nerve (defect of optic nerve, usually congenital)

- Congenital glaucoma has been described (www.emedicine.com/PED/topic482.htm)

Developmental and cognitive delays predominate in individuals with de Lange syndrome. A severe speech delay is typical. Only about 50 percent of the children 4 years of age or older combine words into sentences, and 33 percent have no words, or possibly one or two words. Only 4 percent have normal or low-normal language skills. Severe speech delays are likely to co-occur with intrauterine growth retardation, hearing impairment, upper limb malformations, severe motor delays, and poor social interactions. Typical IQ ranges from 30 to 85, with an average IQ of 53. Those with higher IQs tend to be those who have normal cephalometric measures and high birth weight.

The degree of occurrence of behavioral characteristics tends to vary with the degree of mental retardation and the presence of autistic-like behaviors. In terms of prevalence, hyperactivity occurs in approximately 40 percent, a self-injurious behavior occurs in around 44 percent, and daily aggression is noted in approximately 49 percent.

In spite of the vision problems, visuospatial memory, along with perceptual organization and fine motor skills, are relative strengths. Activities that provide stimulation for the vestibular system are typically pleasant to individuals who have de Lange syndrome. Speech-language therapy should focus on feeding problems, behavioral issues, articulation errors, apraxia, language delays, cognitive impairments, and AAC for those who are nonverbal (Percy et al., 2007; www.emedicine.com/PED/topic482.htm).

Cephalometric measures. Measurements of the size of the head.

Apraxia. A neurological deficit in the cortex that hinders one's ability to make voluntary motor movements even when the muscles function normally.

think about it

We have talked about a variety of syndromes. All involve some degree of cognitive, language, and/or speech deficits. What do you think would be the hardest issues you would face if you were working with this population? Why? Would you work with this population? Why or why not?

MOTOR AND SENSORY DEFICITS

Motor and sensory deficits can contribute to language deficits in children because they affect the degree to which children can explore their environment and, hence, learn language through this exploration. Children who have motor deficits have limited abilities to move about in their environment. The limited mobility may, in turn, restrict some of the environmental exploration that helps them learn about the various properties of specific objects. Similarly, children with sensory deficits face limitations in their ability to explore all properties of an object. For example, a child with a hearing impairment may not be able to hear the music from a music box or to hear and process spoken language. A child with a visual deficit may not be able to distinguish between objects based on appearance alone. These issues are expanded on in the following sections.

Static Encephalopathy

Historically referred to as cerebral palsy, static encephalopathy is not consistently associated with any particular or specific language disorders. Because of abnormal muscle tone and reflexes, a child who has moderate or severe static encephalopathy experiences his or her environment in a different way than a child who does not have mobility, motility, and sensory deficits. For example, if a child has hypotonic musculature and hypotonic reflexes (a low-tone, "floppy" baby), it is likely that he or she is not as responsive to tactile stimulation as a child without such deficits. Thus, concepts based on kinesthetic feedback, such as hot–cold and smooth–rough, may be more difficult to learn because tactile sensation is not as intact. Likewise, a child who has hypertonia and hyperreflexia (a high-tone, "tight" baby) may exhibit an abnormal startle response to noise, leading his or her parents to create a more subdued acoustic environment and limiting the child's exposure to noise. For example, if the child startles and becomes neurologically disorganized when exposed to a vacuum cleaner, the parent is more likely to use the vacuum cleaner when the child is not at home. Therefore, it is possible that the child would not correctly identify certain specific sound sources when exposed to common environmental sounds. In such a case, it is not anticipated that every child with static encephalopathy has the same difficulty with language concepts based on kinesthetic and auditory input; rather, the child has an altered experience of these sensations depending on (1) the degree of sensorimotor impairment and (2) how the environment has been structured specific to his or her needs.

Kinesthetic. Relating to the sensation of movement of joints, muscles, and tendons.

Hypertonia. Abnormally high muscle tone; sometimes referred to as spasticity

Hyperreflexia. Abnormally high reactions when reflexes are stimulated.

think about it   Co-treatment is a critical component of intervention with children who have static encephalopathy. Who should be on the intervention team, and what role would each person play?

Hearing Impairment

ASHA defines *hearing disorder, deaf,* and *hard of hearing* as follows:

- A hearing disorder is the result of impaired auditory sensitivity of the physiological auditory system. A hearing disorder may limit the development, comprehension, production, and/or maintenance of speech and/or language. Hearing disorders are classified according to difficulties in detection, recognition, discrimination, comprehension, and perception of auditory information. Individuals with hearing impairment may be described as deaf or hard of hearing.

- *Deaf* is defined as a hearing disorder that limits an individual's aural and/or oral communication performance to the extent that the primary sensory input for communication may be other than the auditory channel.

- *Hard of hearing* is defined as a hearing disorder, whether fluctuating or permanent, which adversely affects an individual's ability to communicate. The hard-of-hearing individual relies on the auditory channel as the primary sensory input for communication.

Depending on the degree of the hearing loss and the age at which the child becomes hearing impaired, the language disorders associated with hearing impairment are quite variable. Other hearing factors associated with the degree of language impairment are (1) whether or not the hearing loss is stable or progressive, (2) whether it is unilateral or bilateral, (3) what type of hearing loss the child demonstrates, (4) how much intervention the child has had, and (5) the attitude of the family members. Most of these questions and concerns are best addressed by an audiologist who evaluates the hearing of the child and determines if a disorder is present. Audiologists are the best qualified individuals to determine if hearing amplification (using hearing aids or other assistive listening devices) is a viable alternative for the child and, if so, what type of amplification is best.

Types of Hearing Loss

The deficits in the auditory system are categorized in a number of ways. Based on a child's ability to process linguistic information, and taking into account audiometric findings, a child is diagnosed as hard of hearing or deaf. Hearing is typically measured at 500, 1000, 2000, and 4000 Hz. The hearing level of pure tones at 500, 1000, and 2000 Hz (the speech frequencies) is averaged in the better ear. If the loss is 70 dB or more, the individual is considered to be deaf. If the loss is in the 35- to 69-dB range in the better ear, the individual is considered to be hard of hearing (Northern & Downs, 1984).

Conductive hearing losses are those that occur due to a breakdown in the ability of the middle ear to receive acoustic signals from the

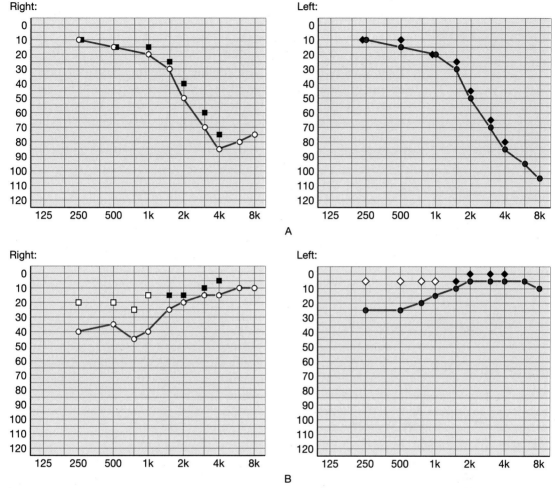

FIGURE 2–8   Audiograms illustrating two types of hearing loss. A. Sensorineural hearing loss. B. Conductive hearing loss. *(Delmar/Cengage Learning)*

environment and then to transmit the acoustic information to the inner ear (see Figure 2–8). Sensorineural hearing losses refer to those that occur in the inner ear. Sensorineural losses are divided into those due to damage to the inner ear (sensory loss), and those due to damage to the eighth cranial nerve (neural loss).

Another method used to categorize hearing loss is through the use of the terms peripheral hearing loss and central deafness. Conductive hearing losses and losses related to malfunction of the inner ear make up the losses associated with peripheral hearing loss. Damage to the eighth nerve in the brain stem or to the cortex is frequently referred to as central deafness. A child also may demonstrate a mixed hearing loss, which means that

Sensorineural hearing loss. Hearing loss due to malfunctioning of the inner ear damage to the acoustic nerve.

Peripheral hearing loss. Conductive hearing losses and losses related to malfunction of the inner ear.

Central deafness.
Damage to the eighth
nerve in the brain
stem or to the cortex.

the child has components of a conductive and of a sensorineural hearing loss, both peripheral deficits.

Prelingual and Postlingual Hearing Loss

It is not unusual for a child with prelingual hearing impairment to exhibit disorders of language content, use, and form, as outlined in Table 2–8. Prelingual hearing impairment means the hearing loss was acquired before the child developed language. Early detection is absolutely critical because it enhances the opportunity to provide early intervention to help the child use any residual hearing that may be present. Crystal and Varley (1993) reported that 95 percent of babies born deaf have some residual hearing, and their prognosis for development of speech increases with early detection. This figure certainly supports the need for routine screening of hearing in all neonates. The extent of the handicap, particularly in the area of the form of the child's language, may be affected by the his or her use of residual hearing, appropriate stimulation in the environment, and use of the proper amplification systems. Typically, children with postlingual hearing loss, who acquire their hearing loss after they develop language, are expected to do better than do children who are prelingually deaf.

Prelingual hearing loss.
The acquisition of a
hearing loss prior to
the development of
speech and language.

Postlingual hearing
loss. The acquisition
of a hearing loss after
the development of
speech and language.

Levels of Hearing Loss

If a child has a mild hearing loss, it is particularly important to determine if the loss is permanent or fluctuating. Children who are prone to

TABLE 2–8 Impact of hearing loss on language development and use

Amount of Loss	Degree of Impact	Characteristics
15–30 dB	Mild	Can still hear all vowels and most voiced consonant sounds; may miss voiceless consonants, which has an impact on morphology
30–50 dB	Moderate	Vowels heard more clearly than consonants; has difficulty understanding spoken language; misses word endings and unstressed words; form is the most severely impacted feature of language
50–70 dB	Severe	Does not hear most speech sounds; conversational speech is delayed; hears own voice and loud noises in environment; content, form, and use of language are disrupted
70 dB+	Profound	Cannot hear spoken language; may hear own vocalizations, rhythmic patterns, and extremely loud noises; form, content, and use are significantly disrupted

Source: Adapted from *Hearing in children* (4th ed.), by H. L. Northern and M. P. Downs (1991). Baltimore, MD: Williams & Wilkins. Copyright 1991 Williams and Wilkins.

repeated occurrences of otitis media and otitis media with effusion experience fluctuating hearing losses depending on the presence of fluid in the middle-ear system. These children should be followed to be sure they are acquiring all their speech sounds and language concepts as expected, but it is rare that extensive intervention is needed. However, if a child has a permanent mild hearing loss, it is worth doing some level of intervention, which may range from environmental manipulation to parent training to direct speech-language therapy. These children may be missing some of the subtleties in our speech and language, so early prevention intervention is warranted.

A child with a moderate hearing loss is very likely to benefit from amplification to facilitate the understanding of conversational speech. It is expected that a child with a moderate hearing loss will have trouble with auditory perception, auditory discrimination, and auditory memory, as many speech signals are distorted or absent. Auditory perception refers to the child's ability to hear specific environmental and speech sounds.

Auditory discrimination is the child's ability to identify specific sounds by their source, their acoustical features, or both. Auditory sequential memory refers to the child's ability to remember sounds in their proper sequence. Auditory memory deficits affect a child's capabilities with regard to remembering how sounds are sequenced in particular words, a deficit that certainly hinders a child's speech and language abilities.

Speech and language skills are likely to be delayed or disordered (or both) in children with severe hearing loss, even when the loss is identified at an early age and the child is provided with adequate and appropriate amplification. It is likely that the child will experience differences in vocal quality and have trouble with the production of all speech sounds, as he or she will have trouble discerning the acoustic qualities of speech. None of these problems is insurmountable as long as the hearing loss is identified early, appropriate amplification is provided, and speech and language intervention is implemented.

For children with a profound hearing loss, the ability to discriminate speech is greatly hindered, even with amplification. They continue to rely on tactile and visual cues and would most likely benefit from a Total Communication approach, particularly if they are very young.

Regardless of the level of hearing impairment, there is no doubt that it can have an effect on the child's use of the features of language. These effects are summarized in Tables 2–9 through 2–11. Table 2–9 lists the effects of hearing impairment on form, including phonology, syntax, and morphology.

The information in Table 2–10 is a review of the effects of hearing loss on semantics, or the content of language. It is expected that children with hearing loss have more difficulty extrapolating meaning associated with words. Curtiss, Prutting, and Lowell (1979) found that children who are hearing impaired tend to use more talk about location than do hearing children.

Otitis media. Inflammation of the middle ear.

Otitis media with effusion. Inflammation of the middle ear accompanied by the accumulation of infected fluid.

Auditory perception. The ability to hear specific environmental and speech sounds.

Auditory discrimination. The ability to identify specific sounds by their source and/or acoustical properties.

TABLE 2–9 Effects of hearing loss on form (phonology, syntax, and morphology)

Impaired intelligibility

Consonant deletions, particularly final consonants

Impaired production of vowels

Reduced speech rate

Slow articulatory transitions

Frequent pauses

Poor coordination of breathing patterns and syntactic phrasing

Inappropriate use of stressed and unstressed syllables

Delay in developmental syntax

Use of innovative syntactical structures by deaf children

Difficulty with verbs and pronouns

Decreased use of unstressed, final inflectional morphemes (plurals and verb endings)

Decreased use of some parts of speech, including adverbs, prepositions, quantifiers, and indefinite pronouns

Receptive and expressive delays in acquisition of morphological rules

Receptive and expressive delays in acquisition of syntactical rules

Source: Adapted from *Childhood language disorders in context: Infancy through adolescence,* by N. Nelson, 1993. New York: Merrill.

TABLE 2–10 Effects of hearing loss on semantics (vocabulary comprehension and production)

Difficulty understanding and using concept words

Difficulty with figurative meanings of words and phrases

Difficulty with multiple-meaning words

Difficulty with connected discourse in oral language

Difficulty with connected discourse in written language

Source: Adapted from *Childhood language disorders in context: Infancy through adolescence,* by N. Nelson, 1993. New York: Merrill.

In Table 2–11 the effects of hearing loss on the use domain, or pragmatic domain, of language are described. Infants and toddlers use a greater variety of pragmatic methods than do many school-age children. In fact, Curtiss, Prutting, & Lowell (1979) found that pragmatic skills were not as

TABLE 2–11   Effects of hearing loss on use (pragmatics)

Communication skills which exceed their semantic abilities

Use of gestures, some invented, to convey linguistic function

Better response to questions than comments

Lack of complexity in discourse

Source: Adapted from *Childhood language disorders in context: Infancy through adolescence,* by N. Nelson, 1993. New York: Merrill.

delayed or disordered in hearing-impaired preschoolers as were semantic skills (Nelson, 1993).

Cochlear Implants

Thal, DesJardin, and Eisenbeg (2007) conducted a study to determine if the MacArthur-Bates CDI is a valid tool for assessing the language development of young children who have profound hearing loss and have received cochlear implants. The children in their study were 32–86 months old. The CDI is a parent-report measure with two sections: words and gestures (8–16 months) and words and sentences (16–30 months). The authors concluded that both had excellent validity for children whose language fell within the range measured by the CDI. The study focused on vocabulary, gestures, and grammar. When examining "the relationship between length of implant use and language skills," there were "significant positive correlations that were large for language sample vocabulary, and moderate for RDLS receptive and expressive scores, offering evidence of a meaningful relationship between the ability to receive acoustic information through the implant device and the development of oral language skills in these children" (p. 59–60).

Several studies have been done to look at language and speech outcomes in children with cochlear implants. Blamey et al. (2001), Svirsky, Robbins, Kirk, Pisoni, & Miyamoto (2000), Tomblin, Barker, Spencer, Zhang, & Gantz (2005) and Thal, DesJardin, and Eisenberg (2007) all conclude that early implantation typically results in better outcomes than later implantation (or no implantation), particularly when combined with intervention and home environments designed to facilitate comprehension and production of language and speech.

think about it — If the parents of a 12-month old girl with a profound hearing loss asked you, "If she were your daughter, would you get a cochlear implant?" what would you reply?

LANGUAGE DISORDERS ASSOCIATED WITH PREMATURITY AND/OR HIGH-RISK INFANCY

Failure to Thrive (FTT) and Premature Babies

Some infants are diagnosed as "failure to thrive" babies because they are physically small or delayed in their overall development. Although this syndrome is due to a variety of factors, emotional or physical abuse (or both) and neglect (i.e., lack of provision of a balanced diet with adequate caloric intake) are often responsible for the developmental defects. Premature babies may be classified primarily into one of three categories: appropriate for gestational age (AGA), small for gestational age (SGA), and very low birth weight (VLBW) (Rossetti, 1986), with differing outcomes with regard to physical, cognitive, and language development. Normally, children are born after 38 weeks of gestation and weigh more than 2500 grams. Full-term infants who do not weigh at least 2500 grams are considered SGA babies, and they may be at risk for developmental disabilities. Even though some of these SGA babies may have relatively normal IQs, research indicates that they frequently have major neurological deficits and have an increased frequency of placement in special education or related services when they reach school age (Rossetti, 1986).

Babies who are born too early (i.e., those who are preterm and SGA) are frequently categorized as VLBW babies. These babies vary in their development, with those who weigh more than 1500 grams doing significantly better than those who weigh less than 1500 grams (Rossetti, 1986). In 1973, Fitzhardinger and Ramsey found that 15–35 percent of VLBW infants had delayed speech and language development when they were 24 months old.

A baby may fail to thrive due to his or her body's being unable to effectively use the calories that he or she takes in, excessive expenditure of calories, or insufficient intake of calories. Failure to thrive can also result from fetal alcohol syndrome (FAS). According to the American Academy of Pediatrics (1993), children with FAS often are born at term, but 80 percent have low birth weight, falling below the 10th percentile. Furthermore, "about 70% of these children have severe feeding problems, often leading to failure to thrive. Children with FAS tend to remain thin and short in childhood but by late adolescence may have attained typical height and weight" (Wunsch, Conlon, & Scheidt, 2002, p. 112).

Another population of babies who may exhibit signs of FTT is those born to mothers with HIV. Even if the infant does not have HIV, he or she is likely to have shorter mean length and lower mean birth weight when compared to babies born to mothers who do not have HIV. However, children who do not have HIV eventually develop normally with regard to height and weight. Those who do have HIV have poor growth due to a variety of reasons, including poor diet and inadequate intake, malabsorption in the gastrointestinal tract, acute infections, overutilization of energy, and stress related to psychosocial factors (Spiegel & Bonwit, 2002).

TABLE 2–12   Normal growth patterns

Age	Size
Full-term newborn	Average weight is 7.5 pounds
4–6 months	Birth weight doubled
12 months	Birth weight tripled
13 months–9 or 10 years	5 pounds per year
Birth	Average length is 19.5 inches
Birth–1 year	Length increases by 50%
Birth–4 years	Length doubles
Birth–13 years	Length triples
Birth–12 months	Head circumference increases by 3 inches
Birth–2 years	Brain weight doubles

Source: Isaacs, J. S., Nutrition and Children with Disabilities. In M. L. Batshaw, L. Pelligrino, and N. J. Roizen (Eds.), *Children with Disabilities* (6th edition), 2007.

Often, failure-to-thrive children are the babies of teenage parents, many of whom have their own physical and emotional needs unmet for a variety of reasons. In such instances it is difficult to isolate one factor that is responsible for the developmental delays. Malnutrition before and after birth can lead to decreased neurological development, with some babies having undersized brains. In fact, lack of stimulation in an otherwise healthy brain also can lead to brains with less intricate neural connections (Fewell, personal communication, 1996). The clinical criteria used to diagnose children who fail to thrive include weight below the third percentile followed by weight gain in the presence of normal nurturing. Also, the failure to grow has to be present in the absence of evidence of systemic diseases or other abnormalities based on physical examination and laboratory studies. Initially, babies who fail to thrive may show signs of developmental retardation, although acceleration in subsequent development may occur with appropriate stimulation (Barbero, 1982). Table 2–12 delineates normal weight gain by infants and toddlers.

Cytomegalovirus Infection

Cytomegalovirus (CMV) infection is a viral disease from the herpes viral strain that results in brain damage to babies who become infected during childhood. The infection can lead to destruction of brain tissues and result in mental handicapping conditions. It can also result in miscarriage. Children born with CMV typically have low birth weight and physical abnormalities. CMV infections can be contracted prenatally and postnatally, with the more devastating effects being seen when it is contracted prior to birth.

Postnatally, CMV is contracted through breast-feeding, blood transfusions, and sexual contact. It is the most common viral disease in fetuses and newborn babies, with approximately 3,000 infants affected annually (Johnson, 1996). CMV can be detected prenatally by fetal blood sampling or amniocentesis (Hill & Haffner, 2002).

Infants who are born with a CMV infection and survive have a high rate of mental handicaps, sensory deficits, motor disabilities, and seizure disorders (Johnson, 1996). Eighty percent of infants who are born with CMV that can be verified clinically have manifestations in the nervous system, including hearing loss (Herer, Knightlyn & Steinberg, 2002). In developed countries where rubella has been eradicated, CMV is probably the most common causative factor of nonhereditary congenital hearing loss, and the loss is usually sensorineural. Jung (1989, p. 261) writes that otoneurological complications secondary to CMV include "extensive invasion of the cochlea and semicircular canals as well as structures of the central auditory nervous system, including the cochlear nuclei, brainstem nuclei, and cerebral cortex." The illustration in Figure 2–9 depicts the physical facial characteristics of a child with CMV.

PRENATAL EXPOSURE TO ALCOHOL AND OTHER DRUGS

The effects of alcohol, cocaine, nicotine, and other drugs on the developing fetus is the focus of much research. The following sections discuss some of the suspected and known relationships between prenatal drug exposure, including alcohol and nicotine, which are also drugs. It is important to recognize that 75 percent of individuals who abuse one of these drugs probably abuse others. Also, the lifestyle of individuals who abuse drugs is typically not conducive to good prenatal, perinatal, and postnatal care. Most likely, it is also an environment that is not enriching, stable, and nurturing, which significantly impacts the child's development.

Fetal Alcohol Syndrome (FAS) and Alcohol-Related Neurodevelopmental Disorder (ARND)

Although recent news reports have focused more on the effects of drugs such as cocaine on a fetus, research clearly shows that alcohol is the worst drug in terms of pervasive, lifelong effects on the fetus (Trace, 1993). Full-blown fetal alcohol syndrome has a prevalence of 0.6–3 in 1,000, although in some communities it may be higher. Statistics indicate that fetal alcohol syndrome and ARND are found in 9.1–10 of every 1000 live births (Nulman, Ickowicz, Koren, & Knittel-Keren, 2007). Wunsch, Conlon, and Scheidt (2002) note that, combined, FAS and ARND "account for about 5% of congenital anomalies, and for 10–20% of all cases of mild mental retardation" (p. 111).

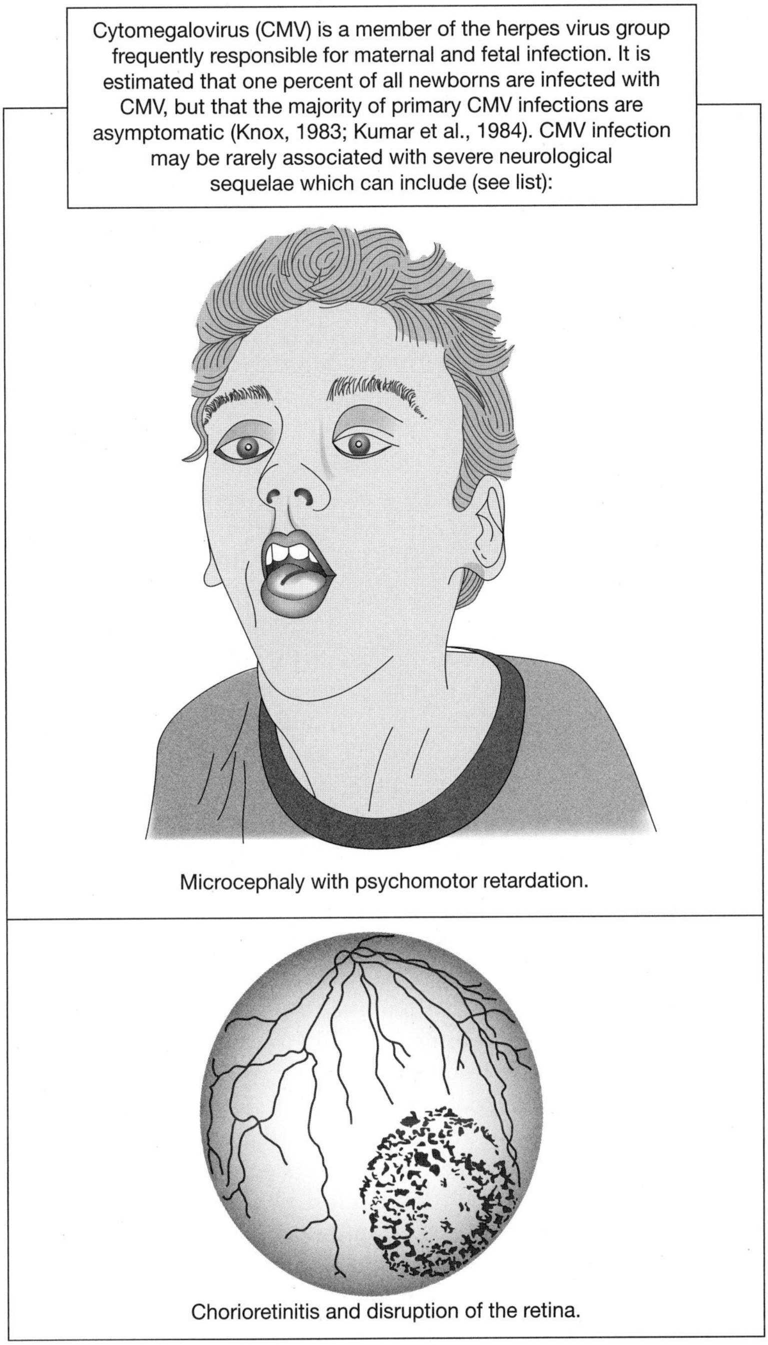

Cytomegalovirus (CMV) is a member of the herpes virus group frequently responsible for maternal and fetal infection. It is estimated that one percent of all newborns are infected with CMV, but that the majority of primary CMV infections are asymptomatic (Knox, 1983; Kumar et al., 1984). CMV infection may be rarely associated with severe neurological sequelae which can include (see list):

Microcephaly with psychomotor retardation.

Chorioretinitis and disruption of the retina.

FIGURE 2–9 Characteristics of children with fetal cytomegalovirus syndrome. (*Source:* Based on *Genetic Syndromes in Communication Disorders.* Austin, TX: Pro-Ed, 1988.)

Fetal alcohol syndrome is one of the leading causes, and the most preventable cause (100% preventable), of intellectual disabilities in the United States (Gerber, 1998). The estimated cost of treating a child with fetal alcohol syndrome over the course of a lifetime is $2 million (Nulman, Ickowicz, Koren, & Knittel-Keren, 2007).

In order to be diagnosed as having fetal alcohol syndrome, maternal drinking during pregnancy must be documented, and the child must exhibit three primary symptoms: growth retardation, facial anomalies, and central nervous system deficits. If a child does not exhibit symptoms in all three categories, he or she may be diagnosed as having alcohol-related neurodevelopmental disorder (ARND), which is diagnosed three times as often as fetal alcohol syndrome. In ARND, the child usually exhibits signs of central nervous system dysfunction but probably does not have signs of growth retardation and facial anomalies.

Numerous physical characteristics are associated with fetal alcohol syndrome. Both prenatal and postnatal growth deficiencies are present, including insufficient development of the head circumference, which can impact completeness of brain development. This is particularly significant because it has been documented that if head circumference is below the fifth percentile, a child is at high risk for developmental disabilities. Other physical anomalies include short stature (from birth), small fingers and toes that are bent or webbed, abnormal palmar creases, hip dislocations, and kidney defects. Club feet, minor genital abnormalities, abnormal pigmentation ("strawberry" birthmarks), heart defects, and generalized failure to thrive also have been noted. Drawings depicting the physical characteristics of FAS are found in Figure 2–10.

As stated earlier, a child with full-blown fetal alcohol syndrome also exhibits characteristic facial features. These features include eyes that appear slanted, small, or squinty, with short eye slits and droopy eyelids. Typically, the eyes are widely spaced or crossed. The upper lip is usually narrow, with no groove between the lip and nose. The nose is flat, and during infancy the child usually has a flat midface with a small rounded chin and jaw. In later childhood, the face appears elongated. Mild to moderate hearing loss and large or malformed ears are frequent anomalies, particularly in fetal alcohol syndrome. Cleft lip and cleft palate also are common.

In addition to the facial and physical characteristics, central nervous system dysfunction is always present in fetal alcohol syndrome and is very common in children with alcohol-related neurodevelopmental disorders. With regard to mental functioning, a child with fetal alcohol syndrome typically functions in the mildly to moderately impaired range of intelligence, with an average IQ around 70. Language deficits and delays are common, including echolalia and perseveration. In addition, their expressive language frequently exceeds their receptive language abilities. However, they may exhibit difficulties with word order and word meanings (Owens, 2004). Behavioral problems, including attention deficit disorder, are also common.

Perseveration. Persistent repetition of a vocalization, verbalization, or gesture.

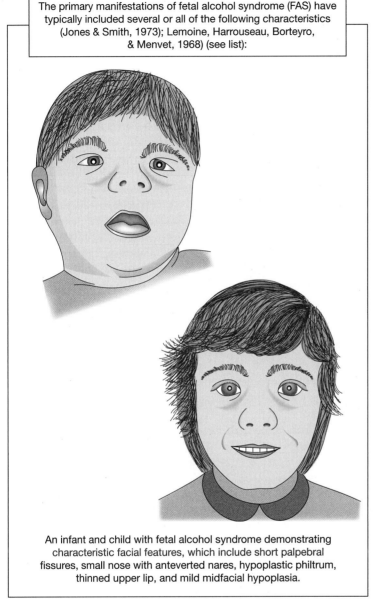

The primary manifestations of fetal alcohol syndrome (FAS) have typically included several or all of the following characteristics (Jones & Smith, 1973); Lemoine, Harrouseau, Borteyro, & Menvet, 1968) (see list):

An infant and child with fetal alcohol syndrome demonstrating characteristic facial features, which include short palpebral fissures, small nose with anteverted nares, hypoplastic philtrum, thinned upper lip, and mild midfacial hypoplasia.

FIGURE 2–10   Characteristics of children with fetal alcohol syndrome.
(*Source:* Based on *Genetic Syndromes in Communication Disorders.* Austin, TX: Pro-Ed, 1988.)

Subtle learning problems due to cognitive deficits often are exhibited by children with fetal alcohol effects, including poor attention skills, poor judgment, and memory deficits. These characteristics often carry over to adulthood, and children and adults with either of these disorders frequently are considered underachievers. The picture is further complicated by the frequent presence of impulsivity and hyperactivity, tremors, restlessness, and frequent temper tantrums.

Academic problems are characteristic of FAS and ARND. These are the result of conceptual deficits (such as difficulties with time and space), difficulties with comprehension of spoken and written materials, deficits in basic problem solving, and visual and spatial memory deficits (Ratner & Harris, 1994).

Behavioral problems, including attention deficit disorder, are also common. In the classroom, these children can be somewhat disruptive. Subtle learning problems due to cognitive deficits, including poor attention skills, poor judgment, and memory deficits are often exhibited by children with fetal alcohol effects (Owens, 2004). Poor development of interpersonal skills also affects children with FAS and ARND. For example, they typically have problems with the reciprocal nature of a conversation. In addition, they have difficulty understanding the expectations and rules associated with social language interactions and generally have poor communication that "lacks substance, cohesion, meaning, and relevance" (Larson & McKinley, 1995, p. 9). The picture is further complicated by the frequent presence of impulsivity and hyperactivity, tremors, restlessness, and temper tantrums. Adolescents with FAS or ARND often have sexual difficulties. They may be depressed (possibly due to social isolation from their peers), and they frequently drop out of school (Ratner & Harris, 1994).

The above characteristics compound the problems of adolescents trying to demonstrate the growth typically experienced during the teenage years. In addition, the same problems typically carry over into adulthood, and children and adults with either of these disorders are frequently considered to be underachievers. Their impulsiveness, poor judgment, and attentional deficits create problems for those who are either in school or who are employed (Ratner & Harris, 1994).

Cocaine or Polydrug-Exposed Infants

Polydrug exposure. The use of multiple drugs, including alcohol, by a pregnant mother.

It is a difficult task to separate the effects of specific drugs on developing babies because, in numerous cases, the mother may be abusing a variety of drugs, including alcohol. Therefore, it is probably more correct to talk about polydrug-exposed babies than about specific drugs. Environmental factors also must be considered because many of these women live in substandard situations. Drug-exposed babies are more vulnerable to other developmental deficits and disorders owing to undesirable conditions such as prematurity, poor nutrition, lack of prenatal health care, and poor to no environmental stimulation. In fact, Griffith (1992) points out that there are three erroneous assumptions about babies exposed to drugs: "(1) That all cocaine-exposed children are severely affected, (2) that little can be done for them, and (3) that all the medical, behavioral, and learning problems exhibited by these children are caused directly by their exposure to cocaine" (p. 30). In actuality, not enough long-term data are available to determine how severely or extensively affected the children are. Also, as pointed out previously, because it is likely that the mothers of these children do not limit their drug use to cocaine, it is a misnomer to call these children "cocaine babies."

Prenatal drug exposure causes some changes in the function and organization of the central nervous system. Typically, babies who have been exposed to cocaine or other drugs have poorly organized nervous systems, resulting in a state of physiological disorganization. In these babies, basic functions such as body temperature and arousal states become disorganized and erratic. The infants also tend to have low thresholds of tolerance for visual and auditory stimulation. In fact, they spend so much time and energy trying to maintain some level of internal organization that they have no stamina with which to interact or react to healthy stimulation from the environment (Griffith, 1992).

This disorganized state is often misinterpreted as an apparent inability to form attachments. In reality, it may be that one of the most important stimulations a mother shares with her baby—eye contact—is too much stimulation for a baby with a low threshold for sensory input. The complexity of the human face may be more input than a physiologically disorganized baby can handle. Thus, at feeding time, the child may not be able to use a coordinated sucking pattern to receive adequate nutrition. In a state of frustration, the mother may interpret the child's attempts to avoid eye contact and physical closeness as signs of rejection (Griffith,1992).

By 1 month of age, most babies can learn to control the environment, and the mother and baby work in synchrony to recognize the meaning behind different vocalizations. For example, a mother quickly learns to interpret her baby's cries as indicating hunger, loneliness, or discomfort. Accordingly, the mother learns what response to make and how to grade the amount of stimulation the baby needs according to the baby's reaction.

An intervention program conducted by Griffith and colleagues at the National Association for Perinatal Addiction Research and Education studied the interactions between mothers who had abused cocaine, with or without other drugs, and their infants. As part of their findings, Griffith pointed out that the differences between babies who were and were not exposed to drugs prenatally are greatest during the first few weeks of life (Griffith, 1992). The investigators found that very simple interventions helped the babies to become neurologically organized and improved the interactions between the mothers and their babies. For example, simply patting the baby at the rate of one pat per second (approximately the same rate as a normal heart beat) helped the baby to coordinate his or her sucking pattern. If this were paired with having the mother divert her face from the baby, the infant's internal organization continued to improve. Gradually, the mothers were able to reintroduce the stimulation associated with eye contact without having the baby react in a negative manner. Vertical (as opposed to the more typical horizontal) rocking also was shown to improve the babies' physiological states.

We cannot ignore the fact that other factors exist that may prolong or aggravate the long-term effects of drug use during pregnancy. For example, it is likely that the mother continues to abuse drugs after the birth of the baby. This may be part of a cyclical pattern that interfaces with the baby's disorganized state. It is also possible that the mother's childhood experiences may affect her own child-rearing practices. Other environmental factors common in the homes of mothers who abuse drugs include poor postnatal nutrition and lack of postnatal health care for the baby and the mother.

Triggers for Behavioral Withdrawal or Increased Impulsivity

Clearly, the environment plays a role in the development of any child. For the child in an inconsistent environment, the amount of stimulation that is provided may be too little to facilitate cognitive, emotional, and social growth. Yet the same degree of stimulation might be too much for a baby with a disorganized nervous system.

Lack of structure in the home environment can lead to inappropriate and ineffective stimulation for a newborn baby. In an attempt to develop self-regulation, the infant is likely to express numerous signals of distress that can exacerbate the mother's feelings of distress and frustration. One way the baby may try to cope with his or her physiological distress is through gaze aversion. By shifting his or her own gaze away from the mother, the baby is systematically decreasing the amount of stimulation he or she is receiving from the mother. However, in addition to this behavioral phenomenon, the baby can exhibit a number of physiological distress signals, such as yawning, hiccoughing, sneezing, color changes, increased movement, crying, and increased rate of respiration.

As the baby gets older, he or she will have difficulty adjusting to new environments, with much the same type of difficulty as in the initial months of life. At a time when he or she should be learning basic cognitive processes through developmental tasks, the infant may have trouble learning through environmental stimulation, particularly those skills that lead to the ability to master complex tasks at the later stages of development. Finally, it is possible that babies who are not able to organize themselves in a disorganized environment will also have difficulty shifting tasks and handling change as they get older. When drug-exposed children attain school age, their language is typified by word retrieval problems and poor pragmatics (Rivers & Hedrick, 1992). Weak pragmatic skills can be further confounded by frequent changes in living arrangements and care settings. This is particularly important when we consider that many babies born to addicted mothers may experience numerous shifts in their environments if they have to be moved from one care setting to another. The good news is that numerous techniques can be used to help the baby organize internal systems so he or she can benefit from normal environmental stimulation. These techniques are discussed in Chapter 6.

Exposure to Nicotine

Babies born to mothers who smoked during their pregnancy are at increased risk for low birth weight, typically less than 2500 grams. In addition to intrauterine growth retardation, these babies have inadequate fetal lung development and poor pulmonary functioning. They are also at a higher risk for the development of childhood asthma. There are several neurotoxic effects of in utero exposure to nicotine and carbon monoxide in the cigarette smoke that have effects on neurobehavior. These babies are subject to increased excitability and increased hypertonia. They may show stress/abstinence symptoms in the central nervous system, the gastrointestinal system, and the visual field. They have a lower IQ, increased development of attention deficit disorder (with or without hyperactivity), and adverse effects on learning, memory, problem solving, and eye-hand coordination. That there are effects of in utero exposure to tobacco on language development is evidenced by decreased responsiveness on auditory-related items on the Bayley Scales of Infant Development at ages 12 and 24 months. These delays still persist at age 4 years. Cognitive deficits are still evident in early adolescence, affecting verbal intelligence, language, and reading (Belcher & Johnson-Brooks, 2008). Other problems that have been noted include antisocial outcomes, greater risk of criminal arrest, and greater likelihood of hospitalization for substance abuse (Percy, 2007).

INTELLECTUAL DISABILITIES

The American Association on Intellectual and Developmental Disabilities delineates the following descriptive criteria to label a child as having an intellectual disability:

- Difficulty learning social rules
- Delays in oral language development
- Memory deficits
- Lack of social inhibitors
- Delay in development of adaptive behaviors such as self-help or self-care skills

The *Diagnostic and Statistical Manual of Mental Disorders* (DSM-IV) (American Psychiatric Association, 1994) lists the following criteria:

- IQ less than 70
- Significant limitations in two or more adaptive behaviors
- Limitations apparent before age 18

These criteria are in contrast with the Developmental Disabilities Assistance and Bill of Rights Act of 1984 (P.L. 98-527), in which a developmental disability is defined as

> a severe chronic disability of a person which (a) is attributable to a mental or physical impairment; (b) is manifested before a person attains age 21; (c) is likely to continue indefinitely; (d) results in substantial limitations in three or more of the following areas of major life activity: (i) self-care, (ii) receptive and expressive language, (iii) learning, (iv) mobility, (v) self-direction, (vi) capacity for independent living, (vii) economic self-sufficiency; and (e) reflects the person's need for a combination and sequence of special, interdisciplinary, or generic care, treatment, or other services which are of lifelong or extended duration and are individually planned and coordinated.

Traditionally, intellectual disabilities are classified by severity according to the child's IQ status (see Table 2–13). Regardless of the preferred definition, children who are intellectually disabled (or any related term such as *mentally challenged, cognitively challenged, developmentally delayed,* or *developmentally disabled*) demonstrate intellectual functioning, personal independence, and social responsibility that are below those expected on the basis of their chronological age. If a child does not demonstrate deficits in each of these three areas, the term *intellectually disabled* is inappropriate. However, we also must look at the age of the person when determining the appropriateness of the diagnosis. Developmental scales that delineate the skills and expectations of children beyond age 6 years are quite sparse and inconsistent in their content.

Generally speaking, speech acquisition by children with intellectual disabilities may parallel that of children with specific language impairment in that they acquire the linguistic features in a normal sequence but at a slower rate, and may plateau before all are acquired. Also, the children may have multiple handicaps that interfere with the coordination of oral motor skills for speech production.

TABLE 2–13 Classification by IQ level

Level	IQ Range
Borderline	70–80
Mild	50–69
Moderate	35–49
Severe	20–34
Profound	Below 20

Source: Based on information from the DSM-IV-TR, ICD-10, and the American Association on Intellectual and Developmental Disabilities.

Children with profound or severe intellectual disabilities typically have an etiological history of genetically inherited disabilities, chromosomal deficits, brain injury (either pre-, peri-, or postnatal), head injury, infections, prematurity, gestational disorders, or drug or alcohol abuse by the birth mother. Etiologically, individuals considered to be mildly or moderately intellectually disabled can trace their deficits to cultural and environmental deprivation, familial patterns, nutritional deficits, or a combination of these.

With regard to expectations associated with severity classifications, mildly intellectually disabled preschoolers typically have delayed social and communication skills and minimal delay in sensorimotor areas of functioning. Many children in this category may not have deficits that are recognized until they reach school age.

During the preschool years, the child who has moderate intellectual disabilities experiences delays in learning to talk and communicate but, as a rule, eventually develops adequate language skills. The child typically displays poor social awareness and fair motor development (Nelson, 1993).

In contrast, the child who has severe intellectual disabilities typically has minimal speech development during the preschool years and continues to have severely limited communication skills as he or she matures. Children at this level of functioning typically have difficulty acquiring self-help skills and have poor motor development.

Children who are profoundly intellectually disabled show very little development of communication, sensorimotor integration, or self-help skills. These children have complete dependence on adults. Sensorimotor skills include cognitive concepts such as object permanence, visual pursuit, object relations, spatial relations, means-end, causality, imitation, and gestures. Table 2–14 lists the developmental stages, and an explanation of each of these domains is given in Table 2–15. Examples of activities used to assess the domains are listed in Appendix B. An explanation of sensorimotor assessment is given in Chapter 5.

It is worth noting that 75 percent of all cases of severe intellectual disabilities are due to biological factors. Thirty-three percent of all identifiable cases of severe intellectual disabilities are due to fragile X syndrome, Down syndrome, and fetal alcohol syndrome (Batshaw, Shapiro, & Farber, 2007).

Children with intellectual disabilities usually follow the same path of acquisition in the various features of language as do typically developing children, but at a slower rate. In approximately 50 percent of the children with intellectual disabilities, there is no gap between their language abilities and their cognitive skills. Many school districts use this as criteria for placement in school-based speech-language therapy (Miller & Chapman, 1984). A sample criterion may be that a child must demonstrate a gap of 12 months between his or her language and cognitive skills in order to be enrolled in therapy.

With regard to the features of language, the delays indicate that the child with an intellectual disability acquires the features in the same

TABLE 2–14 Sensorimotor stages of development

Stage/Age	Skill	Description
Stage 1 Birth–1 month	Use of reflexes	Organizes motor and perceptual responses to the environment
Stage 2 1–4 months	Primary circular reactions	Use motor schemes without intention
Stage 3 4–8 months	Secondary circular reactions	Use motor schemes with intention
Stage 4 8–12 months	Coordination of secondary circular reactions	Can organize and sequence behaviors to achieve a desired response
Stage 5 12–18 months	Tertiary circular reactions	Discovery of new means to accomplish a given objective
Stage 6 18–24 months	Representation and foresight	Mental problem-solving skills

Source: Adapted from *Ordinal scales of psychological development*, by I. C. Uzgiris and J. M. Hunt, 1978. Urbana: University of Illinois Press.

TABLE 2–15 Domains assessed in sensorimotor testing of preschool language disorders

Assessment Domain	Description
Visual pursuit and object permanence	Ability to maintain perceptual contact with an object that undergoes various transformations
Means-ends	Ability to use own body and objects to obtain goals in the immediate environment and to use foresight in simple problem solving
Causality	Strategies used to reactivate objects which create an interesting spectacle
Object relations	Ability to use and understand spatial relationships
Schemes	Use of complex behaviors and discriminative use of objects, with recognition of their functional and socially appropriate use

Delmar/Cengage Learning.

sequence as those who do not have a cognitive handicap, but with a delay in terms of onset times. Owens (2004) studied the pragmatic skills of children with intellectual disabilities and found that, in the preschool years, children with intellectual disabilities used gestures to express intent at approximately the same rate as nondisabled children. However, asking for clarification and asking other questions were problematic for children with intellectual disabilities (Owens, 2004; Mundy, Seibert, and Hogan, 1985). Generally, the early expressive language skills of preschool children with intellectual disabilities are on par with their cognitive abilities. These children do, however, tend to be less assertive when engaged in conversations (Bedrosian & Prutting, 1978).

In 1973, Brown found that when the mean length of utterance is below 3, "children with MR display few differences in the sequence of learning grammatical rules when compared with mental-age mates" (Paul, 2001, p. 119). However, the syntactic and morphological features of their language are reflective of a child with an intellectual disability, and they do not develop forms of language as fully as those of nondisabled children. Specifically, their sentences lack complexity and are shorter than those of their age-level peers. While the sequence of the acquisition of morphemes is similar to that of nondisabled age peers, the rate in which syntax and morphology are learned is slower (Paul, 2001).

With regard to the content of the language of children with intellectual disabilities, these children tend to use more concrete words such as nouns and verbs than adjectives and adverbs (Owens, 2004). Again, in the early stages, the child's sequence of acquisition of words tends to follow that of his or her age-level peers, with delays becoming more evident as the child advances in age. Layton (2001) found that it appears that semantics develop more easily than syntax in the language of children with intellectual disabilities, particularly in children with Down syndrome.

Severe to Profound Intellectual Disabilities

Children with profound intellectual disabilities have difficulty mastering the basic skills needed for academic success. Their curriculum should focus on the development of fundamental skills such as self-help skills, basic communication, and motor development. Instruction for these children should also include efforts to teach functional reading and math skills needed to participate safely in the environment. These children typically need complete care and supervision even into adulthood.

Children who have severe intellectual disabilities have significant difficulties when they reach school age. As a rule, these children do not develop functional academic skills. They may learn to talk and communicate at a rudimentary level, frequently being limited to single words and basic communication via an alternative or augmentative communication device.

Education of these children often focuses on the development of early cognitive skills such as means-end, causality, imitation, and symbolic play schemes. This is in keeping with Piaget's theories with regard to the interaction between innate cognitive precursors to language and the development of language through organization of a child's world and environmental opportunities. Education of these children requires systematic, focused, repetitive training. For example, photos of key objects in the child's environment should be posted in the appropriate areas of the classroom or therapy room. The child should be encouraged (and assisted if necessary) to point to the appropriate picture when the object is being used. When the child is given a cup of water to drink, he or she should point to a picture of the cup. In addition, the development of sensorimotor skills that require the integration of feedback from the sensory system and the resultant motor behaviors should be a curricular focus as these may help lay a foundation for the development of early cognitive and language skills.

Sensorimotor skills. Skills involving the integration of sensory feedback and motor behaviors.

Mild to Moderate Intellectual Disabilities

Preschoolers with IQs of 55 to 69 fall in the mild range of intellectual disabilities and typically have delayed social and communication skills. Actually, mild intellectual disabilities may not even be noticed until the child begins school or later. However, their academic skills usually do not progress beyond the sixth-grade level, at which time these children need special education and may be labeled as educable intellectually disabled. As adults, they may have some social and vocational independence but need guidance in times of social and economic stress.

Children with moderate intellectual disabilities (IQ in the 40–54 range) usually do not progress beyond the fourth-grade level in regard to their academic growth. As adults, they "may be able to work independently at unskilled or semiskilled occupations but often need supervision and guidance under conditions of even mild social or economic stress" (Nelson, 1993, p. 99).

ACQUIRED LANGUAGE DISORDERS

Meningitis. An inflammation of the meninges lining the brain and/or spinal column.

Hypoxia. Absence of adequate oxygen to tissues and organs of the body.

Acquired language disorders are due to a variety of reasons, with the most frequent being illnesses such as meningitis, convulsive disorders, and head trauma. It is difficult to describe a typical language pattern in children with acquired language disorders because the damage is not consistent across patients owing to variations in the area of the brain that is injured by the trauma or illness. Common after-effects of traumatic brain injury that can influence the degree of damage and subsequent recovery include edema, hypoxia, hemorrhage, and seizure activity (Blosser & DePompei, 1994). The causes of trauma in infants are most frequently reported as accidental dropping of the baby, the infant's rolling off the changing table, and physical abuse. In toddlers and preschoolers, motor vehicle accidents, falls, and physical abuse are the major causes of injury (Blosser & DePompei, 1994). Regardless of the cause, the long-term impact of the injury or illness must be considered, including cumulative effects that develop as heavier developmental demands are placed on the child. In these cases, failure to fully recover some of the basic cognitive skills may eventually lead to an overtaxing of the system as the child progresses through school. Thus, a deficit may not become apparent until the child reaches school age (Blosser & DePompei, 1994).

Generally, the younger the child, the better the chance for recovery. If the injury or illness occurs before 3 years of age, the child may seem to regress to a point of being mute and unresponsive, then regain his or her linguistic ability, progressing back through normal development. If the damage occurs after 3 years of age, the child may regress, but not as drastically as a younger child. However, the recovery may be slower and less complete and the child typically has residual word-finding problems.

SUMMARY

To understand language disorders in the preschool population more fully, a clinician must develop a sense of what constitutes age-appropriate language behavior. That is to say, a clinician should have a thorough understanding of language development before beginning to assess and treat language disorders. If he or she does not understand the depth and breadth of normal language development, it is impossible to provide effective and accurate diagnosis and treatment. In the preschool population, this understanding influences a clinician's own bias with regard to whether or not language precedes cognition or cognition precedes language. It also affects the clinician's approach to labeling a disorder without understanding the impact of doing so. It is critical to remember that the child is at the center of the philosophical pull, and that it is his or her life that is most affected by the clinician's decisions.

CASE STUDY

History

Landon is a 5-year-old boy with Down syndrome. He lives at home with his mother (age 39), who is a nurse, and his father (age 42), who is a salesman. He also has two older brothers (ages 8 and 10) who live in the home. His mother reports no problems with the pregnancy. She took daily prenatal vitamins, but no other medications during the pregnancy.

From 18 months of age until this year, Landon attended school at the Early Intervention Program. This year he is in a self-contained varying exceptionalities kindergarten class. He receives occupational therapy for one 30-minute session per week at school.

He also receives group speech therapy for two 30-minute pull-out sessions per week. The speech-language pathologist also spends two 45-minute sessions per week with Landon in the classroom as part of an approach encompassing his goals from speech, occupational therapy, and education.

Landon has all the physical characteristics typically associated with Down syndrome. He has hypotonic musculature, and he is a mouth-breather. Landon has had recurrent ear infections since he was 6 months old. He had PE tubes inserted when he was 26 months old. An audiological evaluation revealed a mild (25-dB) hearing loss in the right ear and normal hearing in the left ear.

(continues)

CASE STUDY *(continued)*

Evaluation

Landon has an expressive vocabulary of approximately 15 single words. He does not combine words. Landon's cognitive and language skills were assessed using the Communication and Symbolic Behavior Scales—Developmental Profile (Wetherby & Prizant, 2002). The results yielded a receptive language age score of 21 months. Landon takes turns when playing with toys. He demonstrates the concept of object permanence by looking for an item that has been hidden under one of three screens. He enjoys looking at a picture book with an adult and attends to this activity for about two minutes. Occasionally Landon imitates a sound produced by the clinician, and he imitates gestures such as "so big," pointing, and clapping hands, and signs such as "more," "eat," "drink," and "play." He engages an adult in communication by hand-leading the adult to obtain an object or action and declaring an intent to communicate by giving the adult an object. Landon understands and responds appropriately to simple commands such as "Go find Daddy."

Summary

Landon has a receptive language age equivalent of approximately 21 months, and an expressive language age of 17 months. A summary of Landon's strengths and weaknesses is a follows:

	Strengths	Weaknesses
Communicative	Pragmatic skills (turn taking, eye contact, joint attention)	Delayed and limited vocabulary development (expressive and receptive)
	Means-end and causality	Does not combine words
	Likes books	Mild unilateral hearing loss
	Attempts to communicate using single words and gestures; engages adult in communication	
	Sound imitation emerging; imitates gestures and signs	
Noncommunicative	Supportive family	Hypotonia
	Has had early intervention	Poor eye-hand coordination
	Personable	Attention span limited to 2–3 minutes on most tasks
	Feeds and dresses self and is toilet trained	

Recommendations

Landon should continue to receive speech-language therapy in the school, and additional one-on-one therapy outside the school setting, with the school-based clinician and the private therapy clinician sharing goals and procedures to facilitate language and communication growth. Therapy should focus on expanding his receptive language skills and facilitating communication through speech and sign.

REVIEW QUESTIONS

1. An etiological classification of language disorders is
   a. Often used when it is necessary to label a child for educational placement
   b. Based on defining a language disorder in terms of causative factors
   c. Focused on the specific features of language in order to define the disorder
   d. Both b and c
   e. Both a and b

2. Intrauterine growth retardation, pulmonary problems, and increased possibility of hypertonicity are characteristic of
   a. Robin sequence
   b. Intrauterine nicotine exposure
   c. Intrauterine cocaine exposure
   d. Fetal alcohol syndrome

3. Which of the following signs must be present for a child to be diagnosed as having fetal alcohol syndrome?
   a. Growth retardation
   b. Central nervous system deficits
   c. Facial anomalies
   d. All of a, b, and c
   e. Both b and c
   f. Both a and b

4. The number one cause of congenital hearing loss, as well as brain damage, in babies who become infected during childhood (prenatally or postnatally) is
   a. Autism
   b. Cytomegalovirus

    c. Fragile X syndrome

    d. Encephalitis

5. The primary etiological factors for children who are mildly to moderately cognitively challenged are environmental and cultural deprivation, familial patterns, and/or nutritional deficits.

    a. True

    b. False

6. In Robin deformation sequence, the problems are intrinsic to the baby.

    a. True

    b. False

7. Children with velo-cardio-facial syndrome usually have a mild language delay but typically catch up with their peers by 36 to 48 months of age.

    a. True

    b. False

8. A sequence is defined by Shprintzen as "the presence of multiple anomalies in the same individual with all of those anomalies having a single cause."

    a. True

    b. False

9. In children with Down syndrome, expressive language is usually more intact than receptive language.

    a. True

    b. False

10. All children with static encephalopathy have some type of language deficit.

    a. True

    b. False

REFERENCES

Accardo, P. J. (2008). *Capute & Accardo's Neurodevelopmental disabilities in infancy and childhood. Volume I: Neurodevelopmental diagnosis and treatment* (3rd ed.). Baltimore: Paul H. Brookes Publishing Company.

Accardo, P. J. (2008). *Capute & Accardo's neurodevelopmental disabilities in infancy and childhood. Volume II: The spectrum of neurodevelopmental disabilities* (3rd ed.). Baltimore, MD: Paul H. Brookes Publishing Company.

Acs., G., Ng, M. W., Helpin, M. L., & Rosenberg, H. M. (2002). Dental care: Promoting health and preventing disease. In M. Batshaw, L. Pelligrino, and N. J. Roizen (eds.), *Children with disabilities* (5th ed.) (pp. 567–578). Baltimore, MD: Paul H. Brookes.

Acs., G., Ng, M. W., Helpin, M. L., Rosenberg, H. M., & Canion, S. (2007). Dental care: Promoting health and preventing disease. In M. Batshaw, L. Pelligrino, and N. J. Roizen (eds.), *Children with disabilities* (6th ed.) (pp. 499–510). Baltimore, MD: Paul H. Brookes.

Alvares, R. L., & Downing, S. F. (1998). A survey of expressive communication skills in children with Angelman syndrome. *American Journal of Speech-Language Pathology, 7*, 1–24.

American Academy of Pediatrics, Committee on Substance Abuse and Committee on Children with Disabilities (1993). Fetal alcohol syndrome and fetal alcohol effects. *Pediatrics, 91*, 1004–1006.

American Psychiatric Association (1994*). Diagnostic and statistical manual of mental disorders* (4th ed., rev.). Washington, DC: Author.

American Speech-Language-Hearing Association. (1993). Definitions of communication disorders and variations. [relevant paper]. Available from www.asha.org/policy.

Barbero, G. (1982). Failure to thrive. In M. H. Klaus, T. Leger, and M. A. Trause (eds.), *Maternal attachment and mothering disorders: Pediatric round table: 1*. Skillman, NJ: Johnson & Johnson Baby Products Company.

Batshaw, M. L. (2002). Chromosomes and heredity: A toss of the dice. In M. Batshaw (ed.), *Children with disabilities* (5th ed.) (pp. 3–26). Baltimore, MD: Paul H. Brookes.

Batshaw, M., Shapiro, B., & Farber, M. L. Z. (2007). Developmental delay and intellectual disability. In M. Batshaw, L. Pelligrino, and N. J. Roizen (eds.), *Children with disabilities* (6th ed.) (pp. 245–262). Baltimore, MD: Paul H. Brookes.

Bedrosian, J., & Prutting, C. (1978). Communicative performance of mentally retarded adults in four conversational settings. *Journal of Speech and Hearing Research, 21*, 79–95.

Belcher, H. M. E., & Johnson-Brooks, S. (2008). Children born to drug-dependent mothers. In Accardo (Ed.), *Caputo and Accardo's neurodevelopmental disorders in infancy and childhood. Volume I: Neurodevelopmental diagnosis and treatment* (3rd ed.). Baltimore, MD: Paul H. Brookes Publishing Company.

Berk, L. E. (2004). *Development through the lifespan* (3rd ed.). Boston: Allyn & Bacon.

Bigby, C. (2007). Aging with an intellectual disability. In I. Brown and M. Percy (ed.), *A comprehensive guide to intellectual and developmental disabilities* (pp. 607–618). Baltimore, MD: Paul H. Brookes Publishing Company.

Blamey, P. J., Sarant, J. Z., Paatsch, L. E., Barry, J. G., Bow, C. P., Wales, R. J., Wright, M., Psarros, C., Rattigan, K., & Tooher, R. (2001). Relationships among speech perception, production, language, hearing loss, and age in children with impaired hearing. *Journal of Speech, Language, and Hearing Research, 44*(2), 264–285.

Blosser, J. L., & DePompei, R. (1994). *Pediatric traumatic brain injury: Proactive intervention*. San Diego, CA: Singular Publishing Group.

Brown, I., & Percy, M. (2007). *A comprehensive guide to intellectual and developmental disabilities*. Baltimore, MD: Paul H. Brookes.

Buckley, S. (1993). Language development in children with Down's syndrome: Reasons for optimism. *Down Syndrome Research and Practice, 1*, 3–9.

Buckley, S. (1995a). Improving the expressive language skills of teenagers with Down syndrome. *Down Syndrome Research and Practice, 3*(3), 110–115.

Buckley, S. (1995b). Teaching children with Down syndrome to read and write. In L. Nadel & D. Rosenthal (eds.), *Down syndrome: Living and learning in the community* (pp. 158–169). New York: Wiley-Liss.

Calculator, S. N. (2002, November). Use of enhanced natural gestures to foster interactions between children with Angelman syndrome and their parents. *American Journal of Speech-Language Pathology, 11,* 340–355.

Carneol, S. O., Marks, S. M., & Weik, L. (1999, February). The speech-language pathologist: Key role in the diagnosis of velocardiofacial syndrome. *American Journal of Speech-Language Pathology, 8,* 23–32.

Carr, J. (1995). *Down's syndrome: Children growing up.* New York: Cambridge University Press.

Caselli, M. C., Vicari, S., Longobardi, E., Lami, L., Pizzoli, C., & Stella, S. (1998, October). Gestures and words in early development of children with Down syndrome. *Journal of Speech, Language, and Hearing Research, 41*(5), 1125–1135.

Chapman, R. S. (1995). Language development in children and adolescents with Down syndrome. In P. Fletcher and B. MacWhinney (eds.), *The handbook of child language* (pp. 641–663). Oxford, UK: Blackwell.

Chapman, R. S., Seung, H.-K., Schwartz, S. E., et al. (1998). Language skills of children and adolescents with Down syndrome II: Production deficits. *Journal of Speech, Language, and Hearing Research, 41,* 861–873.

Crystal, D., & Varley, R. (1993). *Introduction to language pathology* (3rd ed). San Diego, CA: Singular Publishing Group.

Curtiss, S., Prutting, C. A., & Lowell, E. L. (1979). Pragmatic and semantic development in young children with hearing impairment. *Journal of Speech and Hearing Research, 22,* 534–552.

Fabbretti, D., Pizzuto, E., Vicari, S., & Volterra, V. (1997). A story description task in children with Down syndrome: Lexical and morphosyntactic abilities. *Journal of Intellectual Disability Research, 41,* 165–179.

Faires, W., Topping, G., & Cranford, J. L. (1993). The long-term effects of chronic otitis media with effusion on language and auditory sequential memory. *Journal of Medical Speech-Language Pathology, 1,* 163–169.

Fenson et al. (1993). *MacArthur Communicative Development Inventories: User's guide and technical manual.* San Diego, CA: Singular Publishing Group.

Fewell, R. (1996). Personal communication.

Fitzhardinger, P., & Ramsey, M. (1973). The improving outlook for the small prematurely born infant. *Developmental Medicine and Child Neurology, 15,* 447.

Flenthrope, J. L., & Brady, N. C. (2010, May). Relationship between early gestures and later language in children with Fragile X syndrome. *American Journal of Speech-Language Pathology, 19,* 135–142.

Fowler, A. E. (1990). Language abilities in children with Down syndrome: Evidence for a specific syntactic delay. In D. Cicchetti and M. Beeghly (eds.), *Children with Down syndrome: A developmental perspective* (pp. 302–328). Cambridge, UK: Cambridge University Press.

Fowler, A., Doherty, B., & Boynton, L. (1995). The basis of reading skill in young adults with Down syndrome. In L. Nadel and D. Rosenthal (eds.), *Down syndrome: Living and learning in the community.* New York: John Wiley & Sons.

Gerber, S. E. (1998). *Etiology and prevention of communicative disorders* (2nd ed.). San Diego, CA: Singular Publishing Group.

Goldberg, R., Motzking, B., Marion, R., Scambler, R. J., & Shprintzen, R. J. (1993). Velo-cardio-facial syndrome: A review of 120 patients. *American Journal of Medical Genetics, 45,* 313–319.

Golding-Kushner, K., Weller, G., & Shprintzen, R. J. (1985). Velo-cardio-facial syndrome: Language and psychological profiles. *Journal of Craniofacial Genetics and Developmental Biology, 5,* 259–266.

Gravel, J. S., & Wallace, I. F. (1996). Early otitis media, auditory abilities, and educational risk. *American Journal of Speech-Language Pathology, 4*(3), 89–94.

Griffith, D. R. (1992, September). Prenatal exposure to cocaine and other drugs: Developmental and educational prognoses. *Phi Delta Kappan,* pp. 30–34.

Herer, G. R., Knightlyn, C. A., & Steinberg, A. G. (2002). Hearing: Sounds and silences. In M. Batshaw (ed.), *Children with disabilities* (5th ed.) (pp. 193–227). Baltimore, MD: Paul H. Brookes.

Hill, J. B., & Haffner, W. H. J. (2002). Growth before birth. In M. Batshaw (ed.), *Children with disabilities* (5th ed.) (pp. 43–53). Baltimore, MD: Paul H. Brookes.

Johnson, B. A. (1996). *Language disorders in children: An introductory clinical perspective.* Albany, NY: Delmar Publishers.

Jolleff, N., & Ryan, M. (1993). Communication development in Angelman syndrome. *Archives of Disease in Childhood, 69,* 148–150.

Jung, J. H. (1989). *Genetic syndromes in communication disorders.* Boston: College-Hill.

Kay-Raining Bird, E., Cleave, P. L., & McConnell, L. (November, 2000). Reading and phonological awareness in children with Down syndrome: A longitudinal study. *American Journal of Speech-Language Pathology, 9,* 319–330.

Kay-Raining Bird, E., Cleave, P. L., McFarlane, H., & Hackett, A. (1998, July). Written language abilities in children with Down syndrome. Poster presented at the XVth biennial meetings of ISSBD, Bern, Switzerland.

Kay-Raining Bird, E., & McConnell, L. (1994, November). Language and literacy relationships in children with Down syndrome. Poster presented at the Annual American Speech-Language-Hearing Association Convention, New Orleans, LA.

Kumin, L. 2003. *Early Communication Skills in Children with Down Syndrome: A Guide for Parents and Professionals.* Woodbine House, Bethesda, MD.

Kumin, L., Councill, C., & Goodman, M. (1998). Expressive vocabulary development in children with Down syndrome. *Down Syndrome Quarterly, 3,* 1–7.

Larson, V. L., & McKinley, N. (1995). *Language disorders in older students: Preadolescents and adolescents.* Eau Claire, WI: Thinking Publications.

Layton, T. (2001). Young children with Down syndrome. In T. Layton, E. Crais, and L. Watson (eds.), *Handbook of early language impairment in children: Nature* (pp. 302–360). Albany, NY: Delmar Publishers.

Lefler, C. T. (2008). Visual impairment. In Accardo (ed.), *Caputo and Accardo's neurodevelopmental disabilities in infancy and childhood. Volume I: Neurodevelopmental diagnosis and treatment* (3rd ed.), pp. 501–518. Baltimore, MD: Paul H. Brookes Publishing Company.

Lewis, B.A., Freebairn, L., Heeger, S. & Cassidy, S.D. (2002). Speech and language skills of individuals with Prader-Willi Syndrome. *American Journal of Speech-Language Pathology, 11,* 1–10.

Lipkin, P. H. (2008). Attention-deficit/hyperactivity disorder mimic disorder. In Accardo (ed.), *Capute and Accardo's neurodevelopmental disabilities in infancy and childhood. Volume II: Neurodevelopmental diagnosis and treatment* (3rd ed.) (pp. 677–691). Baltimore, MD: Paul H. Brookes Publishing Company.

Mazzocco, M. M. M., & Holden, J. J. A. (2007). Fragile X syndrome. In I. Brown and M. Percy (eds.), *A comprehensive guide to intellectual and developmental disabilities* (pp. 173–188). Baltimore, MD: Paul H. Brookes Publishing Company.

Meyer, G. A. (2007). X-linked syndromes causing intellectual disability. In M. Batshaw, L. Pelligrino, and N. J. Roizen (eds.), *Children with disabilities* (6th ed.) (pp. 275–284). Baltimore, MD: Paul H. Brookes.

Meyer, G. A., & Batshaw, M. L. (2002). Fragile X syndrome. In M. Batshaw (ed.), *Children with disabilities* (5th ed.) (pp. 321–331). Baltimore, MD: Paul H. Brookes.

Miller, J. (1988). The developmental asynchrony of language development in children with Down syndrome. In L. Nadel (Ed.), *The psychobiology of Down syndrome* (pp. 167–198). Cambridge, MA: MIT Press.

Miller, J., & Chapman, R. (1984). Disorders of communication: Investigating the development of mentally retarded children. *American Journal of Mental Deficiency, 88,* 536–545.

Montgomery, T. R. (2008). The dysmorphology examination. In Accardo (ed.), *Capute and Accardo's neurodevelopmental disabilities in infancy and childhood. Volume I: Neurodevelopmental diagnosis and treatment* (3rd ed.) (p. 311–320). Baltimore, MD: Paul H. Brookes Publishing Company.

Mundy, P., Seibert, J., & Hogan, A. (1985). Communication skills in mentally retarded children. In M. Sigman (ed.), *Children with emotional disorders and developmental disabilities: Assessment and treatment* (pp. 45–70). Orlando, FL: Grune and Stratton.

Nelson, N. W. (1993). *Childhood language disorders in context.* New York: Merrill Publishing Company.

Northern, H. L., & Downs, M. P. (1984). *Hearing in children* (3rd ed.). Baltimore, MD: Williams and Wilkins.

Nulman, I., Ickowicz, A., Koren, G., & Knittel-Keren, D. (2007). Fetal alcohol spectrum disorder. In I. Brown and M. Percy (eds.), *A comprehensive guide to intellectual and developmental disabilities* (pp. 213–228). Baltimore, MD: Paul H. Brookes Publishing Company.

Nyhan, W. L. (1983). Cytogenetic diseases. *Clinical Symposia, 35*(1). West Caldwell, NJ: Ciba.

Owens, R. E. (2004). *Language disorders: A functional approach to assessment and intervention* (4th ed.). Needham Heights, MA: Allyn and Bacon.

Papolos, D. F., Faedda, G. L., Veit, S., Goldberg, R., Morrow, B., Kucherlapati, R., & Shprintzen, R. J. (1996). Bipolar spectrum disorders in patients diagnosed with velo-cardio-facial syndrome: Does a hemizygous deletion of chromosome 22q11 result in bipolar affective disorder? *American Journal of Psychiatry, 153,* 1541–1547.

Paul, R. (2001). *Language disorders from infancy through adolescence: Assessment and intervention.* St. Louis, MO: Mosby.

Penner, K., Johnson, J., Faircloth, B., Irish, P., & Williams, C. (1993). Communication, cognition, and social interactions in the Angelman syndrome. *American Journal of Medical Genetics, 46,* 34–39.

Percy, M. (2007). Factors that cause or contribute to intellectual and developmental disabilities. In I. Brown and M. Percy (eds.), *A comprehensive guide to intellectual and developmental disabilities* (pp. 125–148). Baltimore, MD: Paul H. Brookes Publishing Company.

Percy, M., et al. (2007). Other syndromes and disorders associated with intellectual and developmental disabilities. In I. Brown and M. Percy (eds.), *A comprehensive guide to intellectual and developmental disabilities* (pp. 229–268). Baltimore, MD: Paul H. Brookes Publishing Company.

Percy, M., Brown, I., & Lewkis, S. Z. (2007). Abnormal behavior. In I. Brown and M. Percy (ed.), *A comprehensive guide to intellectual and developmental disabilities* (pp. 309–334). Baltimore, MD: Paul H. Brookes Publishing Company.

Philofsky, A., Fidler, D. J., & Hepburn, S. (2007, November). Pragmatic language profiles of school-age children with autism spectrum disorder and Williams syndrome. *American Journal of Speech Language Pathology, 16,* 368–380.

Pore, S. G., & Reed, K. L. (1999). *Quick reference to speech-language pathology.* Gaithersburg, MD: Aspen.

Pueschel, S. M. (1987). Health concerns in persons with Down syndrome. In S. M. Pueschel, C. Tingey, J. E. Rynders, A. C. Corcker, and D. M. Crutcher (eds.), *New perspectives on Down syndrome.* Baltimore, MD: Paul H. Brookes.

Ratner, V., & Harris, L. (1994). *Understanding language disorders: The impact on learning.* Eau Claire, WI: Thinking Publications.

Raven, J. C. (1995). *Raven's Progressive Matrices Test.* San Antonio, TX: PsychCorp/Harcourt Assessment, Inc.

Reber, M. (2002). Dual diagnosis: Mental retardation and psychiatric disorders. In M. Batshaw (ed.), *Children with disabilities* (5th ed.) (pp. 347–364). Baltimore, MD: Paul H. Brookes.

Riski, John. (1999, October). VCF: Neurological findings impacting speech. *Proceedings from 12th Annual Symposium on Cleft Lip and Palate and Related Conditions.* Atlanta, GA.

Rivers, K. L., & Hedrick, D. (1992). Language and behavioral concerns for drug-exposed infants and toddlers. *Infant-Toddler Intervention: The Transdisciplinary Journal, 2*(1), 63–71.

Robb, A., & Reber, M. (2007). Behavioral and psychiatric disorders in children with disabilities. In M. Batshaw, L. Pelligrino, and N. J. Roizen (eds.), *Children with disabilities* (6th ed.) (pp. 297–312). Baltimore, MD: Paul H. Brookes.

Roberts, J. E., Mirrett, P., & Burchinal, M. (2001). Receptive and expressive communication development in young males with fragile X syndrome. *American Journal on Mental Retardation, 106,* 216–231.

Roberts, J. E., Mirrett, P., Anderson, K., Burchinal, M., & Neeve, E. (2002, August). Early communication, symbolic behavior, and social profiles of young men with fragile X syndrome. *American Journal of Speech-Language Pathology, 11*(3), 295–304.

Roizen, N. J. (2002). Down syndrome. In M. Batshaw (ed.), *Children with disabilities* (5th ed.) (pp. 307–320). Baltimore, MD: Paul H. Brookes.

Rondal, J. A. (1978). Maternal speech to normal and Down syndrome children matched for mean length of utterance. In E. Meyers (Ed.), *Quality of life in severely and profoundly mentally retarded people: Research foundations for improvement* (Monograph Series No. 3., pp. 193–265). Washington, D.C.: American Association on Mental Deficiency.

Rondal, J. A. (1993). Down's syndrome. In D. Bishop and K. Mogford (eds.), *Language development in exceptional circumstances*. East Sussex, UK: Lawrence Erlbaum Associates, Ltd.

Rose, M. (2002). Appendix D: Resources for children with disabilities. In M. Batshaw (ed.), *Children with disabilities* (5th ed.) (pp. 795–816). Baltimore, MD: Paul H. Brookes.

Rosner, J., & Simon, D. P. (1971). The auditory analysis test: An initial report. *Journal of Learning Disabilities, 4,* 384–392.

Rossetti, L. (1986). *High risk infants: Identification, assessment, and intervention.* Boston: College-Hill Publications.

Scacheri, C. (2002). Syndromes and inborn errors of metabolism. In M. Batshaw (ed.), *Children with disabilities* (5th ed.) (pp. 749–773). Baltimore, MD: Paul H. Brookes.

Scharfenaker, S. (1990). The fragile X syndrome. *ASHA, 32,* 45–47.

Schopmeyer, E., & Lowe, F. (1992). *The fragile X child.* San Diego, CA: Singular Publishing Group.

Shprintzen, R. J. (1997). *Genetics, syndromes, and communication disorders.* San Diego, CA: Singular Publishing Group, Inc.

Shprintzen, R. J. (2000). *Syndrome identification for speech-language pathology: An illustrated pocket guide.* San Diego, CA: Singular Publishing Group.

Sloper, P., Cunningham, C., Turner, S., & Knussen, C. (1990). Factors related to the academic attainments of children with Down syndrome. *British Journal of Educational Psychology, 60,* 284–298.

Sparks, S. N. (1984). *Birth defects and speech-language disorders.* San Diego, CA: College-Hill Press.

Spiegel, H. M. L., & Bonwit, A. M. (2002). HIV infection in children. In M. Batshaw (ed.), *Children with disabilities* (5th ed.) (pp. 123–139). Baltimore, MD: Paul H. Brookes.

Spiridigliozzi, G., Lachiewicz, A., Mirrett, S., & McConkie-Rosell, A. (2001). Fragile X syndrome in young children. In T. Layton, E. Crais, and L. Watson (eds.), *Handbook of early language impairment in children: Nature* (pp. 258–301). Albany, NY: Delmar Publishers.

Stoel-Gammon, C. (1981). Speech development of infants and children with Down syndrome. In J. Darby, Jr. (ed.), *Speech evaluation in medicine* (pp. 341–360). New York: Grune & Stratton.

Svirsky, M. A., Robbins, A. M., Kirk, K. I., Pisoni, D. B., & Miyamoto, R. T. (2000). Language development in profoundly deaf children with cochlear implants. *Psychological Science, 11,* 153–158.

Thal, D., DesJardin, J. L., & Eisenberg, L. S. (2007, February). Validity of the MacArthur–Bates Communicative Development Inventories for measuring language abilities in children with cochlear implants. *American Journal of Speech-Language Pathology, 16,* pp. 54–64.

Tomblin, J. B., Barker, B. A., Spencer, L. J., Zhang, X., & Gantz, B. J. (2005). The effect of age at cochlear implant initial stimulation on expressive language growth in infants and toddlers. *Journal of Speech, Language, and Hearing Research, 48,* 853–867.

Towbin, K. E., Mauk, J. F., & Batshaw, M. L. (2002). Pervasive developmental disorders. In M. Batshaw (ed.), *Children with disabilities* (5th ed.), pp. 365–388. Baltimore, MD: Paul H. Brookes.

Trace, R. (1993, June 21). Fetal alcohol syndrome. *Advance for Speech-Language Pathologists and Audiologists.*

Wetherby, A. M., & Prizant, B. M. (2002). *Communication and symbolic behavior scales developmental profile.* Baltimore, MD: Brookes.

Wolf-Schein, E. G., Sudhalter, V., Cohen, I. L., Fisch, G. S., Hanson, D., Pfadt, A. G., Hagerman, R., Jenkins, E. C., & Brown, W. T. (1987). Speech-language and the fragile X syndrome: Initial findings. *ASHA, 29,* 35–38.

Woodcock, R, W, (1987). *Woodcock reading mastery tests-revised.* Circle Pines, MN: American Guidance Service.

Wunsch, M. J., Conlon, C. J., & Scheidt, P. C. (2002). Substance abuse: A preventable threat to development. In M. Batshaw (ed.), *Children with disabilities* (5th ed.) (pp. 107–122). Baltimore, MD: Paul H. Brookes.

www.cdlsusa.org/CdLS%20Diagnostic%20Criteria%202007%20_3_.pdf, retrieved February 20, 2010.

www.emedicine.com/PED/topic482.htm, retrieved December 28, 2009.

www.ghr.nlm.nih.gov/condition=praderwillisyndrome, retrieved March 10, 2010.

www.news-medical.net/health/What-is-Angelman-Syndrome.aspx, retrieved March 13, 2010.

www.revolutionhealth.com/articles/cornelia-de-lange-syndrome/nord30?msc=ehdlp_cornelia-delange-syndrome, retrieved February 20, 2010.

Chapter 3

Pervasive Developmental Disorders

LEARNING OBJECTIVES

After completion of this chapter, the reader will be able to:

1. Discuss the early signs of autism.

2. Identify the defining characteristics of autism.

3. Discuss three etiological theories regarding the cause of autism.

4. Identify the functions of the Vaccine Program/Office of Special Masters.

5. Describe the social interaction patterns of children on the autism spectrum.

6. Discuss theory of mind.

7. Discuss the components of intervention to develop emergent literacy in children with autism.

8. Discuss strategies to facilitate the development of reading in children with autism.

9. Differentiate between the various pervasive developmental disorders.

10. Identify screening and assessment tools appropriate for use in assessing autism spectrum disorders.

11. Describe the various treatment methodologies for autism spectrum disorders.

INTRODUCTION

First identified by Leo Kanner in 1943, autism is one of several neurogenetic pervasive developmental disorders. "Pervasive developmental disabilities" (PDD) includes the following: "Autistic Disorder, Asperger's Disorder, Rett's Disorder, and Childhood Disintegrative Disorder (CDD). Pervasive Developmental Disorder—Not Otherwise Specified (PDD-NOS) is a classification used when symptoms are present but specific criteria for one of the other diagnoses in this category are not met" (Hyman &Towbin, 2007, p. 325). Owens (1995) states that symptoms of autism often become more pronounced around 18 months of age. These early symptoms include frequent tantrums and extreme reactions to certain stimuli. The child may exhibit a lack of social play and have communication deficits. He or she may also start to demonstrate ritualistic play and repetitive movements. According to the criteria for diagnosis of autism as set forth in the *Diagnostic and Statistical Manual of Mental Disorders-IV* (DSM-IV), the symptoms of autism must be evident prior to age 3 years. In some children, the diagnosis is evident from infancy, while other children may not be identified until age 2 or 3 when they begin to regress in language, social, and play skills previously demonstrated. Even when this later onset is documented, parents often say that, in retrospect, they had noticed some of the characteristic behaviors but just did not "put two and two together" at the time. This chapter addresses the most prevalent pervasive development disability (PDD) category—autism—but also provides information on four additional conditions that the American Psychiatric Association maintains as belonging to the category of PDDs: Asperger syndrome, pervasive developmental disorder—not otherwise specified (PDD-NOS), childhood disintegrative disorder (CDD), and Rett disorder.

ETIOLOGY OF AUTISM

Much confusion exists regarding the etiology of autism. Tiegerman-Farber (1997) divides the various theories regarding the etiology of autism into three categories: a psychological-psychoanalytic perspective, a psychological-cognitive approach, and a central language disorder category. The psychological-psychoanalytic perspective is based on the theory that autism is a problem of maternal distance and/or the child's reaction to the attitudes of his or her mother. The psychological-cognitive approach focuses on the variety of ways in which children with autism "process and organize information" (Tiegerman-Farber, 1997, p. 526). This approach implies that there is a general cognitive deficit that goes beyond the knowledge and use of linguistic information. Tiegerman-Farber goes on to explain that "the psychological-cognitive approach views the autistic child's language as a productive result of limited and less flexible processing abilities. Although different, the autistic child's idiosyncratic language behaviors should be addressed from the child's perspective of his or her environment" (p. 526).

The Central Language Disorder Category

The central language disorder category is based on the work of Churchill (1978). Tiegerman-Farber writes that Churchill "hypothesized that psychotic children with a psychiatric diagnosis of autism have a central language deficit that is more severe than that found in children with central language disorders. In addition, the three most prominent and clinically significant features of childhood psychosis are impairment of communicative interaction, of social interaction and of appropriate object manipulation" (Tiegerman-Farber, 1997, p. 527). Churchill also posited that each child with autism is unique, implying that children with autism form a heterogeneous group.

It is probably safe to say that the majority of cases of autism have unknown etiology. The central language theory helps to explain the nature of language as exhibited by a child with autism and places the root of the problems at the level of a central language deficit. The psychological-psychoanalytic perspective has been debunked in most of the literature addressing the causes of autism, with current research indicating a neurological basis for the disorder. The psychological-cognitive approach still has some merit and has an impact on some of the treatment approaches employed with children who have autism. These approaches are discussed later in this chapter.

Cortical Dysfunctions

Developmental neurobiology has tried to shed some light on the genesis of autism. In the first trimester, formation of the face occurs. Atypical facial features are typically associated with the existence of more than one disorder, such as ASD with cognitive challenges, tuberous sclerosis complex (43–86% of individuals with tuberous sclerosis complex have a PDD), or a related disorder such as Rett disorder or Angelman syndrome. It is theorized that children who have these atypical facial features may have a susceptible gene for autism. The second trimester is marked by formation of the brain. Neurodevelopmental errors leading to autism may occur during this time, but typically occur no later than 28 to 30 weeks gestation. The hallmark of the third trimester is the development of the central nervous system (CNS), but few individuals with ASD have CNS deficits (Hall, 2009). So, while it is a strong area of focus in the study of autism, "most of the developmental neurobiology of autism remains speculative and unconfirmed" (Minchew, Sweeney, Bauman, & Webb, 2005, p. 473).

Cortical dysfunctions that influence speech and language processing are hypothesized by researchers to be at the root of autism and its related syndromes. Other suspected or associated etiological factors include tuberous sclerosis, maternal rubella, fragile X syndrome, perinatal trauma, and seizure disorders (Hewitt, 1992). Other less specific research points to a malfunctioning of some aspects of the neurological system.

Some research into the causes of autism is focusing on structural and functional differences in the brain. Some posit that there is premature overgrowth of the brain resulting in increase in cerebral volumes and in the number of neurons. Others think it is a disorder of growth regulation of the brain. Five of the 11 children in Kanner's original study of autism had large heads. Increased head circumference corresponds to the increase in brain volume that normalizes by adolescence. However, in the children with autism, the head circumference remained enlarged. Abnormalities in the cerebellum, temporal lobes, amygdala, and brain stem have been documented in autopsy studies of individuals with autism. Functions of these structures correlate with problem areas for individuals with autism. The amygdala functions in affective behavior and helps regulate primary emotions such as rage, fright, and arousal, and the temporal lobes are involved with auditory processing. Frontal lobe damage is another possible explanation. The frontal lobe is responsible for memory formation and emotional expression. Patients with frontal lobe damage have a decreased ability to respond to environmental stimuli. Other functions such as "planning, organizing, self-monitoring, inhibition, flexibility, and working memory" (Hall, 2009, p. 10) are under the control of the frontal lobe, and these are areas that are problematic for older children, adolescents, and young adults who have autism.

Neuroimaging studies have documented the following observations:

1. On tasks of object perception, typical subjects had the most brain activity in the prefrontal regions, whereas those with ASD had more activity in areas of the brain associated with object perception.

2. The neurological systems that underlie face and voice processing function abnormally in the brains of individuals with ASD.

3. During voice and face processing tasks, there is hypoactivation of the amygdala that is interpreted as reflecting less emotional arousal and interest in the subjects with ASD (Hall, 2009).

Environmental Factors: The Measles-Mumps-Rubella (MMR) Vaccine

The MMR vaccine was originally implicated in 1996. A lawyer hired a British gastroenterologist to do research to support litigation against the MMR vaccine. In 1998, a study was published in a British medical journal *The Lancet* indicating that there may be a connection between the MMR vaccine and autism and saying that 12 children with ASD developed inflammation of the intestines when given the MMR. The Medical Research Council set up a panel to study the link between ASD and the MMR vaccine and found no association. In 1999, a study was done that found that thimerosal (a mercury-containing preservative used in the MMR vaccine at that time) "caused several infants to have levels of mercury in their blood that exceeded the guidelines recommended by the Environmental Protection Agency" even though there were no data to indicate any harm occurred as a result of the exposure (Hall, 2009, p. 11). Regardless of the lack of evidence, a decision was made to remove the preservative just in case. In the March 6, 2004 issue of *The Lancet*, researchers associated with the 1998 study retracted their findings, citing a lack of enough evidence, and noted a rise in the outbreaks of measles following a drop in the number of British children receiving the MMR.

There continues to be anecdotal evidence that vaccines are causative factors in the development of autism in some children. For the most part, support for this theory comes from parents, not from scientific research. It should be pointed out that the age at which autistic characteristics are most likely to appear coincides with the timing of MMR vaccinations. Therefore, many physicians believe there is a coincidence based on the timing; the vaccine is not causative. Others say that the vaccine is causative in regressive autism (in which the child develops normally for approximately 18 months, then regresses). There has been discussion that some vaccines trigger an existing genetic predisposition for autism.

At the direction of the Centers for Disease Control and Prevention and the National Institute of Health, the Institute of Medicine (IOM) studied the safety of vaccines, particularly the MMR vaccine, and developed a theory as to whether or not vaccines cause autism. The IOM stated that there is insufficient evidence to say the vaccines cause autism, but further study is needed. In 1986, the National Vaccine Injury Compensation Program (VICP) was enacted, administered by the U S. Court of Federal Claims/ Office of Special Masters. The VICP

> was designed to resolve a perceived crisis in vaccine tort liability claims that threatened the continued liability of childhood vaccines nationwide. In mandating that vaccine injury claims to be considered first under VICP, the statute was intended to reduce lawsuits against physicians and manufacturers, while providing those claiming vaccine injuries a reduced burden of proof. Claimants under the VICP need not prove negligence, failure to warn, or other tort causes of action; they must only prove that a covered vaccine caused injury. (www.uscfc.uscourts.gov/ vaccine-programoffice-special-masters).

Through the Vaccine Program/Office of Special Masters, there was an intention to reduce lengthy and expensive litigation. The Special Masters have two primary functions: "case management, which involves overseeing the collection of information and setting time frames for its submission; and decision making, which involves determining the types of proceedings necessary for presenting the relevant evidence and ultimately weighing the evidence in rendering a final enforceable decision" (www.uscfc.uscourts.gov/vaccine-programoffice-special-masters). The VICP reported the filing of over 12,500 cases as of May 2008. Of that 12,500, 5,365 filings represented cases of autism.

Environmental Factors: Diet

Another environmental factor that has attracted attention is the role of diet. Many children with autism have been found to have yeast in their gut, and the primary culprits are gluten (wheat) and casein (found in milk). The hypothesis is that the child does not digest the gluten and casein and they pass through the stomach to other parts of the body, including the brain. The children experience discomfort, and many display behaviors that are often associated with ASD. There have been enough anecdotal reports that research on the roles of diet and vaccines has come to the forefront. However, no science-based evidence supporting diet as causative of ASD has emerged.

A Neurochemical Disorder

One theory published in 1994, based on results from a small study by DeLong and colleagues at Duke University (Trace, 1996), holds that non-neurologic autism may be an inherited, early onset form of manic depression. The researchers at Duke University studied 40 children diagnosed as having autism or autism spectrum disorder, of whom 14 had normal neurological examinations. In those 14 children there was a strong family history of depression, manic depression, or both. At the time of the study, the prevalence of these two disorders in the general population was 1 percent for manic depression and 8–10 percent for depression. However, in families of the 14 children studied, 26.8 percent prevalence was found across three generations of parents, grandparents, aunts, uncles, and cousins. In these children with higher-level autism, the researchers were able to isolate a neurochemical disorder in the absence of physical signs of brain damage. They concluded that autism in higher-functioning children with apparently normal brains possibly is an inherited psychiatric disorder— probably a neurochemical imbalance—rather than a destructive brain disorder. The idea of a neurochemical basis is certainly an interesting hypothesis and deserves further study with larger numbers of children and more controlled methodology.

The Role of Genetics

A frequent research topic pursued is the role of genetics in autism, particularly looking at families where more than one offspring has the same or a different disorder. Perry, Dunlap, and Black (2007) report that approximately 2–3 percent of disordered siblings of children with autism have disorders related to autism, 5–8 percent have some type of PDD, and 25 percent have a learning disability and/or language disorder. Studies at the University of North Carolina at Chapel Hill (and other affiliated centers) have found genetic markers on chromosome 13 and chromosome 7 that may play a causative role in autism. Other suspected or associated etiological factors (including previously mentioned causes) include tuberous sclerosis, maternal rubella, fragile X syndrome, pregnancy complications, perinatal trauma, seizure disorders, CMV, food allergies, and vaccines (Hewitt, 1992; Paul, 2001; Prelock & Contompasis, 2006). No more than 10 percent of individuals with autism have genetic disorders, such as fragile X syndrome, that result in developmental disabilities in addition to autism (Perry, Dunlap, & Black, 2007).

DEFINING CHARACTERISTICS

Autism is defined according to the presence or absence of a variety of behaviors. The *DSM-IV* (1994) lists the following criteria for a diagnosis of autism:

1. Qualitative impairment in social interaction—This includes impairment in the use of nonverbal behaviors such as eye-to-eye gaze and gestures, lack of spontaneous sharing, lack of social and emotional reciprocity, and failure to develop peer relationships.

2. Qualitative impairment in communication: The child with autism typically has a delay or lack of development of spoken language and gestures, impairment in the ability to initiate and/or maintain a conversation, lack of pretend play, and repetitive and idiosyncratic use of language.

3. Restricted, repetitive, and stereotyped repertoire of behaviors, activities, and interests: The child displays a preoccupation with restricted patterns of interest, inflexible adherence to routines, repetitive movements, and preoccupation with parts of objects (for example, the wheels on a toy car).

The child must show "delays or abnormal functioning in at least one of the following areas with onset prior to age 3 years: (1) social interaction, (2) language as used in social communication, or (3) symbolic or imaginative play" (DSM-IV, p. 70).

Perry, Dunlap, and Black (2007) describe the social interaction patterns of children with autism as follows: "This social deficit does not necessarily involve withdrawing from social contact, but there is difficulty with other people. Children with autism may prefer isolation and ignore other people, may be unresponsive or aloof when others try to interact with them, often show no interest in playing with other children, and rarely initiate social contact" (p. 189). They also point out that nonverbal social skills such as establishing joint attention, making eye contact, showing facial expression, and respecting the feelings and thoughts of others may be deficient, as well.

Batshaw (2002) writes that "the primary feature of all PDDs is impairment in social reciprocity. In addition, impairment in communication and restricted behaviors such as repetitive behaviors, narrow interests, rituals, or stereotypies (repetitive simple movements, e.g., hand flapping) are usually present. Limitations in social motivation and emotional regulation result in profound limitations in play skills" (p. 365). Batshaw, Shapiro, and Farber (2007) compare delays in five developmental disabilities as shown in Table 3–1. Perry, Dunlap, and Black (2007) point out that most children with autism do not engage in pretend play, do not have symbolic language actions, and show little imagination.

The disruptive behavior most characteristically associated with autism is the failure to develop normal responsivity to other persons (varying degrees of social withdrawal). The emotional devastation felt by family members is compounded by the typical failure to develop normal verbal and nonverbal communication (i.e., an inability to interact appropriately with the environment). Failure to use objects functionally and abnormal fixations on inanimate objects also are widely described characteristics. Under- or overreaction to certain sensory stimuli may be observed, leading clinicians and researchers to believe that the sensory thresholds of children with autism are significantly different from those of people in the general population.

TABLE 3–1 Developmental delays in various developmental disabilities during preschool years

Disorder	Developmental area			
	Motor	Language	Nonverbal Reasoning	Social-Adaptive
Mental Retardation	Variable	2	2	2
Autism	N/A	3	Variable	3
Cerebral Palsy	3	Variable	Variable	2
Deafness	N/A	2	N/A	Variable
Blindness	1	N/A	Variable	1

Key: 3, severe impairment; 2, moderate impairment; 1, mild impairment; N/A, not affected

Source: Mental Retardation by M. L. Batshaw, B. Shapiro, & M. L. Z. Farber in *Children with disabilities* (5th ed.). M. L. Batshaw, L. Pelligrino, & N. J. Roizen, p. 253. Copyright 2007 by Paul H. Brookes Publishing Company. Reprinted with permission.

WARNING SIGNS

As more and more is learned about symptoms and signs associated with autism, and through retroactive studies, a series of warning signs has emerged. Specifically, parents should be on the alert if their child exhibits the following characteristics:

- No big smiles or other joyful expressions by 6 months of age
- No back-and-forth sharing of sounds, smiles, or facial expressions by 9 months
- No back-and-forth gestures such as pointing, showing, reaching, or waving bye-bye by 12 months
- No babbling at 12 months
- No single words at 16 months
- No two-word spontaneous (nonecholaic) phrases by 24 months
- Failure to attend to human voices by 24 months
- Failure to look at the face and eyes of others by 24 months
- Failure to orient to name by 24 months
- Failure to demonstrate interest in other children by 24 months
- Failure to imitate by 24 months
- Any loss of any language or social skill at any age

Even if a child cannot be definitively diagnosed as being on the autism spectrum, early intervention for a child demonstrating the above characteristics is warranted. The same approaches used to facilitate language and communication in children with ASD can be implemented.

SYMBOLIC ABILITIES AND SOCIAL ASPECTS OF COMMUNICATION

Wetherby et al. (1998) summarized several studies in identifying impaired symbolic abilities and social aspects of communication as falling into three primary categories: communicative means, communicative functions, and symbolic play. The primary purpose of communication by a child with autism is to regulate the behavior of others, such as requesting others to perform or stop performing a specific action. Their study supports these descriptions, and has implications for early identification and early intervention. Some early indicators of autism and other PDDs include the following:

1. Lack of joint attention

2. Lack of complex gestural communication

3. Lack of reciprocal interaction

4. Poor rate of communication

5. Lack of repair strategies in communication

6. Absence of gaze shifts

7. Poor language comprehension

8. Deficits in symbolic play

Implications for intervention planning based on the work of Wetherby et al. (1998) is that the easiest skill to teach to children with autism and other PDDs is behavior regulation, and the most difficult to teach is joint attention. "Communicating for social interaction to draw attention to self may be viewed as a transition between communication for behavior regulation to achieve an environmental end and joint attention to draw attention to an object or event" (Wetherby et al., 1998, p. 89). The use of contact gestures should be stressed as a way to enhance communication. Finally, the use of constructive play as a means to develop language and functional use of objects should be incorporated into therapy for children with autism or other PDDs.

Social deficits are at the core of the diagnosis of autism. Schopler and Mesibov (1986) have found that when children with autism reach adolescence, they appear to demonstrate an increased awareness and interest in other people. They state that these children's problems seem to be a "lack of social skills rather than a lack of social interest" (p. 5). Thus, implications for treatment suggest that the clinician target pragmatic skills in therapy. Children and adults with autism also may demonstrate splinter skills representing unusual abilities such as being able to memorize the phone directory (Nelson, 1998).

Young children with autism are usually unresponsive to others, and they engage in solitary activity during the early years. As Schopler and Mesibov (1986) found, as the children get older, they show interest in interacting with others socially, but find such interaction difficult. Volkmar et al. (1997) found that older children with autism have difficulty establishing a shared frame of reference with their social partner, frequently speaking tangentially without providing background information needed for the listener to understand the conversation. They are also somewhat impulsive in their language, failing to adhere to accepted social norms. For example, they may blurt out, "That's an ugly dress." Volkmar et al. also found that these children use stereotypical phrases as the norm for social interaction, and fail to recognize and use nonverbal cues when interacting with others.

Stereotypical phrases Fixed, unvarying utterances that are often heard produced by others and used in excess by children with social interaction deficits.

Paul (2001) points out that we tend to dwell on those things that children with autism find difficult or impossible to do. On a more positive side, individuals with autism usually have normal scores on tests of discrimination and short-term memory. They also do well on tasks requiring differentiating features (even small ones) between two or more stimuli. Paul (2005) stresses that the existence of a communication disability is part of the diagnostic criteria for autism, but a structural language disorder is not.

THE DEVELOPMENT OF SPEECH

As stated earlier in this chapter, the criteria for the diagnosis of autism include language deficits as well as qualitative impairments in social interaction and communication. Many children with autism go through a period of mutism, or silence, in the early years. However, when the child does begin to speak, he or she typically has excellent articulation. In fact, this is one differentiator in the diagnosis of ASD as opposed to intellectual disabilities. Children with intellectual disabilities typically have articulation that is delayed along with their language and cognition.

Mutism Not speaking; may be selective, meaning a child does not talk in certain settings, or elective, meaning there is no organic or physical disability that prevents the child from talking.

Hurford (1991) writes that if a functional language system has not developed by age 5 years, there is little likelihood of its developing. DeMyer, Barton, DeMeyer, Norton, Allen and Steele (1973) found that approximately 65 percent of children with autism who were mute at age 5 remained mute several years later in their development. As the child with autism progresses through the developmental period, there appear to be periods of rapid growth and development as opposed to the slow consistent development exhibited by normally developing children.

IS AUTISM CURED OR OUTGROWN?

Paul (2001) and Lord and Paul (1997) indicate that that the majority (maybe as high as 80%) of individuals with autism test out as being mentally deficient on cognitive tests by the time they are school aged, and that approximately 40 percent do not develop expressive language by the time they are 5 years of age (school age). For individuals who do not develop a system of expressive language, the prognosis as adults is guarded. However, for the 15–20 percent of individuals with autism who are cognitively within normal limits (based on intelligence testing), the outlook is more positive. Paul (2001) writes the following:

> A few of these individuals seem to "outgrow" their autism by mid-childhood, but most remain autistic or at least very odd as adults. They may be able to live on their own; they can learn functional job skills, and some can graduate from college in fields such as mathematics or computer science. But even these very bright individuals who have autism continue to have difficulty with human relationships, social judgment, and appropriate use of language. (p. 108) Other researchers indicate that for more than 95% of the individuals who are diagnosed as autistic, the disorder is a lifelong disorder (Volkmar, Carter, Grossman, and Klin, 1997; Grandin, 1997). However, with increased understanding of the behaviors associated with ASD and improved intervention, some children are making significant progress.

THEORY OF MIND

Theory of mind is the ability to understand another's perspective, a skill typically lacking in children who are autistic or on the autism spectrum. These individuals also have trouble recognizing that people can have more than one emotion centered on a particular experience or event. Prelock (2006) summed up the work of Howlin, Baron-Cohen, and Hadwin (1999), who identified three "mental state concepts" that they taught to children on the autism spectrum:

1. Informational states (from simple perspective taking to false-belief understanding)

2. Emotion (from recognition of pictures to belief-based emotions)

3. Pretense (from sensorimotor to pretend play)

Prelock wrote that

> basic principles underlying these mental state concepts include (a) perception leads to knowledge (i.e., individuals will know something if they saw it or heard about it); (b) actions or objects satisfy desires (i.e., if individuals want something, they will be delighted to receive it, and if they do not receive it, they will be unhappy): and (c) pretense involves the substitution of objects

or the suspension of an outcome (i.e., when pretending, an individual does so for fun and with no expectation of using an object in a typical way). (p. 523)

Howlin and colleagues found that children had improved understanding of the perspectives of others upon completion of their training protocol. Much research has focused on the relationship between theory of mind and social skills. The research has typically demonstrated that children with autism can learn theory of mind through a variety of tasks with some success (Swettenham, 1996; Ozonoff & Miller, 1995). Other studies have shown that training in social skills does not result in significant improvement, and yet others have studied the relationships between theory of mind and social interaction (Hadwin, Baron-Cohen, Howlin, & Hill, 1997; Chin & Bernard-Oritz, 2000) and found that mental state teaching does not result in significant change in either theory of mind or social skills. A prevailing thought resulting from these studies is that children with autism have impaired acquisition of theory of mind as evidenced by their poor interactive behaviors. For example, children with autism typically are unable to appreciate the feelings of others or to take on the perspective of their conversational partners. They tend to dominate a conversation, frequently perseverating on a topic of interest to them without regard to the partner's level of interest in the topic. Thus, while it has been shown that children can be taught theory of mind, it is evident that the children do not necessarily generalize that learning to social situations.

Chin and Bernard-Oritz (2000) found in their study that some of the children did improve in their social skills (such as joint attention and eye contact) during conversations, but also found that theory of mind instruction did not generalize. Their theory as to why theory of mind does not generalize well to daily activities is that most theory of mind instruction relies on false belief tasks. In false belief tasks, children are read a story or see a scenario acted out, and then must predict what the character—which has false information—will do. Chin and Bernard-Oritz theorized that the differences between this type of task and the skills needed to infer what a conversational partner is thinking or feeling are vastly different. They also proposed that perhaps false belief tasks are not effectively generalized, but that other types of tasks may be more readily synthesized into daily interactions. Chin and Bernard-Oritz concluded that children with autism can be trained to improve their communication skills, and that possibly they learn some theory of mind skills incidental to that teaching. But they caution that, even when conversational improvement occurs, "performance on False Belief tasks remains constant. Hence, together with findings of past studies, we conclude that caution should be exercised when inferring an individual's social behaviour on the basis of his/her performance in False Belief tasks" (p. 581).

DEVELOPMENT OF READING IN CHILDREN ON THE AUTISM SPECTRUM

The relationship between oral language and reading is discussed in Chapter 10. That relationship also holds up in children with ASD. Traditional views on when to begin reading instruction consider the presence of spoken language and letter identification skills as necessary prerequisites to reading instruction. In 2003, Koppenhaver and Erickson wrote, "Emergent literacy comprises all of the actions, understandings, and misunderstandings of learners engaged in experiences that involve print creation or use" (p. 284). They found not only improvement in emergent literacy, but also some improvement of oral language abilities when children with autism were provided with an enriched environment designed to facilitate emergent reading and writing skills. Mirenda (2003) also found that children with autism, even if nonverbal, could be taught to read through the provision of interventions that use multiple instructional strategies. Mirenda proposed specific strategies for teaching reading to children with autism based on stages of reading (Ehri, 1991, 1994, 1995) and the strategies children use to learn to read words (Ehri & McCormick, 1998).

Providing an Environment to Facilitate Emergent Literacy in Children with Autism

One of the most important endeavors in the facilitation of emergent literacy skills is the provision of adequate and appropriate opportunities for children with autism (in fact, all children) to experience reading and writing activities. Koppenhaver and Erickson (2003) conducted a study in a public school preschool classroom for children with autism in which they documented the change in preliteracy behaviors and skills of three 3-year-old children with severe communication impairments. All three used nonlinguistic communication such as pointing, vocalizing, gesturing, and crying. Prior to implementation of the intervention, the classroom provided few opportunities for the children to engage in literacy activities. Writing materials were available only for specific activities; at other times they were put away. A reading corner consisted of only 20 books to which the children had a few minutes of access between lunch and when the teacher read aloud to the class. The librarian also read aloud to the students one or two times a week. An interview with the teacher revealed that she did not really believe the children, particularly the three children who were the focus of the study, could engage in emergent literacy activities.

Koppenhaver and Erickson (2003) wanted to study the effects of an environment rich in emergent literacy activities and materials on the three children with autism and severe communication deficits. Intervention was provided twice a week for 60–90 minutes for 5 months. Before intervention began, the researchers introduced supports for emergent writing and emergent reading into the classroom. The materials were available at all times throughout the day. There were some structured, teacher-directed periods each day interspersed with times when the children could choose their own activities in the play centers. Intervention occurred during these play center times in groups of one to three students. The intervention was child-directed and included modeling of written language activities (such as writing their name on the attendance sheet at the beginning of the session), comprehension activities, reading, and parallel play in which the instructor would think aloud and model appropriate play. Materials introduced into the environment to encourage emergent writing included a desktop computer (which was already in the room but unused) that was loaded with a "basic children's writing and publishing program" (p. 287), a laptop with a basic word processing program (all caps in 24-point font), a video-painting toy on which the children could write or draw on a membrane keyboard and watch the process and end result on a TV monitor, and less sophisticated tools such as an Etch-A-Sketch, a Magna-Doodle, a Glo-Doodler, crayons, paper, chalk and a chalkboard, a whiteboard and dry-erase markers, a manual typewriter, letter stamps, and Play-Doh with cookie-cutters.

Emergent literacy supports that were introduced to the classroom included a variety of new reading materials, a table, and more shelves. The reading materials included "books with sound effects, board books, wordless picture books, comic books and children's magazines, newspapers, stories with repeated lines, books on tape and computer diskettes, touch-and-feel books, and homemade picture books that included Mayer-Johnson Picture Communication Symbols (PCS)" (Koppenhaver & Erickson, 2003, p. 287). The researchers also integrated text into classroom routines through the use of flipcharts with titles and lyrics of the songs sung during music time, the use of name cards and students' photos for the attendance activity, labels on centers, and six low-tech communication devices used during snack and storybook interactions. In addition, they had typically developing verbal students record messages specific to classroom activities.

The results showed improvement in the interest in books and print activities in all three children. All three typically chose print activities in the play center. There was an increased interest in writing and drawing and improvement in their ability to write their names. One student, the one who was the biggest challenge initially, learned to produce his name on the computer and with letter stamps, naming the letters as he went through the written production of his name. But perhaps the most important lesson learned from this study is that we do not have to "teach" interest in literacy. Introducing appropriate, adequate, and varied materials into a child's natural environment, and having them available for use on a consistent basis, facilitates growth of interest and abilities in emergent literacy behaviors. The researchers were quick to note that it is important to recognize that the children's interests and skills tend to vary from day to day (and sometimes situation to situation). They also pointed out that there is a need for controlled studies "to determine what constitutes the best natural emergent literacy learning environment and opportunities for children with autism" (Koppenhaver & Erickson, 2003, p. 291).

Strategies to Facilitate the Development of Reading in Children with Autism

Lanter and Watson (2008) summed up multiple research studies to note the following language and literacy behaviors in children with ASD:

1. Children with ASD typically have an "uneven profile" in the development of skills that are predictive of reading success. Even though children with ASD typically have some language problems, they often know the alphabet, and some can read in spite of their language problems.

2. There is a discrepancy between nonverbal mental ages and vocabulary levels, with vocabulary being severely delayed in comparison to what would be expected, although this is not always as evident in older children with high-functioning autism.

3. Students and adults with autism "were more likely to include bizarre or inappropriate utterances during story retellings than were individuals with Down syndrome who were matched on verbal age" (p. 34)

4. Children who are diagnosed as being on the autism spectrum have difficulty with personal narratives (more so than with storybook narratives), possibly due to the need to generate the story rather than to retell a story.

Lanter and Watson (2008) suggested that teachers and speech-language pathologists not exclude children with ASD who do not have spoken-language and letter-identification skills from emergent literacy activities. At the emergent literacy stage, they also suggested the following strategies for children on the autism spectrum:

1. Engage the child in shared book reading using both narratives and expository stories. Lantner and Watson cite several studies, noting that some students with ASD who are consistently engaged in shared book reading demonstrate a decrease in echolalia, verbal outbursts, and stereotypic behaviors and an increase in attending skills and oral language skills.

2. Encourage story retelling using visual aids to improve comprehension, story sense, and development of their own narratives. The effects of story retelling instruction on the improvement of language and development of reading in children with ASD has not been addressed in this population, but there is abundant evidence that children with ASD have good visual-cognitive processing abilities. Hence, the use of visual aids in facilitating story retelling is a strategy that is worth trying and researching.

3. Create dialogue around storybooks. The authors encourage the use of strategies such as "think alouds" (originally described by Baker in

2002) in which speech-language pathologists and teachers demonstrate how to answer questions about narratives throughout the book-reading process. Answering questions requires interpreting the information and making inferences. Think alouds can also be used to teach repair strategies and to teach the students to apply the narrative to their own experiences. Again, this strategy has not been explored in the population of students with ASD.

4. Teach literacy in natural contexts. This is consistent with all the research that shows that language and reading activities need to be integrated into the child's daily activities. The children should observe the adults in their environment engaging in reading and writing activities, and the adults should include the children in the activities. For example, if the mother is making out a grocery list, the child could observe her reading the recipe book to see what is needed to make the food, reading the can labels in the pantry to determine what needs to be purchased, writing down the items needed from the store, then going to the story and matching what is on the list with what is on the shelf. The child can be given a crayon or pencil to make his or her "shopping list" and imitate the mother's actions through the whole sequence.

5. Label objects and pictures to promote sight-word reading. This activity facilitates the development of picture-to-text matching, a fundamental reading skill.

6. Have the children read and write about their activities. Having children write narratives about their experiences helps them link their experiences with their knowledge, a critical skill to facilitate comprehension of text. To model writing narratives about their experiences for the children, the speech-language pathologist can create a story about an event in which the children are going to participate, such as a field trip to the fire station.

Children at the conventional stage of reading (typical of children in first and second grade) focus on phonological awareness, decoding, and learning to extract meaning from what they have read. Some children with ASD reach this level. Strategies that are helpful for typically developing children at the conventional stage are (1) promoting phonological awareness, (2) using computer software, (3) assisting students in constructing meaning through dialogue, and (4) matching the text with the language strategy (Lanter & Watson, 2008). These strategies are discussed in more detail in Chapter 10.

Few children with ASD reach the level of being skilled readers. Children who are skilled readers have word-reading skills and good comprehension of what they read. As a rule, typically developing children achieve this level in third grade. Comprehension requires good language skills, strong vocabulary, good general knowledge, and strategies such as questioning, inferencing, analyzing, synthesizing, summarizing, and clarifying. Lanter and Watson (2008) summarized the research and stated that issues in ASD that interfere with becoming skilled readers can be "related to three prominent neuropsychological theories proposed to explain ASD" (p. 39):

1. Theory of mind has been discussed earlier in this chapter, but the difficulty students with ASD have in inferring meaning significantly interferes with text comprehension.

2. Weak central coherence interferes with their ability to make inferences and to derive meaning from the text.

3. Executive function deficits make it difficult for children with ASD to adapt to new situations and interfere with their ability to handle changes in materials they are reading.

As they did with the emergent and conventional stages, Lanter and Watson (2008) suggested teaching strategies for children with ASD at the skilled reading level:

1. Match text with ability: Use narratives and expository texts at a language and cognitive level commensurate with the child's functioning levels.

2. Focus on deep structure, not surface structure: Using fact-based questions is important, but children with ASD need focused intervention that employs comprehension questions to help them draw inferences and better interpret the information they have read.

3. Use group reading and discussion groups with typically developing peers to provide a scaffolding format through which children with ASD learn peer interactions and learn *from* their peers as well.

4. Build background knowledge to facilitate text comprehension.

5. Link texts with prior knowledge: Based on a 2004 study by Wahlberg and Magliano, Lanter and Watson proposed this strategy. Wahlberg and Magliano studied text comprehension in adults with high-functioning autism. Those adults who were given concrete titles and abstracts to read before they read the corresponding text had better recall of information from the material they had read. Thus, having the prior knowledge from the title and abstract enhanced their ability to remember what they had read.

6. Use visual aids: This has been used at every level. At the skilled reading level, visual aids can be expanded to story maps, framed outlines, Venn diagrams, and other text analysis methods to preteach the content.

7. Promote text monitoring: The use of think alouds and the interspersing of questions throughout the text also facilitated comprehension.

OTHER DIAGNOSES ON THE AUTISM SPECTRUM AND ASSOCIATED DISORDERS

Asperger Syndrome and High-Functioning Autism (HFA)

Asperger syndrome was first described by Hans Asperger, a German psychiatrist, in 1944 as a condition in "children with higher cognitive skills and overall functioning but with the specific challenges in social understanding" and in which children exhibit "significant social problems despite their essentially appropriate verbal abilities" (Prelock, 2006, p. 5). Individuals with Asperger disorder have many of the same social and behavioral characteristics as do children with autism, but the individuals with Asperger syndrome do not have the cognitive and language deficits typical of individuals with autism (Towbin, Mauk, & Batshaw, 2002).

Asperger syndrome is a label used to identify children who are at the higher end of the autism spectrum. Typically, these children demonstrate no significant delay in their general language skills and have intelligence scores ranging from average to above average. Individuals with Asperger syndrome usually have difficulty making friends in school, in some part because they have difficulty comprehending nonverbal communication behaviors, and they lack spontaneity in their communication endeavors. Their interests and extracurricular activities typically are narrowly focused (Sicile-Kira, 2004). Organization of information is also problematic, which can significantly impact their academic success. Thus, this should be a major focus of therapy for children with Asperger syndrome. Prelock (2006) summarized the general criteria for a diagnosis of Asperger syndrome based on the characteristics identified by the American Psychiatric Association:

1. No significant delays in language development

2. No significant delays in cognitive development prior to age 3 years

3. Severe and sustained deficits in social interactions

4. Development of restricted, repetitive, and stereotyped patterns of behavior, interests, or activities

5. Significant deficits in social, occupational, or other areas of functioning.

Gillberg (1991) developed a set of six criteria for Asperger syndrome diagnosis. Specifically, Gillberg defined Asperger as being impairment in

1. Reciprocal social interaction

2. Interest development

3. Self-imposed routines

4. Speech and language development

5. Nonverbal communication

6. Motor performance

Children who have Asperger syndrome often demonstrate splinter skills at a high level, such as proficiency in music or mathematics, but at the same time have difficulty with organizational skills and the generalization of skills learned in one setting to a novel setting. An illustration of this is that the child may be able to comprehend complex mathematical or scientific principles, but fail to bring his or her homework home at the end of the school day due to lack of organizational skills. In addition, these children may have temper tantrums, but not as a manipulative effort; rather, the tantrums are usually in response to fear, stress, and/or frustration.

The classroom for children with autism or Asperger syndrome should stick to a regular schedule as much as possible because these children typically have difficulty with transitions to new activities and schedules. The classroom should not be overstimulating in terms of noise and visual distractions. In fact, the child with Asperger syndrome shares many of the characteristics of children with attention deficit disorder.

Remaining seated for an extended period of time and being able to focus on the task at hand are quite taxing for children who fall on the autism spectrum. They may have auditory processing problems, leading to failure to comprehend instructions provided by teachers and therapists, so the students benefit from having directions broken down into small steps and using visual cues when possible.

Comprehension may lag behind expression in children with Asperger syndrome. This certainly interferes with the progression of their academic skills once in school. Likewise, poor organization skills and possible auditory processing deficits may impact their ability to achieve academic success. Children who fall on the autism spectrum often have dysgraphia, or difficulty writing, making it difficult to listen to the teacher and take notes simultaneously. It is helpful to the student to have the teacher make copies of his or her notes for the child or to assign a fellow student as his or her notetaker in the class.

The development of friendships with other students is a big problem for children with Asperger syndrome. As mentioned earlier, they often lack comprehension of basic social skills, and this interferes with the ability to establish and maintain friendships. It may be helpful for the family members, the teacher, and other professionals who interact with the child to lead a classroom discussion with the students in the child's class in order to explain the nature of the disorder and solicit their help in forming relationships with the student. Communication characteristics of individuals with Asperger syndrome primarily focus on disorders in the area of pragmatics. Discussions with these individuals tends to be one-sided and somewhat pedantic. There is typically no attempt to involve the conversational partner's viewpoints, experiences, or ideas. Individuals with Asperger syndrome react to others' attempts to enter the

Attention deficit disorder The presence of behavior that typically includes inattention, hyperactivity, and impulsivity that exceed that expected by children at a given age.

Dysgraphia Impaired ability to write, usually due to brain damage.

conversation with annoyance, lack of interest, or lack of acknowledgement. As a result, the "interactions" are monologue- or lecture-like. They abruptly change topics and introduce unexplained personal associations into conversations. Typically, there is a total lack of conversational reciprocity (Bregman, 2005).

Recently, there have been questions as to whether Asperger syndrome and high-functioning autism are separate entities or not. Baron-Cohen (2000) described two levels of theory of mind: (1) being able to infer one's own mental state and (2) mental states about other people's mental states. Spek, Scholte, and Van-Berckelaer-Onnes (2010) cited Baron-Cohen and wrote that children with high-functioning autism and children with Asperger syndrome demonstrate impairments in functioning on Baron-Cohen's first- and/or second-level theory of mind tasks, but that the adults in each diagnostic group did not show impairments at either level. But, as mentioned before, Ozonoff et al. (1991) found that success on theory of mind tasks did not translate to successful integration of the skills in daily interactions. There is a suggestion that there may be an advanced theory of mind level that "involves interpreting complex social situations, based on subtle information" (p. 281). Spek and colleagues conducted a study to determine the validity of theory of mind tasks and self-reports in differentiating between HFA and Asperger syndrome. They found no difference in performance between the two groups, which lends support to the school of thought that there is little justification for differentiating between HFA and Asperger syndrome. It is important to note that they also found that both groups "have more self-knowledge and introspective abilities" than commonly believed based on earlier studies (p. 287).

Miller and Ozonoff (2000) cited Wing (1991) in writing that both groups have "social isolation, lack of interest in others' feelings, difficulty relating to others, and a lack of flexible imaginative play...abnormalities in communication, including difficulty using language socially, idiosyncratic phrases, and repetitive questioning" (p. 227). Both groups are impaired with regard to nonverbal communication, both exhibit stereotypical behaviors, both have narrow interests, and both want stable routines. Some have found differences between the two groups in the areas of language motor skills, cognition, and visuospatial development. Earlier in this chapter, the criteria for a diagnosis of autism were presented. A diagnosis of Asperger syndrome also includes the presence of repetitive behaviors, narrow interests, and social deficits, but those with Asperger syndrome are defined by the DSM-IV and ICD-10 as having normal language acquisition and normal cognitive development. Also, individuals who have been diagnosed as autistic cannot later be diagnosed as having Asperger syndrome (Miller & Ozonoff, 2000).

In an effort to determine if there were enough differences to justify separate labels, Miller and Ozonoff compared individuals diagnosed with HFA to individuals diagnosed as Asperger syndrome on four domains: intelligence, motor skills, visuospatial abilities, and executive functions. They found that those diagnosed with Asperger syndrome had significantly higher

IQ scores, verbal and full scale, than those with HFA. However, there were no differences on the other three measures when the authors controlled for the higher IQ abilities of the subjects with Asperger syndrome (although they did note slightly poorer performance on fine motor tasks by those with Asperger syndrome). They concluded that the only significant differences between the two groups (HFA and Asperger syndrome) were the IQ levels and the severity of the symptoms. Symptoms long considered to be unique to each group were found in both groups. For example, those with Asperger syndrome showed echolalia, pronoun reversals, and neologisms that are typically associated with autism, and those with autism demonstrated the motor delays and normal language development typically considered to be consistent with Asperger syndrome. Thus, based on their findings, it appears that Asperger syndrome is a "high-IQ autism" (p. 235).

With regard to a prognosis for children with autism, Paul (1987) suggested their language skills and their performance on intelligence tests are two markers. Those children who fall within or close to the normal range of intelligence quotients are more successful in achieving independence in adulthood. Also, the development of speech by age 5 is indicative of a more promising prognosis. Those children who have a relatively normal developmental history followed by a regression have a poorer prognosis than children who do not regress (Watson & Ozonoff, 2001). Some children with autism who have a normal to high IQ may attend college, live independently, and become employed. However, they remain socially handicapped, having difficulty with pragmatics, empathy, and other social skills (Schroeder, LeBlanc, & Mayo, 1996; Paul, 2001).

Rett Disorder

Rett disorder (also known as Rett's syndrome) is a progressive process that only affects girls. The overall clinical presentation of Rett disorder closely resembles that of autism. The girls have typical development for the first few months of life, then demonstrate a loss of skills (including communication). The usual age of onset is 6–18 months of age (Towbin, Mauk, & Batshaw, 2002). Of particular note is the loss of functional use of the hands and the development of persistent hand wringing. The girl also demonstrates poor coordination in walking and other motor skills, often exhibiting a severe delay of psychomotor skills (Sicile-Kira, 2004). Cognitive deficits are typical, along with acquired microcephaly (Towbin, Mauk, & Batshaw, 2002). Batshaw (2005) summarizes the development and progression of Rett disorder as follows:

> At variable ages older than 1 year, children with Rett disorder experience rapid deterioration of behavior, language, and mental status; lose purposeful hand movements; and develop ataxia and seizures. A prominent feature is continuous "hand washing"

TABLE 3–2 Symptoms frequently seen in Rett disorder

Breathing dysfunction

EEG abnormalities

Seizures

Muscle rigidity or spasticity

Scoliosis

Bruxism

Small feet in relation to stature

Growth retardation

Peripheral vasomotor disturbances

Abnormal sleep patterns and agitation

Dysphagia and nutritional deficits

Decreased mobility with age

Constipation

Source: Based on information from *Autism spectrum disorders: Issues in assessment and intervention,* by P. Prelock. Copyright 2006 by Pro-Ed.

movements, often accompanied by hyperventilation. By 6 years of age, an affected girl generally has mental retardation requiring extensive to pervasive support, spasticity, and seizures. The condition then stabilizes over a period of many years. (p. 371)

There is a long list of related symptoms that frequently occur but are not required for diagnosis of Rett disorder. These symptoms are listed in Table 3–2. Prelock (2006) cited the research of many investigators in stating that there are four periods of development in children who have Rett disorder:

- Stage 1: An initial onset of unclear symptoms and developmental stagnation

- Stage 2: A period of rapid deterioration and loss of previously acquired skills

- Stage 3: Stabilization

- Stage 4: "some improvement in social skills, although motor deterioration usually occurs" (p. 8)

Childhood Disintegrative Disorder (CDD)

Children in this diagnostic category show normal development of verbal, nonverbal, social, adaptive, and play skills and behaviors until at least age 2 years and often 3 to 5 years of age, then show a significant loss of those skills

(Towbin, Mauk, & Batshaw, 2002; Prelock, 2006; Sicile-Kira, 2004; Hyman & Towbin, 2007). As cited by Prelock (2006), Volkmar did an extensive

> review of the literature, including case reports of CDD, (that) suggests that this disorder differs from classic autism in four specific areas: reported age of onset (mostly 3 to 4 years of age); clinical features (e.g., loss of previously acquired skills following a course of normal development; course (deterioration in development, sometimes progressive); and prognosis (usually lifelong challenges and high level of care required). (p. 9)

The decline exhibited by children with CDD affects "language, social reciprocity, play, motor skills, and basic adaptive functions such as bowel and bladder skills" (Hyman & Towbin, 2007, p. 326).

Co-Occurrence of Cognitive Disabilities with Autism

Prior to 1980, many studies placed the incidence of cognitive disabilities among individuals with autism at 90 percent. However, with the expansion of the autism spectrum and the diagnosis of milder cases in more recent years, the incidence is now set at approximately 50 percent. Furthermore, there is an increasing tendency to label individuals with moderate to severe cognitive challenges as showing classic characteristics associated with the autism spectrum. That is to say, there is some evidence of co-morbidity of intellectual disabilities and autism (Buckendorf, 2008). According to Lord and Paul (1997), 80 percent of children who are diagnosed with autism score in the mental retardation range on tests of intelligence and adaptive behavior. Generally speaking, the majority of individuals who have cognitive deficits do not have autism.

ASSESSMENT AND DIAGNOSIS OF AUTISM SPECTRUM DISORDERS AND RELATED DISORDERS

There has been an emergence of assessment tools dedicated to the assessment and diagnosis of autism that can be used along with some of the traditional speech and language measures. Hall (2009) wrote that "diagnostic instruments have been most accurate at identifying autism in individuals with some oral language and mild to moderate cognitive disabilities who are school age." Some of the assessment tools that are specific to ASD are as follows:

1. The *Adolescent and Adult Psychoeducational Profile* (AAPEP) (Mesibov, Schopler, Schaffer, & Landrus, 1988) is designed to develop therapy goals for adolescents and adults over the age of 12 years with ASD.

It consists of two interview scales, one for home and one for school or work. There is one observation scale and two interview scales. There are six functional areas on each scale: functional communication, leisure skills, vocational skills, vocational behavior, interpersonal behavior, and independent functioning.

2. The *Checklist for Autism in Toddlers* (CHAT) (1992) was developed by British researchers as a tool to be used by pediatricians to screen for autism. It consists of 14 items, takes 5 minutes to administer, and is administered to children when they are 18 months old. The CHAT assesses social-communicative behaviors, focusing on imaginative play and joint attention (Bregman, 2005). The CHAT is highly effective in predicting autism, PDD, Asperger syndrome, and other developmental syndromes (Baron-Cohen et al., 1992).

3. The *Australian Scale for Asperger Syndrome* (ASIS) was developed by Garnett and Attwood in 1998. It is a questionnaire and rating scale based on six categories: (1) social and emotional abilities, (2) communication skills, (3) cognitive skills, (4) specific interests, (5) movement skills, and (6) other characteristics (Gabovitch & Wiseman, 2005).

4. The *Gilliam Autism Rating Scale 2* (GARS2) (Gilliam, 2006) has three subscales: (1) stereotyped behaviors, (2) communication, and (3) social interaction.

5. The *Assessment of Basic Language and Learning Skills* (ABLLS) (Partington & Sundberg, 1998) is an assessment and curriculum guide for children with autism and other developmental disabilities. It has assessment items and skill tracking grids to guide individualized education program (IEP) development. It has four sections: (1) basic learner skills (cooperation, imitation, receptive language, play, and following classroom routines); (2) academic skills (reading, math, writing, and spelling); (3) self-help skills; and (4) motor skills. The ABLLS is based on the analysis of verbal behavior espoused by Skinner (Zager & Shamow, 2005).

6. The *Autism Spectrum Screening Questionnaire* (ASSQ) (Ehlers, Gillberg, & Wing, 1999) is a screening questionnaire for Asperger syndrome and other high-functioning ASDs in the school-age population. The items are scored on a three-point scale and address (1) social interaction, (2) communication, (3) restricted or repetitive behavior, (4) motor clumsiness, and (5) other associated symptoms (Ehlers, Gillberg, & Wing, 1999; Gabovitch & Wiseman, 2005).

7. The *Modified Checklist for Autism in Toddlers* (M-CHAT) (Robins, Fein, & Bartlett, 1999) is a screener to identify children aged 16–30 months who are at risk for ASD. It consists of 23 yes/no items. If the child fails three items total, or two critical items, he or she should be referred for

a full diagnostic work-up. The M-CHAT can be downloaded from two websites: www.firststeps.org or hwww2.gsu.edu.

8. The *Asperger Syndrome Diagnostic Scale* (ASDS) (Myles, Jones-Bock, & Simpson, 2000) has 50 items and takes about 15 minutes for someone familiar with the child or adolescent to complete. Five behavior areas are examined: (1) cognitive, (2) maladaptive, (3) language, (4) social, and (5) sensorimotor. The ASDS can be used to "document behavior progress as a result of intervention or to target goals on the student's IEP" (Psychological Corporation, 2010).

9. The *Autism Diagnostic Observation Schedule* (ADOS) (Lord, Rutter, DiLavore, & Risi, 2000) is a standardized protocol that can be used to observe social and communicative behaviors of toddlers through adults. Some consider it to be the "gold standard" of tests for ASD. It has four modules for use with individuals of varying developmental and language levels: (1) preverbal/single words, (2) phrase speech, (3) fluent speech—child/adolescent, which overlaps with module 2 but adds friends and marriage, loneliness, emotions, and creating a story, and (4) high-functioning adolescents and adults, which includes daily living and plans and hopes. It has 93 items that are linked to the DSM-IV and the ICD-10 codes. It takes 2 hours to administer the ADOS (Bregman, 2005; Gabovitch & Wiseman, 2005; Western Psychological, 2010).

10. The *Functional Emotional Assessment Scale* (FEAS) (Greenspan, DeGangi, & Weider, 2001) was developed by the same team that developed the Floortime intervention approach. The FEAS "provides a framework for observing and assessing a child's emotional and social functioning" (Psychological Corporation, 2010). There is a clinical version that can be used only as a descriptive measure to organize clinical thinking. There are six functional developmental levels: (1) self-regulation and interest in the world; (2) forming relationships, attachment, and engagement; (3) two-way, purposeful communication; (4) behavioral organization, problem solving, and internalization; (5) representational capacity (elaboration); and (6) representational differentiation.

11. The *Gilliam Asperger's Disorder Scale* (GADS) (Gilliam, 2001) is for individuals aged 3–22 years and is used to determine the probability of Asperger syndrome. There are 32 items on subscales of social interaction, restricted patterns of behavior, cognitive patterns, and pragmatic skills. There are also six yes/no questions for parents to answer. The GADS is norm referenced.

12. The *Pervasive Developmental Disorders Screening Test II* (PDDST II) (Siegel, 2004) is used for screening children aged 12–48 months. Stage I is a checklist completed by the parent(s) and takes about 5 minutes. The odd-numbered items are the critical questions; if three or more of them are checked as "Yes, usually true," the results are considered positive

for needing further evaluation for autism. The even-numbered items are used to differentiate between ASD and other mild developmental disorders. (Psychological Corporation, 2010; Brock & Slone, n.d.)

13. The *Diagnostic Interview for Social and Communication Disorders* (DISCO) (Leekam, Libby, Wing, Gould, & Taylor, 2002) is in its ninth edition. It is an interview format that provides ratings on the degree of delay in developmental milestones and the severity of the untypical behaviors. It can be used for diagnosis and the development of intervention plans for individuals with ASD and other developmental disorders (Bregman, 2005).

14. The *Childhood Asperger's Syndrome Test* (CAST) (Scott, Baron-Cohen, Bolton, & Brayne, 2002) is for children aged 4–11 years. It consists of 37 items with six control items to assess general development.

15. The *Autism Diagnostic Interview—Revised* (ADI-R) (Lord, Rutter, & LeCouteur, 1994) is a semi-structured interview for caregivers. It has three subscales: (1) communication, (2) social reciprocity, and (3) seven restricted, repetitive behaviors. The ADI-R can be used with children whose mental age is greater than 2 years (Bregman, 2005; Gabovitch & Wiseman, 2005).

16. The *Social Communication Questionnaire* (SCQ) (Rutter, Lord, & LeCouteur, 2004) consists of two forms. The current form assesses the child's behavior in the last 3 months, looking at everyday experiences and evaluating treatment and education plans. The lifetime form looks at the child's entire developmental history and can be used to decide if a full assessment is needed. The SCQ's first item documents the child's speaking ability and "determines which items will be used to calculate the score" (Brock & Slone, n.d.). The SCQ differentiates between autism and other disorders, but not between the various ASDs (Gabovitch & Wiseman, 2005).

17. The *Psychoeducational Profile* (PEP) (Schopler, Lansing, Reichler, & Marcus, 2005) was designed by the TEACCH program (see Treatment section) to identify strengths and weaknesses of individuals with ASD in the 6 months to 7 years age range. It consists of a caregiver report and a performance profile. The caregiver report provides a developmental history, problem behaviors, personal care and self-care skills, and adaptive behavior skills. It identifies diagnostic categories and the degree to which the categories interfere with development. The performance profile consists of six subtests measuring developmental abilities and four subtests focusing on maladaptive behaviors (Brock & Slone, n.d., ; Hall, 2009; Bregman, 2005).

18. The *Monteiro Interview Guidelines for Diagnosing Asperger Syndrome* (MIGDAS) (Monteiro, 2005) is a three-step approached used to assess

school-aged children, adolescents, and verbal preschoolers. It includes a checklist for parents and teachers and a student interview. It provides a qualitative description of the student's (1) language and communication, (2) social relationships and emotional responses, and (3) sensory use and interests.

19. The *Assessments for Educational Planning and Intervention* (ASIEP-3) (Krug, Arick, & Almond, 2008) was initially designed to help school personnel identify individuals with autism aged 2 years old to 13 years and 11 months. There are five standardized subtests for diagnosis, placement, educational program planning, and progress monitoring. The five subtests are (1) an autism behavior checklist (ABC) that has 57 items for teachers and parents to describe the child; (2) a sample of vocal behavior; (3) an interaction assessment; (4) an educational assessment; and (5) a prognosis of learning rate. The ABC is good for documenting change, but some feel it has limitations as a screener. The interaction assessment record form is used in the observation of social interaction and constructive play. The vocal behavior sample and prognosis of learning rate require recording the child. The educational assessment is usually done by the teacher and assesses receptive language, expressive language, body concept, and speech imitation.

20. The *Childhood Autism Rating Scale* (CARS2) (Schopler, Van Bourgondien, Wellman, & Love, 2010) consists of two 15-minute rating scales addressing functional areas that are completed by the clinician and an unscored checklist for parents or caregivers. It is designed to assess children over 2 years of age and covers the entire spectrum. The CARS2 can be used to identify children with autism and, using quantifiable ratings that are based on observation of the child, can determine symptom severity. It can be used to design intervention, give parents feedback, and determine the child's functional capabilities.

General guidelines in the assessment of young children who may be on the autism spectrum follow those of any good assessment of preschoolers. As much as possible, it is a good idea to assess the child in his or her natural settings in order to minimize the effect of being in a new environment. The child should be observed (and recorded) in the presence of/interacting with parents, siblings, and peers. Assessment of older children and adolescents should be based on a sensitivity as to the impact of the diagnosis and undertaken with respect for their attitudes and feelings with regard to being tested.

TREATMENT

As mentioned previously, Tiegerman-Farber (1997) proposed three etiological categories. One of them was a psychological-cognitive approach. In describing that approach, she maintained that the language delays and/or disorders displayed by a child with autism need to be addressed in relation to the child's environment. She wrote that

> these language differences should provide a basis for developing therapeutic goals that generate from the child and his or her individual language needs. Perhaps a critical component to this theoretical approach is the utilization of the autistic child's language behavior in the therapy process rather than its elimination. (p. 527)

Home programs should be developed as an integral part of a child's therapy. Children with autism are not likely to generalize treatment goals to everyday environments without heavy participation from those who manage those environments (i.e., the teacher in his or her classroom; the parents at home). These home lessons should be built around the naturally-occurring events in the child's daily routines, not structured language lessons conducted as an imitation of a therapy lesson in an office or classroom. In other words, the lessons should be semantically and pragmatically related to the daily experiences and interests of the child.

Applied Behavior Analysis (ABA)

Based on the principles of operant conditioning as espoused by B. F. Skinner, Applied Behavior Analysis (ABA) was one of the first formalized therapy approaches for autism. Skinner's philosophy on teaching behaviors was based on the supposition that every behavior has an antecedent and a consequence. The antecedent is what happens directly before the behavior, and the consequence is what happens after the behavior occurs. For example, in teaching eye contact, the antecedent may be the clinician's saying, "I see you. Now you look at me," and the consequence could include the clinician's clapping her hands and saying "Good looking at me!" if the child establishes eye contact. Shaping is a technique frequently employed in ABA. Shaping is the rewarding of successive approximations to the target behavior. Prompts can also be used to facilitate the child's achieving the desired behavior. However, prompts should be phased out as quickly as possible.

One may hear the term "the Lovaas Method" used synonymously with ABA. In 1978 at UCLA, Dr. Ivar Lovaas and his colleagues developed an intensive adaptation of ABA that was specifically implemented with preschoolers who had a diagnosis of autism. Lovaas and colleagues provided treatment to two groups of toddlers and preschoolers; one group received intensive treatment for at least 40 hours per week, and the other group received behavioral intervention for approximately 10 hours per week. Treatment in both groups was one-on-one, and the focus was on the development of social and communication skills. These children were followed and assessed up until age 11 years. Forty-seven percent of the children who received the intensive treatment were in the normal range with regard to educational and intellectual functioning when they entered first grade and were included in regular education classrooms. When these children were retested at age 11 years, the improvements were maintained. None of the children who were in the group who received less intensive treatment improved to the extent that the children who received treatment 40 or more hours per week did. These are remarkable results, but one should keep in mind the following factors:

1. The children who showed the most improvement were also those who had a higher mental age when treatment began.

2. Provision of the intensive treatment is a tremendous time and financial strain that most families cannot handle.

3. There was no true control group.

ABA encompasses several principles long associated with behavioral training:

- Positive reinforcement

- Negative reinforcement

- Shaping

- Fading

- Prompting

- Generalization

- Discrete trial teaching

- Incidental teaching

- Pivotal response training

- Incorporating peers and parents

These techniques and principles are defined in Chapter 6, as they are frequently employed in the provision of educational and therapeutic interventions. Parents are informed about goals and progress, and they are involved in implementing the strategies at home so that expectations and contingencies are consistent across all settings in which the child participates. Hall (2009) summarizes ABA as follows:

> The environment would be arranged to facilitate stimulus control for relevant and natural cues. Multiple forms of prompts would be in place...as well as plans for fading those prompts so that the stimulus control is transferred to the cues used in the natural environment....Communication skills would be targeted and many opportunities to practice would be provided. (pp. 86–87)

think about it

Is ABA realistic as far as the demands on the family's time? Do you think the results obtained in therapy would generalize to the child's natural environment? Explain your answers.

Pivotal Response Training (PRT)

PRT was previously known as Natural Language Paradigm (NLP), and was developed by Koegel, Koegel, and Shreibman. Koegel (1995) wrote, in reviewing the effectiveness of Discrete Trial Training, "not only did language fail to be exhibited or generalize to other environments, but most behaviors taught in this highly controlled environment also failed to generalize" (p. 23). Koegel and colleagues developed PRT using the principles of ABA and Discrete Trial Training, but applying them in naturalistic settings. PRT addresses a variety of skills (communication, social, academic, and language) and also works to decrease self-injurious and destructive behaviors. PRT is child-focused, and the program is tailored to fit the family's routines and schedules. Because everyone in the child's environment needs to implement the strategies, "PRT has been described as a lifestyle adopted by the affected family" (www.autismspeaks.org/treatment/prt.php).

One pivotal area is increasing the child's self-initiations. The child is taught to ask *wh-* questions and questions to gather information and gain assistance. A second pivotal response is improving the child' self-motivation. When the child requests an item, he or she receives it, thereby increasing his or her motivation to continue to initiate requests. A third pivotal area in PRT is teaching the child to respond to multiple cues and stimuli in order to facilitate generalization. The fourth pivotal area is increasing the child's ability to self-manage (Koegel, Koegel, Harrower, & Carter, 1999).

Language, social, and communication skills are taught in structured and unstructured sessions in the child's natural environment. PRT has been shown to be an effective approach, particularly in the areas of self-initiation, social communication, and expressive language (Koegel, Koegel, Harrower, & Carter, 1999; Koegel, Koegel, Shoshan, & McNerney, 1999; Jones, Carr, & Feely, 2006; Baker-Ericzen, Stahmer, & Burns, 2007).

Treatment and Education of Autistic and Related Communication Handicapped Children (TEACCH)

The TEACCH program is a structured, highly organized teaching approach "designed to provide the environmental and instructional adaptations necessary for an individual with ASD to function well within the larger social structure" (Hall, 2009, p. 134). It focuses on providing individuals with autism the modifications that they need to function throughout their lifetime in the culture of autism. The developers of the TEACCH program view autism as a culture of individuals who are different, not damaged. In the TEACCH program, parents work collaboratively with educators to identify their child's interests and strengths, and then to work within the cultural realm of autism to address the problem areas. Some of the factors that define the culture of autism are these children's limited play skills, adherence to routines, restricted social skills, lack of initiation, and noncompliant behaviors. Techniques employed in the approach are based on the characteristics associated with the autism culture. These include focusing on irrelevant details, distractibility, concrete thinking, impairment of organizational and sequencing skills, atypical sense of time, different learning styles, hyper/hyposensitivity, impulsivity, and high levels of anxiety (Hall, 2009). The TEACCH program utilizes ABA as part of the teaching strategy.

TEACCH pairs typically developing peers of the same age with the child with autism to teach conversation skills. Adults participate in the group to provide reinforcement and support as needed. The groups are very structured, utilizing charts, checklists, and scripts, and they focus on the interests and understanding of the conversation partners. This approach was the first one to teach social skills to adolescents with ASD, but there has not been any research to determine if the children with ASD are able to generalize their socialization skills beyond the structured groups (Hall, 2009).

Peer-Mediated Interactions

With regard to school placement, most professionals recommend that children with autism be in an inclusive setting in order to have good language and communication peer models throughout their school day. Some children may be so severely involved that placement in a regular education classroom may not be possible. In that event, it is still important that the child receive some regular interaction with typically developing children in order to have the aforementioned models. Typically developing children should be "in-serviced" in the characteristic behaviors of children with autism and how to interact with the child with autism.

SCORE

SCORE (Vernon, Schumaker, & Deschler, 1996) is a curriculum designed to teach social skills to higher-functioning adolescents on the autism spectrum. Through a series of steps such as having the skill introduced and modeled, practicing through role play, reviewing, and using the skills in natural settings (Prelock, 2006), the adolescents are taught five social skills:

1. Sharing ideas

2. Complimenting others

3. Offering help and encouragement

4.   Recommending changes nicely

5.   Exercising self-control

The training takes place over a 10-week period in group settings.

Floortime/Developmental Individual-Difference Relationship-Based Model (DIR)

DIR was developed at the George Washington University School of Medicine by Greenspan and Wieder (1997). Influenced by Piaget, DIR is an early intervention program that focuses on the development of relationships based on a developmental model. It has a curriculum to be implemented in the home in addition to the therapeutic setting. Prelock (2006) describes Floortime as an intervention model "designed to facilitate affect, attachment, and a sense of relatedness between a child with special needs and a caregiver or interaction partner" (p. 481). As described on their website, (http://soaringeagleacademy.org/DIRcurriculum.pdf,) Floortime provides instruction in the following six developmental milestones:

1.   Shared attention and regulation: the child's ability to take in sensory information and remain organized and attentive

2.   Engagement: the ability of the child to sustain mutual engagement with another individual while experiencing a broad range of emotions

3.   Affective reciprocity and gestural communication: the ability of the child to initiate and respond using circles of communication in a back-and-forth exchange that is driven by affect (intent)

4.   Complex presymbolic shared social communication and problem solving: the ability of the child to extend circles of communication by creating a continuous flow of circles; problem-solving abilities emerge at this level

5.   Symbolic and creative use of ideas, including pretend play and pragmatic language

6.   Logical and abstract use of ideas and thinking, including the capacity for expressing and reflecting on feelings and having insights into self and others

A complete description of elements of each milestone can be found in Table 3–3. There are four stages for mastery of social and cognitive growth: engagement (sharing attention with another person), two-way communication (intentional communication), shared meanings (relating behavior, sensations, and gestures to the world), and emotional thinking (organizing ideas or experiences and learning how to connect ideas). Caregivers are taught to follow their child's lead and to bring their child into a shared world (Buckendorf, 2008). The primary goal is "to enable the child to form a sense of himself or herself as an intentional, interactive individual" (Hall, 2009, p.117).

TABLE 3–3 The Developmental, Individual Difference Relationship Based Floortime (DIR/F) model: Six developmental milestones

1. **SHARED ATTENTION AND REGULATION:** the child's ability to take in sensory information and remain organized and attentive.
   - Use the child's individual sensory and motor profile to draw him or her into shared attention
   - Harness all the available senses, as well as motor capacities and affects (e.g. involve the child in interactions that involve vision, hearing, touch, and movement), coupled with highly enjoyable activities.
   - Use both constructive and playful obstructive strategies.
   - Stretch the child's capacity for shared attention by increasing interactive circles of communication rather than trying to get the child to focus on a particular object or toy.

2. **ENGAGEMENT:** the ability of the child to sustain mutual engagement with another individual while experiencing a broad range of emotions.
   - Follow the child's lead in order to engage in interactions that bring pleasure and joy.
   - Build on these pleasurable interactions.
   - Join in the child's rhythm in terms of affect, visual, auditory and motor movements.
   - Join with physical objects of the child's pleasure.
   - Attempt to deepen the warmth and pleasure by giving priority to his or comfort and closeness.
   - Use playful obstruction to entice him or her to focus on you.

3. **AFFECTIVE RECIPROCITY AND GESTURAL COMMUNICATION:** the ability of the child to initiate and respond using circles of communication in a back-and-forth exchange that is driven by affect (intent).
   - Be very animated and attempt to exchange subtle facial expressions, sounds, and other gestures.
   - Open and close circles of communication by building on natural interests.
   - Treat everything that the child does as purposeful and meaningful.
   - Encourage initiative by avoiding doing things for the child.
   - Support initiative by enticing the child to do things to you.
   - Over time build obstacles to increase the number of circles communicated in order for him or her to achieve a goal.

4. **COMPLEX PRESYMBOLIC SHARED SOCIAL COMMUNICATION AND PROBLEM SOLVING:** the ability of the child to extend circles of communication by creating a continuous flow of circles; Problem-solving abilities emerge at this level.
   - Create problem-solving opportunities for the child.
   - Lengthen chains of interaction to beyond 10 circles of communication in a row.
   - Support the beginning of symbolic play in the form of simple schemes and representational ideas.

5. SYMBOLIC AND CREATIVE USE OF IDEAS, INCLUDING PRETENT PLAY AND PRAGMATIC LANGUAGE

- Role play and puppet play.
- Use toys and dress up in pretend fashion; the toy or costume is elevated to the level of an "idea."
- Themes of aggression and power will emerge.
- Expand range of themes.

6. LOGICAL AND ABSTRACT USE OF IDEAS AND THINKING, INCLUDING THE CAPACITY FOR EXPRESSING AND REFLECTING ON FEELINGS AND HAVING INSIGHTS INTO SELF AND OTHERS.

- Ask why questions.
- Ask for opinions.
- Compare and contrast different points of view.
- Ask the child to predict or put him- or herself in someone else's position.
- Reflect on feelings and ideas.

Source: http://soaringeagleacademy.org/DIRcurriculum.pdf. Reprinted with permission.

SCERTS

Developed in 2005 by Prizant, Wetherby, Rubin, Laurent, and Rydell, SCERTS is a developmental approach to intervention that emphasizes the use of functional communication (nonverbal and verbal) in natural settings in activities that occur as part of daily routines. *SCERTS* is an acronym for the three main areas of attention: Social-Communication, Emotional Regulation, and Transactional Supports. It is a hybrid approach based on developmental theory, learning theory, and family systems theory. Following assessment of the child's social-communication and emotional regulation abilities, goals and objectives are set in one of three stages: social partners stage, language partner stage, and conversational partner stage. In the social partners stage, adults are quite active. Gestures and vocalizations are used within social exchanges. In the language partner stage, there is an increased range of intentions including requesting assistance, greeting others, showing off, taking turns, and commenting about actions or events. At the conversational partner stage, there is a focus on language abilities, social awareness of others, and increasing sensitivity to others' perspectives and emotional states (Buckendorf, 2008).

Wetherby, Rubin, Laurent, Prizant, & Rydell (2006) summarized the research that has assessed the evidence supporting the use of the SCERTS model in "A Matrix of Reference for the 4 Levels of Research Evidence and 3 Domains" found in Chapter 6 of their clinical manual.

Responsive Teaching

Responsive Teaching, developed by Mahoney and McDonald in 2005, is a developmental approach to intervention. It is designed to be done by caregivers or parents to maximize the potential of routine interactions. It has three domains: (1) cognition, (2) communication, and (3) social-emotional development. It "promotes development by encouraging children to use 'pivotal behaviors' such as initiation, social play, joint attention, problem solving, conversation, trust, and feelings of competence" (Hall, 2009, p. 120).

Relationship Development Intervention (RDI)

Developed by Gutstein, Sheely, and their associates, RDI is a social-relational approach that focuses on the quality of life. Other approaches start with what the child does well. RDI facilitates those aspects of the brain that do not work well. It has an aim of "spotlighting communication" through a variety of techniques. These techniques include pausing prior to communicating, whether through a gesture or words, altering the pace of the communication, exaggerating one's facial expressions, and leaning toward the child. The primary focus of RDI is on providing parents with an approach that enables them to establish a social-emotional relationship that resembles a master–apprentice relationship. It develops "mindfulness" by focusing on emotions, roles, ideas, perspectives, and levels of complexity. RDI is unique in that its focus is actually on quality of life of the child and his or her family.

The Hanen Approach

The Hanen approach was developed by Sussman in 1999 as a family-focused program (Hanen pamphlet "More Than Words"), and it has enjoyed a broad appeal among professionals working with families of children who are on the autism spectrum. The 11-week program is facilitated by a Hanen-certified speech-language pathologist. "More Than Words" is targeted toward teaching parents of children with ASD ways to help their child communicate. It teaches parents ways to set up opportunities to communicate, and then to help their child interact during these daily routines and activities. Parents or caregivers and the clinician co-treat, with the therapist often being in a coaching role as he or she guides the parents or caregivers in interacting with their child in a manner that encourages communication (see Figure 3–1). Clinicians videotape the parent and child together, and then the clinician and parent(s) critique the videotape and discuss how to implement the strategies of the Hanen approach. There are four goals of the Hanen program: (1) improved two-way interaction; (2) more mature and conventional ways of communicating; (3) better skills in communicating for social purposes, and (4) improved understanding

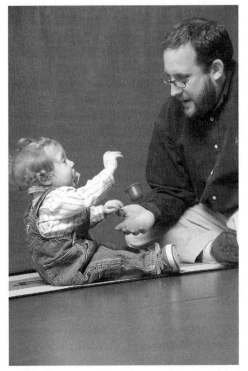

FIGURE 3–1 Social-pragmatic approaches to therapy emphasize the role of the caregivers or parents in stimulating language and communication development in their children. (*Delmar/Cengage Learning*)

of language (www.hanen.org). "More Than Words" emphasizes two sets of strategies: OWL and the 4 I's. OWL stands for Observing/Wait time/ Listening. While observing, the parent, caregiver, or clinician watches the child to determine objects or events that are of interest to the child. Wait time is important because it gives the child a chance to communicate his or her message in the way that best suits the child. Listening helps the parent, caregiver, or clinician understand what the child is trying to communicate and how he or she communicates. The four I's are designed to support the child's initiations:

- **Include:** Incorporate the child's interests into the communicative exchange. Comment on interests that were identified in the Observing activity.

- **Interpret:** Make the child's vocalizations and actions meaningful by interpreting communicative intent.

- **Imitate:** Imitate the child's vocalizations and actions to help maintain any communicative attempt and engage the child.

- **Intrude:** When the child is not participating with the communicator, or if the child begins to engage in repetitive behaviors, intrude in order to re-engage the child.

In summary, the Hanen approach "includes child-oriented strategies (e.g., observe the child, follow the child's lead, be face-to-face), interaction-promoting strategies (e.g., use routines, take a turn and pause for a response, cue the child to take a turn), and language-modeling strategies (e.g., interpret child's actions, label, expand)" (www.txautism.net).

RT, DIR/Floortime, Hanen, and SCERTS are similar in several ways:

1. The emphasis is on building communication and relatedness.

2. They are all social-pragmatic interventions.

3. The focus is on developing a relationship, not completing a task.

4. Motivation is the pleasure of the activity.

5. "Instead of looking at the child as someone to be 'taught', the focus is on respectful engagement and on building reciprocal interactions—a relationship" (Buckendorf, 2008, p. 81).

Overall, the research on treatment methods based on milieu models that are child-directed and provided in the child's natural environments is supportive (National Research Council, 2001; Aldred, Green, & Adams, 2004; Barry, Klinger, Lee, Palardy, Gilmore, & Bodin, 2003; Charman, Swettenham, Baron-Cohen, Cox, Baird, & Drew, 1997; Kaiser, Hancock, & Nietfeld, 2000; Wetherby, Prizant, & Hutchinson, 1998).

Picture Exchange Communication System (PECS)

Developed by Andy Bondy and Lori Frost (1998), PECS is based on the child's forming a sentence by unprompted selection of pictures or a series of pictures. In the early stages of PECS, the child gives a picture of an object to his or her communication partner in an effort to express his or her wants. The child progresses from single pictures to series of pictures in the form of sentence strips. PECS uses some of the same behavioral techniques found in ABA, using shaping, prompting (as minimal as possible), fading, and modeling to facilitate the child's learning. The PECS system has six phases:

- Phase I: Teaching the Physically Assisted Exchange

- Phase II: Expanding Spontaneity

- Phase III: Simultaneous Discrimination of Pictures

- Phase IV: Building Sentence Structure

- Phase V:Responding to "What do you want?"

- Phase VI: Commenting in Response to Questions

PECS differs from pointing to pictures because there is an exchange of the picture with a communication partner in a social context. Initially, the child is physically assisted in making the exchange of the picture of a highly preferred item. The child is then guided to increasing levels of independence and to requesting and responding to less preferred items. The PECS method is easily implemented, functional, and replicable. Although "teaching speech" is not considered by the developers to be a goal of PECS, Bondy and Frost found that children may begin to develop speech in the higher phases (IV–VI). Nonetheless, a criticism of PECS is that it does not teach a variety of communication functions.

Flippin, Reszka, and Watson (2010) reviewed the literature on PECS that was published between 1994 and June 2009. The purposes of the analysis were to

1. assess the quality of the research evidence on the PECS method

2. identify "pretreatment characteristics of children who responded to PECS training" (p. 178)

3. identify "program characteristics that may support the development of speech in children through the PECS program" (pp. 178–179).

Their two research questions centered around the effects PECS training would have on communication outcomes and speech of children with ASD. Communication outcomes examined in the literature on PECS were frequency of PECS exchanges, requests, and initiations. Flippin and colleagues concluded that single-subject studies and group studies demonstrated "increases in communication outcomes following PECS training" (p. 186). Although PECS seems to be "fairly effective" as a method for teaching communication to young children with ASD, there is little research on whether the improvements in communication during PECS training are maintained and generalized. The few studies that did evaluate maintenance and generalization yielded mixed reviews.

With regard to speech outcomes, Flippin, Reszka, and Watson (2010) were careful to point out that the developers of PECS do not claim that children with autism improve their speech as a result of PECS training; nonetheless, it is a frequent subject of research on PECS. The analysis of single-subject studies yielded the finding of "questionable effectiveness of the PECS approach for increasing speech for young children with autism" (p. 187). Only one study (out of five) looked at maintenance and generalization of a child's speech beyond the PECS training, and that child did demonstrate maintenance of the speech gains one year later, but there was limited generalization of speech. Analysis of group studies on speech outcomes also yielded variable results.

With regard to their hope to identify characteristics of children who would be responsive to PECS training, Flippin and colleagues concluded that the children who would be successful with PECS would have "a) limited joint attention, b) relatively stronger object exploration, and c) limited motor imitation" (p. 188).

Flippin, Reszka, and Watson (2010) had a third aim—to identify characteristics of the PECS program that support speech development. Much as Bondy and Frost claimed, Flippin and colleagues found Phase IV to be the apparent crucial phase with regard to speech. Some research has been done looking at variables (and combinations of variables), such as the provision of a verbal model and the introduction of a time delay. Early studies seem to have focused primarily on the effects of time delay. However, they made the point that much more research focusing on speech gains in children trained in the PECS model is needed.

As a result of their meta-analysis, Flippin, Reszka, and Watson (2010) concluded that although PECS is promising as an intervention method for developing communication in children with autism, evidence of the effectiveness of the intervention method has not been established in children aged 1–11 years with autism.

Are There Factors That May Affect Language Development Outcomes in Children Receiving Early Intervention?

The possible effects of cognition and social-affective skills on language behaviors of children with autism have been discussed elsewhere in this chapter. Bopp, Mirenda, and Zumbo (2009) studied problem behaviors to see if they might be predictive of language growth. They conducted their study because of the lack of heterogeneity in outcomes of early intervention, which led them to believe that perhaps there were variables affecting the outcome of early intervention that had not been identified. They questioned whether some of the behaviors existing pre-intervention might be predictive of children's response to early intervention. Specifically, they studied five behaviors:

1. Inattentiveness

2. Socially unresponsive behavior

3. Repetitive, stereotypic motor behaviors

4. Acting-out behavior

5. Insistence on sameness

They asked two questions regarding these behaviors:

1. Do scores in one or more type of child problem behavior at the onset of intervention predict changes in the developmental trajectories of vocabulary and language skills in young children with ASD over two years?

2. Do changes in scores related to one or more types of child problem behavior over a 6-month period predict changes in developmental trajectories of vocabulary and language skills in young children with ASD over two years? (p. 1109)

The 69 children in the study had a mean age of 4.2 years at the first testing. They were tested with the CARS to determine the severity of the autism, with several standard language tests, and with behavioral measures. The mean score on the CARS was 36.3. Of the 69 children, 55 were diagnosed as having autism, and the other 14 were identified as having PDD-NOS. They were tested at the beginning of intervention, 6 months after early intervention had been initiated, 12 months after early intervention began, and finally 24 months after the initiation of early intervention. Each child received 15–20 hours per week of (typically) one-on-one intervention for two years. The intervention was based on the principles of ABA. Thirty-nine of the children received intervention in one of three early intensive behavior intervention sites. The other 30 received intervention from behavior consultants and other professionals who were hired by the families. Occupational therapists, speech-language pathologists, and other professionals also provided intervention for some of the children. Some of the children (87%) also attended preschools.

Bopp and colleagues summed up their findings as follows:

1. High scores for inattentive behavior at the first testing (beginning of intervention) were predictive of "lower rates of change in vocabulary production and language comprehension" over the 2-year period of the study (p. 1106).

2. High scores for social unresponsiveness (i.e., not looking at faces of others, avoiding eye contact, not responding to their name, rarely smiling) at the first testing were predictive of "lower rates of change in vocabulary comprehension and production and in language comprehension" over the 2 years (p. 1106).

3. "Insistence on sameness" behaviors, repetitive stereotypic motor behaviors and acting-out behaviors documented at the initial testing were not significant predictors of future language development "after differences in NVIQ and CARS scores were considered" (p. 1116). The authors note that these findings were unexpected given the results of other studies, and perhaps their results were artifacts of how

they chose the variables in these areas and/or the range of behaviors in their study.

4. Changes in problem behaviors between the initiation of intervention and the testing at 6 months were not predictive of language and vocabulary outcomes after 2 years.

5. Autism severity scores prior to intervention were predictive only of language production over time; they were not predictive of the development of other language skills.

6. Nonverbal IQ prior to intervention was predictive of the development of expressive and receptive vocabulary and of the development of expressive language.

Bopp and colleagues stated that the implications of their findings on early intervention are that we need to provide "focused instruction on attending skills early in the treatment process" (p. 1115), which is consistent with the therapy models of ABA, PRT, and TEACCH. They also stated that training in early social behaviors (i.e., imitation, joint attention, turn taking) is critical for future language development. This type of training is consistent with the child-directed and family-centered therapies found in SCERTS, the Hanen approach, DIR, and Responsive Teaching.

Diet Management

Management of a child's food intake has received much attention in recent literature. Some of the diets that are being studied are the specific carbohydrate diet (SCD), the gluten and casein-free diet, and the Candida diet (removal of sugars that may exacerbate growth of Candida in the digestive tract) tied with the Feingold diet (elimination of foods with preservatives and salicylate) (Oller & Oller, 2010). There is much anecdotal evidence that some children with autism see an improvement in behaviors and defining characteristics when they are placed on one of these diets. All of them involve the removal of specified food items from the diets of the children. According to a survey of parents of children with autism by the Autism Research Institute, 69 percent of children on the specific carbohydrate diet, 66 percent of the children on the gluten/casein-free diet, 56 percent of children on the Candida diet, and 56 percent of the children on the Feingold diet showed improvement.

PROGNOSIS

Paul (2001) writes the following:

> A few of these individuals seem to "outgrow" their autism by mid-childhood, but most remain autistic or at least very odd as adults.

They may be able to live on their own; they can learn functional job skills, and some can graduate from college in fields such as mathematics of computer science. But even these very bright autistic individuals continue to have difficulty with human relationships, social judgment, and appropriate use of language. (p. 107–108)

Children who have developed functional speech by the time they are 6 years old typically have a better prognosis than those who do not. Furthermore, children who had regression of skills following period of normal development tend to have a poorer prognosis (Paul, 2001).

In a study that looked at the presence of behaviors associated with autism in adolescents and adults, Seltzer, Krauss, Shattuck, Orsmond, Swe, and Lord (2003) attempted to determine if behaviors seen at age 4–5 years persisted into adolescence and adulthood. Using the ADI-R, they interviewed parents to identify behaviors that were present at age 4–5 years, or any time during the developmental years ("lifetime" score), then documented the presence or absence of the behaviors in an adolescent cohort (age 10–21 years with a mean age of 15.71 years) and an adult cohort (age 22 years and older with a mean age of 31.57 years) ("current" score). Selzer and colleagues did extensive analyses of the results, summarized here.

Seltzer and colleagues studied behaviors associated with the communication domain, the reciprocal social interaction domain, and the restricted, repetitive behaviors and interests domain. In the communication domain, they studied the presence of nonverbal communication behaviors such as pointing to show interest, nodding "yes," and using conventional gestures by the adolescents and the adults. The adolescents were not as impaired in nonverbal communication skills than the adult cohort. Adolescents were also more able to participate in reciprocal conversations, but the adult cohort outperformed the adolescents with regard to verbal symptoms (particularly in the use of inappropriate language behaviors). Overall, both groups had a decrease in the use of repetitive, stereotypic, and/or idiosyncratic speech and improvements in nonverbal communication skills and use of language. Developing the ability to speak in phrases of at least three words is considered to be a significant gain, due partially to the abatement of some early symptoms. The least likely area to improve over time was "having friendships" (p. 565).

Findings on 13 items comprising the domain of reciprocal social interaction were that the adults were more impaired than the adolescents when compared to their lifetime scores. Both groups showed "improved ability to regulate social interactions, develop social relationships, share enjoyment with others, reciprocal socioemotionality, and sustain friendships" (p. 573). A significant number of the adolescents became asymptomatic in the areas of social overtones, offering comfort, seeking to share enjoyment, interest in people, range of facial expressions, offering to share, and having friendships. The adults were more impaired in all domains but use of other's body, using appropriate social response, and inappropriate facial expressions. Further study of the ability to develop and maintain friendships showed that adolescents age 16 and older were better able to sustain friendships than adolescents at age 10–15, and the adult cohort was worse in sustaining friendships at the earlier time and the current time.

Both groups showed a decrease in symptoms associated with restricted, repetitive behaviors and interests over time. The greatest improvement was reflected by the fact that 46 percent of the subjects were asymptomatic on "repetitive use of objects, 33.1 percent of the subjects who had used complex mannerisms in the early years were asymptomatic as adolescents and adults, and 23.8 percent demonstrated a decrease in displaying hand and finger mannerisms." However, fewer than 20 percent of the subjects who had a history of being symptomatic in "unusual preoccupation, unusual sensory interests, verbal rituals, compulsions/restricted and circumscribed interest" (p. 577) were no longer symptomatic.

Selzter and colleagues also studied whether symptoms identified as lifetime behaviors were still present in the adolescents and adults in their study. All of the individuals studied had communication impairment as children, but communication impairment was apparent in only 75 percent of the adolescents and adults. Specific findings were that:

1. 60.2 percent of the subjects who did not use three-word phrases when they were 4–5 years old could do so as adolescents and adults.

2. 45.5 percent who had reversal of pronouns as children were asymptomatic in the follow-up as adolescents and adults.

3. 38.8 percent of the population who had used neologisms and idiosyncratic language no longer exhibited these language behaviors.

4. 24.6 percent of the subjects who could not indicate "yes" with a head nod could do so as adolescents and adults.

5. 8.3 percent of the subjects who had used inappropriate questions no longer did so.

Further comparison of communication behaviors exhibited by the adolescent cohort and the adult cohort found that a significantly greater proportion of the adolescent cohort became asymptomatic in nodding the head "yes" and shaking the head "no" than did the adult cohort.

Selzter and colleagues concluded that, overall, the adolescents were less impaired than the adults on measures of reciprocal social interactions, and the adults were less impaired than the adolescents on measures of repetitive, restricted behavior and interests. The results were mixed regarding communication, as explained earlier. One hypothesis for future consideration in the research is whether there is an abatement of abnormal behaviors associated with autism (i.e., the use of abnormal verbal behaviors and the presence of restricted, repetitive behaviors and interests) between adolescence and adulthood. Also, further study is needed as to why the adolescents demonstrated less impairment in communication and social interaction than the adults. Selzer and colleagues hypothesized that three processes may have resulted in the outcome that the adolescents were less impaired than the adults in prosocial behaviors:

1. Developmental intensification of symptoms: The limited prospective studies that are available "indicate that adults with autism show gains in interpersonal behavior and communication" (p. 578) and it is reasonable to expect this improvement to continue into adulthood (as opposed to the poorer functioning of the adults in the study).

2. Improvement in educational, therapeutic, and social services available to younger cohorts.

3. Changes in the diagnostic process (i.e., the emergence of the autism spectrum results in the inclusion of individuals with autistic disorder who are higher-functioning that those historically identified as having autism).

All three of these factors show evidence of improved outcomes, and hence a better prognosis, for children, adolescents, and adults on the autism spectrum. Further research on the effectiveness of various treatment procedures, the validity of assorted diagnostic tools, and generalization and maintenance of learned skills over time is needed.

SUMMARY

The subject of autism has been introduced in this chapter, but it would take volumes to fully explore this enigmatic disorder that affects so many individuals and families. Questions about etiology still abound, and our ability to differentially diagnose autism and other developmental disorders is increasing. Oftentimes, autism and other PDDs are not diagnosed until a child is 2.5 to 3 years of age (Sigman & Capps, 1997). Because of this, there is very little research on children with autism under the age of 2.

There are many approaches to treatment, a few of which are summarized in this chapter. The reader is encouraged to read some of the books listed in Appendix E—biographies and memoirs written by families of children with autism and by adults who are diagnosed as being on the autism spectrum—to understand better the impact of autism and related disorders on individuals and their families.

CASE STUDY

Sammy is a 4-year old boy with autism. His main difficulties involve communication and social interaction. Sammy has minimal communication and uses behaviors to express himself. For example, when he does not like an activity or food he turns away or resists. Occasionally he communicates using some single words, the Picture Exchange Communication System (PECS), and some sign language. He occasionally leads people by pulling to indicate his wants or to initiate interaction. Sammy makes limited eye contact and has difficulty participating in play with fellow peers. Although he has the ability to engage in a variety of activities, Sammy prefers and perseverates on tasks involving letters and numbers. He also benefits greatly from daily, consistent routines paired with visual schedules.

Sammy is currently enrolled in a regular education pre-K class at Redwood Elementary School. He receives group speech and language therapy at school twice a week for 30 minutes, and two individual therapy sessions at a local private practice. These sessions last 45 minutes. Family history is significant for the fact that Sammy has an older brother who also has a diagnosis of autism.

Assessment

Based on Sammy's case history and parent interview, the *Peabody Picture Vocabulary Test—3rd Edition (PPVT-III)* (Dunn & Dunn, 1997) was administered. This test provides a measurement of receptive vocabulary for standard American English and screens verbal ability. No reading or writing is required, making it useful for individuals with autism who have communication difficulties. During the first administration attempt, Sammy did not respond or participate in the assessment. He did not look at the stimulus pictures, even after many prompts from the clinician. Based on his lack of response and general inability to participate, administration of the test ended and no reliable score was obtained.

The *Preschool Language Scale—4th Edition (PLS-4)* (Zimmerman, Steiner, & Pond, 2002) measures both receptive and expressive language skills. The test provides information about strengths and weaknesses in the areas of sensory discrimination, logical thinking, grammar, memory span, temporal/spatial relations, and self-image. Similar to the PPVT-III, Sammy was unable to participate and did not respond to the clinician. Administration of the assessment was terminated.

Since formal, standardized testing did not provide valuable information about Sammy's communication, a parent questionnaire was used as the main method of assessment. *The Functional Communication Assessment: Informant Interview* was selected and given to Sammy's parents to complete. This questionnaire obtains information about all aspects of communication, including nonverbal functions such as facial expressions and gestures. It also gives parents and caregivers an additional opportunity to express their personal goals for their child and desired therapy outcomes.

Results of the *Functional Communication Assessment: Informant Interview* are illustrated in the following chart:

Communicative Function	Sammy's Example
Expressing emotions	Facial expressions; behaviors; occasional verbal request
Requesting	Pulling; sign language; PECS; behaviors; brings object to adult's attention; facial expressions
Protesting	Behaviors
Responding	Inconsistent responding; difficulty with wh-questions; no yes/no responses
Acknowledging others	Pulling; facial expressions; behaviors; initiates play; occasional turn taking
Commenting	Occasionally comments on words, letters, and animals
Noncommunicative language	Occasional self-talk
Vocabulary	Diverse single word vocabulary

Treatment

Report Period Goals – Projected Outcome	Initial Status	Ending Status (4 months later)
1. Sammy will attend to same object/activity as communication partner 5 times within a 45 minute session when given verbal prompts for 6 consecutive sessions.	1. Joint attention skills emerging.	1. Met objective.
2. Sammy will use an overlay to follow the sequence of events of a book to identify core vocabulary words with 80% accuracy.	2. Used overlays to follow sequence of events during *Buddy Bear Opposites: Animals* with 69% accuracy.	2. Met objective.
3. Sammy will take turns with communication partner 5 times within a 45 minute session when given verbal prompts for 6 consecutive sessions.	3. Would not engage in turn taking.	3. Sammy took turns with communication partner 5 times within a 45 minute session when given verbal prompts for 3 consecutive sessions.
4. While participating in an interactive activity, Sammy will follow 1-step directions with 75% accuracy when prompted by the clinician.	4. Sammy would respond to verbal directions with multiple prompts 60% of the time.	4. Met objective.
5. Sammy will follow a 2–3 sequence visual schedule with 80% accuracy in 3 consecutive sessions with minimal prompting from the clinician.	5. Sammy followed a 3 sequence visual schedule with 67% accuracy with maximum prompting from the clinician.	5. Met objective.

(continues)

CASE STUDY (continued)

All objectives will be addressed in a playful, interactive setting. They will be integrated into functional activities such as cooking, shopping, and building.

Recommendations

Sammy demonstrated an improvement in joint attention skills and met the stated goal. Continued support and prompting should be used to maintain these skills. Sammy appropriately identified core vocabulary with an overlay in a story. However, as he continues to approach school age, it is important to continue to address vocabulary building. Turn-taking skills improved but the stated objective was not met. To continue the development of this emergent skill, continue to target this as a therapy objective. Sammy met the objective of following one-step directions. In the future, increasing to two- to three-step directions is recommended. Sammy met the objective for following a visual schedule. He benefits from daily, consistent routines paired with visual schedules. These should continue to be implemented in the future.

REVIEW QUESTIONS

1. According to the DSM-IV, children with autism must show regression in one of three areas of development. Which one of the following is not one of those three areas?

    a. Social interaction

    b. Language as used in social communication

    c. Motor skills

    d. Symbolic or imaginative play

2. Which approach focuses on the variety of ways in which children with autism process and organize information?

    a. Psychological-psychoanalytic perspective

    b. Psychological-cognitive approach

    c. Central language disorder category

3. Imitation by children with autism follows the same pattern as imitation by neurotypical children since symptoms of autism frequently do not emerge until age 2–3 years.

    a. True

    b. False

4. Like all children on the autism spectrum, children with Asperger syndrome show significant language delays.

a. True

b. False

5. Pragmatics is a primary focus in therapy for children with Asperger syndrome.

a. True

b. False

6. At what age do children with childhood disintegrative disorder typically begin to show loss of skills?

a. Age 1–3 years

b. Age 3–6 years

c. Age 2–5 years

d. Age 4–7 years

7. Which one of the following is not a social-pragmatic approach to intervention?

a. PECS

b. Floortime

c. SCERTS

d. Hanen

8. The Lovaas Method is associated with which one of the following therapy programs?

a. Picture Exchange Communication System

b. Floortime

c. Facilitated Communication

d. Applied Behavioral Analysis

e. SCORE

9. Loss of functional use of the hands and poor gross motor coordination are characteristic of which of the following?

a. Autism

b. Asperger syndrome

c. Childhood disintegrative disorder

d. Rett disorder

e. PDD-NOS

10. Autism is characterized by regression in language, social, and play skills around the age of 2–3 years.

a. True

b. False

REFERENCES

American Psychiatric Association. (1994). *Diagnostic and statistical manual of mental disorders* (4th ed.). Washington, D.C.: American Psychiatric Association.

Baron-Cohen, S. (2000). Is autism necessarily a disability? *Development and Psychopathology,* 12, 489–500.

Baron-Cohen, S., Allen, J., & Gillberg, C. (1992). Can autism be detected at 18 months? The needle, the haystack, and the CHAT. *British Journal of Psychiatry, 161,* 839–843.

Barry, T. D., Klinger, L. G., Lee, J. M., Palardy, N., Gilmore, T., & Bodin, S. D. (2003). Examining the effectiveness of an outpatient clinic social skills group for high-functioning children with autism. *Journal of Autism and Developmental Disorders, 33*(6), 685–701.

Batshaw, M. L. (ed.) (2002). *Children with disabilities* (5th ed.). Baltimore, MD: Paul H. Brookes Publishing Company.

Batshaw, M., Shapiro, B., & Farber, M. L. Z. (2007). Developmental delay and intellectual disability. In M. Batshaw, L. Pelligrino, and N. J. Roizen (eds.), *Children with disabilities* (6th ed.) (pp. 245–262). Baltimore, MD: Paul H. Brookes.

Bondy, A. S., & Frost, L. A. (1998). The picture exchange communication system. *Seminars in Speech and Language, 19*(4), 373–388.

Bopp, K. D., Mirenda, P., & Zumbo, B. D. (Oct., 2009). Behavior predictors of language development over two years in children with autism spectrum disorders. *Journal of Speech, Language, and Hearing Research,* 52(4), 1106–1120.

Bregman, J. D. (2005). Definitions and characteristics of the spectrum. In D. Zager (ed.). *Autism spectrum disorders: Identification, education, and treatment* (pp. 3–46). Mahwah, NJ: Lawrence Erlbaum.

Brock, S. E., & Slone, M. (n.d.). Autism spectrum disorders (Part 1): Case finding and screening. In-service at Irvine Unified School District.

Buckendorf, G. R. (2008). Child-directed social-pragmatic developmental approaches. In G. R. Buckendorf (ed.), *Autism: A guide for educators, clinicians, and parents* (pp. 79–96). Greenville, SC: Thinking Publications.

Charman, T., Swettenham, J., Baron-Cohen, S., Cox, A., Barid, G., & Drew, A. (1997). Infants with autism: An investigation of empathy, pretend play, joint attention, and imitation. *Developmental Psychology, 33*(5), 781–789.

Chin, H. Y., & Bernard-Optiz, V. (2000). Teaching conversational skills to children with autism: Effect on the development of a theory of mind. *Journal of Autism and Developmental Disorders, 30,* 569–583.

Churchill, D. (1978). *Language of autistic children.* New York: Wiley.

DeMyer, M., Barton, S., DeMeyer, E., Norton, J., Allen, J., & Steele, R. (1973). Prognosis in autism: A follow-up study. *Journal of Autism and Childhood Schizophrenia, 3,* pp. 199–216.

Dunn, L. M., & Dunn, L. M. (1997). *The Peabody Picture Vocabulary Test—III.* Circle Pines, MN: American Guidance Service.

Ehlers, S., Gillberg, C., & Wing, L. (1999). Autism spectrum screening questionnaire. *Journal of Autism and Developmental Disabilities,* 29, pp. 129–141.

FlippinL, M., Reszka, S., & Watson, L. R. (2010, May). Effectiveness of the Picture Exchange Communication System (PECS) on communication and speech for children with autism spectrum disorder: A meta-analysis. *American Journal of Speech-Language Pathology, 19*, pp. 178–195.

Gabovich, E. M., & Wiseman, N. D. (2005). Early identification of autism spectrum disorders. In D. Zager (ed.), *Autism spectrum disorders: Identification, education, and treatment* (pp. 145–172). Mahwah, NJ: Lawrence Erlbaum.

Garnett, M. S., & Attwood, A. J. (1998). Australian scale for Asperger's syndrome. In T. Attwood (Ed.), *Asperger's syndrome: A guide for parents and professionals* (pp. 17–19). Philadelphia, PA: Jessica Kingsley.

Gillberg, C. (1991). Clinical and neurobiological aspects of Asperger syndrome in six family studies. In J. Frith (ed.), *Autism and Asperger syndrome* (pp. 122–146). New York: Cambridge University Press.

Gilliam, R. (2001). *The Gilliam Asperger's disorder scale.* Austin, TX: Pro-Ed.

Gilliam, R. (2006). *The Gilliam autism rating scale 2.* Austin, TX: Pro-Ed.

Grandin, T. (1997). A personal perspective on autism. In D. Cohen and F. Volkmar (eds.). *Handbook of autism and pervasive developmental disorders* (2nd ed.) (pp. 1032–1042). New York: John Wiley & Sons.

Greenspan, S. I., DeGangi, G., & Wieder, S. (2001). *Functional Emotional Assessment Scale.* Interdisciplinary Council on Developmental and Learning Disorders. www.icdl.com

Greenspan, S. I., & Wieder, S. (1997). An integrated developmental approach to interventions for young children with severe difficulties in relating and communicating. *Zero to Three, 17,* 5–17.

Hadwin, J. A., Baron-Cohen, S., Howlin, P., & Hill, K. (1997). Does teaching Theory of Mind have an effect on the ability to develop communication in children with autism? *Journal of Autism and Developmental Disorders, 27,* 519–537.

Hall, L. J. (2009). *Autism spectrum disorders: From theory to practice.* Upper Saddle River, NJ: Pearson.

Hewitt, L. E. (1992, March). *Facilitating narrative comprehension: The importance of subjectivity.* Paper presented at the Conference on Pragmatics: From Theory to Therapy, State University of New York, Buffalo.

Howlin, P., Baron-Cohen, S., & Hadwin, J. (1999). *Teaching children with autism to mind-read: A practical guide.* New York: Wiley.

Hurford, J. (1991). The evolution of the critical period for language acquisition. *Cognition, 40,* 159–201.

Hyman, S. L., & Towbin, K. E. (2007). Autism spectrum disorders. In M. Batshaw, L. Pelligrino, and N. J. Roizen (eds.), *Children with disabilities* (6th ed.) (pp. 325–343). Baltimore, MD: Paul H. Brookes.

Jones, E. A., Carr, E. G., & Feely, M. K. (2006). Multiple effects of joint attention for children with autism. *Behavior Modification, 30,* 782–834.

Koegel, L. (1995). Communication and language intervention. In R. Koegel and L. Koegel (eds.), *Teaching children with autism* (pp. 17–32). Baltimore, MD: Paul H. Brookes.

Koegel, R. L., Koegel, L. K., Harrower, & Carter. (1999). Pivotal response intervention I: Overview of approach. *Journal of Association for Persons with Severe Handicaps, 24,* 174–185.

Koegel, L. K., Koegel, R. I., Shoshan, Y., & McNerney, E. (1999). Pivotal response intervention II: Preliminary long-term outcome data. *Journal of the Association for Persons with Severe Handicaps, 24,* 186–198.

Koppenhaver, D., & Erickson, K. (2003). Natural emergent literacy supports for preschoolers with autism and severe communication impairments. *Topics in Language Disorders, 23*(4), 283–292.

Krug, D. A., Arick J. R., & Almond, P. J. (2008). *Assessments for educational planning and intervention.* Austin, TX: Pro-Ed.

Lanter, E., & Watson, L. R. (2008). Promoting literacy in students with ASD: The basics for the speech-language pathologist. *Language, Speech, and Hearing Services in the Schools, 39,* 33–43.

Leekham, S. R., Libby, S. J., Wing, L., Gould, J., & Taylor, C. (2002). Diagnostic interview for social and communication disorders. *Journal of Child Psychology and Psychiatry, 43*(3), pp. 327–342.

Lord, C., & Paul, R. (1997). Language and communication in autism. In D. Cohen and F. Volkmar (eds.), *Handbook of autism and pervasive developmental disorders* (2nd ed.) (pp. 195–225). New York: John Wiley & Sons.

Lord, C., Rutter, M., DiLavore, P. C., & Risi, S. (2000). *Autism diagnostic observation schedule.* Los Angeles, CA: Western Psychological Services.

Lord, C., Rutter, M., & LeCouteur, A. (1994). Autism Diagnostic Interview – Revised. A revised version of a diagnostic interview for caregivers of individuals with possible pervasive developmental disorders. *Journal of Autism and Developmental Disorders, 24*(5), 659–685.

Mesibov, Schopler, Schaffer, & Landrus, (1988) *Adolescent and adult psychoeducational profile (AAPEP).* Austin, TX: Pro-Ed.

Miller, J. N., & Ozonoff, S. (2000). The external validity of Asperger disorder: Lack of evidence from the domain of neuropsychology. *Journal of Abnormal Psychology, 109,* pp. 227–238.

Minchew, N. J., Sweeney, J. A., Bauman, M. L., & Webb, S. J. (2005). Neurological aspects of autism. In F. Volkmar, R. Paul, A. Klin, and D. Cohen (eds.), *Handbook of autism and pervasive developmental disorders* (pp. 473–514). New York: John Wiley & Sons.

Mirenda, P. (2003). "He's not really a reader. . .": Perspectives on supporting literacy development in individuals with autism. *Topics in Language Disorders, 23*(4), 271–282.

Monteiro, M. J. (2005). *Monteiro interview guidelines for diagnosing Asperger syndrome.* Los Angeles, CA: Western Psychological Services.

Myles, B. S., Jones-Bock. S., & Simpson, R. L. (2000). *Asperger syndrome diagnostic scale.* Austin, TX: Pro-Ed.

National Research Council (2001). *Educating children with autism.* Committee on Educational Intervention for Children with Autism, Division of Behavioral and Social Sciences and Education. Washington, DC.: National Academy Press.

Nelson, N. W. (1998). *Childhood language disorders in context: Infancy through adolescence* (2nd ed.). Boston, MA: Allyn & Bacon.

Oller, J. W., & Oller, S. D. (2010). *Autism: The diagnosis, treatment, and etiology of the undeniable epidemic.* Sudbury, MA: Jones and Bartlett.

Owens, R. E. (1995). *Language disorders: A functional approach to assessment and intervention* (2nd ed.). Needham Heights, MA: Allyn & Bacon.

Ozonoff, S., & Miller, J. N. (1995). Teaching theory of mind: A new approach to social skills training for individuals with autism. *Journal of Autism and Developmental Disorders, 25*, 415–433.

Ozonoff, S., Pennington, B. F., & Rogers, S. J. (1991). Executive function deficits in high-functioning autistic individuals: Relationship to theory of mind. *Journal of Child Psychology and Psychiatry, 32*(7), 1081–1105.

Partington, J. W., & Sundberg, M. L. (1998). *Assessment of basic language and learning skills.* Los Angeles, CA: Western Psychological Services.

Paul, R. (1987). *Language disorders from infancy through adolescence: Assessment and intervention.* St. Louis, MO: Mosby.

Paul, R. (2001). *Language disorders from infancy through adolescence: Assessment and intervention* (2nd ed.). St. Louis, MO: Mosby.

Paul, R. (2005). *Language disorders from infancy through adolescence: Assessment and intervention* (3rd ed.). St. Louis, MO: Mosby.

Perry, A., Dunlap, G., & Black, A. (2007). Autism and related disorders. In I. Brown and M. Percy (eds.), *A comprehensive guide to intellectual and developmental disabilities* (pp. 189–203). Baltimore, MD: Paul H. Brookes Publishing Company.

Prelock, P. A. (2006). *Autism spectrum disorders: Issues in assessment and intervention.* Austin, TX: Pro-Ed.

Prelock, P., & Contompasis, S. H. (2006). Autism and related disorders: Trends in diagnosis and neurobiologic considerations. In P. Prelock (ed.), *Autism spectrum disorders: Issues in assessment and intervention.* Austin, TX: Pro-Ed.

Robins, D., Fein, D., & Barton, M. (1999). The modified checklist for autism in toddlers (M-CHAT). Storrs, CT: Self-published.

Schopler, E., Lansing, M. D., Reichler, R. J., & Marcus, L. M. (2005). *The psychoeducational profile -3.* Los Angeles, CA: Western Psychological Services.

Schopler, E., & Mesibov, G. B. (eds.). (1986). *Communication problems in autism.* New York: Plenum Press.

Schopler, E., Van Bourgondien, M. E., Wellman, G. J., & Love, S. R. (2010). *Childhood autism rating scale—2.* Austin, TX: Pro-Ed.

Scott, F., Baron-Cohen, S., Bolton, P., & Brayne, C. (2002). Childhood Asperger's syndrome test. *Autism, 6*(1), pp. 9–31.

Seltzer, M. M., Krause, M. W., Shattuck, P. T., Orsmond, G., Swe, A., & Lord, C. (2003, Decemeber). The symptom of autism spectrum disorder in adolescence and adulthood. *Journal of Autism and Developmental Disorders, 33*(6), 65–581.

Sicile-Kira, C. (2004). *Autism spectrum disorders.* New York: Perigee.

Siegel, B. (2004). *Pervasive developmental disorders screening test.* San Antonio, TX: Psychological Corporation.

Sigman, M., & Capps, L. (1997). *Children with autism: A developmental perspective.* Cambridge, MA: Harvard University Press.

Spek, A. A., Scholte, E. M., & Van-Berckelaer-Onnes, I. A. (2010). Theory of mind in adults with HFA and Asperger syndrome. *Journal of Autism and Developmental Disorders, 40*, 280–289.

Swettenham, J. S. (1996). Can children with autism be taught to understand false belief using computers? *Journal of Child Psychology and Psychiatry, 37*, 157–166.

Tiegerman-Farber, E. (1997). Autism: Learning to communicate. In D. K. Bernstein and E. Tiegerman-Farber (eds.), *Language and communication disorders in children* (pp. 524–569). Boston, MA: Allyn & Bacon.

Towbin, K. E., Mauk, J. E., & Batshaw, M. L. (2002). Pervasive developmental disorders. In M. L. Batshaw (ed.), *Children with disabilities* (5th ed.). Baltimore, MD: Paul H. Brookes.

Trace, R. (1996, January 8). Research links infantile autism, manic depression. *Advance for Speech-Language Pathologists and Audiologists*, pp. 3, 14.

Vernon, D. S., Schumaker, J. B., & Deshler, D. D. (1996). *The SCORE skills: Social skills for cooperative groups*. Lawrence, KS: Edge Enterprises.

Volkmar, F., Carter, A., Grossman, J., & Klin, A. (1997). Social development in autism. In D. Cohen and F. Volkmar (eds.), *Handbook of autism and pervasive developmental disorders* (pp. 173–194). New York: John Wiley & Sons.

Watson, L.R., & Ozonoff, S. (2001). In T. Layton, E. Crais, & L. Watson (Eds.), *Handbook of early language impairment in children: Nature* (pp. 177–257). Albany, NY: Delmar.

Wetherby, A. M., Prizant, B. M., & Hutchinson, T. A. (1998, May). Communicative, social/affective, and symbolic profiles of young children with autism and pervasive developmental disorders. *American Journal of Speech-Language Pathology, 7*(2), 79–91.

Wetherby, A. M., Rubin, E., Laurent, A. C., Prizant, B. M., & Rydell, P. J. (2006). Summary of research supporting the SCERTS model. Chapter 6 in *Clinical Manual of the SCERTS program*. Baltimore, MD: Paul H. Brookes.

Zager, D., & Shamow, N. (2005). Teaching students with autism spectrum disorders. In D. Zager (ed.), *Autism spectrum disorders: Identification, education, and treatment* (pp. 295–326). Mahwah, NJ: Lawrence Ehrlbaum.

Zimmerman, I. L., Steiner, V. G., & Pond, R. E. (2002). *The preschool language scale—4* (PLS-4). San Antonio, TX: The Psychological Corporation.

www.autismspeaks.org/treatment/prt.php, retrieved May 26, 2010.

www.txautism.net, retrieved March 10, 2010.

www.uscfc.uscourts.gov/vaccine-programoffice-special-master, retrieved September 15, 2010.

Chapter 4

Setting the Stage in the Preschool Years for Linguistic and Literacy Success

LEARNING OBJECTIVES

After completion of this chapter, the reader will be able to:

1. Discuss the role socio-economic status plays in the development of language and literacy.

2. Describe the growth of language in preschoolers.

3. List and discuss common signs of language disorders exhibited by preschoolers.

4. Discuss the role of oral language in the acquisition of literacy.

5. Compare and contrast written and spoken language.

6. Discuss the development of discourse.

7. Discuss the development of narratives.

INTRODUCTION

The preschool years are fun years that are rich with opportunities to stimulate language and literacy development. Good oral language skills and phonemic awareness are considered to be strong foundational skills that predict success in school. Along the same lines, children who have speech and language deficits in the preschool years are frequently proven to have language learning disabilities when they reach school age. This chapter focuses on how to facilitate language and literacy in preschool-age children.

ASHA has stated the roles and responsibilities for speech-language pathologists with regard to reading and writing in children and adolescents. They include the following:

1. *Prevention.* This role addresses the goal of preventing written language problems by fostering language acquisition and emergent literacy.

2. *Identification.* This role addresses the goal of identifying children and adolescents with (or at risk for) reading and writing problems so that they may receive appropriate attention.

3. *Assessment.* This role addresses the goal of assessing reading and writing abilities and relating them to spoken communication, academic achievement, and other areas.

4. *Intervention.* This role addresses the goal of providing effective intervention for problems involving reading and writing and documenting the outcomes.

5. *Other roles.* Other roles include providing assistance to general education teachers, families, and students; advocating for effective literacy practices; and advancing the knowledge base. (www.asha.org/policy).

In this chapter, we discuss the speech-language pathologist's role in prevention and identification with regard to emergent literacy and preparation of young children for their school-age years. The reader is encouraged to read the guidelines developed by ASHA that describe our role in oral and written language in order to become familiar with the knowledge and skills ASHA sees as critical to functioning in these roles (see ASHA, 2001). Speech-language pathologists and audiologists have extensive knowledge of the development of receptive and expressive language, processing skills, communication, interaction abilities, reading, writing, and a host of other skills and abilities critical to academic, social, and vocational success, which enables us to identify children who are delayed or disordered in these area and therefore are at risk for poor performance in academic and social environments.

THE EMERGENCE OF LANGUAGE

Toddlers and preschoolers see a rapid growth of language and communication skills during the developmental years. The developmental achievements related to early language can be affected by numerous variables including neurophysiological factors, emotional and environmental factors, early language sequences, synergistic demands, and developmental domains. Billeaud (1998) summarizes these factors as shown in Table 4–1.

Risk Factors Affecting Language Growth in the Preschool Years

There are several risk factors that may be seen in this age group that can predict difficulty with language and literacy and, potentially, school success. One risk factor is low socio-economic status (SES, which is based on a ratio of the number of individuals in a household and the income of the household). Many children in homes of poverty are not exposed to as many words in discourse, books, or opportunities to "play" with language. Research by Hart and Risley (1995) shows that children from low-income homes are exposed to fewer words per day than those in working-class and professional homes. Their study yielded the following facts:

- At age 3, children of low-SES (welfare) parents produce 500 words.

- At age 3, children of working-class parents produce 700 words.

- At age 3, children of professional parents produce 1100 words.

TABLE 4–1 Elements affecting early language development*

Neurophysiologic Factors	Early Language Sequences	Synergistic Demands	Developmental Domains
Regulatory capacity	Perception of stimuli	Sensory integration	Sensory integration
Sensory integrity	Memory for experiences	Phonation dynamics	Physical growth
Brain structure integrity	Presymbolic (R) (e.g., sound discrimination)	Resonation dynamics	Gross and fine motor control
Myelination process	Presymbolic (E) (e.g., babbling, vocal play)	Articulation dynamics	Emotional adjustment
Cortical integrity	Symbolic, nonverbal (E, R)	Gross and fine motor control	Cognitive skills
Physical health		Cognitive processing	Social skills
Emotional and Environmental Factors	Communication skills	Executive function (e.g., intonation, stress)	Communication skills
Attachment and emotional security	Symbolic, first word and holophrasis (E)	Integration of social and cultural conventions	
Experimental exposure	Symbolic complexity (E, R) (e.g., semantics, syntax, and morphology)		
Need and motivation to communicate			
Opportunity to communicate			
Impact of effort to communicate (i.e., choices, rewards, and power to affect others or the environment)			

E = expressive modality; R = receptive modality.

*Language development, both typical and atypical, occurs in conjunction with simultaneous maturation and development across many parameters. Anything that disturbs development in one area has the potential to affect development in other areas (transactional theory of development).

Source: Communication disorders in infants and toddlers: Assessment and intervention (2nd ed.), by F. P. Billeaud,. Copyright Elsevier (1998). Boston, MA: Butterworth-Heinemann.

- Children of professionals hear a ratio of six encouraging (affirmative) statements to one discouraging (prohibitive) statement per hour. Children of working-class parents hear a ratio of two encouraging statements to one discouraging statement per hour, and children of welfare parents hear a ratio of one encouraging to two discouraging statements per hour. This means that, by age 4 years, children of professionals hear 560,000 more instances of encouraging statements than discouraging; working-class parents say 100,000 more encouraging statements than discouraging; and welfare children hear 125,000 more discouraging statements than encouraging statements.

Various factors lead to the decrease in the quantity and quality of language activities provided to children in low-SES situations. Self-esteem and feelings of self-worth are lower in parents who feel unsuccessful and/or unable to provide for their families, and children of welfare-status parents are more likely to exhibit these same feelings than are children of working-class and professional parents (Polakow, 1993).

Sometimes, life circumstances affect the amount of exposure to language children receive at home. For example, the child's parent(s) may be working two jobs and have little time to interact with their child. Nonetheless, hour-by-hour measurements show that in an hour of interaction, children from low SES homes are exposed to fewer words (Hart & Risley, 1995).

A study done by LaPoro, Justice, Skibbe, and Pianta (2004) studied maternal characteristics (sensitivity and depression), child characteristics (health history and behavior), and demographic factors (SES and maternal education) present when the children were age 3 years. Based on review of previous research, LaPoro and colleagues believed that those characteristics and factors might be relevant to the persistence of specific language impairments (SLI) in young children. With regard to maternal characteristics, the presence of maternal depression and low or absent maternal sensitivity were associated with the persistence of SLI. Children in the resolved group (those who were identified at age 3 years as having had speech-language pathology services but scored within normal ranges at age 5.5 years) had mothers who demonstrated sensitivity toward their children and had less depression than the mothers of the children in the persistent group. The role of demographic factors highlights the findings of Hart and Risley (1995) presented above. LaPoro and colleagues noted that 61.5 percent of the children in the group of children whose language impairments persisted at age 54 months were from low-SES families, compared to 15.5 percent of the Caucasian children. They cited a database developed by the National Institute of Child Health and Human Development (NIHCD, 1999) that documented a higher incidence of maternal depression and less maternal sensitivity among the mothers who were from low-SES environments. Thus, LaPoro and colleagues expressed that their findings and those in the NIHCD database suggest that there is an important "interaction among three environmental factors—namely, SES, maternal sensitivity, and maternal depression—and the persistence of language difficulties in young children of language impairments" (p. 298). They go on to say that further exploration is needed of the roles of "poverty, maternal health, and developmental stability of language impairments" (p. 300).

Late Talking as a Risk Factor

Another risk factor is being a late talker. Children who are not combining words by 3 years of age or who have limited vocabularies are more prone to language disorders than neurotypical children. McLaughlin (2006) summarized the growth of language in toddlers as follows:

1. Toddlers produce their first true word—that is, an approximation that is recognizable as an attempt at an adult word and is used consistently and meaningfully.

2. Toddlers combine words with gestures to accomplish an increasing variety of goals—requesting objects and actions, labeling objects and actions, imitating, and so forth.

3. Topics expand as toddlers' experiences and vocabularies grow, but dialogue is limited to a few brief turns during each "conversation" with caregivers.

4. Toddlers' growing vocabularies are composed of words that signal basic semantic categories and relationships that encode objects, persons, events, and their locations.

5. Toddlers begin to produce utterances that are initially trial-and-error attempts at combining words and gradually become reliable word orders that represent syntax.

6. Toddlers increasingly use the language they have learned to obtain more information about the world from those around them.

7. Toddlers become increasingly aware of the connection between various symbols they are consistently exposed to—signs, logos, and familiar words—and the way caregivers read them (p. 221).

These developmental factors represent growth in primarily semantics, syntax, and pragmatics. Any child who does not master these skills should be considered at risk for language deficits. Pence and Justice (2008) listed the common signs of language disorders in preschoolers. These signs are found in Table 4–2.

Paul (1996) conducted a small longitudinal study in which she followed 31 children with slow expressive language development (SELD). She first saw the children when they were between 20 and 34 months of age and followed them through first grade. SELD was defined as a "small (usually less than 50 words) expressive vocabulary size during the second year of life" (Paul, 1996, p. 6). In toddlers, one of the first aspects of language to resolve is the size of his or her expressive vocabulary, and all of the children in Paul's study who were determined to have SELD at age 2 had normal expressive vocabularies by age 3 years. However, there was some persistence of phonological deficits. Thirty-five percent of the children with SELD at age 2 scored below average on articulation tests at age 4 years and at the low end of the normal range at age 5 years. Syntactic production problems also persisted, but these, too, steadily progressed to normal throughout the preschool years.

TABLE 4–2   Common signs of language disorders: Preschool

- Omission of grammatical inflections, including present progressive (-*ing*), plural (-*s*), possessive ('*s*), past tense regular and irregular verbs, and auxiliary verbs
- Slow development of and errors with pronouns
- Shorter sentence length
- Problems forming questions with inverted auxiliaries
- Immature requests resembling those of younger children
- Difficulty with group conversations (conversing with more than one child)
- Difficulty with oral resolution of conflicts
- Longer reliance on gesture for getting needs met
- Difficulty initiating with peers
- Difficulty sustaining turns in conversation
- Difficulty comprehending complex directions and narratives

Source: From *Language development from theory to practice*, by K. L. Pence and L. M. Justice. p. 326. Copyright 2008 by Pearson Education, Inc.

Children with syntactic and articulatory deficits at age 3 typically had one or the other, but not both, at age 4.

Paul (1996) presented outcomes of the 31 middle-class children in kindergarten and first grade. Both years they were assessed in the areas of school readiness, oral language abilities, cognitive functioning, reading achievement, and articulation (using a 10-minute speech sample). A narrative sample was also collected using a wordless picture book, *A Boy, A Dog, and a Frog* (Mayer, 1967) in kindergarten and the standardized *Bus Story Language Test* (Renfrew, 1991) in first grade. Developmental sentence scores (DSS) (Lee, 1974) were assigned to each speech sample based on the first 50 unique noun-verb utterances. The percentage of consonants correct score was calculated using the middle 100 words of the speech sample, and the narratives were assigned to one of five stages of development (heaps, sequences, primitive narratives, chains, or true narratives) and were assigned an information score based on Renfrew's instructions on the *Bus Story Language Test*.

The children were divided into two groups based on test results: the Hx group, who were children with a history of SELD but who were functioning within normal range (at or above the 10th percentile for age) in terms of the DSS score, and the ELD group (for "chronic expressive language delay"). The ELD group consisted of the students with a history of slow language development who were still showing DSS scores below normal (below the 10th percentile for age in kindergarten or first grade). There was also a control group (NL) consisting of age-, gender-, and SES-matched children who scored above the 10th percentile on the DSS. The results for children in kindergarten are summarized as follows:

- 74 percent of the children with a history of SELD scored within normal range on the DSS.

- There were no differences in nonverbal cognitive scores as toddlers or kindergartners.

- The NL and HX groups scored significantly higher on the verbal portions of the McCarthy, TOLD-P, and Developmental Skills Checklist; the ELD group continued to have verbal deficits by comparison, but were still within normal range (but on the low end).

- The speech of all three groups was determined to be intelligible, but the ELD group received more "fair" ratings than the NL and Hx groups.

- The ELD and Hx groups ranked significantly lower than the NL group on narrative scores. The narrative maturity ratings of the ELD and Hx groups were in the third stage (primitive narrative) and the ratings for the NL group were the fourth stage (chain).

- The NL and Hx groups scored significantly higher than the ELD group on narrative information scores.

In first grade, the students presented the following profile:

- DSS scores that were deficient in kindergarten continued to be deficient in first grade.

- On the TOLD-P, the NL group scored significantly higher than the Hx group, and the Hx group scored significantly higher than the ELD group (who were at the low end of the normal range).

- There were statistically significant differences in intelligibility in free speech, but not clinically significant with regard to articulatory ability.

- There were no significant differences between the three groups in percent correct consonants scores.

- There were "no statistically significant differences in the proportions of subjects in each of the three groups with high enough decoding skills to allow a measure of reading comprehension to be computed" (p. 11). (The reading comprehension test could only be administered to those subjects who achieved a raw score of 18 on reading recognition.).

- The narrative stage in kindergarten persisted in first grade.

- There was no significant difference between the three groups on narrative information scores.

Paul compared her results to those of Whitehurst and Fischel (1994) and agreed with them that "SELD in toddlers is a risk factor rather than a *bona fide* disorder, since the majority of the affected children will go on to have language skills broadly within the normal range by school age" (Paul, 1996, p. 12). Paul summed up the work of Rescorla (1993), who also studied SELD and found that children with a history of SELD had poorer performance than their peers on "measures of verbal short-term memory, auditory processing of complex verbal material, word retrieval, and elaborated verbal expression" (Paul, p. 12). In her own subjects, Paul found that some weaknesses in oral language persisted in the ELD and Hx groups, specifically less mature narrative macrostructures and less semantically complex narratives. Paul's results also compare favorably with the results obtained by Rescorla (2002), who looked at the effects of late talking up to age 9 years. All of the late talkers in Rescorla's (2002) study had normal nonverbal ability and age-adequate language at age 5 years. At age 6–7 years there was no difference in reading skills exhibited by the late talkers compared to the controls, but at age 8–9, the late talkers were slightly behind the control group on reading. Rescorla (2002) made two important conclusions, both of which are supported by the Paul (1996) and Whitehurst and Fischel (1994) studies:

1. "Slow early language development reflects a predisposition for slower acquisition and lower asymptomatic performance in a wide range of language-related skills into middle childhood" (p. 360).

2. "Vocabulary skills at ages 2–3 years may be a better index of underlying language endowment for late talkers than are grammatical skills measured in the preschool period" (p. 370).

I have dedicated this much space to Paul's 1996 study because her results, discussions, and conclusions raise important questions with regard to how we handle children who are slow talkers. During Paul's study, each time the parents brought the child in for testing, they were provided with language stimulation and literacy facilitation activities. If their child scored below the normal range on any tests of speech or expressive language, parents were offered a referral to one of three intervention programs or services. Of the 31 children in the study, 34 percent received some type of intervention during the preschool years; 39 percent of the children were still below normal range on subsequent testing, and 29 percent were in the normal range. There were no significant differences in DSS scores between those who did get therapy and those who did not.

Any time one deals with children demonstrating delays, there is concern about the long-term impact. The evidence on SELD shows that many of the language and speech problems resolve by the time they reach school age. There is no support that suggests long-term significant academic problems for children with SELD. Indications are that they are not likely to be academic superstars, but they do not appear to have significant academic disabilities, either. However, facilitative therapy may help lessen or avoid potential problems or help children move from the low end of the normal range to the middle of the normal range. The second grade children Whitehurst and Fischel studied were not considered to be "at any increased risk for reading disability, although reading was an area of underachievement" (Paul, 1996, p. 12). Taking into account public policy, education law, ethics, and evidence-based knowledge about SELD, Paul recommended "careful and consistent monitoring" with re-evaluations on a regular basis. Paul stated that she felt safe in taking a "watch and see" stance because there is over a 70 percent chance that the oral language problems resolve without intervention by school age. Paul recommended recommending 2–3 year old children every 3–6 months and 3–5 year old children every 6–12 months. However, Paul cautioned that this stance only applies if expressive language is the *only* concern, the child is progressing with regard to "sentence length and complexity, intelligibility, and conversational skill," and the child's speech at age 3 is intelligible to family, friends, and peers.

Even children who do not get a complete resolution of symptoms still meet the curricular demands of the early school years. Therefore, Whitehurst and Fischel (1994) recommended that children with SELD not receive intervention until kindergarten, and then only if delays persist. However, they and others have stated that if there are other risk factors present, such as poverty, a dysfunctional home, disadvantaged backgrounds, or co-morbidity with other delays or disorders, intervention is warranted.

One reason to provide early intervention is to reduce any frustration that may exist (the child's and/or the parent's) (Vinson, 2007). Therapy could also increase the child's awareness of language elements that could impact the acquisition of "higher-level language skills associated with literacy" (Paul, 1996, p. 11). Based on the data of Paul and the others, if a child with SELD does receive intervention, it is recommended that therapy focus on the development of narrative skills, phonological awareness, and phonological processing because these skills are so critical to reading and thus to academic performance.

As a follow-up to Paul's own study, Paul, Murray, Clancy, and Andrews (1997) studied the progress of this cohort of children when they were in second grade. In this study, the subgroups were:

- HELD: originally classified as SELD and with DSS scores at or above 8.11 (10th percentile for children aged 6:6) ($n = 27$; 84% of original 31)

- ELD: same criteria as 1996 study ($n = 5$; 16% of original 31)

- NL: DSS above 8.11 in second grade; never SELD

In kindergarten, 26 percent of the children in the HELD cohort were assigned to subgroup ELD based on having a history of SELD and achieving a raw score below 8 on the DSS. In second grade, only 16 percent of the original cohort was still in the ELD cohort. Even so, Paul and colleagues wrote that the "children with persistent ELD and lower generalized performance intelligence still operate within the normal range of school achievement at the primary level" (p. 1043). On retesting, there were no significant differences between the cohorts on measures of reading recognition, reading comprehension, or spelling achievement, all of which are preliteracy skills. There were significant differences between the NL and ELD cohort on the TOLD speaking quotient (a composite of scores on expressive syntax, semantics, and phonology), mathematics, the Lindamood Auditory Conceptualization test (LAC), and general information, but all the children in the ELD group were still within the normal range. The LAC scores were the only ones that were predictive of word identification performance and reading comprehension in the later school years.

As Paul and colleagues expressed, the bottom line is that the second graders with a history of SELD achieved scores "within the normal range on standardized measures of language and school achievement" (p. 1043). None of the children with SELD were able to meet the definition of learning disabled because there were "no significant discrepancies among verbal, nonverbal, and achievement performances' (p. 1043), and the performance of the ELD group was in keeping with the fact that they had lower general cognitive levels (but, again, at the lower end of the normal range). Paul did, however, hypothesize that these children may face academic difficulties as the curriculum progressed. This hypothesis was informally supported by the findings on follow-up phone interviews with the parents of children in the ELD cohort when the children were in fourth grade (Abild-Lane, 1996). Four of the five "had received some special services in school, and three of the five were currently eligible for special education or speech/language services" (p. 1043).

> **think about it**
> How can an enriching environment be established that facilitates a child's exposure to higher quantity and quality vocabulary on a daily basis?

THE EFFECTS OF SPECIFIC LANGUAGE IMPAIRMENT ON SUCCESS IN SCHOOL

Specific language impairment (SLI) is discussed extensively in Chapter 9 but merits mention here in regard to the resolution or persistence of SLI prior to kindergarten. Bishop and Edmundson (1987) conducted an historic study in which they hoped to identify the variables involved in the persistence of SLI in children as well as characteristics of language behaviors in children who had resolved SLI between ages 4 years to 5.6 years. They tested vocabulary, grammar, and discourse skills in 87 children at ages 4 years, 4.6 years, and 5.6 years. A "good outcome" was defined as a child having no score in the impaired range and no more than one score below the satisfactory range (p. 161). For example, children whose only deficit was a phonological impairment were more likely to have a good outcome at age 5.6 years (78% had a good outcome) than a child with language problems across multiple domains. Fifty-six percent of the children whose impairments were restricted to phonology, syntax, and morphology also experienced a good outcome. Only 14 percent of the children who had receptive and expressive disorders with impairment in all four areas of language (phonology, morphology, semantics, and syntax) had a good outcome, and 13 percent of the children who had all disorders in all expressive functions had a good outcome. There was a 33 percent good outcome for all other patterns of impairment encountered in the 87 subjects. The determining factors as to whether a language impairment persisted or resolved were found to be the type of impairment and the severity of the impairment.

Bishop and Edmundson (1987) found that phonological competence at age 4 years did not relate to outcome. A probable explanation for this is that if the child uses phonological processes that are typically seen but are persistent for longer than usual, he or she can be expected to have a better outcome than a child who uses atypical processes, which is a more severe phonological impairment. They also found that the ability to retell a simple story with pictures was the best predictor of a child's resolving his or her language impairment by the time school enrollment occurred. Specifically, Bishop and Edmundson found that, with regard to story retelling,

- "A child who, at 4 years of age, is unable to give even a simplified account of a sequence of events in a story accompanied by pictures is likely to have a poor outcome" (p. 169).

- "The ability to relate the main events from a story in the correct sequence is a good prognostic sign in a 4 year old, even if the syntax, morphology, and phonology used by the child are very immature" (p. 169–170).

Children whose preschool language impairments persisted into the school years were more likely to have reading, spelling, writing, and other academic difficulties.

In 1990, Bishop and Adams found that preschoolers with SLI whose language problems resolved by age 5.5 typically did well with reading at age 8.5 years. The found that only 4 percent of the children with SLI who had resolved at age 5.5 years struggled with reading at age 8.5. In contrast, 25 percent of the children who had persistent language impairment at age 5.5 struggled with reading at age 8.5 years.

THE ROLE OF ORAL LANGUAGE IN THE ACQUISITION OF LITERACY

Oral language forms the primary foundation for literacy comprehension skills. "Aside from the oral language demands of classroom discourse, oral language plays a second crucial role in school success: it lays the foundation for acquiring literacy" (Paul, 2001, p. 397). In the 1970s, recognition of the psycholinguistic aspects of the reading process emerged. Reading was no longer considered to be just a visual-perceptual skill. Recognition dawned that reading and writing are language-based skills that use visual input to access the language-processing system. Because of our background in oral language development, it is logical that speech-language pathologists be involved in the teaching of reading as well as the treatment of reading and spelling disorders. Understanding text requires knowledge of form, content, and use, just like understanding oral language. Based on the work of Gerber, Paul (2001) made the statement that decoding of text is the first step, and after the decoding is completed, the intended message is treated cognitively just like oral language input would be (p. 397). This statement has two major implications:

> Intact, well-developed oral language skills in syntax, semantics, and pragmatics are necessary to comprehend written texts, just as they are to comprehend classroom discourse. Second, assessing a student's comprehension of oral semantic, syntactic, and pragmatic structures will build toward comprehension of both oral and written language. (Paul, 398)

The Relationship Between Oral and Written Language

Both speech and reading are based on the processes of identification and discrimination. Kamhi and Catts (1999) differentiate between discrimination needed for speech and reading as follows:

- Discrimination in speech: "the ability to hear the difference between two sounds that differ acoustically and phonetically" (p. 6).

- Discrimination in reading: "the ability to see the differences between letters" (p. 7).

While there are distinct differences between reading and spoken language at the perceptual stage, there are similarities at the word recognition stage. The mental lexicon is accessed via the features that were identified during the perceptual stage. When the individual hears or sees a word, he or she must access the concepts that are stored in memory. Thus, reading and speech at the word recognition stage go through the same process with regard to the

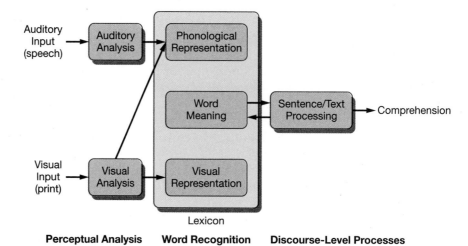

FIGURE 4–1 A model of spoken and written language comprehension.
(*Source:* Language and reading: Convergence and divergence, by A. G. Kamhi and H. W. Catts. In *Language and reading disabilities*, by H. W. Catts and A. G. Kamhi (eds.), Figure 1-1, p. 6. Needham Heights, MA: Allyn & Bacon, 1999.)

individual's mental lexicon. Both speech and reading rely on recognition of the phonological representation of the word, but reading also demands that one be aware of the phonological structure and phonemic segments of the words on the (Kamhi & Catts, 1999). Speech and reading suppositions of Kamhi and Catts are summarized in Figure 4–1.

While there are similarities in how spoken and written languages are processed, it should be pointed out that there are physical, situational, functional, formal, contextual, and grammatic differences between them. Unless it is recorded, speech is referential, and it is heard once and must be remembered to be of use. Speech and oral language typically take place in an environment in which the conversation partners draw information from cues in their surroundings (such as events, activities, signs, and objects) to augment the words being spoken by the conversation partner. Since speech involves face-to-face interactions, the conversant can draw information from the gestures, facial expressions, intonation, pitch, loudness, and vocal quality of those involved in the exchange. Hence, oral language is highly contextualized and is used primarily for social purposes, although it has functions that include giving and getting information. The participants share linguistic and nonlinguistic circumstances, so there is immediate feedback on whether the message was understood or not and clarification of the message or information can be provided immediately (Kamhi & Catts, 1999; Paul, 2001; Westby, 2001).

Written language is more permanent, can be read over and over again, and is functional. Reading and writing are generally used to learn and convey information. A person writes something and another person reads it at a later time, but there is no immediate feedback with regard to the understandability of the message as there would be with a spoken exchange of information. Therefore, literate language is considered to be highly decontextualized in comparison to spoken language (Kamhi & Catts, 1999; Paul, 2001; Westby, 2001).

Boudreau and Hedberg (1999) assessed the general categories of language processing, narrative abilities, phonological awareness, and print-related skills of 36 preschool children aged 56–70 months ($M = 63$, $SD = 3.6$). Eighteen of the children were typically developing, and 18 were diagnosed as having specific language impairments. Specifically, the investigators assessed the children's receptive and expressive rhyme skills, their understanding of print conventions, their knowledge of alphabet letters and letter-sound association, and their narrative abilities. The children with SLI performed worse than the typically developing children on all tasks related to phonological awareness, print conventions, and processing.

The narrative abilities were evaluated using a story retelling task based on the wordless storybook *Frog, Where Are You?* (Mayer, 1969). The examiner read a script that followed the book to each child (the script was not in the children's line of sight), then asked the child to take the book and retell the story. The researchers analyzed the children's narratives in terms of what and how many linguistic structures the children used, the amount of relevant information they recalled, and the structure of the narrative. The stories told by the children with SLI were less complex semantically and syntactically and contained a smaller amount of information than the stories told by the typically developing children. On one measure, the number of key events that were critical to the plot line, the children with SLI recalled as many events as the typically developing children.

Overall, the children with SLI in Boudreau and Hedberg's study (1999) performed "poorly on some early developing skills that are strongly correlated with later reading achievement" (p. 255). Skills such as letter-name knowledge, expressive and receptive rhyming, and metalinguistic tasks that are predictive of decoding and comprehension abilities were poorly developed in the young children with SLI; this has implications for treatment objectives for preschool children who are at risk for reading outcomes in school.

EMERGENT LITERACY

According to Justice, Skibbe, and Ezell (2006), emergent literacy is the "children's developing knowledge about print and sound in the years prior to receiving formal reading and writing instruction" (p. 390). According to ASHA,

> The components of emergent literacy can each be used to draw a child's attention to print: (a) joint-book reading,

(b) environmental print awareness, (c) conventions/concepts of print, (d) phonology and phonological processing, (e) alphabetic/ letter knowledge, (f) sense of story, (g) adult modeling of literacy activities, and (h) experience with writing materials. (2001)

Early and substantial exposure to books correlates with many verbal skills, including the acquisition of knowledge and growth in vocabulary (Stanovich, 1994). Direct and dedicated instruction on phonemic awareness can prevent the reading, spelling, and writing failures that are often associated with reading disabilities (Goldsworthy, 1996; Livesay, 1995). Goldsworthy (1996) outlined several early interventions that can be used for children getting ready to read. These interventions are delineated in Table 4–3.

We know that children who are exposed to stories (e.g., those who are read to by their parents) have better language, reading, and spelling skills

TABLE 4–3 Activities to promote reading readiness

Promoting Emergent Literacy	1. Play word games with letter sounds and syllables.
	2. Expose the child to the printed word, reading aloud to the child a variety of books and encouraging his or her participation.
	3. Have the child construct stories using household events and items, as well as by "reading" books without words.
	4. Encourage the child to draw and write.
Enhancing Listening Skills, Concentration, Memory, and Selective Attention	1. To encourage listening, have the child indicate by raising his hand, ringing a bell, etc. when he or shehears a specific word as a story is read to him or her.
	2. Have the child participate in activities such as finding hidden pictures or words and matching patterns, letters, words, and pictures.
	3. Alert the child when you are beginning to say something by saying the child's name and asking if he or she is ready to listen.
	4. Have the child retell a paragraph and answer specific questions about what he or she has heard and gradually increase the length and complexity of the auditory input.
	5. Have the child focus his or her attention on an interesting object and challenge him or her to see how long he or she can concentrate on the object.

6. Vary the rate of presentation of material, gradually try to increase the time interval between presentation of material and response from the child, introduce visual and auditory distracters through which a child must concentrate on the primary material, and vary directions.

7. Play games with the child.

8. Help the child organize his or her school work, homework, desk, room, etc.

9. Encourage children to "stop, look, and listen" before providing a response to a question or request.

10. Encourage memorization and recitation of songs, rhymes, riddles, story sections, and tongue twisters.

Phonological Awareness	1. Read aloud to the child on a regular basis.
	2. Encourage story telling and "reading" wordless books.
	3. Sing songs.
	4. Have the child answer questions about what has been read.
	5. Pose a question to the child prior to reading the story and then have the child listen for information needed to answer the question.
	6. Use puns, idioms, and riddles to enhance manipulating sounds and words.
	7. Teach the child to discriminate pitch, volume, and rhythms of auditory information.
	8. Point to words and letters as you read to the child.
	9. As you read to the child, omit words and have him or her guess what the word should be.
	10. Provide the child with word cards that can be arranged to formulate a sentence.

Source: Compiled from information in *Developmental reading disabilities: A language-based treatment approach* (pp. 127–170) by C. L. Goldsworthy. Copyright 1996 by Delmar, Cengage Learning.

than those who are not read to by their parents or others. In fact, children who enter school with good narrative skills are more likely to succeed on tasks addressing comprehension and production of the decontextualized language of writing and reading (Owens, 2004). Good books to encourage the development of pre-reading skills and narrative development are *Go, Dog, Go* (Eastman, 1961), *Goodnight, Moon* (Brown, 1947), *Brown Bear, Brown Bear, What Do You See?* (Martin, 1995) and *The Very Hungry Caterpillar* (Carle, 1987), as well as other books by these authors. Wordless books such as *A Boy, A Dog, and a Frog* (Mayer, 1967) and *What Next Baby Bear* (Murphy, 1983) facilitate narrative development when the adult encourages the child to create the story to go along with the pictures.

Catts, Fey, Zhang, and Tomblin (2001) conducted a study in which they assessed 604 kindergarten children on language abilities, narrative abilities, phonological awareness, rapid automatized naming, letter identification, and nonverbal cognition. They then retested the children at the end of second grade to determine which factors identified in kindergarten were predictors of reading outcomes in second grade. The second graders who were identified as poor readers were those who were more than one standard deviation below the mean on a composite measure of reading comprehension.

Catts and colleagues (2001) cited several previous studies that found that a history of oral language problems, phonological awareness, rapid naming ability, vocabulary, grammar, and narrations were predictive of reading ability in children. They found that letter identification, rapid naming, sentence imitation, phonological awareness, and mother's education were predictors of reading performance in second grade and made several recommendations for assessment and intervention based on their findings. These are discussed later in this chapter.

Also, the role of phonological awareness, vocabulary size, and speech perception cannot be overemphasized when looking at causative factors in reading and spelling disorders. When determining a preschooler's level of phonological awareness, ASHA recommends that one assess "the awareness of syllables and rhymes, rather than phonemes, in the context of verbal play and tapping or clapping out syllables. This may include identifying rhyming words as well as generating new rhymes." (ASHA, 2002, p. 14). Stanovich (2000) was one of the first to prove the relationship between phonological awareness and reading ability. Snowling, Bishop, and Stothard (2000) found that phonological awareness deficits are seen in children who have dyslexia, specific language impairment, and/or speech-sound disorders.

Snowling, Bishop, and Stothard (2000) and Storch and Whitehurst (2002) found that the development of a child's vocabulary is a critical factor in the development of a child's ability to decode and hence of reading comprehension. Bird, Bishop, and Freeman (1995) and Larrivee and Catts (1999) found that children with expressive phonological delays or disorders are at risk for developmental reading problems. Several studies have shown that a relationship between phonological awareness and articulation abilities seems to exist, with children with speech-sound deficits having more difficulty with phonological awareness than their peers who do not have a speech impairment (Carroll, Snowling, Hulme, & Stevenson, 2003; Rvachew, Ohlberg, Grawburg, & Heyding, 2003; Larivee & Catts, 1999).

Rvachew (2006) tested 47 children who had speech sound disorders; they were tested in the spring before they began kindergarten and again at the end of kindergarten. She assessed speech perception, vocabulary, articulation, and phonological awareness. Her results showed that speech perception and receptive vocabulary were predictors of unique phonological awareness variances at the end of kindergarten. In her study, articulation ability was not predictive.

The role of speech-sound disorders in reading is inconclusive. Some studies have found that children with speech-sound disorders are at risk for inadequate development of their phonological awareness skills (Webster, Plante, & Couvillion, 1997; Rvachew, Ohberg, Grawburg, & Heyding, 2003). As seen in Rvachew's study (2006), articulation alone is not predictive. Some researchers maintain that the persistence of speech delays or disorders until the child begins school is a risk factor for the development of phonological awareness and reading (Nathan, Stackhouse, Goulandris, & Snowling, 2004: Raitano, Pennington, Tunick, Boada, & Shriberg, 2004). Rvachew (2006) cited several researchers in making the assertion that speech perception difficulties, which are often experienced by children with speech-sound disorders, seem to be the key factor in predicting difficulty in developing phonological awareness.

Auditory awareness is comprised of listening to and understanding sounds. Initially this is based on environmental sounds but then advances to sound awareness. Semantic awareness is comprised of awareness of words, including breaking compound words down into their root words and breaking down sentences into words. Semantic awareness also includes matching written words (as in books) to spoken words (as when read to) (Ukrainetz. 2006) and can facilitate vocabulary growth in children.

"Developing phonological awareness requires that one play with the sounds of the language by identifying and producing rhyme, segmenting sentences into words and words into syllables, and segmenting and blending sounds within syllables" (Goldsworthy, 1996, p. 147). Goldsworthy has delineated a phonological awareness training program that is outlined in Table 4–4.

Children should be taught to group words on the basis of common sounds. For example, a list of 10 to 15 words could be provided with approximately half of the words containing the sound /a/. The children would then be asked to write the words from the list that contain the /a/ sound. They should also learn to segment words into phonemes. Other phoneme games include rewriting words by reversing the phonemes and deleting phonemes. As an example, the child could be asked to rewrite a one-syllable word by reversing the first and last phoneme in the word, or to rewrite the words leaving out all the /b/ sounds (Blachman, 1994).

TABLE 4–4 A phonological awareness training program outline

1. Program levels
   a. Level I. Increasing word awareness: dividing sentences into words
   b. Level II. Increasing syllable awareness: dividing words into syllables
   c. Level III. Increasing sound awareness: dividing syllables into sounds

2. Level sections
   a. Level I. Listening activities for increasing word awareness
   b. Level I. Deliberate manipulation of words in sentences
   c. Level II. Listening activities for increasing syllable awareness
   d. Level II. Deliberate manipulation of syllables in words
   e. Level III. Listening activities for increasing sound awareness
   f. Level III. Deliberate manipulation of sounds in syllables

Source: Developmental reading disabilities: A language-based treatment approach (p. 154) by C. L. Goldsworthy. Copyright 1996 by Delmar, Cengage Learning.

There is no doubt that phonemic awareness and exposure to books play a role in the literacy of school-age children. Thus, it makes sense that these activities should be a substantial part of early childhood education geared toward preparing children for school.

think about it

How does the absence of phonological awareness impact the development of reading?

Figure 4–2 is an observation tool for emergent literacy. It is a checklist "for guiding preventive interventions with infants and toddlers and assessment and intervention activities with preschool-age children" (Nelson, 2010, p. 326). Basically, we want children to learn to be exposed to and engaged in books during the preschool years and to feel good about interactions centered on books.

There are many activities in which parents can engage with their child to encourage literacy. One is to read books that are developmentally appropriate for the child. Reading repetitive texts to preschoolers helps in basic decoding. *Goodnight, Moon* (Brown, 1947) and *Brown Bear, Brown Bear, What Do You See?* (Martin, 1995) are examples of such books. If a book is not available, simple pictures (e.g., labeling a baby in an advertisement) can be used to "read" to the child. Exposure to written language does not have to be limited to books. Parents can model writing by making shopping lists and reading signs. "Writing" letters to family members is another way to expose

Components of Emergent Literacy	Observational Evidence (example, date observed)

The child demonstrates knowledge about:
❑ Books:
  ❑ Held in certain way and read from front to back
  ❑ Describe events outside of real time
  ❑ Represent fictional world
  ❑ Chosen for repeated reading by adult
  ❑ Used for pretend reading by child
❑ Pictures and printed words in books:
  ❑ Are for pointing and naming
  ❑ Represent other things
  ❑ Can represent events even though they are static
 	
The child demonstrates metalinguistic awareness about:
❑ Environmental symbols (e.g., golden arches, stop signs)
❑ Print representing words (e.g., *What does this say?*)
  ❑ Scribbling as means for creating print messages
  ❑ Dictating stories for adult to write down and reread
❑ Alphabetic letters:
  ❑ Some letter names (especially in their names)
  ❑ Some sounds that letters make
 	
The child demonstrates narrative knowledge about:
❑ Components of story grammar episodes:
  ❑ Main characters
  ❑ Feelings (emotional states of main characters)
  ❑ Selling (time and place of story action)
  ❑ Complicating action (problem facing main characters)
  ❑ Dialogue (reported speech of story characters)
  ❑ Coda (ending resolving action of story)
❑ Cohesive devices for connecting parts of discourse:
  ❑ Additive (using and comprehending conjunctions, such as *and*, that link clauses through addition)
  ❑ Temporal (using and comprehending conjunctions, such as *then*, *next*, that link clauses temporally)
  ❑ Causal (using and comprehending conjunctions, such as *because*, *so*, that relate clauses causally)	

FIGURE 4–2   Observation tool for emergent literacy. (*Source: Language and literacy disorders: Infancy through adolescence,* by N. W. Nelson. Needham Heights, MA: Allyn & Bacon, 2010.)

children to writing. These letters may consist of nothing but scribbles, but they underline the idea that written language is a form of communication. Manipulating magnetic letters on the refrigerator and working puzzles consisting of letters are other preliteracy activities. Stapling papers together to make a book and having the child "write" a story is another way to encourage literacy (Paul, 2001).

The phonemic and phonological awareness skills that are learned through these types of activities are highly correlated with reading:

> Evidence of phonemic awareness is observed when children can manipulate individual phonemes, usually in a progression that starts with awareness of initial phonemes, followed by awareness of final phonemes, then phoneme blending, and later segmentation of single-syllable words into component phonemes. The early forms of these abilities can be observed among typically developing children in the preschool years, but research suggests that at least some phonemic awareness develops in the process of learning to read and write, rather than preceding it. (Nelson, 2010, p.p 328–329)

Metalinguistic Skills

The development of metalinguistic skills is another component of emergent literacy. Metalinguistic skills enable a child to think about language and include such skills, in the preschool years, as sound play and word play, which are critical steps in the development of literacy. Rhyming activities, such as learning nursery rhymes, playing rhyming games, and reading repetitive books, help to develop metalinguistic skills and facilitate the development of reading (Paul, 2001; Nelson, 2010). Reading predictable texts to preschoolers also facilitates the ability to develop anticipatory hypotheses. Anticipating what will happen in the story is often problematic for children who develop language learning disabilities and/or reading disabilities.

Phonological awareness is a type of metalinguistic knowledge that is first seen during the preschool years. Phonemic awareness, a subset of phonological awareness, is the understanding that sounds make up words, and it comes to fruition as children learn to segment words during the later preschool years. This knowledge of syllables, along with rhyming skills, forms the basis of phonemic awareness. "These skills are predictive of early word recognition and spelling, but are not directly related to these alphabetic skills" (Ukrainetz, 2006, p. 431).

In summary, Paul (2001) cites Watson Layton, Pierce, and Abraham's 1994 study in listing six components of emergent literacy:

- Print awareness
- Book awareness

- Story sense

- Phonological awareness

- Matching speech to print

- Practicing prereading and prewriting.

WRITING SYSTEMS

There are three types of writing systems: pictographic, syllabary, and alphabetic. Pictographic writing systems are also called ideographic or logographic. Each symbol stands for a whole word, as in the Chinese language. This system does not require decoding, but it requires more memory than do syllabary and alphabetic systems because one must remember a symbol for each word.

In syllabary systems, each symbol represents a syllable, and syllables are combined to make words (as in kana forms of Japanese). This system has a heavier memory load than the alphabetic principle but less than the pictographic.

The third system, and the one on which the English language is based, is the alphabetic system. Phonological awareness is necessary to learn letter–sound correspondences, and it must be developed in order to understand and use the alphabetic system. In this system, each symbol represents a phoneme. This system does not need much memory but it does require decoding skills. The alphabetic system, which relies on phonological awareness, is key to reading. Phonological awareness is made up of

> the ability to break words down into component sounds, to realize that these units of sound can be represented by letters, to learn letter-sound correspondence rules, to analyze words into component sounds (for spelling), and to synthesize sounds represented by letters into words (for reading)." (Paul, 2001, pp. 399–400)

Direct teaching of phonological awareness and letter-sound correspondences to nonreaders enhances reading and spelling development. Speech-language pathologists can be instrumental in providing early intervention to at-risk children who do not have reading readiness skills and in training parents to provide opportunities in the child's natural environment to facilitate phonemic awareness and phonological awareness.

think about it

Knowing that phonological awareness and letter–sound correspondences are critical to literacy, how would you set up a program in a preschool to facilitate a child's learning of these skills?

THE DEVELOPMENT OF DISCOURSE GENRES

The first phase in the development of discourse is oral discourse. Oral discourse is informal, spontaneous, and conversation or dialogue based. Moving along a continuum of discourse growth, narrative discourse is the next phase. Narrative discourse is the telling of a story. It is more of a structured monologue shared through an informal conversation. It should be noted that narrative skills are predictors of success in school (Paul, 2001).

Literate discourse, which is formal written discourse, is next to develop. It consists of communication in the form of papers, essays, lectures, and sermons. Literate discourse differs from basic oral discourse in degree of contextualization. Oral discourse is highly contextualized; information supporting the exchange such as body language, gestures and facial expressions, is available in the immediate environment. Literate information for comprehension is in the linguistic signal itself with little support available outside of it (Paul, 2001).

Expository discourse relies most heavily on linguistic processing. Expository discourse lies at the literate end of the continuum and offers the least contextual support. Expository discourse does not consist of a contextualized story. Rather, it is the relaying of descriptions consisting of facts and information that usually are new to the receiver. Top-down strategies (applying previous knowledge to comprehend the text) used in earlier forms of discourse do not work in expository discourse. Rather, one has to use a bottom-up strategy of "attending to the individual facts and details to get the meaning...[which] puts an extra load on memory and information-integrating processes" (Paul, 2001, p. 394).

The last to develop is argumentative discourse, which is used to debate and persuade others to see one's viewpoint or persuade others to take desired actions (Paul, 2001).

THE DEVELOPMENT OF NARRATIVES

The development of narratives is noted in Figure 4–3. Heap stories, used by children aged 2–3 years old, contain labels and descriptions of events or actions. The sentences of heap stories are simple declaratives. There is no organization of the components of the story, and there is no central theme.

Sequence stories involve the labeling of events around a central theme, character, or setting. First used by children 3 years of age, sequence stories have no plot. Rather, they are a description of what the character has done. There are no temporal or causal relationships between the events in the story (Paul, 2001).

Primitive narratives, used by children 4–4.6 years of age, have a core person, object, or event. These stories contain three of the story grammar elements (initiating event, an attempt or action, and some consequence)

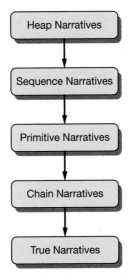

FIGURE 4–3   The progression of development of narratives.
(*Delmar/Cengage Learning*).

and develop around a central theme. There is no real resolution or ending, and there is little evidence of motivation of characters (Paul, 2001).

Used by children 4.6 to 5 years of age, chain narratives show some evidence of cause-effect and temporal relationships. There is a weak plot, but it does not build on attributes and motivations of the characters. It contains the three story grammar elements found in chain narratives. However, the consequence develops around a central theme, and there is some early notion of the plan or characters' motivation affecting the consequence. Nonetheless, the plot does not build on attributes and motivations of characters. The ending is not necessarily logical based on the events of the story, and it may be very abrupt, almost as if the child got tired of telling the story and ended it (Paul, 2001).

True narratives develop around 5–7 years of age. They contain a central theme, character, and plot. There are motivations behind the characters' actions; and the events are logical and temporally sequenced. True narratives contain at least five story grammar elements (all of above and a resolution) (Paul, 2001).

think about it

You are asked to provide a presentation to a Parents of Toddlers club on achieving school readiness. What would you tell parents to do in order to facilitate the development of oral and written narratives?

> **think about it**
>
> In tough economic times, some may question expanding public school services to progressively younger children. How would you justify the expense of providing early education for children who are at risk for failure in school?

SUMMARY

The preschool years can have a tremendous impact on a child's academic success when he or she reaches school age. Children who are exposed to print through a variety of means are less likely to have language learning disabilities and/or reading or spelling deficits. Children need to be taught the different ways in which written and spoken language are used and processed, along with the fundamental skills of literacy. These include phonological and phonemic awareness, understanding of rhyming, being able to develop anticipatory hypotheses, and understanding the structures of narratives. Children go through a specific developmental sequence in their progression in story telling, and caregivers and interventionists need to be aware of this progression in order to best facilitate the child's growth in the production and comprehension of oral and written language.

REVIEW QUESTIONS

1. Until the 1980s, reading was considered to be primarily a visual-perceptual task.

   a. True

   b. False

2. Vocabulary skills at ages 2–3 years may be a better index of underlying language endowment for late talkers than are grammatical skills measured in the preschool period.

   a. True

   b. False

3. The evidence on SELD shows that many of the language and speech problems resolve by the time they reach school age.

   a. True

   b. False

4. Which of the following is/are true?

   a. Written language is more lexically dense than spoken language.

   b. Spoken language is more lexically dense than written language.

   c. Writing is more functional whereas speech is more referential.

   d. Writing is more referential whereas speech is more functional.

   e. Both a and c.

   f. Both a and d.

   g. Both b and c.

   h. Both b and d.

5. Phonemic awareness is a _____ skill.

   a. Metapragmatic

   b. Metanarrative

   c. Metaphonological

   d. Metalinguistic

6. The Chinese language is an example of a syllabary system.

   a. True

   b. False

7. Literate discourse relies more on linguistic processing than does expository discourse.

   a. True

   b. False

8. Cause-effect and temporal relationships are first evident in what type of narratives?

   a. Heap

   b. Sequence

   c. Primitive

   d. Chain

9. Children in what age group use primitive narratives?

   a. 2–3 years

   b. 3.5–4 years

   c. 4–4.5 years

   d. 4.5–5 years

10. The first phase in the development of discourse is oral discourse.

   a. True

   b. False

REFERENCES

Abild-Lane, T. (1996). Children with early language delay: A group case study of outcomes in the intermediate grades. Unpublished Master's thesis, Portland State University, Portland, OR.

American Speech-Language-Hearing Association. (2001). *Role and responsibilities of speech-language pathologists with respect to reading and writing in children and adolescents [Guidelines]*. Available from www.asha.org/policy.

American Speech-Language-Hearing Association. (2002). *Knowledge and skills needed by speech-language pathologists with respect to reading and writing in children and adolescents [Knowledge and Skills]*. Available from www.asha.org/policy.

Billeaud, F. P. (1998). *Communication disorders in infants and toddlers: Assessment and intervention* (2nd ed.). Boston, MA: Butterworth-Heinemann.

Bird, J., Bishop, D. V. M., & Freeman, N. H. (1995). Phonological awareness and literacy development in children with expressive phonological impairments. *Journal of Speech and Hearing Research, 38,* 446–462.

Bishop, D. V. M., & Adams, C. (1990). A prospective study of the relation between specific language impairment, phonological disorder, and reading retardation. *Journal of Child Psychology and Psychiatry, 31,* 1027–1050.

Bishop, D. V. M., & Edmundson, A. (1987). Language-impaired 4-year-olds: Distinguishing transient from persistent impairment. *Journal of Speech and Hearing Disorders, 52,* 15–173.

Blachman, B. A. (1994). What we have learned from longitudinal studies of phonological processing and reading and some unanswered questions: A response to Torgeson, Wagner, and Rashotte. *Journal of Learning Disabilities, 27*(5), 287–291.

Boudreau, D. M., & Hedberg, N. L. (1999). A comparison of early literacy skills in children with specific language impairment and their typically developing peers. *American Journal of Speech-Language Pathology, 8,* 249–260.

Brown, M. W. (1947), *Goodnight, Moon.* New York: Harper & Row.

Carroll, J. M., Snowling, M. J., Hulme, C., & Stevenson, J. (2003). The development of phonological awareness in preschool children. *Developmental Psychology, 39,* 913–923.

Catts, H. W., Fey, M. D., Zhang, X., & Tomblin, J. B. (2001). Eliminating the risk of future reading difficulties in kindergarten children: A research-based model and its clinical implementation. *Language, Speech, and Hearing Services in the Schools, 32,* 38–50.

Eastman, P. D. (1961). Go, dog, go. New York, NY: Random House.

Goldsworthy, C. L. (1996). *Developmental reading disabilities: A language-based treatment.* San Diego, CA: Singular Publishing Group, Inc.

Hart, B., & Risley, T. (1995). *Meaningful differences in the everyday experience of young American children.* Baltimore, MD: Paul H. Brookes.

Justice, L. M., Skibbe, L., & Ezell, H. (2006). Using print referencing to promote written language awareness. In T. A. Ukrainetz (ed.), *Contextualized language intervention: Scaffolding preK-12 literacy achievement* (pp. 389–428). Eau Claire, WI: Thinking Publications.

Kamhi, A. G., & Catts, H. W. (1999). Language and reading: Convergence and divergence. In H. W. Catts and A. G. Kamhi (eds.), *Language and reading disabilities* (pp. 1–24). Needham Heights, MA: Allyn & Bacon.

LaPoro, K. M., Justice, L., Skibbe, L. E., & Pianta, R. G. (2004, November). Relations among maternal, child, and demographic factors and the persistence of preschool language impairments. *American Journal of Speech-Language Pathology, 13,* 291–303.

Larivee, L. S., & Catts, H. W. (1999). Early reading achievement in children with expressive phonological disorders. *American Journal of Speech-Language Pathology, 8,* 118–128.

Lee, L. (1974). *Developmental sentence analysis.* Evanston, IL: Northwestern University Press.

Livesay, Y. (1995). Dyslexia and reading instruction: Presented to the California educators, legislators, and advocates. *Answers, 1,* 1–8.

Martin, B. (1995). *Brown bear, brown bear, what do you see?* New York: Henry Holt & Company, LLC.

Mayer, M. (1967). *A boy, a dog, and a frog.* New York: Dial Books for Young Readers.

Mayer, M. (1969). *Frog, where are you?* New York: Dial Books for Young Readers.

McLaughlin, S. (2006). *Introduction to language development* (2nd ed.). Clifton Park, NY: Delmar Cengage Learning.

Nathan, L., Stackhouse, J., Goulandris, N., & Snowling, M. J. (2004). The development of early literacy skills among children with speech difficulties: A test of the "critical age" hypothesis. *Journal of Speech, Language, and Hearing Research, 47,* 377–391.

Nelson, N. W. (2010). *Language and literacy disorders: Infancy through adolescence.* Boston: Allyn & Bacon.

NICHD Early Child Care Research Network. (1999). Chronicity of maternal depressive symptoms, maternal sensitivity, and child functioning at 36 months. *Developmental Psychology, 35,* 1297–1310.

Owens, R. (2004). *Language disorders: A functional approach to assessment and intervention* (4th ed.). Boston: Allyn & Bacon.

Paul, R. (1996, May). Clinical implications of the natural history of slow expressive language development. *American Journal of Speech-Language Pathology, 5,* 5–21.

Paul, R. (2001). *Language disorders from infancy through adolescence: Assessment and intervention* (2nd ed.). St. Louis, MO: Mosby.

Paul, R., Murray, C., Clancy, K., & Andrews, D. (1997). Reading and metaphonological outcomes of late talkers. *Journal of Speech, Language, and Hearing Research, 40,* 1037–1047.

Pence, K. L., & Justice, L. M. (2008). *Language development from theory to practice.* Boston: Pearson Education, Inc.

Polakow, V. (1993). *Lives on the edge: Single mothers and their children in the other America.* Chicago: University of Chicago Press.

Raitano, M. A., Pennington, B. F., Tunick, B. F., Boada, R., & Shriberg, L. D. (2004). Pre-literacy skills of subgroups of children with speech sound disorders. *Journal of Child Psychology and Psychiatry, 45,* 821–835.

Renfrew, C. (1991). *The bus story: A test of continuous speech.* Old Headington, Oxford, England: Author.

Rescorla, L. (1993). Language Development Survey (LDS). The use of parental report in the identification of communicatively delayed toddlers. *Seminars in Speech and Language, 14*(4), 264-277.

Rescorla, L. (2002). Language and reading outcomes to age 9 in late-talking toddlers. *Journal of Speech, Language, and Hearing Research, 45,* 360–371.

Rvachew, S. (2006, May). Longitudinal predictors of implicit phonological awareness skills. *American Journal of Speech-Language Pathology, 15,* 165–176.

Rvachew, S., Ohlberg, A., Grawburg, M., & Heyding, J. (2003). Phonological awareness and phonemic perception in 4-year-old children with delayed expressive phonology skills. *American Journal of Speech Language Pathology, 12,* 463–471.

Snowling, M. J., Bishop, D. V. M., & Stothard, S. E. (2000). Is preschool language impairment a risk factor for dyslexia in adolescence? *Journal of Child Psychology and Psychiatry, 41,* 587–600.

Stanovich. K. E. (1994). Romance and reality. *The Reading Teacher, 47,* 280–290.

Stanovich. K. E. (2000). *Progress in understanding reading: Scientific foundations and new frontiers.* New York: Guilford Press.

Storch, S. A., & Whitehurst, G. J. (2002). Oral language and code-related precursors for reading: Evidence from a longitudinal structural model. *Developmental Psychology, 38,* 934–947.

Ukrainetz, T. A. (2006). *Contextualized language intervention: Scaffolding preK-12 literacy achievement.* Eau Claire, WI: Thinking Publications University.

Vinson, B. P. (2007). *Language disorders across the lifespan: An introduction (2nd ed.).* San Diego, CA: Singular Publishing Group.

Watson, L., Layton, T., Pierce, P., & Abraham, L. (1994). Enhancing emergent literacy in a language preschool. *Language, Speech, and Hearing Services in the Schools, 25,* 136-145.

Webster, P. E., Plante, A. S., & Couvillion, M. (1997). Phonologic impairment and prereading: Update on a longitudinal study. *Journal of Learning Disabilities, 30,* 365–374.

Westby, C. (1994). The effects of culture on genre, structure, and style of oral and written texts. In G. Wallach and K. Butler (eds.) *Language learning disabilities in school-age children and adolescents* (pp. 180–218). New York: Merrill-Macmillan College Publishing Company.

Whitehurst, G., & Fischel, J. (1994). Early developmental language delay: What, if anything, should the clinician do about it? *Journal of Child Psychology and Psychiatry, 5,* 613–648.

Chapter 5

General Considerations in Assessment of Language Deficits in Infants and Preschool Children

LEARNING OBJECTIVES

After completion of this chapter, the reader will be able to:

1. Describe the etiological-categorical and the descriptive-developmental approaches to assessment.

2. Discuss the four basic assumptions for assessment from a social interaction theoretical perspective.

3. Discuss the application of the seven steps of the scientific model to the diagnostic process.

4. Identify and differentiate between the different types of validity and reliability with regard to language testing.

5. Describe the various types of receptive assessment tasks including the features of language that can be assessed with each type.

6. Describe the various types of expressive assessment tasks including the features of language that can be assessed with each type.

7. Discuss the process of dynamic assessment and its use to differentially diagnose children as being language delayed, language disordered, or language different.

INTRODUCTION

For many reasons, the identification of children under the age of 5 years who have language abnormalities is not the easiest job in the world. One of the biggest problems is that there is no universal screening of preschool children. Pediatricians do not routinely do screenings of speech and language. Most day-care centers and preschools do not have a regular means of screening and assessment, so even enrolling a child in a preschool or day-care setting does not guarantee that speech and language abnormalities will be identified prior to the child's attending school. A tendency exists to take a "wait and see" approach, hoping that any suspected problems resolve by the time the child enters school. Both of these problems were partially remedied with the passage of P. L. 99-457, the Education of All Handicapped Children's Act amendments, in 1976. However, one major problem is the lack of uniformity in testing procedures and programming for preschool children.

Regardless of the age of the child being assessed and the nature of the assessment, specific questions need to be answered. Some of these questions are directed toward the parents or primary caregivers, whereas others may be better addressed by the referral source if it is someone other than the child's family. Furthermore, the clinician must be aware of his or her own personal biases regarding children from different cultural or socio-economic backgrounds. Personnel associated with any educational institution, including preschool settings, must be careful about racial and cultural bias when considering children with nonstandard English as being language impaired.

> The issue of readiness, interlaced with the unquestioned assumption that the child must "fit" the classroom rather than the classroom made to "fit" the child, makes for a rigid, formalized curriculum and turns the developmental kindergarten into a training ground for compliance. More significantly, the developmental kindergarten seems to have become a receiving room for poor children whose economic disadvantage marks them as cognitively and socially deficient; they are being acculturated into monocultural passive learning norms in preparation for formal schooling. (Polakow, 1993, p. 135)

This is an important concept to keep in mind because one of the primary objectives of assessment of preschool children is to ensure that any absence of readiness skills is identified and remedied prior to having the child enter school.

In Chapter 2, the classification of disorders by etiology was presented. In this chapter, a descriptive/developmental approach is discussed. This is in keeping with the two approaches to language assessment outlined by Bernstein and Tiegerman-Farber (2009). Bernstein and Tiegerman-Farber's two approaches are etiological-categorical and descriptive-developmental. The five causative categories Bernstein and Tiegerman-Farber suggested in the etiological-categorical approach are motor disorders, sensory deficits, central nervous system damage, severe emotional-social dysfunctions, and cognitive disorders. Similarly, these same two authors (2009) list five descriptors of language problems in the descriptive-developmental approach based on the work of Bloom and Lahey (1978):

1. Problems learning linguistic form, including rules of phonology, morphology, and syntax

2. Semantic difficulties, including conceptualizing and formulating ideas about objects, events, and relations

3. Pragmatic disorders, including difficulty in using language for a wide variety of functions and adapting language to different speakers or events

4. Difficulties integrating the form, content, and use of language

5. Delayed language development, with the usage of language resembling that of younger, normally developing children

Regardless of whether one prefers the etiological-categorical approach or the descriptive-developmental approach, the process as described in the remainder of this chapter is essentially the same. How the outcome is expressed is where the process is different. Both approaches rely on essentially the same procedures in that language is assessed through case history information, observation, standardized and nonstandardized assessment tools (including language scales), and language samples (Shipley & McAfee, 1998).

OBJECTIVES OF THE ASSESSMENT AND DIAGNOSTIC PROCESS

As outlined in Table 5–1, Lund and Duchan (1988) list five major objectives of the assessment process.

Does the Child Have a Problem?

Assessment process. The process of interviewing, observing, and testing an individual to determine the nature, extent, and severity of his or her language disorder, delay, or difference.

The major objective of the assessment process is to determine whether or not the child has a language problem of any type. That is, is the child's language different, disordered, or delayed in comparison to that of his or her peers?

Typically, a child is referred for evaluation because someone (e.g., parents, teachers, neighbors, child-care workers) believes that the child's language does not compare favorably with the language used by his or her peers. Sometimes, a child is evaluated for possible behavioral or learning problems by a psychologist, who then refers the child to a speech-language pathologist for an evaluation. In those cases, children who have scored one or more standard deviations below their age group on standardized tests, or whose language performance falls at a level 6 months or more below their chronological age in language production, should be referred for testing.

TABLE 5–1 Five major objectives of the assessment process

1. Determine whether or not the child has a language disorder, a language delay, or a language difference
2. Identify etiological factors
3. Identify weaknesses in the child's use of language
4. Describe the strengths in the child's language behaviors
5. Make the appropriate recommendations for the child

Source: Adapted from *Assessing children's language in naturalistic contexts*, by N. Lund and J. Duchan, 1988, Englewood Cliffs, NJ: Prentice Hall, as cited in *An introduction to children with language disorders*, by V. Reed, New York: Merrill, 1994.

Furthermore, any child who is at risk for developing language problems also should be referred for testing. This includes children who are born with disabling conditions, such as hearing impairment, cerebral palsy, or a variety of syndromes and sequences; children who are born addicted to alcohol or other drugs; and children who are at risk due to poverty or trauma in their histories. A sample of a nonstandardized checklist of language development from birth through age 7 is provided in Appendix 5A.

What Caused the Problem?

A second objective is to identify the cause of the problem. Although this is not always important, it is helpful information if the child has a condition that causes progressive deterioration, such as muscular dystrophy, or a genetic condition, such as fragile X syndrome (see Chapter 2), that may affect decision making in the family about future children. For example, a child who was enrolled in a local public school had pervasive developmental disabilities as well as unique facial characteristics and ataxia. It was eventually determined that she had Angelman syndrome, a genetic condition that could be passed on to other biological siblings or to the children of her siblings who did not have the syndrome. In this case, the diagnosis did not change anything being done in therapy, but it did affect family planning decisions by her siblings.

Hearing loss (fluctuating or chronic) can affect a child's speech and language development, so it should always be one of the first tests done in order to rule out that it could be causing (or contributing to) the child's deficits. With the advent of neonatal hearing screenings, the congenital hearing loss is identified much earlier than it used to be, so early intervention can be implemented to minimize the speech and language deficits traditionally associated with hearing loss in children.

Other etiological factors are discussed elsewhere in this book, but one should keep in mind that it is not always possible to determine the cause of a child's speech and language deficits.

> *think about it*
>
> What are some environmental factors that could predispose a child to have a language disability?

What Are the Child's Deficits?

A third purpose of the assessment process is to identify deficit areas in the child's production and comprehension of language. In the preschool population, these deficits are described most frequently in terms of the features of language that the child exhibits or does not exhibit and relative to the child's level of functioning in comparison to his or her peers.

As expressed in Chapter 1, it is preferable to describe a child's language deficits in terms of the features of language that are affected or in terms of a comparison of the child's abilities and deficits to normative development. In other words, it is critical to review the child's language in terms of content, form, and use in relationship to normative data. It is also important to review a child's cognitive and sensorimotor skills and how they affect the child's language.

Based on the research of Erickson, Nelson (1993) lists four basic assumptions that serve as an efficient and effective basis for assessment on a social interaction theoretical perspective:

1. Language is a symbolic, generative process that does not lend itself easily to formal assessment.

2. Language is synergistic, so that any measure of the part does not give a picture of the whole.

3. Language is a part of the total experience of a child and is difficult to assess as an isolated part of development.

4. Language use (quality and quantity) varies according to the setting, interactors, and topic. (p. 228)

Taking this perspective, a clinician can focus on a child's ability to use language to communicate in an efficient and effective manner. This allows a functional description of the child's language abilities and disabilities that can be used as the basis for an intervention program.

What Are the Child's Abilities?

Task analysis. The breaking down of a task into small steps that must be accomplished individually before the whole task can be completed.

Functional outcome. Terminology coined to define environmentally based results of therapy that can be generalized to the patient's natural settings.

Closely tied to the third objective is a fourth goal of the assessment process. It is just as important to identify a child's abilities as it is to identify his or her deficits. This is particularly important when interpreting the assessment findings and deciding what to recommend for the child. A careful review of a child's abilities can be used to provide "stepping stones" to follow in remediation of the deficits. This process of comparing abilities and deficits is part of task analysis, and it forms the foundation for effective therapy. The abilities the child demonstrates must be examined in order to build a task-analyzed program to help the child develop the areas that are revealed as deficits in the assessment process. Therapy should always be focused on a functional outcome, with treatment being provided in the most expedient and effective manner possible.

In order to plan therapy, the clinician needs to know the skills in the child's repertoire that can serve as a foundation for developing skills that are absent. Therefore, the need to know what the child can do as well as what he or she cannot do is of paramount importance.

think about it

Why is it just as important to report what a child *can* do as it is to report what the child *cannot* do?

What Are the Correct Recommendations?

It is critical for the beginning clinician to understand that diagnosis of a language disorder is a process, not an event. Too often, the assessment process is viewed as the 2 to 3 hours that a clinician spends giving a set of tests that were chosen to answer specific questions. However, should it be determined that the child needs intervention, assessment is an ongoing process that continues throughout the delivery of services to the child. The initial diagnostic meeting is only the first step in the assessment process.

The final step in the diagnostic process before beginning therapy is to make the appropriate recommendations for the child. In some cases, this may mean a referral to another professional; in others it is the beginning of the therapeutic relationship between the child and the clinician. Either way, a good referral delineates the child's abilities and deficits in a clear, comprehensive manner.

APPLICATION OF THE SCIENTIFIC MODEL TO THE DIAGNOSTIC PROCESS

Nation and Aram (1984) put forth a model for the diagnostic process that likens the procedure to the scientific model taught in basic science courses. It is an excellent model for all clinicians to follow but is particularly useful for neophyte clinicians who are learning the diagnostic process. By following such a model, the clinician is prepared to implement the diagnostic process for any disorder. This approach is much more useful for the beginning clinician than disorder-specific approaches.

think about it

Why is it logical to apply the scientific model to a clinical process?

Step 1: Defining the Problem

In Step 1 (Table 5–2), the clinician is attempting to understand the subject matter. Some of this understanding comes about as a result of the preassessment discussion with the client, his or her caregivers, or both. During this

TABLE 5–2 Step 1 in the diagnostic process based on the scientific model: Definition and delineation of the problem area

---

What is the problem?

What is being diagnosed?

What fund of knowledge does the clinician need as a diagnostician?

How does the clinician acquire the knowledge needed to make the diagnosis?

How may the diagnostician organize this knowledge?

How much does theory rule the diagnostician's job?

Since the diagnostician is confronted with so many different speech and language disorders, does he or she need a broader base of knowledge than the researcher?

How does the diagnostician use his or her general fund of knowledge for the purpose of diagnosing an individual patient?

Source: Adapted from *Diagnosis of speech and language disorders*, by J. E. Nation and D. M. Aram. Clifton Park, NY: Delmar, Cengage Learning. Copyright 1984.

stage, the clinician begins to assume the role of a diagnostician by asking questions that form the foundation for the other six steps of the process. This is the beginning of the application of academic knowledge in the clinical setting. After obtaining the child's developmental history, the clinician makes decisions as to what knowledge he or she has about the child's needs, what additional information is needed, and how that information will be applied in a diagnostic manner.

The initial evaluation session usually is the first contact between a clinician and the client and his or her family, and it serves as the first step in the diagnostic process. Typically, the session consists of a preassessment interview, observation and testing of the child, and a postassessment conference in which the initial findings are shared with the family.

Case History and Interview Questions

Every assessment should begin with an interview of the parent(s) or the person(s) designated to convey information about the child at the initial assessment session. The first and most critical questions to be addressed are, "Why are you here?" and "What questions do you expect me to answer as a result of this session today?" These questions serve several purposes for the clinician. First, they give the clinician a good baseline of information for determining the family's understanding of a possible language deficit.

Second, these questions provide the clinician with a guideline to direct the testing so that the clinician can be sure to provide an answer to the

Baseline. The preintervention measurement of a patient's skills.

family's most pressing questions. This is also an excellent time to empower the family to be a part of the diagnostic process. No matter how much knowledge a clinician has, it is important to remember that the clinician's knowledge relates to the disorder and the academic aspects of the process. Just as important is the fund of knowledge the family has about their child. The family needs to be encouraged to share as much information about the child and his or her environment as possible, so that the clinician can make the appropriate decisions as to what testing to use during the next phase of the diagnostic process. If the clinician is to empower the family to be a part of the therapeutic process, a good first step is to answer the family's primary questions. It can be difficult to get information from the family, so active listening skills, clinical observations, and tactful questioning skills are critical. The clinician also should be prepared to explain the purpose of each question in case the family challenges the need for the information. A good rule of thumb is to ask only questions for which there is a clear use for the answer.

The hallmark of a good relationship between a clinician and his or her pediatric client's family is an ability to relate to the family. By understanding what the family wants to know, the clinician can be sure to include procedures in the diagnostic protocol that provide answers to the family's primary questions.

The third critical question is, "How does the child communicate now?" It is important to know this information before beginning the diagnostic session to improve the effectiveness of the communication exchanges between the clinician and the child. To answer this question fully and meaningfully, it is helpful to assess the environment using the questions outlined in Table 5–3. The family needs to be encouraged to share as much information about the child and his or her environment as possible so that the clinician can make the appropriate decisions as to what testing to use during the next phase of the diagnostic process. An example of a case history for a pediatric language patient is in Appendix 5B.

TABLE 5–3   Questions to determine the communication environment and status of a child

---

1. What are the child's communication abilities at this time?

2. For what purposes does the child communicate at this time?

3. What are the demands and expectations in the child's daily environments?

4. How does the child interact with his or her environments?

5. Is there any difference in how the child communicates in one environment as opposed to other environments?

Delmar/Cengage Learning

Step 2: Developing the Hypotheses

Table 5–4 delineates the questions to be addressed in Step 2 when the diagnostician begins to formulate the questions that will be tested throughout the diagnostic process. At this point, the clinician begins to apply theoretical knowledge to form a preliminary supposition as to the nature of the child's language deficits. This hypothesis becomes the foundation for the selection of tests to be used in Step 3.

Step 3: Planning the Diagnostic Process

When the clinician progresses to Step 3 (Table 5–5), the driving question is, "What tests and procedures will be used to determine the nature and extent of the child's language abilities and deficiencies?" Using the predetermined hypotheses, the clinician develops questions that must be answered and decides which tools will best provide those answers. In the scientific model, these questions are the research design—how to find out what the researcher wants to know. In many ways, the diagnostician becomes a researcher at this point. It is critical to choose the correct tools to get the desired answers. Otherwise, at the conclusion of the diagnostic process, the hypotheses will remain untested and the questions will remain unanswered.

Based on the information gleaned from the case history and pre-assessment interview, the clinician identifies a set of questions that

TABLE 5–4 Step 2 in the diagnostic process based on the scientific model: Development of hypotheses to be tested

What are the purposes of diagnosis?

How can hypotheses be formulated by the diagnostician that fit the concept of the use of the hypotheses in research or in the use of the method of science?

Are statements of hypotheses appropriate for studying the individual?

How is a clinical hypothesis stated?

How do hypotheses relate to the problem presented by the patient or by the referral source?

What relationships should be expressed in a clinical hypothesis?

Can clinical hypotheses be unbiased?

A researcher is generally free to study hypotheses of specific interest to him or her; hypotheses that are as narrowly defined as he or she feels warranted for predicting events in his or her field of knowledge. Does the diagnostician have this freedom?

Source: Adapted from *Diagnosis of speech and language disorders*, by J. E. Nation and D. M. Aram. Clifton Park, NY: Delmar, Cengage Learning. Copyright 1984.

TABLE 5–5   Step 3 in the diagnostic process based on the scientific model: Development of procedures for testing the hypotheses (research design)

What clinical tools does the diagnostician need?

How are the tools of diagnosis selected for the purposes of diagnosis for the individual patient?

How does the diagnostician evaluate the appropriateness of his or her tools?

Can the diagnostician exert control in testing sessions by selection of tools?

Do clinicians have tools for diagnosis that meet the requirements for measuring instruments that are so important for research? Do they have to be concerned about precision, reliability, and validity?

Since the diagnostician does not know his or her patient personally before the time of the diagnosis, how can he or she consider control over the variables that may be present?

How much time should be allotted for testing procedures?

Is there an order for presenting testing procedures in diagnosis? Are clinicians concerned about the effect one procedure may have on another?

Source: Adapted from *Diagnosis of speech and language disorders,* by J. E. Nation and D. M. Aram. Clifton Park, NY: Delmar, Cengage Learning. Copyright 1984.

need to be answered at the conclusion of the testing. In most cases, a combination of standardized and nonstandardized procedures is needed to adequately address all of the questions that have been identified. Standardized tests or procedures include formal tests that are based on data gathered from normative samples. Nonstandardized procedures include criterion-referenced tests and observations of the child in a variety of contexts.

In addition, a variety of developmental checklists can be used to organize observations. Some of these checklists can be completed by the parents or caregivers, whereas others are used by the clinician while interacting with the child. These developmental checklists are particularly useful in the preschool population because a variety of factors make formalized testing more difficult with children in this age group.

The clinician's job is to analyze the information gathered in the interview or case history stage of the process, decide which questions to address, and then determine the best tools to use to answer the questions in an efficient manner. Identifying the most important questions and the most appropriate tools is critical; asking the wrong questions, or using the wrong tools so that the needed answers are not obtained, destroys the value of the assessment process.

> **Standardized test.** A test that has been evaluated using a sample of individuals that represents a broad cross-section of cultural groups. Standardized tests offer norms that allow a comparison of a child's performance on a test with those in the standardization sample.

Questions Preceding Test Selection

As stated previously, the evaluation should consist of interviews, standardized tests, nonstandardized measurements, and observation. Literally hundreds of assessment devices are available, so before giving any test a clinician should ask the questions outlined in Table 5–6. It is very important that the clinician have the answers to these questions when selecting the tests and testing procedures to be used in the initial evaluation session.

Although Question 1 seems obvious, many tests that claim to test a person's language skills may test some aspect of cognition but not necessarily a specific dimension of language. For example, a test that has the word *comprehension* in the title may be testing recognition, memory, identification skills, or a combination of these areas rather than language comprehension per se.

Statistics related to the validity and reliability of a test are in the test's manual. The clinician should read the information in the test manual carefully to determine whether or not the tool tests what it claims to test and whether or not it gives reliable data.

Validity A major mistake made with regard to standardized testing is ignoring the validity and reliability information on the test. Validity may be of different types, and it serves the clinician well to understand the differences among the types. Validity is concerned with what the test measures and how well it does so.

One type of validity is content validity, which is a "systematic examination of the test content to determine whether it covers a representative sample of the behavior domain to be tested" (Anastasi, 1968, p. 100). Content validity looks at the relevance of the responses instead of the relevance of the test items in an attempt to answer two questions:

1. Does the test contain an adequate sampling of relevant items to assess the behavior?
2. Are the responses relatively free from the influence of irrelevant variables?

Validity. The degree to which a test measures what it is designed to measure, and how well it does so.

Content validity. A systematic examination of the relevance of the responses given to the test items in order to ascertain how well the test covers a representative sample of the skills to be assessed.

TABLE 5–6 Questions preceding test selection

What is the purpose of the test?

Has the test been validated for this purpose?

What is the standardization group?

Are the characteristics of the patient similar to those of the sample group?

Are there any data or experiences to support differing performances across cultural groups (age, sex, socioeconomic status, geographic location)?

Would different values, experiences, behaviors, or other factors affect any of the responses?

Delmar/Cengage Learning

A second type of validity is face validity, which addresses the relevance of the test items. For example, a test designed to assess adults with language impairments caused by a stroke (aphasia) may cover some skills and concepts the clinician desires to test in a child with learning disabilities. However, the vocabulary of the test items on the aphasia test may not be applicable for an elementary school–age child. Therefore, the test would not have face validity for the purpose of testing a child for learning disabilities. Face validity answers the questions, "Are the items relevant and applicable in the setting in which they will be used?"

A third type of validity is criterion-related validity, which is sometimes called predictive validity. Criterion-related validity determines how effectively a test predicts an individual's behavior, abilities, or both in specific situations. For example, the Graduate Record Examination (GRE) is used to predict success in graduate school.

Finally, construct validity is the degree to which the test measures a theoretical construct or trait (Anastasi, 1968). Theoretical constructs include intelligence, fluency, anxiety, aptitude, and other similar concepts. Table 5–7 illustrates the concept of test validity.

Reliability A test's reliability coefficients define the consistency of the test in measuring what it claims to measure in the same individual on reexamination. Statistical measures that can be used to determine a test's reliability include the correlation coefficient, test-retest reliability, and alternate-form reliability. For example, the *Peabody Picture Vocabulary Test III* (PPVT III) (Dunn & Dunn, 1997) is available in two forms. The clinician could test reliability by having the child take each form and then comparing the child's

> **Face validity.** How well test items represent what they claim to test.
>
> **Criterion-related validity.** How effectively a test predicts an individual's behavior, abilities, or both in specific situations.
>
> **Construct validity.** The degree to which a test measures a theoretical construct or trait.
>
> **Reliability.** The consistency of a test in measuring what it claims to measure in the same individual on reexamination.

TABLE 5–7 Illustrative examples to compare and contrast validation procedures

Purpose of Testing	Illustrative Question	Type of Validity
Achievement test in elementary school language arts	How much has Jim learned in the past?	Content
Aptitude test to predict performance in middle school language arts	How well will Jim learn in the future?	Criterion-related: Predictive
Technique for diagnosing brain damage	Does Jim belong in the normal group or in the group of children with neurological deficits?	Criterion-related: diagnostic
Measure of logical reasoning	How can we describe Jim's cognitive processes?	Construct

Source: Adapted from Psychological testing, by A. Anastasi. New York: Macmillan. Copyright 1968 by Macmillan Publishing Company.

Correlation coefficient. A number that represents the degree of the relationship between two sets of scores.

Test-retest reliability. Evaluating the reliability of a test by having the child take the same test on two separate occasions (usually within a 6-month period) and comparing the child's performance on each test.

Alternate-form reliability. Evaluating the reliability of a test by having the child take two different forms of the same test, then comparing the child's performance on each form.

Identification tasks. Tasks in which the child is asked to identify a picture or object that is named by the clinician.

Acting-out tasks. Tasks in which the clinician offers a set of instructions on what the child must complete; the clinician needs to ascertain that the child is truly responding to the examiner's questions and not performing tasks that he or she knows due to real-world familiarity with the item.

performance on each form (alternate-form reliability); alternatively, the same form could be administered on two separate occasions (test-retest reliability). Usually some fluctuations occur in the performance due to random chance factors. However, these are accounted for through the test's standard error of measurement, which enables the clinician to factor in chance circumstances that may cause some variation in an individual's scores (Anastasi, 1968).

The information on the standardization sample should be perused carefully to be sure that the child to be tested is represented in the standardization sample. Newer tests tend to have broader standardization samples, as professionals have become more aware of the effects of different cultures and backgrounds on testing children's language abilities. However, many older tests do not have representative samples and should be used cautiously with underrepresented groups of children. Examples of culturally biased responses include the response of a child who was shown drawings of four different facial expressions and asked to show the examiner the one that represents "delight." Instead of selecting one of the four pictures, the child pointed toward lights on the ceiling.

Test Objectives

A common mistake made by beginning, and some experienced, clinicians is to give a test without being clear about the objectives to be accomplished with the test data. This is why, when planning a testing session, the clinician's first job is to determine what questions need to be answered about the child. Then the clinician should carefully review his or her arsenal of tests to determine which ones (whether standardized tests, nonstandardized tests, or observational checklists) will help to answer the questions. If a test does not contribute to answering a question about the child, it should not be used. Specifically, the clinician should ask, "What question does this test answer, and do I have any use for the answer?"

Receptive Language Tasks

The clinician should also keep in mind that no one test is right for every situation. Also, there are problems inherent in almost all standardized testing. For example, on identification tasks, the child is asked to identify a picture or object that is named by the clinician. Typically, three or four choices are given from which the child must make a selection. The child could get the correct answer by guessing or through the process of elimination. Therefore, identification tasks could be as much a test of recognition as they are of an ability to identify specific language constructs.

In acting-out tasks, the clinician offers a set of instructions on what the child must complete. However, the clinician needs to ascertain that the child is truly responding to the examiner's questions and not performing tasks that he or she knows due to real-world familiarity with the item. For example, the clinician may give the child a cookie and a figurine of a boy. If the clinician asked the child to show "The boy eats the cookie," possibly the child would not understand the task but would have the boy eat the cookie because that is what would be expected. In other words, the child could perform the most probable action without comprehending the word order in the test question. However, if the clinician asked, "Show me the cookie eats the boy," and the child responds by making the cookie eat the boy or saying, "That is silly," the clinician could feel more convinced that the child responded to the request instead of what would be expected to occur.

Another factor in determining whether a test is appropriate for a situation is to look at the level of the task. A judgment task requires that the child make a determination of the accuracy or reasonableness of a statement made by the clinician. To complete such a task, the child must have developed his or her metalinguistic skills because the clinician is asking the child to interpret the language. For children under age 4 years, this may be an inappropriate task because it requires processing of the word's or sentence's form independent of the meaning, and the metalinguistic skills needed to accomplish this task do not usually evolve in a child's language until sometime after 48 months of age. The uses and difficulties with different types of test tasks are listed in Table 5–8 (receptive language tasks) and

Judgment tasks. Tasks that require the child to make a determination of the accuracy or reasonableness of a statement made by the clinician.

TABLE 5–8 Types of receptive tasks

Type	Used For	Potential Limiting Factors
Identification tasks: child selects a picture in response to the examiner's questions	Lexicon Morphology	Child can use guessing or use a process of elimination; may be more a test of recognition than comprehension
Acting out using schemes, role play, and scripts; child manipulates toys and objects in response to the examiner's directions	Semantics Morphology Pragmatics Syntax Comprehension	Have to be careful that the child is truly responding to the examiner's questions and not performing tasks that he or she knows due to real-world familiarity with the item (the monster scared the boy scared the monster)
Judgment tasks: child makes formal judgment of the suitability of a word or sentence—examiner makes a statement, and the child responds if the statement is wrong or right, silly or OK, and so forth	Semantics Syntax Lexicon Morphology	Very difficult for children under age 4 years as it requires processing of the word or sentence's form independent of the meaning (requires metalinguistic skills)

Delmar/Cengage Learning

TABLE 5–9 Types of expressive tasks

Type	Used For	Potential Limiting Factors
Elicited imitation tasks: examiner says a sentence and the child repeats it	Semantics Syntax Morphology Rule out auditory memory problems	Works on the assumption that if a child does not use a particular construction in his or her speech, he or she will omit it in imitation
Delayed imitation tasks: examiner shows child two pictures and says, "The man sees the boy; the man sees the boys. Which one is this?"	Semantics Syntax Morphology	Works on the assumption that if a child does not use a particular construction in his or her speech, he or she will omit it in imitation
Carrier phrase task: child completes incomplete sentences spoken by the clinician	Semantics Morphology Lexicon	Child can fail if there is an auditory memory deficit
Parallel sentence production tasks: examiner places two pictures in front of child. Examiner describes first one, and child describes second one using a similar format	Semantics Syntax Lexicon Morphology	Works on the assumption that if a child does not use a particular construction in his or her speech, he or she will omit it in imitation
Analysis of spontaneous language sample: child and clinician engage in spontaneous conversation, which is recorded mechanically and later analyzed by the clinician	Semantics Syntax Lexicon Morphology	Getting a sample with an adequate number of utterances

Delmar/Cengage Learning

Table 5–9 (expressive language tasks). In addition to the tables, Figure 5–1 depicts a continuum that ranks tasks used to assess receptive and expressive language as requiring the most to the least contextual support.

Step 4: Collecting the Data—Testing and Observing

In the scientific model, collecting the data is the fourth step of the scientific process (Table 5–10). In the diagnostic model, this is the actual testing of the patient. However, many factors need to be considered in this stage of the process. It is imperative, particularly with children, to get the most responses possible in the least amount of time. Therefore, the diagnostician must plan the data collection phase carefully to minimize distractions and maximize responses. The diagnostician also needs to select behavioral procedures carefully,

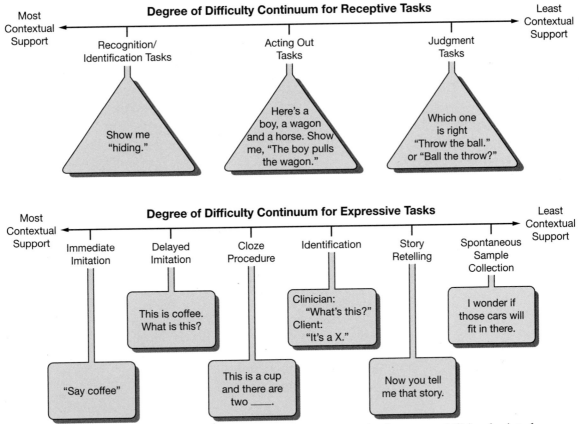

FIGURE 5–1 Tasks typically used to assess receptive and expressive language abilities depicted on a continuum representing most to least contextual support. (*Source:* From *Diagnosis in speech-language pathology* (2nd ed.), by J. B. Tomblin, H. L. Morris, and D. C. Spriestersbach, p. 142. Clifton Park, NY: Delmar, Cengage Learning, 2002)

considering the timing of the presentation of the pertinent stimuli as well as what reinforcements and reinforcement schedules will be used to facilitate the testing process. Some children can be sustained throughout the session with verbal praise. Others may need more tangible reinforcement such as stickers. It is a good idea to avoid the use of food because it can be messy; in addition, eating extends the length of the evaluation session because the clinician must wait for the child to finish eating before progressing to the next item.

Standardized Measures

Evaluation of a preschool child should consist of standardized tests, nonstandardized measurements, and observation. Most tests for children are norm referenced, meaning that there is a standardization sample against which the child's performance can be measured. In other words, the abilities of the child being tested are compared to those from a normative sample of children with similar characteristics to those of the child being assessed. It is the norms that give meaning to the raw scores. By definition, a standardized test

TABLE 5–10 Step 4 in the diagnostic process based on the scientific model: Collection of the data

What are the clinical procedures of diagnosis?

Can the diagnostician control all the variables during the testing session?

How does he or she account for variables that he or she cannot control?

What happens if the diagnostician is not able to use the procedures initially selected? Does this invalidate the diagnosis?

Young children present significant testing problems. What can a diagnostician do during the testing to assure that the data that are obtained are recorded accurately?

Can the diagnostician be as systematically in collecting the data needed for diagnosis as the researcher who has control over his or her experiment? Can the word systematically be interpreted in such a way as to apply to the diagnostic process?

How can the diagnostician observe and record verbal information objectively?

Source: Adapted from *Diagnosis of speech and language disorders,* by J. E. Nation and D. M. Aram. Clifton Park, NY: Delmar, Cengage Learning. Copyright 1984.

allows comparison of a child's performance against that of age-level peers in the standardization sample. Therefore, norm-referenced tests frequently yield an intelligence quotient (IQ) or a developmental quotient (DQ).

Spontaneous Language Samples

The gathering of a spontaneous language sample is a valuable tool that can provide assessment of the child's play skills and analysis of all aspects of the child's language. This can be done even when more formalized tests cannot be successfully administered. The clinician can make note of the type of words the child uses in addition to gathering a phonologic inventory. For example, with regard to types of words, does he or she use nominals ("shoe"), action words ("eat"), negation ("no juice"), pronouns ("me eat") and modifiers ("big ball")? What combinations of words does the child utter? Hegde and Pomaville (2008) summarized the work of Bloom and Lahey (1978), Brown (1973), and Schlesinger (1971) in developing a table to delineate the semantic relations found in children's two-word early utterances. This table is replicated here as Table 5–11. With regard to the phonologic inventory, it is helpful to analyze the child's speech in a spontaneous sample even when a standardized articulation or phonology test is administered because the child's use of sounds in connected, spontaneous speech may differ from that demonstrated in single-word, noncontextual articulation tests. Even when there is a sounds-in-sentences subtest (as on the Goldman-Fristoe Test of Articulation), modeling is provided to some degree because the clinician reads the story to the child and the child then tells the story back to the clinician. Intelligibility percentages of words and utterances can be calculated. Voice and fluency can also be assessed via a spontaneous language sample.

TABLE 5–11   Semantic relations and children's two-word utterances

Semantic Relation	Linguistic Structures	Example of Two-Word Utterance	Possible Intended Meaning*
Nomination	Demonstrative + Noun	That baby!	That is a baby.
Nonexistence	Negative + Noun	No kitty	There is no kitty here.
Agent-object	Noun + Noun	Doggie food	The dog is eating his food.
Agent-action	Noun + Verb	Daddy sleep	Daddy is sleeping.
Action-object	Verb + Noun	Kick ball	Let's kick the ball!
Action-indirect object	Verb + Noun	Drink baby	Give baby a drink.
Action-locative	Verb + Noun or Verb + Locative	Go home Jump here!	Let's go home. Jump right here!
Possessor-possession	Noun + Noun	Mommy hat	That is Mommy's hat.
Entity-locative	Noun + Noun or Noun + Locative	Horsie barn Granma here!	The horse is in the barn. Grandma is here!
Entity-attribution	Noun + Adjective or Adjective + Noun	Dolly pretty Pretty dolly	The dolly is pretty.
Recurrence	Adjective (*more* or *another*) + Noun	More milk!	I want more milk!
Rejection	Negative + Noun	No milk!	I don't want milk!
Conjunction	Noun + Noun	Shoes socks!	I need my shoes and socks.

*Discerned by context.

Source: From *Assessment of communication disorders in children: Resources and protocols,* by M. N. Hegde and Frances Pomaville, p. 201. Copyright 2008 Plural Publishing, Inc.

The clinician can also use the spontaneous language sample to analyze the child's pragmatic functions. Does he or she request ("Get milk?")? Does he or she comment ("hot light")? Does he or she label ("shoe")? Does he or she provide information ("Daddy go")? The Fey and Damico Analysis of a Spontaneous Language Sample is useful in assessing the pragmatic functions and intents of a child's language.

Screenings

Many times, a screening process is administered to a child as part of a routine assessment battery used to determine a child's possible deficit areas prior to beginning school. A screening test is a short test used to determine if a child may have a language deficit or difference. Screening tests are used to determine if a child's language is within normal limits. If the results are not within normal limits, the child should have a full evaluation. A screening

Screening. The administration of short tests in order to determine if a child's language is within normal limits or if he or she needs to be referred for a complete diagnostic process.

test cannot be used to define or delineate a specific diagnosis. It simply serves to determine whether a child may be at risk for deficits in language development and, if so, in need of further, more comprehensive assessment.

Most screening tests use cut-off scores, which can be percentile levels or raw scores. Most diagnostic tests provide this for each age level, with children scoring in the lower percentiles being suspect for a disorder in the area or areas assessed by that test. Percentiles indicate the percentage of children in the standardization sample for an age level who scored below a given raw score. The middle of the scale is usually anchored to an average level of performance for a particular normative group, with the units of the scale being a function of the distribution of scores above and below the average level.

think about it

Explain the statement, "Screening does not result in a diagnosis."

Standard score. A score obtained by converting the raw score to a weighted raw score that takes into account the average score and the variability of scores of children that age.

Standard deviation. A statistical measurement used to document the disparity between an individual's test score and the mean.

Raw scores can be used to determine a standard score by converting the raw score to a weighted raw score, which takes into account the average score and the variability of scores of children that age. Using standard scores, a child who scores 1 standard deviation below the mean is suspected of having a language deficit. A child who scores 2 standard deviations below the mean most likely exhibits a language deficiency relative to his or her peers.

It is critical that any test used be administered, scored, and interpreted according to the directions for that particular test. Any deviation from the prescribed format can destroy the validity and reliability of the test and make the results meaningless.

Receptive and Expressive Tests. Many standardized tests assess either expressive or receptive language, whereas others have subscales that assess both dimensions of language and communication. Receptive tests measure a child's linguistic competence: what he or she knows about language. Expressive tests measure a child's linguistic performance: how well he or she uses the knowledge he or she has about language.

Nonstandardized Measures

Developmental Checklists. Another type of test frequently used with infants and preschool children is the developmental checklist. Most checklists are ordinal, meaning that the behaviors are arranged in a developmental order and are dependent on each other, as in a hierarchy. The child's chronological age is compared to a developmental age based on the number of items passed on the checklist. The extent of the language deficit is based on the discrepancy between the child's chronological age and the developmental age (Dunst, 1980). Developmental checklists can be used to record observations, as a guide for a parent interview, or as a formalized method of assessing a child's developmental level based on behaviors and skills exhibited through play. In other words, some checklists are completed by observation, some are completed by interaction with the child, and some are completed by interaction with the primary caregivers.

Most checklists are descriptive in that they include items that should be passed by children at designated age levels. They can be used to describe the child's language, cognitive, and communicative behaviors, but they do not necessarily yield percentiles or standard scores. They simply provide information on specific skills that are present or absent in the child's repertoire. Many checklists are not limited to language functioning but tend to look at the overall development of the child. They provide excellent information, regardless of whether or not a child can be tested using more standardized measures.

The *Receptive-Expressive Emergent Language Scale–2* (Bzoch & League, 1991) is a standard checklist used to guide the interviewing of parents about their child's speech and language capabilities. Another interview scale that is used in a variety of settings is the *Vineland Social-Emotional Early Childhood Scale* (Sparrow, Balla, & Cicchetti, 1998), in which the clinician checks off behaviors identified by the primary caregiver as typical of the child's communicative behaviors.

The *Symbolic Play Assessment for Preschool Children* (Lombardino & Kim, 1986) (Appendix 5C) can be used for children from presymbolic through symbolic stages of play (12–16 months of age). This test and others similar to it are based on schemes or make-believe scenarios. The child may be asked to act out a doctor scenario or a cooking scheme. The independence the child demonstrates in imitating a variety of behaviors associated with each scheme is then recorded to determine the child's level of symbolic ability. This symbolic ability is critical to the development of metalinguistic and pragmatic skills that guide much of the child's social development throughout the preschool and early elementary ages.

Play can be encouraged at many levels. The shy and withdrawn child should be approached using self-talk and parallel talk. In such a case, clinicians are often uncomfortable with silence in the room. However, it is critical that the clinician learn to wait silently for the child to respond. These periods of silence are needed periodically to give the child a chance to talk. When setting up play opportunities for diagnostic purposes, the clinician should sequence the interaction with the child. Initially, solo play may be the most effective. In the case of a cooking scheme, the clinician and the child could each have their own spoons and own pans to play with on the stove. Using self-talk, the clinician can comment on his or her own perceptions and activities ("I'm stirring my soup. It smells so good!"). After a period of solo play, tangential contact play can begin. During this phase, the clinician may add some food to his or her pan and also add some to the child's pan. Parallel talk in which the clinician comments on his or her own activities as well as those of the child should commence shortly after tangential contact play begins. This should be followed by intersecting play, during which the clinician's toys interact with the child's toys. For example, the clinician could take some food from his or her pan and put it in the child's pan. Finally, cooperative play should ensue in which the clinician assists the child in playing together. In the cooking scheme, this could involve setting the table and eating the good food that they have just cooked.

When working with an aggressive, hyperactive, or uncooperative child, the clinician must gain and retain control of the session. The setting should be structured to reduce stimulation and to help the child focus on the task at hand. Using a firm voice (firm, not loud or threatening), the clinician should let the child know that he or she is not threatened by the child's behavior. Do not reinforce the behavior by pleading, using rambling logic, or cajoling. Be matter of fact, and use self-talk. ("Well, if you want to scream, I'll just keep on with the work and I'll get the sticker for this set of words.") It also helps to do something you know the child likes to do. For example, if you know the child enjoys playing with cars and trucks, set up a garage scheme and use solo play to draw the child into the play.

Another checklist, the *Early Communication Checklist* (Lombardino, Stapell, & Gerhardt, 1987), can be used to evaluate communicative behaviors in infancy (Appendix 5D). Published in the *Journal of Pediatric Health Care*, this checklist was designed to assist nurses and other health care professionals in identifying suspected delays in the early development of communication and in making referrals to speech-language pathologists and audiologists when appropriate.

The *Communication and Symbolic Behavior Scale* (CSBS) was developed by Wetherby and Prizant (1993) and consists of normed developmental checklists that use parent interviews and naturalistic sampling procedures. These checklists are designed not only to test language but also to assess communication functions in children 8–24 months of age. They can also be used to assess the language and communication skills of children up to 72 months who have developmental delays. The communication skills that are assessed include gaze shifts, use of gestures, positive affect, and rate of communicating. The clinician interviews the primary caregiver(s) using the caregiver questionnaire and then videotapes an interaction between the caregiver and the child. The interaction is designed to include shared books, communication temptations, language comprehension tasks, constructive play activities, and symbolic play. There are 22 five-point scales that are divided into seven clusters: communicative function, communicative means—gestural, communicative means—vocal, communicative means—verbal, reciprocity, social-affective signaling, and symbolic behavior. The *CSBS-Developmental Profile* (CSBS-DP) (Wetherby and Prizant, 2002) is also norm-referenced and can be used as a screening and evaluation test. The CSBS-DP provides assessment of symbolic development and communicative behaviors. It is shorter than the CSBS and can be used for children who have a functional communication age of 6–24 months and a chronological age of 9 months to 6 years.

Finally, the *MacArthur Communicative Development Inventories* (Fenson et al., 1993) are parent checklists based on normative data. There are two checklists: Words and Gestures and Words and Sentences. The Words and Gestures checklist is for use with 8- to 16-month-old infants, whereas the Words and Sentences checklist is designed to assess the language of children 16–30 months of age.

The *MacArthur Communicative Development Inventory: Words and Sentences* (Fenson et al., 1993) is a parent report test tool that measures vocabulary development. The CDI includes an "extensive vocabulary checklist containing words that children typically produce in the second and third years of life" (Miller, Sedley, and Miolo, 1995, p. 1037). A study using the CDI was conducted by Miller and colleagues (1995) to determine the validity of the measure in reporting vocabulary development in children with Down syndrome who had a mental age of 12–27 months. The researchers measured the lexicon of 44 children with Down syndrome and 46 normally developing children in a clinical setting. They also evaluated predictive validity by comparing the lexicon of 20 of the children with Down syndrome and 23 of the typically developing children at a mental age of 20 months and then at a mental age of 28 months. The findings in the clinic were compared with those reported by the parents, and they concluded that parent report tools such as the CDI are valid for measuring a child's vocabulary. Miller and colleagues report that parent report tools are advantageous over clinical measures because they allow the clinician to tap into the parents' knowledge about their child's abilities with regard to language, the tools are cost effective and efficient, and they record the child's language in a natural setting as opposed to formal testing, which may be affected by the child's lack of familiarity with the setting and the examiner. In addition, tools such as the CDI can be completed by the parents prior to the clinical assessment, which enables the clinician to better plan subsequent testing, and they empower the parents to be a part of the assessment process.

Ordinal Scales of Development An example of an ordinal scale of development completed through interaction with the child is the *Uzgiris and Hunt Scales of Infant Psychological Development* (Uzgiris & Hunt, 1978). This scale is used to assess children at the presymbolic level of functioning, covering skills children normally develop between birth and 24 months of age. At the presymbolic level, the child does not use conventional words, gestures, or pictures for communication (Owens, 1995). In other words, it is most likely that the child does not use a recognizable communication system beyond a few words and gestures. The Uzgiris and Hunt checklist is divided into seven scales covering six domains that provide an overall picture of the child's cognitive functioning up to the age of 24 months, or during the presymbolic period of the child's life (Table 5–12). These domains can be tested through the establishment of play schemes in which the child is an active participant, as shown in Figure 5–2. Each domain is important in some manner to the assessment of cognitive skills needed for the child's future development.

Presymbolic level. The stage of communication that precedes the use of gestures, words, and actions to denote specific language concepts or words.

TABLE 5–12 Scales of development assessed in the Uzgiris and Hunt Psychoeducational Battery

Scale 1:	Visual Pursuit and the Permanence of Objects
Scale 2:	Means for Obtaining Desired Environmental Events
Scale 3A:	The Development of Vocal Imitation
Scale 3B:	The Development of Gestural Imitation
Scale 4:	The Development of Operational Causality
Scale 5:	The Construction of Object Relations in Space
Scale 6:	The Development of Schemes for Relating to Objects

Source: From *A clinical and educational manual for use with the Uzgiris and Hunt Scales of Infant Psychological Development,* by C. Dunst, 1980. Austin, TX: Pro-Ed.

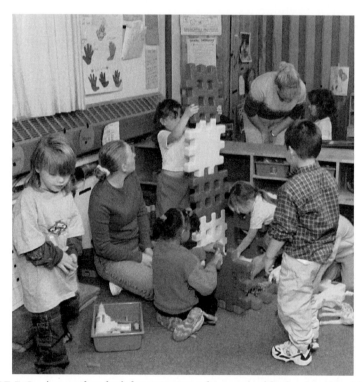

FIGURE 5–2 A preschooler's language can be assessed by having the child play with a variety of toys and observing his or her language and interactive behaviors while engaged in play activities. (*Delmar/Cengage Learning*)

The seven scales represent seven sensorimotor domains that develop parallel to each other. The Ordinal Scales of Psychological Development permit independent assessment of each domain, with the child's highest level of performance being determined for each scale by noting the highest item that is passed on each scale. This permits a clinician to develop knowledge about the child's weaknesses and strengths across several developmental domains (Dunst, 1980).

Criterion-Referenced Tests By definition, a criterion-referenced test is a nonstandardized probe that is individualized for a child in order to examine a specific linguistic skill in greater depth. To use criterion-referenced tests, a clinician must rely on his or her own knowledge of normative data because the tests offer no comparison to children of similar ages. These types of tests provide knowledge about the consistency of a child's problems and the contexts in which the problem occurs.

> **Criterion-referenced test.** A nonstandardized probe used to study a language construct in more depth than is normally associated with standardized tests.

Reed (1994) offered three rationales for using criterion-referenced tests. First, they allow the clinician to examine in more detail features of language that appeared most troublesome for a child on a standardized instrument. For example, if a child demonstrates problems with the verb items on the PPVT, the clinician could construct a criterion-referenced test that examines the child's understanding and use of verbs in a variety of contexts.

Second, Reed stated that criterion-referenced testing examines aspects of language that may be omitted from standardized testing. These tests can be used to determine the scope of a child's difficulty with a particular feature of language. Sometimes criterion-referenced testing can determine if it is the test stimulus that is creating the problem for the child, as opposed to the specific language feature.

Referring again to the PPVT, Penner and Vinson (1981) did a study that looked at performance of adults with intellectual disabilities on the PPVT after noticing that the individuals missed an inordinate number of verbs. On the PPVT, the verbs are actually presented as gerunds ("running"), the noun form of a verb. When the stimulus was presented as a verb ("somebody *verb*-ing"), the number of verbs missed decreased significantly. Therefore, in some of these cases, it was the stimuli, and not the verbs, that were problematic.

However, just as with standardized testing, problems occur associated with criterion-referenced testing. One problem is the choice of behaviors and items to be tested and selecting the criterion levels at which mastery is determined. As a rule, it is not good to have 100 percent mastery, as children often miss items owing to inattention or some other environmental reason, even though the child may know the items. Additional issues relate to validity, reliability, and problems associated with repeated testing, just as with standardized testing. Third, criterion-referenced testing can be used to answer the question, "Did the child fail to demonstrate a skill because of the manner in which the clinician tried to elicit the skill, or does the child not have the skill in his or her repertoire?" Thus, criterion-referenced tests provide an alternative means of assessing a child's language abilities and disabilities.

When developing criterion-referenced testing, care must be taken in deciding what criterion are used to determine if the child has the skill, does not have the skill, or is developing the skill. Also, if using this type of testing to monitor progress in therapy, the clinician must take care to ensure that the skill is completely acquired and not just occurring in response to repeated administrations of the task.

A sampler of tests for language in preschoolers can be found in Appendix 5E. This list includes screening tools, normative tests, and criterion-referenced tests.

Dynamic Assessment

Reuven Feuerstein first introduced the concept of dynamic assessment in 1979. He believed that intelligence could be measured better by observing how a child learns a novel task than by standard tests of intelligence. By combining instrumental enrichment (IE) and dynamic assessment, the clinician constructs an interactive, adult-mediated situation in which to evaluate the child (Nelson, 2010). Nelson wrote that "master clinicians convey confidence in their clients' abilities to acquire new knowledge and skills, while working to support their learning directly and intentionally. This involves identifying missed cues in meaningful contexts and framing them to focus students' attention on those cues" (p. 445).

It is important to note that standard assessment batteries should not be replaced by dynamic assessment; rather, dynamic assessment should be used to augment the clinician's evaluation of a child's learning style and capabilities. Dynamic assessment tells us more about *how* the child learns than standardized assessment instruments do. These instruments typically tell us *what* the child knows. After obtaining baseline information, the clinician uses experiential language situations as mediated learning experiences (MLEs) to determine the child's ability to learn new information and to assess how he or she approaches learning. The MLEs are set up in a tiered fashion, creating a scaffold approach to presenting the new task. The examiner demonstrates the tasks to be learned, then practices the tasks with the child, observing "the child's ability to modify his or her performance" (Kaderavek, 2011, p. 46).

The use of narratives can form the foundation for dynamic assessment of a child's discourse skills. The clinician can assess the child's ability to summarize a narrative and to answer questions designed to determine how well the child comprehended the narrative that has been practiced together. Comparative scoring can be used to determine the amount of learning that has occurred, thus assessing the child's response to intervention (which is discussed in Chapters 9 and 10). This is known as a test-teach-retest process based on experientially based treatment.

"The dynamic assessment process is used to differentiate children with and without disorders, not on the basis of standardized scores but on the basis of their modifiability and generalization to other narrative tasks"

(Nelson, 2010, p. 310). For example, the child could "read" a wordless book, thereby constructing a narrative. The narrative could be analyzed in terms of the number and sophistication of the story elements present in the narrative. Through the employment of contextually based learning experiences, the clinician can provide intervention in a fluid manner, then retest the child to determine his or her progress. This information, along with other data, can then be considered when making decisions about educational placement. The child who needs extensive scaffolding to learn may do better in a smaller, more individualized classroom than in a full-inclusion school (Nelson, 2010).

Dynamic assessment can be useful in the assessment of culturally diverse children. Through dynamic assessment, the clinician can reduce the effects of cultural influences on the performance of children from diverse backgrounds. Although test developers have made substantial progress in reducing cultural bias in standardized tests, a child's culture may influence how he or she responds in the testing situation. For example, Asian children may not be willing to guess at an answer when they are unsure about the answer; some children see guessing as being playful and not understand the concept of a "serious guess" (Curenton, 2011). A child who has low baseline scores but responds favorably to mediated learning may be identified as having a language difference rather than a language disorder as the result of dynamic assessment as opposed to the more traditional static assessment.

Step 5: Analyzing the Data

Analyzing the data involves understanding what test scores mean. The clinician should note the skills the child has and their potential to serve as a foundation for the development of the absent skills. Of course, one of the objectives in using standardized testing is to find out how the child uses language in comparison with his or her peers (Table 5–13).

TABLE 5–13   Step 5 in the diagnostic process based on the scientific model: Analysis of the data

How is the information obtained for analysis?

How does the diagnostician score the information?

How is the information analyzed in the diagnostic process?

Are measures available that are descriptive and predictive?

Can the results obtained in diagnosis be quantified?

Source: Adapted from *Diagnosis of speech and language disorders*, by J. E. Nation and D. M. Aram. Clifton Park, NY: Delmar, Cengage Learning. Copyright 1984.

TABLE 5–14 A four-box system to interpret findings from diagnostic tests and procedures

	Strengths	Weaknesses
Communicative		
Noncommunicative		

Delmar/Cengage Learning

Percentile scores. The percentage of individuals in the standardization sample for an age level who scored below a predetermined raw score.

The percentile scores that can be derived from standardized testing are a tremendous asset in this aspect of the diagnostic process. The percentile scores indicate the percentage of children in the standardization sample for an age level who scored below a given raw score. Most diagnostic tests provide percentile scores for each age level.

Another type of score available from standardized testing is a standard score. Using standard scores, a child's raw score (the actual number of correct) on a test is converted to a weighted raw score, which takes into account the average score and the variability of scores for children of that age. Thus, as with percentiles, a child's performance can be compared to that of children with similar characteristics. Children who score 1 standard deviation below the mean are suspected of having difficulties in language skills.

Any child who scores greater than 1.5 standard deviations below the mean should receive direct intervention. Using a four-box system, the skills that are present and absent in a child's repertoire can be divided easily into those that are communicative, those that are not communicative, those that are strengths, and those that are weaknesses. (Table 5–14). This information, along with the standard scores, can then be used to decide whether to use direct intervention or whether to make some environmental manipulations and recheck the child at a later date.

Step 6: Interpreting the Data

Beginning clinicians should be aware of the existence of many common errors and misconceptions about standardized tests.

First, although some clinicians believe that the way to demonstrate professional accountability is to give a standardized test, there are times when a situation does not warrant standardized assessment. For example, a child may not have the attention span needed to complete a standardized test. Also, it is usually recommended that a test not be repeated within a specified time period. Therefore, if a child has already taken specific standardized tests, the clinician may be better off spending time using nonstandardized measures of assessment.

The second common error, particularly made by new clinicians, is using tests with children not represented in the norming sample. If a speech-language pathologist is working in Montana, for example, there is a good chance that Native American children are part of the population to be tested. Therefore, it is important for the clinician be sure that Native Americans are represented in the norming sample. If not, it might be necessary for the clinician to collect local norms in order to have a representative sample for comparison.

A third common error is the belief that, by reporting the scores a child receives on the standardized tests, the clinician has adequately informed the child's family about the meaning of the scores, the implications for placement in therapy, or the need for a referral to another professional. In actuality, reporting scores does little to help referral sources or the family understand the extent of a child's problems. Scores must always be derived in accordance with the directions in the manual, but the interpretation of these scores is not necessarily explained in the manual. Therefore, it is useful to spend some time analyzing the results in terms of what the child missed and what he or she got correct. This information is much more useful than a numeric score, particularly for preschool children. It is good to share with the parents the skills you believe the child has or has not developed, based on the items missed on the standardized test.

A fourth misconception is that standardized tests can be used as an end rather than as a means to an end in the diagnostic process. The administration of a standardized test is only the beginning of a process that includes scoring and interpretation before that test can be considered complete. Therefore, to administer a test just so a score can be reported is an injustice to the child and to the persons waiting to hear the results of the assessment. Careful interpretation, as outlined in Table 5–15, is essential.

TABLE 5–15   Step 6 in the diagnostic process based on the scientific model: Interpretation of the data (support or reject the hypothesis)

How does the diagnostician interpret the results obtained in the diagnosis?

How can clinicians know if their results are close to the true behaviors they set out to study?

When interpreting the findings of the diagnosis, do the clinicians rely only on the specific test findings?

How is the information organized in relationship to the hypothesis?

How is the information synthesized and summarized?

Source: Adapted from *Diagnosis of speech and language disorders,* by J. E. Nation and D. M. Aram. Clifton Park, NY: Delmar, Cengage Learning. Copyright 1984.

Step 7: Making Conclusions

The Postassessment Conference

After testing the child, the clinician should take the time to meet with the child's family to discuss some of the findings. The clinician is responsible for conducting the postassessment conference. Going into the postassessment conference, the family is likely to be concerned about the diagnosis and the prognosis. They may be grappling with assorted feelings including concern, fear, anxiety, and potential relief from finally having some answers. The clinician brings a body of knowledge gathered from the preassessment interview, the case history, and the individual's performance on the tests. Even though there may not have been time at this point to score and interpret the testing, there is still information that can be shared regarding the child's overall performance. The clinician should give the name of the test, describe what it is designed to test, and explain why he or she chose that particular test. The clinician should review some of the constructs and/or concepts that the child missed and passed and question the parents as to whether this is an accurate reflection of the child's typical abilities.

A description of the child's behavior and communication efforts should be offered to the family. Remember, during the preassessment interview, the family was empowered to be part of the team. Once the clinician has shared the results of the diagnostic session, it is helpful to ask the family, "What do you need to know from me at this point?" The answer to this question will guide him or her as to how much information the family is willing and able to receive. The family and the clinician should use this time to share with each other all the knowledge they have about the child and to then decide the best follow-up procedures to implement in the future (Table 5–16). This is the time to reinforce to the family that they have been empowered to be part of the team, with the focus now moving from the diagnosis to the

TABLE 5–16   Step 7 in the diagnostic process based on the scientific model: Making conclusions from the data

How does the diagnostician interpret and communicate the findings of the diagnosis?

What applications to other patients can be made from the interpretations made on the patient seen? Can this or should this be done?

In what forms is the information from the diagnosis communicated?

Does diagnosis stop at this point?

How does the diagnostician determine appropriate management plans?

Source: Adapted from *Diagnosis of speech and language disorders*, by J. E. Nation and D. M. Aram. Clifton Park, NY: Delmar, Cengage Learning. Copyright 1984.

treatment. Keep in mind that the value of the diagnostic session may very well depend on the quality of the postassessment conference.

The Diagnostic Report

The diagnostic report is a written record that summarizes the relevant information obtained, why this information was obtained, and how this information was obtained. The diagnostic report has several functions. The first is to serve as an official document of the interaction with the child and the family. Information from the case history, the preassessment and postassessment conferences, and the testing session are all incorporated into the diagnostic report. Copies of this report are sent to the family and to any referral sources that the family would like to have notified.

Second, the report serves as an entry point into the clinical service delivery system for the client. The report contains baseline and pretherapy information that is used to develop the goals and procedures for any subsequent therapy the child might receive. Thus, the report can be used to communicate the clinician's questions and findings to other professionals. Because this report may be the primary interaction with another professional, the clinician's professional credibility may be established by his or her report writing. Finally, the diagnostic report serves as a document for research purposes.

A good diagnostic report should contain the most information in the fewest words possible. The author once asked a physician how much of a report he actually reads. The response was, "I read what would fit on the back of an envelope."

Typically, the first information in the report is the identifying information. This includes the child's name, his or her parents' names, and their address and telephone number. Background information should include a statement of the problem. Case history information is often critical in the formation of a diagnosis, so accuracy is paramount. The second primary area of focus in the report is the examination information. This includes a description of how the child approached the task, the tests that were used, the purpose of each test, and the results. Again, the results should not be limited to reporting the scores; rather, they should include information about what items the child missed, what items he or she answered correctly, and a description of the strengths and weaknesses exhibited by the child on the tests. Then the clinician should summarize behavioral observations made during the course of the session. This includes information about how the child approached the tasks, distractibility, and the child's ability to respond and maintain focus on the task.

The next section of the report should include the clinician's summary, conclusions, and recommendations. This consists of clinical impressions and formulation of the diagnosis. All of the information gained from the history, the assessment, and the conferences should be integrated and synthesized

Clinical facts. Statements made about events that actually took place and were observed or measured directly by the clinician.

Clinical assumptions. What clinicians judge to be true, although they may not observe or measure attributes related to these events directly.

into this section of the report. It is very important in this section (and, indeed, throughout the report) to differentiate between clinical facts and clinical assumptions. Clinical facts are statements made about events that actually took place and were directly observed or measured by the clinician. Clinical assumptions are what clinicians judge to be true, although they may not observe or measure attributes related to these events directly.

Both clinical assumptions and clinical facts have their place in a report. However, clinical assumptions should be used only in the summary and conclusions section of the report. Also, clinical assumptions should be labeled as such to avoid any misconceptions by the reader. It is important to remember that the summary and conclusions are often the only section that many people read. Thus, they should be concise, accurate, and the best written section of the report. Finally, the clinician should sign the report.

With regard to the ethics of report writing, the clinician must be honest about what he or she knows and does not know as a result of the assessment. If information was not gathered for whatever reason (e.g., the child was fatigued, the clinician inadvertently omitted it), assumptions cannot be made. Rather, the clinician needs to state honestly that the information was not obtained. Second, the clinician cannot guarantee results. The prognosis and recommendations must be written very carefully from an ethical viewpoint. Third, the clinician must not interpret causes of psychological symptoms and behaviors. To do so could lead to ethical and legal complications. A final warning is to be sure that a release of information has been obtained before sharing the evaluation results with anyone. A copy of the release should be sent with any report requested from or supplied to another individual.

think about it Why is a diagnostic report considered to be the most important document a clinician writes?

SUMMARY

The assessment of preschool children presents a unique challenge for beginning and experienced clinicians. Regardless of the inherent difficulties, accurate determination of a child's abilities with regard to language and communication is critical. If a preschool child is already a frustrated communicator, it is possible that the child will abandon all attempts to communicate and regress to a point where communication intervention is extremely difficult. It is also important to note whether a child is using compensatory skills to accommodate deficits in language or communication skills. This, too, may indicate the level of ability and inability the child has in this critical area of development. For example, if a 36-month-old child relies primarily on gesturing to communicate, the clinician and family should carefully analyze the communicative environment of the child. Is the child gesturing because this is accepted as an adequate attempt without challenging the child to use speech? Or, if the child does not use speech despite adequate environmental stimulation and encouragement, is there an organic reason for this child not communicating as expected? The answers to these critical questions can be obtained only through a complete assessment process in which the child, the family, and the clinician all play a critical role.

CASE STUDY

History

Richard, a 3-year, 8-month-old boy, was initially seen at the Speech and Hearing Clinic (SHC) for a hearing evaluation. Reportedly, Richard has an ongoing history of serous otitis media that is treated with antibiotics. He has had three to four ear infections per year since birth. Richard's hearing was found to be within normal limits bilaterally for speech stimuli. However, his expressive language skills appeared to be below average for a child his age, and his parents advised the clinician that Richard was scheduled for a speech and language evaluation at Memorial Hospital in the near future.

Richard's mother reported that his spontaneous speech was mostly jargon and babble rather than true speech, although occasionally he would produce two- to three-word sentences imitatively. She reported that Richard did not verbally respond appropriately when spoken to but rather babbled a response or repeated what he heard. Richard's mother believed that his language comprehension and language expression were delayed. Richard lives at home with his parents and one older brother. He attends a church-related preschool three mornings per week.

Previous Testing

Richard's speech and language were first evaluated two months ago by a speech-language pathologist in the Division of Child and Adolescent Medicine at Memorial Hospital. The Preschool Language Scale-Revised (PLS-III) was administered to assess auditory comprehension (receptive) skills as well as verbal abilities (expressive). No basal age was obtained for the receptive or the expressive portion of the PLS-III. The child's auditory comprehension skills were reported to be at the 27-month level and his verbal abilities to be at the 24-month level. The Bzoch-League Receptive Expressive Emergent Language Scale (REEL Scale) was completed through a parent interview. On the REEL scale, Richard's expressive language skills were estimated to be at the 12-month level, and his receptive skills were in the 20- to 26-month-old range.

Evaluation at SHC on November 9, 2009

Play Skills. Lombardino and Kim's Symbolic Play Assessment for Preschool Children (1986) was administered to assess Richard's level of nonverbal symbolic play development. During

(continues)

CASE STUDY (continued)

this assessment, Richard was presented with toys for a cooking scheme (i.e., cooking dinner script). Although Richard's play skills were limited, he demonstrated up to two different action schemes carried out in a logical sequence. For example, following a model by the clinician, Richard put play food on a plate and brought the food to his mouth. This corresponds to an approximate age range of 19–24 months. Richard demonstrated object substitution, which was modelled by the clinician, when he pretended to use a dowel to substitute for a spoon. Richard substituted a block for a telephone after the clinician provided a model. This corresponds to an approximate age range of 24–30 months. Agent play, during which the child ascribes agency to an object or assumes another person's role, was modelled by the clinician but not observed during Richard's play. The clinician pretended a doll was crying by imitating crying sounds and pretended the doll could walk and talk. Richard's optimal and modal level of play, which was modelled by the clinician, was object substitution with multistage combinations.

The Uzgiris and Hunt Scales of Infant Psychological Development (1975) assess an infant's cognitive development during the first 24 months of life. The integration and refinement of sensory and motor behaviors to produce adaptive responses during the first 24 months is referred to as sensorimotor intelligence. The acquisition of sensorimotor abilities affords children the critical skills necessary for achieving higher-level thought and adaptive processes. Although Richard's chronological age exceeded 24 months, the clinicians used the Uzgiris and Hunt instrument to better document Richard's status on cognitive and language skills that serve as a foundation for future language development. Richard attained Stage VI, representation and foresight, which is the highest developmental level within this assessment.

Receptive Language

The Peabody Picture Vocabulary Test-III (Dunn & Dunn, 1997) was administered to assess Richard's receptive vocabulary. A basal level was not established because Richard would not point to the pictures the examiner named. However, he spontaneously labelled four pictures.

Expressive Language

The Expressive One Word Picture Vocabulary Test (Gardner, 1981) was administered to assess Richard's expressive vocabulary. Again, a basal level could not be established. However, Richard correctly identified six of the nine pictures in the age range of 3–3.5 years old. During interactions, Richard demonstrated the ability to produce utterances of two words, which were primarily echolalic. Most of his spontaneous speech consisted of single-word utterances such as "ball" and "shoe." Articulation was subjectively judged to be within normal limits.

Behavioral Observations

Richard easily separated from his mother and engaged cooperatively with the clinician during the evaluation session. He demonstrated very little spontaneous speech, and limited imitation of conversation was observed. Richard did not play interactively with the clinicians, and he made no verbal requests to obtain toys and snacks that were placed out of his reach. He rarely made eye contact with the clinicians and did not express curiosity when one of the clinicians left the room.

Summary and Conclusions

Based on the observations made during Richard's symbolic play assessment, his symbolic play behaviors were limited. Following a model, Richard demonstrated the ability to combine two schemes.

One instance of object substitution was observed following a model. These behaviors correspond to an approximate age range of 19–24 months. Results of the Uzgiris and Hunt Scales of Infant Development revealed that Richard has attained sensorimotor stage VI. On receptive and expressive language tests, Richard did not achieve a basal score. During conversational interactions, Richard produced single-word and two-word utterances that were often echolalic. He responded better to the clinicians' requests for action when the verbal requests were augmented with gestures.

Richard has an expressive and receptive language disorder that affects the content and use domains of language. He also demonstrates some autistic-like behaviors. Therapy is recommended, with emphasis on developing naming behaviors and pragmatic skills. Therapy should employ experiential language activities to facilitate contextually appropriate language.

	Strengths	Weaknesses
Communicative	Hearing WNL	Developmentally approx. 18–23 month delayed
	Responds to model of play	
	Responds to model of speech	Unable to attain basal on PPVT, PLS, or EOWPVT
	Spontaneously labels some pictures (verbally)	Does not point to pictures
	Echolalic	Echolalic
	Articulation WNL	Does not initiate conversation
	Responds more accurately when clinician uses gestures and speech	Limited functions of language
		Does not consistently respond to verbal instructions
		MLU below average for chronological age
Noncommunicative	Separates easily	Stage VI on sensorimotor skills
	Attends preschool	Does not play interactively
	Cooperative	

REVIEW QUESTIONS

1. Which of the following groups of tests represent receptive tasks?
   a. Identification tasks, acting out, carrier phrase tasks
   b. Identification tasks, acting out, judgment tasks
   c. Identification tasks, judgment tasks, parallel sentence production tasks
   d. Identification tasks, acting out, delayed imitation

2. Which of the following statements about receptive language tasks is/ are not correct?
   a. Judgment tasks are well suited and easy for children below 4 years of age.
   b. Identification can be achieved on the basis of recognition and superficial comprehension.
   c. Acting out may reveal knowledge of the real world rather than understanding of the linguistic features.
   d. All of the above are incorrect.
   e. None of the above is incorrect.

3. What type of validity is addressed by the question, "How well will Jim learn in the future?"
   a. Criterion-related diagnostic
   b. Construct
   c. Content
   d. Criterion-related predictive

4. The assessment domain that evaluates a child's ability to use foresight in simple problem solving is
   a. Object permanence
   b. Causality
   c. Schemes
   d. Means-end

5. Which of the following represent a set of developmental checklists?
   a. The REEL, the Uzgiris and Hunt, and the Symbolic Play Scale
   b. The REEL, the MacArthur, and the Preschool Language Scale
   c. The CDIS, the Uzgiris and Hunt, and the Peabody Picture Vocabulary Test
   d. All of the above contain at least one test that is not a developmental checklist.

6. Identification tasks are especially useful for assessing pragmatics.

   a. True

   b. False

7. Syntax should be assessed expressively and receptively since comprehension of form precedes production.

   a. True

   b. False

8. Dynamic assessment is less culturally biased than most standardized assessment tools.

   a. True

   b. False

9. By definition, a standardized test is a valid test for all cultural groups.

   a. True

   b. False

10. During the constituent analysis phase of the diagnostic process, the clinician determines the meaning of the results and supports or rejects the hypothesis.

   a. True

   b. False

REFERENCES

Anastasi, A. (1968). *Psychological testing* (3rd ed.). New York: Macmillan.

Bernstein, D. K., & Tiegerman-Farber, E. (2009). *Language and communication disorders in children* (6th ed.). Boston: Allyn and Bacon.

Bloom, L., & Lahey M. (1978). Language development and language disorders. New York: John Wiley and Sons.

Bzoch, K., & League, R. (1991). *The receptive-expressive emergent language scale—2.* Los Angeles: Western Psychological Services.

Curenton, S. M. (2011). Multicultural issues. In J. N. Kaderavek (ed.), *Language disorders in children: Fundamental concepts of assessment and intervention* (pp. 383–412). Boston: Allyn & Bacon.

Dunn, L. M., & Dunn, L. M. (1997). *The peabody picture vocabulary test–III.* Circle Pines, MN: American Guidance Services.

Dunst, C. (1980). *A clinical and educational manual for use with the Uzgiris and Hunt Scales of Infant Psychological Development.* Austin, TX: Pro-Ed.

Fenson, L., Dale, P. S., Reznick, J. S., Thal, D., Bates, E., Hartung, J. P., Pethick, S., & Reilly, J. S. (1993). *MacArthur communicative development inventories: User's guide and technical manual.* San Diego, CA: Singular Publishing Group.

Gardner, M. F. (1981). *Expressive one-word picture vocabulary test.* Novato, CA: Academic Therapy Publications.

Hegde, M. N., & Pomaville, F. (2008). *Assessment of communication disorders in children: Resources and protocols.* San Diego, CA: Plural Publishing, Inc.

Kaderavek, J. N. (2011). *Language disorders in children: Fundamental concepts of assessment and intervention.* Boston: Allyn & Bacon.

Lombardino, L. J., & Kim, Y. T. (1986). *Symbolic play assessment for preschool children.* Unpublished manuscript.

Lombardino, L. J., Stapell, J. B., & Gerhardt, K. J. (1987, September-October). Evaluating communicative behaviors in infancy. *Journal of Pediatric Health Care, 1,* 5.

Lund, N., & Duchan, J. (1988). *Assessing children's language in naturalistic contexts* (2nd ed.). Englewood Cliffs, NJ: Prentice Hall.

Miller, J. F., Sedley, A. L., & Miolo, G. (1995, October). Validity of parent report measures of vocabulary development for children with Down syndrome. *Journal of Speech and Hearing Research, 38*(5), 1037–1044.

Nation, J. E., & Aram, D. M. (1984). *Diagnosis of speech and language disorders* (2nd ed.). San Diego, CA: Singular Publishing Group.

Nelson, N. W. (1993). *Childhood language disorders in context: Infancy through adolescence.* New York: Merrill.

Nelson, N, W. (2010). *Language and literacy disorders: Infancy through adolescence.* Boston: Allyn & Bacon

Owens, R. E. (1995). *Language disorders: A functional approach to assessment and intervention* (2nd ed.). Boston: Allyn and Bacon.

Penner, K., & Vinson, B. P. (1981). Facilitation of verb recognition by MR subjects through syntactic cuing. *Language, Speech, and Hearing Services in the Schools, 12,* 39–43.

Polakow, V. (1993). *Lives on the edge: Single mothers and their children in the other America.* Chicago: University of Chicago Press.

Reed, V. A. (1994). *An introduction to children with language disorders* (2nd ed.). New York: Merrill.

Schlesinger, I. Production of utterances and language acquisition. In D. Sloan (Ed.), The ontogenesis of grammar. New York, NY: Academic Press, 1971.

Sparrow, S. S., Balla, D. A., & Cicchetti, D. V. (1998). *Vineland social-emotional early childhood scales.* Circle Pines, MN: American Guidance Services.

Uzgiris, I. C., & Hunt, J. M. (1978). *Assessment in infancy: Ordinal scales of psychological development.* Urbana: University of Illinois Press.

Wetherby, A. M., & Prizant, B. M. (1993). *Communication and symbolic behavior scales.* Baltimore, MD: Brookes.

Wetherby, A. M., & Prizant, B. M. (2002). *Communication and symbolic behavior scales–developmental profile.* Baltimore, MD: Brookes.

APPENDIX 5A

Assessment of Language Development

Name: _____ Age: _____ Date: _____

Examiner's Name: _____

Instructions: Mark a plus (+) or a check (✓) if the child *does* exhibit the behavior, a minus (–) or a zero (0) if the child *does not* exhibit the behavior, and an *S* if the child exhibits the behavior *sometimes*. This form can be used during informal observation or completed by a parent or knowledgeable caregiver. Because children develop at different rates, avoid using strict application of the age approximations. The time intervals are provided only as a general guideline for age appropriateness.

0–6 Months

____ Frequently coos, gurgles, and makes pleasure sounds

____ Uses a different cry to express different needs

____ Smiles when spoken to

____ Recognizes voices

____ Localizes to sound

____ Listens to speech

____ Uses the phonemes /b/, /p/, and /m/ in babbling

____ Uses sounds or gestures to indicate wants

____ Responds to *no* and changes in tone of voice

7–12 Months

____ Understands *no* and *hot*

____ Responds to simple requests

____ Understands and responds to own name

____ Recognizes words for common items (e.g., cup, shoe, juice)

____ Babbles using long and short groups of sounds

____ Uses a large variety of sounds in babbling

____ Imitates some adult speech sounds and intonation patterns

(continues)

APPENDIX 5A *(continued)*

____ Uses speech sounds rather than only crying to get attention

____ Listens when spoken to

____ Uses sound approximations

____ Begins to change babbling to jargon

____ Uses speech intentionally for the first time

____ Uses nouns almost exclusively

____ Has an expressive vocabulary of one to three words

____ Uses characteristic gestures or vocalizations to express wants

13–18 Months

____ Imitates individual words

____ Uses adult-like intonation patterns

____ Uses echolalia and jargon

____ Omits some initial consonants and almost all final consonants

____ Produces mostly unintelligible speech

____ Follows simple commands

____ Receptively identifies one to three body parts

____ Has an expressive vocabulary of three to 20 or more words (mostly nouns)

____ Combines gestures and vocalization

____ Makes requests for more of desired items

19–24 Months

____ Uses words more frequently than jargon

____ Has an expressive vocabulary of 50–100 or more words

____ Has a receptive vocabulary of 300 or more words

____ Starts to combine nouns with verbs and nouns with adjectives

____ Begins to use pronouns

____ Maintains unstable voice control

____ Uses appropriate intonation for questions

____ Is approximately 25–50% intelligible to strangers

____ Asks and answers "What's that?" questions

____ Enjoys listening to stories

____ Knows five body parts

____ Accurately names a few familiar objects

____ Understands basic categories (e.g., toys, food)

____ Points to pictures in a book when named

2–3 Years

____ Speech is 50–75% intelligible

____ Understands *one* and *all*

____ Verbalizes toilet needs (before, during, or after act)

____ Requests items by name

____ Identifies several body parts

____ Follows two-part commands

____ Asks one- to two-word questions

____ Uses two- to four-word phrases

____ Uses words that are general in context

____ Continues use of echolalia when difficulties in speech are encountered

____ Has a receptive vocabulary of 500–900 or more words

____ Has an expressive vocabulary of 50–250 or more words

____ Exhibits multiple grammatical errors

____ Understands most things said to him or her

____ Frequently exhibits repetitions—especially starters, "I," and first syllables

____ Increases range of pitch

____ Uses vowels correctly

____ Consistently uses initial consonants (although some are misarticulated)

____ Frequently omits medial consonants

____ Frequently omits or substitutes final consonants

____ Uses auxiliary *is* including the contracted form

____ Uses some regular past tense verbs, possessive morphemes, pronouns, and imperatives

____ Maintains topic over several conversational turns

(continues)

APPENDIX 5A (continued)

3–4 Years

____ Understands object functions

____ Understands opposites (stop-go, in-out, big-little)

____ Follows two- and three-part commands

____ Produces simple verbal analogies

____ Uses language to express emotion

____ Uses four to five words in sentences

____ Repeats six- to 13-syllable sentences accurately

____ May continue to use echolalia

____ Uses nouns and verbs most frequently

____ Is conscious of past and future

____ Has a receptive vocabulary of 1200–2000 or more words

____ Has an expressive vocabulary of 800–1500 or more words

____ May repeat self often, exhibiting blocks, disturbed breathing, and facial grimaces during speech

____ Increases speech rate

____ Speech is approximately 80% intelligible

____ Appropriately uses *is*, *are*, and *am* in sentences

____ Tells two events in chronological order

____ Engages in long conversations

____ Sentence grammar improves, although some errors still persist

____ Uses some contractions, irregular plurals, future tense verbs, and conjunctions

____ Consistently uses regular plurals, possessives, and simple past tense verbs

____ Uses an increasing number of compound or complex sentences

4–5 Years

____ Imitatively counts to five

____ Continues understanding of spatial concepts

____ Has a receptive vocabulary of 10,000 or more words

____ Counts to 10 by rote

____ Listens to short, simple stories and can answer questions about them

____ Answers questions about function

____ Uses adult-like grammar most of the time

____ Grammatical errors primarily in irregular forms, reflexive pronouns, adverbial suffixes, and comparative/superlative inflections

____ Has an expressive vocabulary of 900–2000 or more words

____ Uses sentences of four to eight words

____ Answers complex two-part questions

____ Asks for word definitions

____ Speaks at a rate of approximately 186 words per minute

____ Reduces total number of repetitions

____ Significantly reduces number of persistent sound omissions and substitutions

____ Frequently omits medial consonants

____ Speech is usually intelligible to strangers even though some articulation errors may persist

____ Accurately tells about experiences at school, at friends' homes, etc.

5–6 Years

____ Follows instructions given to a group

____ Asks *how* questions

____ Uses past tense and future tense appropriately

____ Uses conjunctions

____ Has a receptive vocabulary of approximately 13,000 words

____ Sequentially names days of the week

____ Counts to 30 by rote

____ Continues to drastically increase vocabulary

____ Uses sentence length of four to six words

____ Reverses sounds occasionally

____ Exchanges information and asks questions

(continues)

APPENDIX 5A *(continued)*

____ Uses sentences with details

____ Accurately relays a story

____ Sings entire songs and recites nursery rhymes

____ Communicates easily with adults and other children

____ Uses appropriate grammar in most cases

6–7 Years

____ Understands *left* and *right*

____ Uses increasingly more complex descriptions

____ Engages in conversations

____ Has a receptive vocabulary of approximately 20,000 words

____ Uses a sentence length of approximately six words

____ Understands most concepts of time

____ Counts to 100 by rote

____ Uses most morphologic markers appropriately

____ Uses passive voice appropriately

Source: The assessment of language development. In K. G. Shipley and J. G. McAfee, *Assessment in speech-language pathology: A resource manual* (4th ed.), copyright 2009 by Delmar Cengage Learning.

APPENDIX 5B

Sample Case History for Pediatric Language Cases
Identifying Information

Child's Legal Name: _____ Nickname: _____

Date of Birth: _____ Age: _____ Date History Form Completed: _____

Parents'/Legal Guardians' Names: _____

Address: _____
           Street   City/State   Zip Code

Mailing Address (if different): _____

Person Completing This Form: _____

Mother's Employer: _____ Job Title: _____

Mother's Daytime Phone #: _____ Evening Phone: _____

Father's Employer: _____ Job Title: _____

Father's Daytime Phone #: _____ Evening Phone: _____

Child's Social Security #: _____

Do you have Medicaid: Yes _____ No _____

If yes, please provide your 8-digit policy/care number: _____

Name of Family Doctor or Referring Physician: _____

Phone # of Family Doctor or Referring Physician: _____

Name of Insured Individual: _____

Name of Person Responsible for Payment: _____

Address/Phone (if different from above): _____

(continues)

APPENDIX 5B *(continued)*

Referral Information

Who referred the child to this clinic:

☐ Pediatrician   ☐ Relative   ☐ Self/Parent

☐ Teacher   ☐ Friend   ☐ Other _____

Would you like the referring individual to receive a copy of the report? Yes _____ No _____

Address: _____
          Street   City/State   Zip Code

Are there others who should receive a copy of the report? Yes _____ No _____

Name: _____

Address: _____
          Street   City/State   Zip Code

Name: _____

Address: _____
          Street   City/State   Zip Code

What is the reason for referral? (Check all that apply)

☐ Diagnosis   ☐ School Placement

☐ Treatment   ☐ Other _____

Present Communication Status

Please describe your child's speech: _____

_____

Have diagnostic or therapeutic services related to the speech problems previously been received?
Yes _____ No _____ If yes, by whom and when? _____

Results of previous diagnosis or therapy: _____

When did the problem first begin? _____

Has the problem: _____ remained the same

                        _____ gradually worsened

                        _____ worsened quickly?

Educational History

Name of Current Preschool/School: _____

Grade: _____ Primary Placement: _____ Regular Ed. Classroom

                                        _____ Self-Contained Classroom (full day)

                                        _____ Special Education (part day)

                                        _____ Other _____

Current Teacher's Name: _____

Describe your child's progress in school: _____

_____

In your opinion, does your child's speech/language problem have an effect on his/her school performance or school placement? Yes _____ No _____ If yes, please explain:

_____

Does your child receive speech-language therapy at school? Yes _____ No _____

If yes, please indicate the following:

Name of Clinician: _____

Length and Frequency of Sessions: _____

Primary Focus of Therapy:_____

Family History

Mother's Name: _____   Age: _____ Highest Degree/Grade: _____

Father's Name: _____   Age: _____ Highest Degree/Grade: _____

Siblings: Name: _____   Age: _____ Highest Degree/Grade: _____

(continues)

APPENDIX 5B *(continued)*

Name: _____ Age: _____ Highest Degree/Grade: _____

Name: _____ Age: _____ Highest Degree/Grade: _____

Name: _____ Age: _____ Highest Degree/Grade: _____

Others in the Home: _____

      Name   Relationship

      _____

      Name   Relationship

Pregnancy and Birth History

Did the mother have any illnesses or accidents during the pregnancy? Yes _____ No _____

Did the mother receive/take any prescribed medications while pregnant? Yes _____ No _____

If yes, what medications and for how long? _____

_____

Were the medications used during the _____ 1st trimester _____ 2nd trimester _____ 3rd trimester

Did the birth mother drink alcohol or use any illegal drugs while pregnant? Yes _____ No _____

Were there any complications during the labor and/or delivery? Yes _____ No _____

Was your baby's birth: _____ premature _____ term _____ late?

Did your baby have difficulty with any of the following in the first 48 hours following birth?

_____ breathing   _____ crying   _____ sleeping

_____ sucking   _____ responding to noise   _____ other

Comments on any of the above:

_____

_____

How long did your baby remain in the hospital following birth? _____

Developmental History

I have never been concerned about my child's developmental patterns. Yes _____ No _____

I am concerned about my child's development because _____

_____

Please indicate the approximate ages at which each of the following occurred for the first time:

_____ Cooing   _____ Ask Questions   _____ Feed Self/Hands

_____ Babbling   _____ Sit Unassisted   _____ Feed Self/Utensils

_____ Single words   _____ Stand Unassisted   _____ Toilet Trained

_____ Combine words   _____ Walk Unassisted   _____ Dress Self

Is English your child's native language? Yes _____ No _____

If not, what is your child's native language? _____

How many languages are spoken in the home? _____ which languages? _____

_____

Medical History

General Health: _____ Excellent   _____ Good   _____ Fair   _____ Poor

Please indicate any ongoing medical conditions: _____

Please indicate any regular medications: _____

Has your child ever been seen by any of the following specialists? Check all that apply:

_____ ENT Physician   _____ Psychologist   _____ Nutritionist

_____ Neurologist   _____ Behavior Specialist   _____ Orthodontist

_____ Psychiatrist   _____ Physical Therapist   _____ Other

_____ Physiatrist   _____ Occupational Therapist   _____

(continues)

APPENDIX 5B *(continued)*

Please list names/approximate dates/reasons for specialists:

Name: _____ Date: _____

Reason: _____

Name: _____ Date: _____

Reason: _____

Name: _____ Date: _____

Reason: _____

Please list previous surgeries/illnesses/injuries:

Problem	Dates	Comments

Please check all that apply and provide clarifying information under "Comment."

Illness	Comments	Yes	No
Allergies			
Recurrent colds/flu/sore throat			
Dizziness			
Dental problems			
Frequent laryngitis/hoarseness			
Epilepsy/seizure disorder			
Reading and/or spelling problems			
Other academic problems			

Attention deficit disorder (ADD)			
ADD with hyperactivity			
Vision problems			
High fevers			
Kidney problems			
Swallowing/digestive disorders			
Respiratory difficulties			
Heart/circulatory problems			
Neurological disorders			
Cancer			
Endocrine/metabolic disorders			
Viruses (HIV, herpes)			
Connective tissue disorders (lupus, arthritis, scleroderma)			
Frequent and/or intense headaches			
Measles			
Mumps			
Chicken pox			
Meningitis			
Unusual fatigue/stress			
Mental illness			
Congenital disorders (list please)			

Audiological History

Please check the appropriate column:

	Yes	No
My child had 3+ ear infections between birth and 12 months of age.		
My child has had at least one ear infection that lasted more than 3 months.		

(continues)

APPENDIX 5B *(continued)*

	Yes	No
My child has been evaluated by an audiologist who determined that his/her hearing is within normal limits. Date of visit:		
My child has failed a hearing screening in school. Date of screening:		
My child has passed a hearing screening in school. Date of screening:		
I suspect that my child has a hearing problem.		
My child has tubes in his/her ears. If yes, when:		
My child prefers one ear to the other. If yes, which ear?		
My child wears hearing aids. If yes, what type and for how long?		

Comments: _____

_____

_____

Speech and Language History

Please check the appropriate column:

	Yes	No
My child follows directions well.		
My child gives directions well.		
My child asks for help when needed.		
My child expresses himself/herself in a coherent manner that is understood by others.		
My child likes to have stories read to him/her. How long does he/she attend to the story?		
My child plays with age-appropriate toys appropriately.		
My child has failed a speech screening in school. Date of screening:		
My child has passed a speech screening in school. Date of screening:		

	Yes	No
My child communicates primarily through whining/crying.		
My child communicates primarily through gesturing/pointing.		
My child tries to communicate through verbalizing, but cannot be understood.		
My child primarily uses one-word utterances to communicate.		
My child primarily uses two-word phrases to communicate.		
My child primarily combines 3+ words to communicate.		
My child uses proper sentence structure for most of his/her utterances.		
Familiar persons easily understand my child's communication efforts.		
Unfamiliar persons easily understand my child's communication efforts.		
My child frequently drools.		
My child has difficulty chewing his/her food.		
I am concerned about my child's speech (how well what he/she says can be understood.)		
I am concerned about my child's language development (the content of what he/she says; how well he/she understands what others say).		

Overall, I would rate my child's speech intelligibility as:

_____ excellent _____ good _____ fair _____ poor _____ completely unintelligible

Comments:

_____

_____

_____

_____

APPENDIX 5C

Guidelines for Symbolic Play Scale Administration

This scale was developed from longitudinal and cross sectional data on the evolution and progression of play behaviors in normally developing children. The primary literature sources used for play levels, ordinal arrangement of play levels, and the corresponding ages were Bretherton (1984), Fenson (1984), McCune-Nicolich (1981), Watson & Fisher (1980), and Wolf, Rygh, & Altshuler (1984).

This scale is not a standardized assessment of play but rather serves as an observational tool for use in approximating levels of nonverbal symbolic play development in language-impaired preschool children. While there are not data to suggest that language-impaired children demonstrate differences in the developmental sequence of their play when compared to their normal developmental peers, studies have reported that language-impaired children are often delayed in their acquisition of play as observed in their restricted diversity of play schemes, shorter play schemes, and limited organization of play sequences (Lombardino, Stein, Kricos, & Wolf, 1986; Terrell & Schwartz, 1983).

Scale Organization

The scale is hierarchically organized for play levels spanning approximately 9 months to 5 years of age. Ages corresponding to each play behavior are only estimates and should be used by the therapist as developmental guidelines rather than as absolute indices. Age levels corresponding to the more advanced symbolic play behaviors (i.e., beyond the 3-year level) are based on very limited pool of empirical information as few studies have delineated ordinal levels of play at these higher stages of development.

Recommended Procedures

No standard procedures have been developed for use with this scale; however, several procedures are recommended to help ensure (1) a representative sample of the child's play behaviors; (2) optimal level of play at which the child is capable of functioning; and (3) some degree of uniformity across test sessions and examiners.

Guidelines

1. Assess the child's play performance over a minimum of two 30–45 minute sessions. (If the child is verbal, this offers an excellent opportunity for collecting a language sample.)

2. Allow for an approximately 10–15 minute preassessment warm-up period in which the child is encouraged to play with a random set

of toys in the presence of the parent and examiner (see list at end for recommended props). The parent and examiner should not actively participate in this play unless the child solicits their participation. The child should be permitted to direct the course of his or her play without restrictions (except in cases of disruptive behavior). If the child shows no initiative in playing with the toys, he or she can be prompted to do so or should be given the opportunity to choose a new set of toys.

3. Present the child with an organized set of toys to facilitate theme-related plays (e.g., cooking, grooming, doctoring). These toys or props allow the child to represent familiar events or scripts in play. Scripts are ordered sequences of actions in which temporal, causal, and spatial links are organized around a goal such as "making dinner," "bathing a baby," or "being examined by a doctor" (see list of recommended props for two scripts). These scripts are only examples of the types of organized play contexts that can be used.

    There is empirical evidence to suggest that organized sets of toys facilitate more advanced action sequences in play (Largo & Howard, 1979; McCune-Nicolich & Fensen, 1985). Also, studies have shown that script contexts facilitate several aspects of language learning (Conti-Ramden & Friel-Patti, 1986; Snow, Perman, & Nathan, 1986; Harrison, Lombardino, & Farrar, 1989).

4. The child should be given the opportunity to play spontaneously with one theme-related set of toys (e.g., cooking set) at a time. The therapist can verbally prompt the child to enact a familiar script by suggesting, for example, that the child cook dinner for the baby. However, the child should not be coerced into following a script. Prompting is often not necessary because children spontaneously enacts a familiar routine.

While the child plays spontaneously, the examiner should note the child's highest level of spontaneous symbolic play. After approximately 15–20 minutes, the therapist should model[1] for the child levels of symbolic play that exceed those observed in the child's spontaneous play. For example, if the child produces multischemes spontaneously in a "dinner preparation" script but does not demonstrate object substitution and agent play behaviors, the examiner should model a "dinner preparation" script incorporating examples of object substitutions and agent play behaviors.

Following approximately 10 minutes of modeling, the therapist should encourage the child to reenact the play scripts for approximately 15 minutes

---

[1]Modeling is an important procedure in the assessment of symbolic play because research has shown that modeling is effective in eliciting levels of play that are within the child's action repertoire but not necessarily demonstrated in spontaneous play (Fenson, 1984). Additionally, children have been shown to simplify a modeled interaction when the model exceeds their level of conceptual development (Bretherton et al., 1984).

while verbally prompting if necessary. It is at this time that the therapist should observe and record diversity of levels in the child's play schemes, diversity and length of play sequences, and optimal levels of play. Symbolic play sequences are defined as one or more schemes or action units uninterrupted by (1) social interaction; (2) object manipulation or exploratory behavior; (3) shift in focus of activity; and/or (4) unrelated or irrelevant activity. For example, "*child pretends to stir milk in a cup*, then *feeds the baby*, then *feeds mother*" is a symbolic gestural sequence comprised of three schemes. *Recording Data on Protocols*

Developmental levels and other observations can be recorded on the scale assessment form during the evaluation session.[2] A summary form is provided as a quick reference for access to the child's most frequent (modal) and highest (optimal) levels of play. Additionally, the child's general developmental level in four major domains—cognitive domains, decentration (roles), decontextualization (objects), and integration (actions)—can be recorded on the three-scheme dimension summary form. This information can be used as one means for developing intervention objectives that target component actions of pretend play in addition to overall levels of play.

Interpreting Performance Information

The child's developmental play level should be examined relative to his or her chronological age (CA) if the child is not showing signs of having a generalized mental retardation. In cases where a child has mental retardation, performance levels should be examined relative to the child's mental age (MA). However, specific information regarding the child's cognitive status may not be available at the time of testing.

Clinical decisions for language intervention should be based on the child's (1) highest level of symbolic play performance; (2) performance in the domains of objects, actions, and roles; (3) diversity of play schemes; and (4) structural complexity of play schemes. If the child is placed in treatment, scripted play formats should provide the contexts for facilitating both advanced nonverbal symbolic behavior and communication.

Note of Caution

Many contextual variables such as type of props (realistic vs. abstract), degree of modeling, complexity of modeled behavior, and immediate interests and preferences of the child can serve to enhance or depress play performance (Bretherton et al., 1984). For example, the child may perform an object substitution spontaneously but reject a substitution modeled by the therapist. Bretherton et al. (1984) suggested that the therapist attempt

---

[2] All child play behaviors occurring during random play, spontaneous organized play, and postmodeling play can be used to assess play performance.

to determine the child's range of symbolic play abilities in context of various types of play contexts. Such information could provide valuable directions for clinical intervention.

Sources for Scale Development

Bretherton, I. (1984). Representing the social world in symbolic play: Reality and fantasy. In I. Bretherton (ed.), *Symbolic play: The development of social understanding.* Orlando, FL: Academic Press.

Brown, R. (1973) *A first language: the early stages.* Cambridge, Mass.: Harvard University Press.

Bretherton, I., O'Connell, B., Shore, C., & Bates, E. (1984). The effect of contextual variation on symbolic play: Development from 20 to 28 months. In I. Bretherton (ed.), *Symbolic play: The development of social understanding.* Orlando, FL: Academic Press.

Conti-Ramden, G., & Friel-Patti, S. (1986). Situational variability in mother-child conversations. In K. Nelson (ed.), *Children's language* (Vol. 6). New York: Gardner Press.

Fenson, L. (1984). Developmental trends for action and speech in pretend play. In I. Bretherton (ed.), *Symbolic play: The development of social understanding.* Orlando, FL: Academic Press.

Harrison, J., Lombardino, L., & Farrar, J. (1989). *Language comprehension strategies used by young children in scripted-routines.* Unpublished paper.

Largo, R. & Howard, J. (1979). Development progression in play behavior of children between nine and thirty months: Spontaneous play and imitation. *Development Medicine in Childhood Neurology, 21,* 229–316.

Lombardino, L., Stein, J., Kricos, P., & Wolf, M. (1986). Play diversity and structural relationships in the play and language of language-normal preschoolers: Preliminary data. *Journal of Communication Disorders, 19,* 475–489.

McCune-Nicolich, L. (1981). Toward symbolic functioning: Structure of early pretend games and potential parallels with language. *Child Development, 52,* 783–797.

McCune-Nicholich, L., & Fenson, L. (1984). Methodological issues in studying early pretend play. In T. D. Yawkey and A. D. Pellegrini (eds.), *Child's play: Developmental and applied.* Hillsdale, NJ: Lawrence Erlbaum Associates, Inc.

Snow, C., Perman, R., & Nathan, D. (1986). Why routines are different: Toward a multiple factors model of the relation between input and language acquisition. In K. Nelson (ed.), *Children's language* (Vol. 6). New York: Gardner Press.

Terrell, B. Y., & Schwartz, R. G. (1983, November). Symbolic play: Is children's play determined by the objects used? Paper presented at the annual convention of the American Speech-Language-Hearing Association.

Watson, M., & Fisher, K. (1980). Development of social roles in elicited and spontaneous behavior during the preschool years. *Developmental Psychology, 16,* 483–494.

Wolf, D., Rygh, J., and Altshuler, J. (1984). Agency and experiences: Actions and states in play narratives. In I. Bretherton (ed.), *Symbolic play: The development of social understanding.* Orlando, FL: Academic Press.

List of Props

Props for Cooking Theme: Cooking Dinner Script

- Baby doll
- Mother doll
- Father doll
- Bear
- Pots
- Bowls
- Large Wooden Spoon
- Regular spoon
- Pretend food
- Pitcher
- Block
- Box
- Book
- Telephone
- (Use imaginary items, e.g., salt, ice cream, refrigerator)

Props for Grooming Theme: Bathing Baby Script

- Baby doll
- Mother doll
- Father doll
- Bear
- Washcloth
- Shoe box on basin
- Shampoo
- Comb/brush
- Block
- Book
- Telephone
- Mirror
- (Use imaginary items, e.g., hairdryer, towel)

Props for Random Play

- Doll
- Bear
- Legos
- Car
- Toy hammer
- Nesting cups
- Tea set
- Blocks
- Telephone

APPENDIX 5D

Early Communication Checklist*†

Linda J. Lombardino, Ph.D., Jamie B. Stapell, M.A.,

Kenneth J. Gerhardt, Ph.D.

Child's Name _____ Date of Birth _____

Examiner _____ Test Date _____

Reactive Primitive Behaviors (1–3 months)
(Early perlocutionary)

____   Arouses from sleep by sudden noises

____   Startles to unexpected loud noises

____   Looks to or fixates on adult's face

____   Looks to or fixates on inanimate objects

____   Responds to adult's facial expressions and vocalizations (cooing sounds)

____   Smiles during face-to-face interactions

____   Responds differentially to familiar vs. unfamiliar, angry vs. happy, male vs. female voices

Purposeful Primitive Behaviors (4–7 months)
(Late perlocutionary)

____   Begins to make rudimentary head turns toward sound source

____   Searches for sound sources that are out of sight

____   Demonstrates a listening attitude

____   Reaches for an object held out to child or close by

____   Pushes away (or turns body away from) undesired object or event

____   Uses global body movements (vocal/gestural/eye contact) as a means to reinstate a desired activity

---

* Indicate whether behavior was directly observed (d) or reported by parent (p)

† Reprinted from Evaluating Communicative Behaviors in Infancy, by L. J. Lombardino, J. B. Stapell, and K. J. Gerhardt, *Journal of Pediatric Health Care, 1*(5), pp. 240–246, © 1987, with permission from National Association of Pediatric Nurse Practitioners. Reprinted from Evaluating Communicative Behaviors in Infancy, by L. J. Lombardino, J. B. Stapell, and K. J. Gerhardt. *The Lancet, 1*, pp. 240–246, © 1987, with permission from Elsevier.

(continues)

APPENDIX 5D (continued)

____ Responds to familiar phrases to reinstate a desired activity

____ Produces syllable repetitions

Transitional/Instrumental Communicative Behaviors (8–11 months)
(Transition from perlocutionary to illocutionary)

____ Turns to out-of-sight sound sources in the lateral plane

____ Enjoys shaking rattle or noise maker

____ Participates in social games such as pat-a-cake and peek-a-boo

____ Gives an object in response to adult's outstretched hand

____ Uses adult's hand to recreate a spectacle (does not look to adult's face as if to bid for help)

____ Reaches for objects at a distance (does not look back at adult)

____ Engages in "showing off" behaviors

____ Extends arms to be picked up

____ Waves "hi" or "bye" (with prompting from parent)

____ Responds to own name

____ Responds to "no" and a few single words

____ Uses "ma-ma" or "da-da" (void of any real meaning)

Intentional/Conventional Communicative Behaviors (11–14 months)
(Illocutionary)

____ Alerts to telephone ring

____ Looks to the television when certain programs or commercials come on

____ Initiates routine games

____ Spontaneously waves "hi" or "bye"

____ Spontaneously gives objects to adult

____ Spontaneously shows objects to adult

____ Spontaneously points to request objects from adult

____ Spontaneously points to request assistance

____ Shakes head "no" to indicate rejection

___ Uses a few words as performatives (proto-words)

___ Responds to a number of single words (names of family members, names of pets, labels for games or social routines, food-related items)

First Words (14–16 months)
(Locutionary)

___ Localizes to sounds in all planes (left, right, down, up, diagonal)

___ Responds to name when called from another room

___ Uses gestures, varying intonation patterns, and/or words to express a number of communicative functions

___ Draws attention to self

___ Draws attention to objects

___ Requests objects

___ Requests actions or social routines

___ Expresses dislikes or protests

___ Expresses pleasure or surprise

___ Greets

___ Answers

___ Uses a few words to refer to objects, events, actions, attributes, and locations

___ Responds to several words in addition to questions such as "Where's daddy?" and "Where's your nose?"

APPENDIX 5E

Sampler of Frequently Used Tests to Assess Language of Preschoolers (Ages birth–4:11)

Test	Author	Ages	Publisher
AGS Early Screening	Harrison et al.	2:0–6:11 years	AGS
Assessment for Persons Profoundly or Severely Impaired	Connard & Bradley-Johnson (1998)	Birth–8 months	Pro-Ed
Bankson Language Test	Bankson (1990)	3:0–6:11 years	Pro-Ed
Birth to Three Assessment and Intervention System, 2nd ed.	Ammer & Bangs (2000)	Birth–3 years	Pro-Ed.
Boehm—3 Preschool	Boehm (2001)	3:0–5:11 years	Psychological Corporation
Bracken Basic Concept Scale—Revised	Bracken (1998)	2.6–7:11 years	Psychological Corporation
Bracken School Readiness Assessment	Bracken (2002)	2.6–7:11 years	Psychological Corporation
Carolina Picture Vocabulary Test for Deaf and Hearing Impaired Children	Layton & Holmes (1985)	4–11:6 years	Pro-Ed
Childhood Autism Rating Scale	Schopler, Reichler, & Renner	2 years and older	Psychological Corporation
Clinical Evaluation of Language Function—Preschool	Wiig, Secord, & Semel (1992)	3–6 years	Psychological Corporation
Comprehensive Assessment of Spoken Language	Carrow-Woolfolk	3:0–21 years	AGS
Communication and Symbolic Behavior Scales	Wetherby & Prizant (1993)	8–24 months	Brookes
Communication and Symbolic Behavior Scales—Developmental Profile	Wetherby & Prizant (2002)	6–24 months	Brookes
Comprehensive Receptive & Expressive Vocabulary Test, 2nd ed.	Wallace & Hammill (2003)	4:0–89:11 years	Psychological Corporation.

Test	Author	Ages	Publisher
Detroit Tests of Learning Aptitude—Primary, 2nd ed.	Hammill & Bryant	3:0–9:11 years	AGS
Developmental Activities Screening Inventory, 2nd ed.	Fewell & Langley (1984)	Birth–60 months	Pro-Ed
Developmental Assessment of Young Children	Voress & Maddox (1998)	Birth–5:11 years	Pro-Ed
Developmental Indicators for the Assessment of Learning (DIAL-3)	Mardell-Czudnowski & Goldenberg	3:0–6:11 years	AGS
Early Language Milestone Scale, 2nd ed.	Coplan (1993)	Birth–36 months	Pro-Ed
Evaluating Acquired Skills in Communication Revised	Riley (1991)	3 months–8 years	Psychological Corporation
Expressive One-Word Picture Vocabulary Test	Brownell (2000)	2:0–18:11 years	Psychological Corporation
Expressive Vocabulary Test	Williams	2:6–90+ years	AGS
First STEP: Screening Test for Evaluating Preschoolers	Miller (1993)	2:9–6:2 years	Psychological Corporation
Fluharty Preschool Speech and Language Screening Test, 2nd ed.	Fluharty (2000)	3:0–6:11 years	Psychological Corporation
Joliet 3-Minute Pre-School Speech and Language Screen	Kinzler (1993)	2:6–4:6 years	Psychological Corporation
Kaufman Assessment	Kaufman & Kaufman	2:6–12:5 years	AGS
Miller Assessment for Preschoolers	Miller (1982)	2:9–5:8 years	Psychological Corporation
Kaufman Survey of Early Academic & Language Skills	Kaufman & Kaufman	3:0–6:11 years	AGS
Kindergarten Language Screening Test, 2nd ed.	Gauthier & Madison (1998)	3:6–6:11 years	Pro-Ed
MacArthur Communicative Development Inventories	Fenson et al. (2003)	8–30 months	Brookes
Mullen Scales of Early Learning	Mullen	Birth–68 months	AGS

(continues)

APPENDIX 5E *(continued)*

Test	Author	Ages	Publisher
OWLS: Listening Comprehension Scale & Oral Expression Scale	Carrow-Woolfolk	3:0–21:11 years	AGS
The Patterned Elicitation Syntax Test—Revised	Young & Perachio (1993)	3:0–7:5 years	Psychological Corporation
Peabody Picture Vocabulary Test—III	Dunn & Dunn	2:6–90+ years	AGS
Preschool Language Assessment Instrument, 2nd ed.	Blank, Rose, & Berlin (2003)	3:0–5:11 years	Pro-Ed
Preschool Language Scale, 4th ed.	Zimmerman, Steiner, & Pond (2002)	Birth–6:11 years	Psychological Corporation
Receptive-Expressive Emergent Language Scale, 3rd ed.	Bzoch, League, & Brown	Infants & Toddlers	Pro-Ed.
Receptive One-Word Picture Vocabulary Test	Brownell (2000)	2:0–18:11 years	Psychological Corporation
Rice-Wexler Test of Early Grammatical Impairment	Rice & Wexler (2001)	3:0–8 years	Psychological Corporation
Sequenced Inventory of Communication Development-Revised	Hedrick, Prather, & Tobin	4 months–4 years	Pro-Ed
Structured Photographic Expressive Language Test, Preschool	Werner & Kresheck (1983)	3:0–5 years	Psychological Corporation
Test for Auditory Comprehension of Language, 3rd ed.	Carrow-Woolfolk (1999)	3:0–9:11 years	Pro-Ed
Test of Early Reading Ability—Deaf or Hard of Hearing	Reid, Hresko, Hammill, & Wiltshire (1991)	3:0–13:11 years	Pro-Ed
Test for Examining Expressive Morphology	Shipley, Stone, & Sue (1983)	3:0–8 years	Psychological Corporation
Test of Early Language Development, 3rd ed.	Hresko, Reid, & Hammill (1999)	2:0–7:11 years	Pro-Ed

Test	Author	Ages	Publisher
Test of Language Development—Primary, 3rd ed.	Newcomer & Hammill (1997)	4:0–8:11 years	Pro-Ed
Test of Word Finding, 2nd ed.	German (2000)	4:0–12:11 years	Psychological Corporation
Test of Written Language, 3rd ed.	Hammill & Larsen (1998)	3:0–11 years	Psychological Corporation
The Token Test for Children	DiSimoni (1978)	3:0–12 years	Pro-Ed
Utah Test of Language Development, 4th ed.	Mecham (2003)	3:0–9:11 years	Pro-Ed
Vineland Adaptive Behavior Scales	Sparrow, Balla, & Cicchetti	Birth–18:11 years	AGS
Wiig Criterion—Inventory of Language	Wiig (1990)	4:0–13 years	Psychological Referenced Corporation
The Wilson Syntax Screening Test	Wilson (2000)	Pre-K and K	Psychological Corporation

Chapter 6

Treatment of Language Delays and Disorders in Preschool Children

LEARNING OBJECTIVES

After completion of this chapter, the reader will be able to:

1. Differentiate between treatment principles, treatment procedures, and treatment goals and write a language goal for a preschooler with language deficits.

2. List characteristics of the perlocutionary stage, the illocutionary stage, and the locutionary stage with regard to pediatric language development.

3. Explain the functional model of intervention and differentiate between the more traditional model and the functional model.

4. Differentiate between the cycles approach to therapy and focused stimulation as explained by Cleave and Fey.

5. Describe at least four considerations when choosing therapy procedures for a child with a language-based delay or disorder.

6. Explain the evaluative planning process and discuss its role in the treatment sequence.

INTRODUCTION

One of the most important questions a clinician can ask when planning therapy is, "What are the reasons the child communicates?" MacDonald (1989) wrote that children communicate for personal reasons, instrumental reasons, and social reasons. Personal reasons include talking for the child's own physical pleasure and, in infants, babbling just to make sounds. Instrumental reasons include communication that occurs in order to get something to meet a need. Socially, communication is used to comment on the environment and create an exchange of information. As the child matures, the early sounds and gestures are replaced with more advanced symbols of language to produce an effective communicative exchange with another individual. But MacDonald made the important point that instrumental communication does not generalize to social use, but social communication does generalize to instrumental communication. Therefore, it is critical in therapy to emphasize the social uses of language in order to facilitate the communication process.

In this chapter, the reader will not find exact treatment procedures other than illustrative examples. Precise treatment procedures always vary from client to client, so to provide the reader with procedures to use with a specific disorder would be of little value in the long run. However, providing theoretical principles on which to base the decision-making process in treatment gives future clinicians the tools needed to deal with the range of language delays and disorders seen in preschool children.

THE THERAPY ENVIRONMENT

Therapy Emphases Over the Years

Historically, language stimulation activities were created in the context of behavioral paradigms. In the 1960s and 1970s, different techniques such as shaping, fading, modeling or imitation, and reinforcement procedures dominated the literature and provided many of the techniques that are still the foundation for many therapies. However, in the 1990s, the emphasis shifted away from behavioral procedures per se to focus on functional outcomes; that is to say, the goal is communication first, followed by expansion and generalization in the natural environment. Currently, the philosophy of communication first dominates many therapies owing to the possibility of fewer therapy sessions and a reliance on functional outcomes that results from the current emphasis in health care reform. It is important that therapy goals can easily be generalized to the child's natural setting. When a functional model of intervention is used, the child has the opportunity to develop an array of language structures as well as communication skills. This learning is based on spontaneous conversations and social interactions with the child. It is beneficial to conduct the therapy in the child's natural contexts (home and preschool) to facilitate the generalization and maintenance of his or her language skills (Owens, 1999).

Organizing the Therapy Environment

In addition to setting functional goals, a concern when planning therapy is structuring the child's environment to facilitate the growth of his or her language and communication skills. An initial area of attention in this structuring is the concept of sensory integration—how much sensory input can the child tolerate? One way to measure this is to notice how distractible the child is and to monitor the visual and auditory stimulation present when the child is in therapy. Distractions that should be monitored include decorations and furnishings in the room, toys and other therapy materials, noise in the vicinity of the therapy room, and the clinician's attire (which should be conservative and businesslike, but comfortable).

> Sensory integration. The organization and interpretation of input from the various sensory systems of the body.

The diagnostic and therapeutic materials available should be selected carefully to be safe, durable, and appropriate to the goals. When on a budget, it is wise to choose toys that can teach a variety of concepts, such as doll houses, play villages, cooking sets, and doctor kits. Regardless of the materials chosen, however, one of the biggest concerns of the clinician should be to keep the intervention procedures uncomplicated. Procedures should be designed to require minimal input from the clinician, to facilitate maximum responses from the child, and to ease the task of data collection. Schemes that involve role-play with family members and other individuals with whom the child has contact are excellent therapy tools.

Use of Peer Interactions to Facilitate Language Growth

Another consideration in the progression of language intervention is the use of peer interactions to facilitate the development, maintenance, and generalization of language skills by children with language delays or disorders. Until the passage of P.L. 94-142, the concept of least restrictive environment had received little attention in the education of children with handicaps. With subsequent expansion of the original legislation, the passing of P.L. 99-457 and the Individuals with Disabilities Education Act further mandated the inclusion principle as the model for school placement of children with handicapping conditions. As part of inclusion, it has become evident that time needs to be spent teaching the typically developing classmates about the handicaps exhibited by their classmates, as well as strategies the child with handicaps may use to communicate and become socially involved with his or her peers.

think about it

Describe an ideal therapy environment.

Encouraging the Family to Facilitate Language Development

Schemes that reflect daily living situations encountered by the child should be the focus of preschool therapy. It is best to pick a few everyday situations to target in therapy and then encourage the family to generalize the concepts and techniques to other situations at home. Also, by using this approach, follow-through at home is more likely to occur because the suggestions made by the clinician can be used to facilitate language in the routine activities of the family, and anecdotal reports from the family (as opposed to specific data collection, which rarely gets done) are sufficient documentation.

One rule of thumb that can be used is to develop intervention strategies that can be done by the family in the car. Parents spend an inordinate amount of time driving family members hither and yon—and this is a great time to facilitate language development. For example, while sitting at a stop light, parents can encourage the children to look around and find all the things that are red, or that start with the letter *l*. Word games involving rhyming and alliteration can be played while riding in the car. The tried-and-true alphabet game in which children look for letters on license plates, trucks, signs, and billboards can also be done to encourage print awareness. The main instruction to the parent is that the adult's level of language should be equal to or slightly more complex than the child's level. This means the parent provides a reachable example for the child as he or she, the parents, and the clinician work toward the ultimate goal: effective communication at any time and any level.

Parent Involvement in Therapy: A Study by Cleave and Fey (1997)

Cleave and Fey (1997) conducted a study in which there were two groups of preschoolers, with one group receiving clinician-directed intervention only and the other group receiving parent intervention only. All children in the study had expressive language deficits, particularly in the area of morphosyntactic development, but they "were judged to be normally responsive and able to play an assertive role in conversation" (p. 23) with adults. Basic goals were defined as general goals of intervention based on the child's social–interactional skills. For each group, three basic goals of intervention were addressed:

1. To increase the frequency and consistency of the child's use of grammatical forms and operations that typically are used infrequently and inconsistently

2. To foster the child's acquisition of new content–form interactions to perform available conversational acts

3. To set the child's existing language-learning mechanisms in motion to promote the acquisition of general linguistic principles and to foster broad, systematic changes in the child's grammar (p. 23)

In treatment, the first basic goal was based on facilitating consistent use of the child's use of structures used inconsistently before therapy. The second goal focused on teaching the child new morphosyntactic constructions that were not previously in the child's repertoire. The final goal was developed to stimulate the child's existing language-learning processes in hopes of facilitating efficient learning of language beyond the clinical setting. Intermediate and specific goals were also developed for each child in the study. The list of specific goals for each child was quite large, and it was unrealistic to expect that all the goals could be focused on in therapy. Thus, intermediate goals that encompassed a large number of specific goals were developed. It was hoped that this would lead to generalization of the skills learned when the intermediate goals were addressed. Within the context of the intermediate goals, four specific goals were selected for each child. A cyclical goal attack strategy, based on the cycles approach developed by Hodson and Paden (1991) for the treatment of phonological disorders, was incorporated into the treatment, along with focused stimulation procedures. In the cycles approach, the treatment focused on one goal per week for four consecutive weeks (e.g., goal 1 in week 1; goal 2 in week 2; goal 3 in week 3; goal 4 in week 4; goal 1 in week 5). Focused stimulation (Fey, 1986) was also used in the treatment protocol. In the focused stimulation procedures, the basis for intervention was natural conversation between the child and the adult. The child was bombarded with a chosen language form "in a variety of semantically and pragmatically appropriate contexts" (Cleave & Fey, 1997, p. 24). The adult modelled the target behaviors, and the child was encouraged to attempt the target.

As a result of their study, Cleave and Fey (1997) suggested that parents should be actively involved in the clinical process by combining the parent program with the clinic program. Although some parents may gain some knowledge about intervention by observing (as they did in the clinician–directed treatment), it is more beneficial to provide training for the parents to facilitate the learning of language beyond the clinical setting. Within the cycles approach and focused stimulation, sentence recasts helped the child meet the target by providing a model of correct productions that maintained the meaning of the child's utterance while simultaneously correcting or modifying the child's utterance (Cleave & Fey, 1997). All of these strategies enhance the preschool child's mastery of grammatical structures and should be considered when planning an intervention program for preschoolers.

How would you involve parents in the therapy process?

EARLY COMMUNICATION

Successful intervention with preschool children frequently hinges on the clinician's ability to determine if the child is at a presymbolic or a symbolic level of communication and on planning appropriate goals and activities based on the child's level.

Cognitive Skills as Foundations for Facilitating Language

Regardless of the approach a clinician chooses, it is critical that he or she look for basic language parameters that serve as precursors to effective communication skills. These parameters, as outlined in the Ordinal Scales of Psychological Development (Uzgiris & Hunt, 1975), include means-end, turn taking, object permanence, use of gestures, requesting behaviors, joint attention, behavior regulation, play schemes, causality, and imitation skills. All of these skills help us to understand how the child relates to his or her environment, including objects and the people in it. The best success in therapy is when social contact, environmental exposures, and intact maturational systems are in place; these are needed for adequate development of language. As written by Dunst (1980),

the description of the child's sensorimotor performance in *qualitative* terms represents the critical and most important step in the

Symbolic level. Communication in which the individual understands the relationships among words and objects and events (i.e., that the words represent the objects and events).

Language parameters. Aspects of language that form the basis of linguistic functioning.

Means-end. A language parameter in which the child has the ability to use foresight in simple problem solving (e.g., using a dowel to obtain an object that is out of reach).

Joint attention. The sharing of visual and auditory attention to the same stimulus.

Causality. The reactivation of a spectacle or event by bodily movement (e.g., turning the key to have a toy car reactivate).

overall clinical-educational process. Procedures used to describe a child's performance in qualitative terms permit an assessment of the extent to which a child is delayed in development, whether or not a child's pattern of development is typical or atypical (disordered), a determination of a child's major strengths and weaknesses, and an identification of appropriate interventions designed to remediate or ameliorate any delays and/or deficits found. (p. vii)

Child-Centered Therapy

When beginning treatment, it is critical to remember that, regardless of the philosophical approach or the techniques chosen to accomplish the stated goals, the child is at the center of the treatment plan. Teachers and speech-language clinicians are usually highly directive individuals, meaning that they tend to give many directions that require specific responses. Although this may be satisfactory in some settings, therapy that is designed to generate maximum responses and facilitate generalization while keeping the child as the primary focus needs to be more experiential than directive. By nature, most preschoolers are exploratory creatures. However, some children have handicaps that limit their ability to explore their environments and, in turn, restrict the development of language.

In addition, many children with disabilities experience learned helplessness because their caregivers, clinicians, or both anticipate their needs and fulfill them before the child has to communicate them using idiosyncratic or conventional means of expression. Whenever a child's needs are met before he or she expresses them overtly, the child may lose motivation to communicate. However, this can be a problem at the opposite end of the spectrum as well. In some cases, children desperately try to communicate their needs but, due to the idiosyncratic nature of their communication signals, their attempts may not be understood. In these cases, as a child is misinterpreted over time, he or she may give up attempting to initiate communication through conventional methods. The goal is to help this child avoid being frustrated by getting him or her to use more conventional signals to communicate needs and to engage in social exchanges for a range of communicative functions.

For example, a child with many autistic behaviors had a communication system that consisted of a gesture for "eat" and arm movements to signal the clinician to restart a spectacle such as a battery-operated toy. In this case, the adults in his environment imitated these movements, always gave food for the gestural request to eat, and always restarted the toy and paired the child's arm movements with the word "more." By doing so, the clinicians validated the child's two primary attempts at communication. In this case, social contact and environmental manipulation were used to increase the child's communicative attempts, despite his underdeveloped communication signals.

> **Learned helplessness** A state of inaction that a child learns because his or her needs are constantly anticipated by his or her caregivers so that there is little or no need for the child to communicate or initiate communication.

Eventually, meaning was assigned to other movements the child made, and within six months, he had a communicative repertoire of approximately 10 gestures that were used in effective communication exchanges. In his case, his social-emotional development was enhanced through appropriate early intervention.

Interactive Environmental Frameworks

Morris (1982) developed a chart that demonstrates the interactive frameworks that affect speech and language development in children with disabilities (Figure 6-1). The critical message of this framework is that assessment and

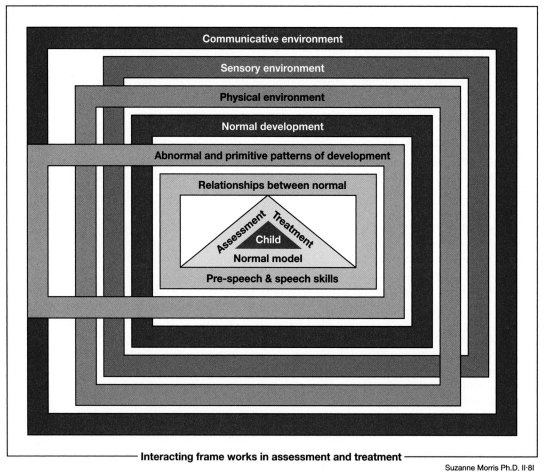

FIGURE 6–1 Interactive frameworks to facilitate communication. (*Source: The normal acquisition of oral feeding skills: Implications for assessment and treatment,* by S. E. Morris. New York: Central Islip. © 1982 by Therapeutic Media, Inc.)

therapy must be child centered and based on the clinician's knowledge of normal development.

As noted previously, the child is at the center of the figure, representing the fact that assessment and treatment are based on the child's abilities and deficits. The next box stresses the relationships among normal prespeech and speech skills. Thus, when studying the sensorimotor stages and social stages of the child's development, a clear correlation is observed among prespeech activities such as gestures, babbling, and jargon and a child's development of normal speech and language patterns.

The third box stresses the importance of looking at abnormal and primitive patterns of development. By doing so, the clinician is able to determine if the child has a delay or a disorder, particularly when considered in the context of the next box, which represents normal development. The outer three boxes emphasize the fact that there must be an analysis and manipulation of the physical, sensory, and communicative environments of the child in order to facilitate growth of speech and language skills. It is particularly important to recognize the fact that the outer box (communicative environment) and the fourth box (normal development) are represented by solid lines, with one break where abnormal and primitive patterns of development interrupt the flow of normal development in the communicative environment. This alerts the clinician to the fact that any abnormal or primitive patterns of development must be eliminated or normalized in order to have complete development of the communicative environment.

> *think about it*
>
> Hypothesize as to why the persistence of abnormal and primitive patterns of development interferes with the development of meaningful, intentional communication.

Social Stages of Development: Considerations in Treatment

Bates, Camaioni, and Volterra (1975) described three social stages of communication development, or pragmatics. The three stages are based primarily on the level of intention that the child demonstrates and on the three functions of the speech act. According to linguists, "*perlocutions* referred to how listeners interpreted the speaker's speech acts; *illocutions* referred to the intentions of the speaker; and *locutions* referred to the meanings expressed in the utterance" (Shulman & Capone, 2010, p. 78).

The first stage, the perlocutionary stage, lasts from birth to 9 months of age. During this time period, children are nonverbal but communicative; however, their communication is unintentional. In this stage, the adult

Perlocutionary stage. The social stage of communication development during which the child is interactive but uses nonverbal and unintentional communication.

assigns meaning to the behaviors of the child. That is to say, the adult interprets the child's smiles, crying, and cooing as if they were intentional communication. Basically, at this stage, the infant has functional communication in that his or her behavior functions as communication even though it is not intentionally goal-directed.

The second stage is the illocutionary stage, which develops around 10 months of age. In this stage, the infant is still nonverbal (he or she does not use any specific words), but the communication efforts are intentional. The infant may use eye gaze, conventional gestures that others would use (e.g., waving "good-bye" and pointing), and vocalizations to convey a message in an organized and coordinated manner. During this stage the use of jargon is noted as the child uses protowords. Protowords are words the child invents that may or may not sound like standard English words Protoimperatives and protodeclaratives also emerge at this stage. Protoimperatives are described by Shulman and Capone (2010) as the "child's use of a means to cause the adult to do something" (p. 145). The protoimperatives represent the child's first attempts to do something for him- or herself (causality). Protodeclaratives are "a preverbal effort to direct the adult's attention to some event or object in the world" (Shulman & Capone, 2010, p. 145). In this stage, the child brings a toy to the adult just to get the adult's interest and attention.

During the third stage, the child starts to use real words, which are primarily nouns and labels. During this locutionary stage, which begins around 12 months of age, the child uses intentional linguistic communication. In the locutionary stage, the child uses conventional words to make things happen. Around 18 months of age, the child combines words and develops an expressive vocabulary of 50 words. However, receptive language (i.e., what the child understands) exceeds expressive language.

Referencing is prerequisite to illocutionary and locutionary behaviors. In referencing, the child uses linguistic means in order to manage and direct the attention of his or her communication partner. That is to say, the child follows the adult's line of regard, searches for the object, then looks at the adult again if he or she does not find the object (Shulman & Capone, 2010).

Referencing is followed in a short time by pointing. When the child points and uses words consistently, he or she can engage in *what* and *where* games. Once a child can reference, he or she can request. There are three types of early requests:

1. Request for an object

2. Invitation or request to an adult to share in play or a game

3. Request for supportive action

Requesting absent objects or requesting help emerges around 18 months. However, in these early stages of requesting, the caregiver has to figure out what object is being requested. Likewise, the caregiver has to figure out what

Illocutionary stage. The social stage of communication development in which the child is interactive and communication efforts are intentional, although some of the communication may still be nonverbal.

Locutionary stage of development. The social stage of communication development during which the child develops intentional, linguistic communication and speech consists primarily of nouns and labels.

the invitation is for when the child wants the adult to participate in his or her ongoing activity. With regard to requests for action, the child attempts to get the adult's ability or skill to help him or her achieve a desired goal. In this instance, the caregiver has to figure out with what the child needs help (Shulman & Capone, 2010).

The implications of the stages of development for therapy are that teaching functional skills, such as pointing to request, that can facilitate communication is key. Knowing the typical developmental progression of intentional communication can facilitate accurate determination of the child's current level and means of communication and help provide a focus in encouraging the child to engage in communicative behaviors.

Although the Bates, et al. model does not explain language acquisition, it does provide a focus on language use that is based on the social interactions between the child and his or her caregiver. It also provides a basis from which to judge if a child may be developing a delay in expressive language. If a child is not using single words by 18 months and is not combining words by 30 months, there is reason to suspect that he or she may have a language deficit.

Again, it is critical to identify children with language deficits early in their development in order to facilitate socially appropriate and effective communication before they become frustrated communicators. In early childhood, the listener provides interpretation of a child's vocalizations and verbalizations to determine the intent of the communicative effort.

Communication Breakdowns

Halle, Brady, and Drasgow (2004) noted that preschoolers with disabilities often have a limited repertoire of communication and social skills. These authors pointed out that a preverbal preschooler who is engaged in an activity but has limited communication skills may begin to cry, with that crying having several possible implications. For example, the child could be bored, frustrated, finished with the activity, requesting another task, lonely, and/or needing attention. It is up to the listener to interpret the cry and respond appropriately. Incorrect interpretation leads to a communication breakdown and the need for the child to initiate a communication repair strategy to meet his or her needs. "Hence, it is important to carefully consider variables affecting communication breakdowns as well as strategies that may be effective in facilitating communication success following a breakdown" (pp. 43–44).

Halle, Brady, & Drasgow (2004) identify three types of communication breakdowns: (1) requests for clarification, (2) nonacknowledgments, and (3) topic shifts. Brady (2003) presented some preliminary data that indicate that when faced with a communication breakdown, beginning communicators are more likely to respond positively to requests for clarification (e.g., the listener asking "What?" or "Do you mean . . . ?") than they do to nonacknowledgments and topic shifts. Nonacknowledgement refers to the listener's lack of response to the child's attempt at communication, which does not adequately communicate to the child that he or she needs to use a repair strategy in order to get a response. Whether the lack of acknowledgment is intentional or not, the child's communication effort is not reinforced, which may lead to frustration, lack of motivation to communicate, and fewer attempts to communicate in the future.

Topic shifts may be an attempt to distract the child from his or her original effort to communicate. Once again, this is a communication breakdown because the child does not achieve his or her communicative goal or intent. Sometimes a topic shift occurs because the listener chooses not to honor the child's request and wishes to distract the child. If the distraction is equally desirable to the child (e.g., the parent offers a cup of juice when the child requested milk), then the child will not be motivated to implement a repair strategy. In other instances, it is possible that the child does not desire the intended outcome enough to make the effort to engage in a repair strategy.

> **think about it**
>
> How would you teach a child to resolve the three types of communication breakdowns: requests for clarification, nonacknowledgments, and topic shifts?

Generally speaking, there are two types of repair: repetition and modification. When using repetition, the initiating communicator simply repeats verbatim the original signal. Modifications can consist of additions (adding information to the original signal), reductions (omitting information in the original communication), and substitutions (providing information in place of any of the original signal) (Halle, Brady, & Drasgow, 2004; Brady & Halle, 2002; Wetherby, Alexander, & Prizant, 1998). Halle and colleagues (2004) listed five factors that determine the response efficiency of the child's communication:

1. Response effort

2. Immediacy of obtaining the desired outcome

3. Consistency of obtaining the desired outcome

4. Quality or magnitude of outcome

5. History of punishment—"any likelihood that reduces the likelihood of the response" (p. 46) such as screaming or throwing materials

All of these factors together help determine what repair strategies the child attempts as well as affecting his or her motivation to continue a communicative exchange. Clearly, the environment plays a significant role in the use of repair strategies and in maintaining a child's desire to communicate.

FUNCTIONAL COMMUNICATION

Later in this chapter we discuss functional goals, defined as those that have meaningful use in the child's natural environment. Functional communication follows the same line of thought in that it is child-centered, child-directed communication in the natural environments of the child. The focus of the therapy is on the process of communicating instead of on isolated goals and skills. Owens (1995) listed five dimensions of communication context: cognitive context, social context, physical context, linguistic context, and nonlinguistic context.

Cognitive context refers to information the communication partners share about their physical surroundings. Essentially, it is factual information about the physical world shared by the communication partners. Social context consists of content about the communication partner, the setting in which the communication occurs, and the rules of engagement practiced by each partner in the communication exchange. Owens (1995) defines the physical context as "each partner's perceptions of people, places, and objects that form the context....Intervention can occur in everyday settings in which training targets are likely to occur" (p. 10). Linguistic features are those that surround verbalizations, primarily emphasizing language form and grammar. Nonlinguistic context, along with paralinguistic features, refers to aspects of communication that are not formal language but are important in the comprehension and expression of one's thoughts in a communicative exchange. This includes such things as intonation, posturing, gestures, and facial expressions (Nicolosi, Harryman, & Kresheck, 2004, p. 225).

> **think about it**
>
> Using child-centered therapy is a proven approach to pediatric language intervention. How would you respond to a parent's saying, "It looks like you are just playing with him"?

THERAPEUTIC PRINCIPLES AND PROCEDURES

Therapeutic Principles

With the development of a scientific approach to assessment and treatment of communication disorders, it has become abundantly clear that learning is not a random process. Rather, learning to be an effective communicator is the result of an organized, data-based program designed to capitalize on strengths to improve deficits. Succinctly put, a therapy program is formulated to delineate the principles and procedures that will be used to achieve the therapy objectives.

Principles. Summary statements of experimental evidence that provide the rules from which treatment procedures are developed.

Principles form the theoretical basis of a therapy program. Principles are conceptual in nature and are relatively broad based compared to procedures. For example, a principle could be how the clinician approaches therapy. A clinician may choose to do either within-discipline therapy, interdisciplinary therapy, or transdisciplinary therapy. Which principle is selected depends on the clinician's philosophy about the need to interact with other professionals treating a client. In within-discipline therapy, the clinician does not interact with other professionals (physical therapy, occupational therapy, social work, nursing, education) who are working with the client. In the interdisciplinary approach, the clinician works within his or her own discipline but participates in regular (usually weekly) meetings with other professionals for the purpose of sharing information about the client's progress in the varying programs of intervention. The transdisciplinary approach takes the interdisciplinary approach a step farther in that the clinicians all learn the various therapy programs a patient is undergoing and incorporate information and procedures from all programs into each therapeutic discipline (see Figure 6–2). Table 6–1 provides an example of combining therapy goals from speech-language pathology, occupational therapy, and physical therapy.

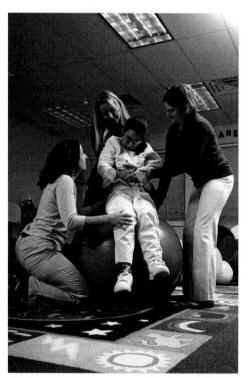

FIGURE 6–2 In the transdisciplinary model, therapists and educators provide co-treatment for children with multiple disabilities. (*Delmar/Cengage Learning*)

TABLE 6-1   Model of a transdisciplinary goal

Physical Therapy Goal: The child will exhibit a protective righting response while on the ball in 8 of 10 attempts.

Physical Therapy Procedures:

1. Place child on stomach on large ball.
2. While holding onto the child's feet, roll the child forward.
3. Have assistant assist the child in extending his or her arms and placing the palms on the floor as if breaking a fall.
4. Roll the child back toward the clinician and repeat the procedure.

Language Therapy Goal: In 8 of 10 trials, the child will choose the correct item from an array of three when asked to select an item based on a description of its function.

Language Therapy Procedures:

1. An array of three items, each with a different function (eat, play, dress, write), will be placed in front of the child.
2. When the function of one of the items is described, the child will select the intended object and give it to the clinician.

Occupational Therapy Goal: The child will use a pincer grasp when picking up objects on 90% of all trials.

Occupational Therapy Procedures:

1. The child will imitate a model of bringing the tips of the index finger and thumb together.
2. The child will pick up a small object using a pincer grasp.

Transdisciplinary Procedures:

1. While on the ball, the child will demonstrate a protective righting response as he or she is rolled forward.
2. As the child extends arms and hands, he or she will select the designated object using a pincer grasp.

Delmar/Cengage Learning

Therapy Goals

The choice of goals is affected by many of the same questions that were answered during the testing portion of the process. One of the determinants of a goal is whether the child is exhibiting a language delay, a language disorder, or a language difference. If the child has a language delay, the focus should be on determining where the child is developmentally with regard to language competence and language performance, and then moving on

Code switching. The ability of an individual to switch dialects or languages depending on the communicative situation.

from that point through a normal progression of language acquisition. If the child is displaying a language disorder, the focus shifts to getting rid of the abnormal behaviors and replacing them with language behaviors that would normally be observed in developing children. Finally, if the child has a language difference, therapy, if provided, concentrates on structuring the environment in such a way as to facilitate the development of both languages and to teach the child to code switch. Code switching is the adjustment of a person's use of a language or dialect to the setting at hand.

Other factors that affect the choice of goals are the severity of the delay or disorder and the presence of organic factors in the etiology. Obviously, the more severe a disorder, the greater the challenge for the clinician. If the child's insurance or Medicaid coverage requires limitations in the number of visits that can be made, this is an additional area of concern. If the child has severe limitations in language, enlisting the support of his or her significant others is critical in structuring the environment so that language learning and use are facilitated on a daily basis. Of course, structuring the environment is important regardless of the level of the severity of the communication and/or language deficit, but as the severity increases, the need for environmental structuring also increases. In addition, certain etiological factors may present obstacles the clinician cannot change that could affect progress. In these cases, it is important to work with interdisciplinary or transdisciplinary teams and the family to facilitate progress and provide opportunities that the child can use to learn despite any etiological factors. For example, if a child has severe oral-motor problems, the likelihood of using speech as a primary communication mode is lessened. The use of an augmentative system may be of paramount importance to help the child be an effective communicator. The timing of the introduction of an augmentative system and the development of a system a child can use in light of other disabling conditions are crucial.

Goals, or objectives, can be long term or short term. Long-term goals are more general in expression than are short-term goals. The long-term goal or objective is broadly expressed in terms of the overall therapy program. For example, a long-term objective may be "improve auditory comprehension" or "increase lexicon." Short-term objectives reflect the specific behavior or skill to be achieved. For example, relating to the long-term goal of improving auditory comprehension, a short-term goal could be "Joseph will accurately answer five questions based on a passage read to him with no prompts with at least 60 percent accuracy for three consecutive sessions." With regard to increasing lexicon, a short-term goal could be "Nicholas will correctly identify 10 common objects presented in context with no prompts with 90 percent accuracy for three consecutive sessions." Typically, short-term objectives have a time specification, whereas long-term objectives are more open ended. Also, short-term objectives should form a sequence of increasing difficulty as a progression toward accomplishment of the long-term objective.

Determination of the child's cognitive level is important. This may be more complex than it appears because the lack of ability to use language effectively can be misinterpreted as a cognitive problem instead of a language problem. Thorough and careful analysis of a child's psycho-educational abilities is critical in determining the long-term goals for a child with multiple deficits.

As said before, goals should be functional; that is, they should have meaningful use in the child's daily routines. This is discussed further in the section later in this chapter on therapy for children with cognitive challenges. Another meaning of *functional* is that each goal serves as a foundation for the next goal. One can envision a flight of stairs in which one must conquer a lower step to reach a higher step. The same concept applies to foundational goals with a gradual increase in the physical, sensory, and cognitive complexity of the objectives as the child progresses toward the final goal.

> **think about it**
>
> Brainstorm some ideas of functional goals for a 3-year-old child who has a receptive language delay of approximately 12 months and is at the single-word level with regard to production.

Therapy Procedures

In contrast to principles, procedures are concrete, measurable, and objective. It is also important that they be replicable, which means that another clinician could implement the plan with results similar to those obtained by the original clinician. Procedures can be thought of as clinical activities based on the experimental evidence that forms the foundation outlined in the principles (Hegde, 1995). Another difference between procedures and principles is that principles are generic, whereas procedures are written specific to the client, the disorder, or both (Hegde, 1995).

When choosing which treatment procedures to use, the clinician should keep in mind the six questions outlined in Table 6–2. The first question addresses the issue of whether or not the technique has been evaluated in a controlled setting. One of the major concerns of the profession relates to the need to have experimental evidence on the abilities of the procedures to create a positive, functional outcome. To gather the data, more structured clinical research is required to evaluate experimentally the procedures used in speech-language therapy. Tied closely to this first question is the second question, which addresses the issue of whether or not the evaluation of the procedures was favorable. In other words, has the evidence from controlled research settings in therapy yielded a positive outcome for the patients?

A third critical question relates to the replicability issue: Can the procedures be used by different clinicians in different settings with results similar

Procedures. Concrete, measurable, and objective clinical activities based on the experimental evidence that forms the foundation for therapy outlined in the principles.

TABLE 6–2 Questions to answer in the selection of treatment procedures

Has the technique been evaluated experimentally?

Have the results been favorable?

Has the technique been replicated across settings, clinicians, and clients?

Is the procedure appropriate for this client?

Can the environment be manipulated to implement the procedure?

Is my client improving?

Delmar/Cengage Learning

to those obtained in the experimental evaluation? A procedure that works only under highly controlled circumstances that cannot be readily replicated in other settings should not be considered part of a clinician's repertoire of therapy procedures.

In some cases, as the fourth question shows, the procedures may be replicable, but they may not necessarily be appropriate for the client. For example, if a piece of equipment is required to use the procedure and the clinician does not have that equipment available, it is not a procedure that can be duplicated in that circumstance with that particular client. Another example is the teaching of eye contact to children of Native American descent. Native American culture teaches children that it is disrespectful to have eye contact with elders. However, a clinician may identify this as a goal for a Native American child. Procedures to teach eye contact are well documented, yet they would be inappropriate as a goal for many Native American children.

The fifth question relates to the clinical environment in which the procedure is being used. Procedures that require a child's total attention would not be appropriate procedures to use in most hospital units for children owing to the presence of other stimulations inherent in that environment. Some activities require more space than others and thus would be impractical to implement in a small therapy room.

Of all the questions, the sixth question is without doubt the most important. A client may fail to progress for many reasons, but one of the easiest to rule out is the choice of incorrect procedures. A common mistake made by beginning (and some experienced) clinicians is to choose a procedure that is too difficult for a child. This often occurs because the clinician has not carefully analyzed the task at hand. Task analysis is a critical clinical tool that must be mastered in order to choose correct procedures. In a task analysis, the clinician works through a task step by step, ensuring that the child has the skills necessary to master the procedure. For example, many sequencing activities require an intact short-term memory. Thus, if a child is unable to remember a simple sequence, he or she cannot be expected to succeed on a task that requires remembering one step before another.

Regardless of the principles and procedures selected by the clinician, the overall goal in therapy is to increase the number of options available to the client to help him or her reach his or her maximum potential. For a 3-year-old preschooler who does not talk, therapy should not focus solely on getting the child to talk. Rather, therapy should concentrate on teaching the child to communicate in some manner, whether by speech, gestures, sounds, sign language, or a communication board. Speech should be modeled in all communication exchanges, but it should not be the sole focus of therapy. Otherwise, it is possible the child will become extremely frustrated and shut down on all communicative attempts. It is important to remember that all children learn to communicate by exploring the use of a variety of systems—cognitive, sensory, and motor—before adapting to the most common form—speech. Clinicians do not help the child by demanding only one form of communication. Children learn speech and language by exploring their environment through a myriad of sensory and motor experiences. Thus, for children functioning below the age level of 24 months, it is critical to guide a child through a variety of sensorimotor experiences to facilitate the neurological maturation needed for effective communication.

Going with the Flow

Another common mistake made by beginning clinicians is not tempering the demand for therapeutic compliance with some flexibility as opportunities present themselves in the clinical setting. A clinician was observed teaching a 3-year-old child the concept of *over* and *under*. The activity required the child to sit in a chair at the table and to identify *over* and *under* on a series of illustrations (a questionable approach with a 3-year old). After doing about 10 cards, the child slid out of his seat and took refuge under the table. The clinician was so determined to complete the task with the illustrations that she completely missed the opportunity to use the fact that the child was *under* the table to reiterate and demonstrate the concept being taught! Children are playful creatures who present clinicians with many opportunities to teach a variety of concepts. It is critical for clinicians not to miss these incidental learning opportunities by adhering to a rigid lesson plan.

THE CLINICIAN–CLIENT INTERACTION

Rapport

In order to set appropriate goals or target behaviors, time must spent on developing the clinician–client interaction. A crucial element is rapport, which is described by Hegde (1995) as "a harmonious connection." Rapport consists of mutual respect and a level of trust between the client and the clinician. It is frequently established through small talk in which the clinician spends time learning about the client as a person. In the process of taking a case history,

Rapport. A harmonious connection between two individuals based on mutual respect and a level of trust.

TABLE 6–3 Elements of rapport (RAPPORT)

Respect: to hold in mutual regard the roles the child, the family, and the clinician play in addressing the communication deficit

Admiration: to hold in esteem the families' efforts to facilitate language and communication in their child

Participation: to develop a therapy program that empowers the child and the family to be active participants in the diagnostic and therapeutic processes

Professional Interaction: to maintain a professional, yet personal, level of interaction with the child and family

Opportunity: to go with the flow and take advantage of situations that present themselves in accordance with the therapy procedures and goals

Restraint: to be less directive and more accommodating of the child's language and communication efforts, thereby encouraging active participation in therapy

Timing: to be cognizant of a family's readiness to receive and accept the fact that their child may have a communication deficit

Delmar/Cengage Learning

the clinician should interject questions that help him or her understand the child as a person, not as a diagnostic and/or therapy case. These questions should include such information as the child's favorite toys, special activities that the child enjoys, whether he or she enjoys books, and other such questions. Above all, the parents of a preschool child need to trust the clinician, who is responsible for telling them if their child has a problem and what can be done about the problem. If a level of respect and trust has not been established, most likely the family will not return to the clinician for intervention.

Another critical element in establishing rapport is the clinician's enthusiasm. No client wants to spend a therapy session with a clinician who is not enthusiastic about his or her work. If clinicians think back over their educational careers, certain teachers stand out as favorites who taught the student in a meaningful and effective manner. Most of these teachers could be described as being enthusiastic about their task. As speech-language pathologists, we deal with many different types of children and families, but the basic skills with regard to establishing a rapport with the child and his or her family remain the same. Actually, the word *rapport* can be described using an acronym, as outlined in Table 6–3.

> **think about it**
>
> What are some ways a clinician could entice a shy, reticent child to interact with him or her?

Analyzing the Child's Temperament

When dealing with the preschool population, clinicians must understand the biological foundations for the behaviors the child exhibits and appreciate how they influence the provision of treatment for a communication deficit. Table 6-4 delineates nine areas that should be considered when analyzing a client's temperament in preparation for therapy.

Activity Level

It is normal for preschoolers to move about and fidget as part of their attempts to explore their world and determine where they fit into the broad picture of life. Beginning clinicians should spend time in a preschool setting to learn about the wide ranges of activity that occur in the process of normal growth and development. This understanding keeps many children from having their normal activity levels diagnosed as hyperactivity. Children need to move around, and therapy should be structured to accommodate that need.

TABLE 6–4   Nine areas of assessment when determining a client's temperament

Category	Description
Activity level	The degree to which the child moves around
Rhythmicity	The child's regularity with regard to sleep patterns, eating, and bowel and bladder functions
Approach or withdrawal	The reaction of the child to any new stimulus, including people, food, places
Adaptability	The child's ability to adapt to a new situation even if the initial response was withdrawal
Intensity of reaction	The child's tendency to scream or whimper when hungry, and shriek with laughter or smile when amused
Threshold of responsiveness	The degree of sensitivity to environmental stimuli and to changes in the environment
Quality of mood	The child's overall disposition, whether pleasant and friendly or grumpy and unfriendly
Distractibility	The ease with which the child can be interrupted in an ongoing activity
Attention span and persistence	The length of time a child pursues an activity or persists despite interruptions

Source: Adapted from *Applied behavior analysis for researchers*, by P. A. Alberto and A. C. Troutman. Columbus, OH: Merrill. Copyright 1986. Merrill Publishing Company.

Rhythmicity

The body has a normal heart rate of about 60 beats a minute, or one per second. Children who have not developed a normal body rhythm, as explained in the discussion of babies suffering the effects of drug and alcohol abuse, need special consideration in developing this rhythm. If an infant is having difficulty coordinating sucking and swallowing, simply patting the baby at a rate of one pat per second can provide external control that, through consistent and persistent application, leads to the establishment of an internal rhythm. This is important because if a child is trying physiologically to determine a normal rhythm, he or she has little energy left to learn the use and power of communication and language.

Approach or Withdrawal

Some children are easily separated from their parents; others are not. To fully participate in therapy activities, a child must learn to separate physically and emotionally from his or her parents. In this category of functioning, the clinician also should analyze carefully how a child reacts to the introduction of new environments and new stimuli. If a clinician is in a facility with several different therapy rooms, he or she may find that a child reacts negatively to being seen in a therapy room other than the one in which therapy is typically received. Other children may need a gradation in presentation of stimuli because they are physiologically incapable of handling multiple stimulations. Generally, approach is considered to be a positive response and withdrawal a negative one (Leith, 1984).

Intensity of Reaction

Along with observing approach or withdrawal of the child, the clinician needs to determine the child's threshold of responsiveness. Is the child reticent in the presence of strangers or in the presence of known adults making specific demands for responses? Is the child overly responsive, which may interfere with his or her attention span on a given task? It is important to be able to "read" the child to determine if he or she is anxious or relaxed about the tasks. The quality of the child's mood is greatly affected by his or her level of reaction to novel and familiar settings and stimuli. Children who are under-responsive or overly responsive may have difficulty exhibiting the persistence and attention span needed to complete a task. All humans, including children, have a level of responsiveness beyond which they cannot be pushed without negative ramifications. The child's temperament needs to be evaluated carefully so the clinician can obtain maximum responses in the therapy setting.

Adaptability

Adaptability is defined as an individual's ability to adjust to new or changing circumstances (Guralnik, 1968). By carefully studying the child's approach and withdrawal systems and the intensity of his or her reactions, the clinician can determine how adaptable a child is. The child's adaptability relies in part on the clinician's ability to motivate the child.

Motivation

Success in therapy cannot occur if the clinician is unable to motivate the child. Motivation is affected by receiving the cooperation of significant others, carefully grading the environmental support and reinforcers for communication attempts, and using the proper contingencies in a variety of settings.

Cause and Effect

A good clinician always thinks in terms of cause-and-effect relationships. Every behavior has a cause, and every behavior has an effect. The question that begs an answer in therapy is how the causes create the desired or undesired effects. For example, if a child has a low sensory threshold, the clinician needs to present stimuli carefully to encourage desired responses. If the child reacts by withdrawing from the stimulus, the cause of this withdrawing needs to be analyzed carefully. Is it a matter of offering too much stimulation in too short a period of time? Is the stimulus too complex for the child to tolerate? Does the stimulus demand a reaction from physiological levels that the child has not fully integrated? Addressing these questions adequately can lead to a better understanding of the causes of the child's responses and lead to more effective therapy planning.

Quality of Mood

Quality of mood is closely related to approach and withdrawal. Is the child excited about attending therapy? Is the child friendly (positive approach) or unfriendly (negative approach or withdrawal)? Is the child grumpy or in a bad mood? All of us have days when we would rather be doing something else, but with maturity comes the ability to alter our mood to the situation at hand. When a child is not in the mood to participate in the therapy activities, it may be necessary for the clinician to alter the lesson plan to facilitate the child's participation. This is part of the "going with the flow" approach mentioned previously.

Distractibility, Attention Span, and Persistence

All of us are distractible under certain conditions, but how well we learn is affected by our ability to attend to and participate in the activities that should be dominating us at any given time. A child with attention deficit disorder has difficulty prioritizing events in the environment in such as way that he or she can stay attuned to the important stimuli and minimize his or her attention to the distracters. For example, a child sitting in a classroom may have difficulty paying attention to the teacher if there is noise on the playground outside the classroom window. The distractible child gives more energy and focus to the extraneous noise than to the primary stimulation being provided by the teacher. More information on this topic can be found in Chapter 8.

THE TREATMENT SEQUENCE

The Evaluative-Planning Process

The treatment sequence consists of two major portions: the evaluative-planning process and the clinical process. The evaluative-planning process includes the evaluation of the client and the determination of behavioral change goals. The clinical process, or what is more commonly referred to as therapy, consists of establishing and habituating the new skills, then generalizing the skills to the client's natural environment (Leith, 1984).

Therapy. The process of establishing and habituating new skills, then generalizing the skills to the client's natural environment.

Evaluate the Client

It cannot be stressed enough that evaluation is the first step of the therapeutic process. It is through a careful analysis of the evaluation results that the clinician makes decisions about the goals, procedures, and principles for the therapy. During the evaluative-planning process, four issues need to be addressed (Table 6–5). Describing the nature of the problem includes identifying whether the child is exhibiting a delay, a disorder, or a difference with regard to language and communicative functioning. Within each category, the current level of functioning the child exhibits should be described. In infants and toddlers this is frequently done in terms of the stages of social communication and sensorimotor development (see additional information in Chapter 5). For the preschool child (age 3 to 4 years old), the child's communication skills are described relative to stages of typical development in expressive and receptive language acquisition.

Defining the severity of the problem is a second critical purpose in the evaluative planning process. The clinician first offers a description of the child's abilities and deficits. In defining the severity of the problem, the clinician applies objective measures to determine how much of a delay is present or how severe a disorder the child exhibits when compared with a normative sample. In other words, the description is based on observation, and judgments on the severity can be based on normative samples.

TABLE 6–5 Four purposes of the evaluative-planning process

1. To describe the nature of the problem
2. To define the severity of the problem
3. To determine the etiology (cause), if possible
4. To make recommendations

Source: Adapted from information in *Handbook of clinical methods in communication Disorders*, by W. R. Leith, 1984. Clifton Park, NY: Delmar, Cengage Learning.

A third purpose of the evaluative-planning process is to identify the etiology, if possible. As discussed thus far, etiologic information is sometimes required to determine if a child is expected to progress or regress, and possibly it is needed to place a child into treatment. Procedural and fiscal needs often dictate the identification of the etiology; thus this information should be obtained whenever possible.

The final purpose of the evaluative-planning process is to make recommendations with regard to treatment. This step entails recommending whether or not therapy should be initiated and defining specific areas of concentration for the therapy program if needed.

Determine Behavioral Change Goals

As already explained, goals are based on the results of the evaluation. One of the questions that needs to be answered in determining goals is, "What does the child need to be able to communicate successfully in his or her environment?" The answer to this question should help determine the mode or method of communication the child will use. Will he or she be taught to rely on speech, or will he or she use an augmentative or alternative communication strategy? In light of the answer to this question, a second important question is, "What skills is the child currently demonstrating?" If the child has an effective gestural system, it may be beneficial to increase the use of gestures while encouraging the child to vocalize with each gesture. Over time, it would be hoped that the vocalizations could be shaped into appropriate words.

A third question in determining goals is, "How do you facilitate the child's use of the newly learned skill in his or her natural environment?" This is the step in which the support of the child's caregivers is critical. No child is going to develop into an effective language user in one hour of therapy per week. The natural environment must be structured to facilitate language exploration and use.

Set Up an Environment to Facilitate Language

In actuality, the child learns in three different environments. First, incidental teaching occurs in his or her daily living. Incidental teaching is done by the caregivers and the clinician as the child presents opportunities to reinforce a language concept. A second environment is the formal therapy setting, in which the clinician plays the primary role in facilitating the child's growth in receptive and expressive language skills. The third teaching strategy based on environment is stimulation in contrived settings, which is followed through by the clinician and the caregivers in formal and informal circumstances.

In all cases, regardless of whether the child has a language delay, disorder, or difference, and regardless of the severity, synergy must occur between therapy and everyday contexts in the child's family and educational settings.

As expressed by Owens (1995), "language facilitators should be trained to recognize the communicative intentions of the child's behaviors, to implement the training program, and to assess functionality and practicality of intervention methods, materials, and adaptations" (p. 119). Success hinges on the ability of everyone in the child's natural environment to recognize opportunities to stimulate language and to structure the environment to facilitate language learning opportunities.

As mentioned previously, therapy should target functional communication. One way to do this is to focus on everyday situations that the child encounters. Through doing this, the clinician can address the aspects of language that are necessary to function in those situations. To facilitate generalization of these skills, the clinician should provide therapy in the child's natural settings whenever possible and educate the caregivers on how to encourage the child to incorporate his or her new knowledge into daily life activities and encounters.

Factors That Interfere with Achieving Therapy Goals

Many years ago I read a statement that has guided my therapy with children who have developmental disabilities. I do not remember the source, but the statement was, "The ultimate goal is to increase the number of options the child can employ to communicate effectively." However, there are several factors that can interfere with achieving the ultimate goal. One is that many clinicians find it difficult to implement child-centered therapy. These clinicians are more comfortable with a lesson plan, organized activities, and being in charge. All of these are counterproductive when implementing child-centered therapy. There are still principles, procedures, and goals, but the difference is that everything is geared toward functionality and letting the child teach us what is important for him or her to interact effectively in his or her daily environments. Another interfering factor is that the child may not be motivated. Sometimes this is due to physical health issues that keep the child from being fully engaged in the therapy. Lack of motivation may be due to emotional impacts of events in the child's life (i.e., death of a family member, abuse, lack of a nurturing home environment). Yet another factor to be considered is that one-third of the homeless population consists of families, so issues of poverty and lack of structure may impact a child's resources that can be used to facilitate the development of communication and language skills. Finally, lack of support from the child's family and other caregivers, such as day-care providers, can interfere with achieving the goals of therapy.

Families

It is absolutely essential to get the family involved in treatment. They are with the child more than the clinician is, so they must be involved if therapy goals are to be met. Family education is critical. This includes educating the family about the delay or disorder that is affecting their child in addition to involving them in clinical decision making. The family should be taught about incidental teaching, learning how to take advantage of opportunities the child presents them to expand language and communication abilities. The family also needs to be instructed on how to structure the environment to stimulate language and communication, and particularly how to teach the child to initiate communication exchanges and not always be a responder.

How could a clinician involve a child's siblings in their brother or sister's therapy?

Efforts to Modify the Environmental Factors of Poverty

Many poor children come from disorganized, unregulated worlds and fail when put into an overly structured school system (Polakow, 1993). During his presidential administration, Lyndon Baines Johnson declared a war on poverty as part of his vision of a "Great Society." In 1965, The Equal Opportunity America program funded the Head Start program in hopes that the provision of cognitive enrichment programs would lead to higher IQs and fewer special education placements for elementary school–age children. The Head Start program differed from other similar programs because it was holistic in its approach, consisting of four components: education, health, nutrition, and social services (parent education) (Polakow). Another major difference between this initiative and others with similar goals was that the programs were justified "in terms of avoidance of future economic costs, rather than on positive humanitarian grounds" (Polakow, p. 101). That is to say, the justification was that, through participation in Head Start, children were less likely to need expensive special education placements once they attained school age. In addition, when children are ready to start school by age 5 years, they are more likely to have successful experiences, which helps ensure that fewer drop out as they progress through the educational system.

What concepts could be stimulated and taught in the produce section of the grocery store?

The Clinical Process

Throughout the clinical process, the clinician is assisting the client in developing new skills. A *skill* is defined as a sequence of responses. The responses are learned through the coordination of various sensory and motor systems that are eventually organized into complex response chains (Hegde, 1995).

Skill. A sequence of responses that are learned through the coordination of various sensory and motor systems and are eventually organized into complex response chains.

Effective therapy occurs only if the clinician and the child understand the relationship between the stimulus presented by the clinician, the response of the child, and the consequence (positive or negative reinforcement) offered by the clinician. The child has to understand that, when a stimulus is presented, he or she is expected to integrate his or her own knowledge to respond appropriately.

Development of New Skills

In teaching a new skill, a logical sequence must be followed. In actuality, a skill is taught in three different stages: the cognitive stage, the fixation stage, and the autonomous stage (Hegde, 1995).

The Cognitive Stage The cognitive stage is also referred to as the acquisition stage because it is the stage at which the child acquires the new skills. Therapy begins as the clinician introduces the goals and procedures to the client. During this stage, the clinician provides information using several different techniques, and the client demonstrates the behavior in response to the techniques and stimuli presented by the clinician. During this stage, the clinician should be aware of the prompting hierarchy outlined in Figure 6–3. At the beginning of the therapy, the clinician may find it necessary to offer physical assistance by actually guiding the child through the expected responses. For example, a clinician may offer an array of three items (stimuli), such as a toy truck, a spoon, and a shirt, and then ask the child to choose the item he or she uses to eat. If the child does not point to the desired item, the clinician could offer verbal assistance by offering a verbal prompt such as, "I eat soup with a spoon. Show me spoon." If the child does not respond correctly, the clinician could offer visual assistance such as moving the spoon a little closer to the child

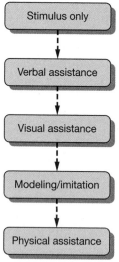

FIGURE 6–3 The prompting hierarchy. (*Delmar/Cengage Learning*)

than the foil items or pretending to use a spoon to eat. Lack of an appropriate response after visual assistance could indicate the need for modeling the desired response. If the child is physically capable of reaching for the spoon but does not, the clinician may model the behavior by pointing to the spoon and having the child imitate the response. If the child still points to the wrong item, the clinician could gently guide the child through the act of pointing to or selecting the spoon. It is important that the clinician move through the prompting hierarchy as quickly as possible so that the child does not come to rely on the clinician's assistance to make the correct response.

The Fixation Stage Otherwise known as the proficiency stage, the purpose of the fixation stage is to stabilize the new skills in the clinical setting. During this stage, the clinician fades out the consequences with the assumption that the use of the new skills provides its own reinforcement. The client works at habituating the new behavior by practicing and perfecting the skill in a controlled clinical setting. The goal is for the client to continue the performance of the new skills after the contingencies have been withdrawn. This is one of the most difficult stages of therapy.

Clinical activities during the fixation stage include varying the stimuli presented to elicit the response, varying the conditions under which the response occurs, and varying the presenter of the stimulus. This is a good time to bring in the caregivers and have them assume the role of the clinician so that the next stage of therapy, the autonomous stage, is facilitated.

The Autonomous Stage Also known as the maintenance stage, the autonomous stage is the phase of therapy in which the goal is getting the new behavior to occur in the client's everyday settings. The client generalizes the skill to make it functional in all settings.

Specific Therapy Procedures Based on a Behavioral Paradigm

Physical Assistance During the cognitive stage of therapy, the clinician can utilize a variety of therapy procedures borrowed from the psychology literature for addressing the creation of new skills. With children, frequently the first step is to have the clinician physically guide the child through making the correct choice from a myriad of stimuli (see Figure 6–3).

Modeling and Imitation A second type of intervention is modeling and imitation. In this approach, the clinician demonstrates a desired behavior in order to prompt an imitative response. Imitation is a powerful teaching tool and forms the foundation for the development of many different skills in normal development.

Modeling. The demonstration of a desired behavior to elicit an imitative response.

However, many children with cognitive disabilities do not have the ability to imitate, which negates this method as a teaching tool. In cases in which the child does not imitate, physical assistance is needed to teach the skill of imitation. Another problem is that some behaviors are difficult to model, although this is more problematic in speech therapy than in language therapy. Research principles support modeling and imitation and indicate that "subjects reinforced for imitating various responses will eventually also imitate unreinforced responses" (Alberto & Troutman, 1986, p. 279).

Shaping. The differential reinforcement of successive approximations to a specified target to create a new behavior.

Shaping   A third technique, shaping, is rarely used in its purest form. Shaping is the differential reinforcement of successive approximations to a specified target to create a new behavior.

In its pure form, no model is offered and the clinician does not tell a client why he or she is being reinforced. When used without other techniques, shaping is a very slow process. To use shaping effectively, the clinician must define the target precisely and grade the steps carefully. If the steps are too small, the therapy is inefficient; if steps are too large, reinforcement is not sufficient to keep the child on task. Similarly, it is important to choose the correct place to start in teaching the sequence of behaviors. Each task should be analyzed carefully and broken into small steps. The starting point should be determined systematically by assessing the child's performance on each small step, with therapy beginning at the step in which the child fails. It is also important for the clinician to know when to progress. If the progression is too slow, the child may plateau; that is, he or she will not continue to progress through the sequence of tasks. If, on the other hand, the progression is too fast, the behaviors may extinguish, or disappear, before the entire sequence can be learned. Shaping can be used if a child does not demonstrate any vocalizations and the clinician wants the child to go from being nonvocal to being able to vocalize appropriately. Initially, each sound the child makes would be reinforced. As the child increases the frequency of vocalizations, the clinician could begin to focus on the quality of the vocalizations and reinforce differentially only those sounds which approximate a specific phoneme or word.

Prompt. A supplementary antecedent that is added to the original stimulus to increase the probability of a correct response.

Prompting with Verbal Assistance   Offering verbal instruction as a prompt is another effective therapy technique. A prompt is also referred to as a supplementary antecedent because it is added to the original stimuli in the hope that it will increase the probability that the child performs the desired response in reaction to the stimulus. Returning to the example in which the child is shown the toy truck, the spoon, and the shirt, if the child did not correctly select the spoon when asked to show the clinician what the child uses to eat, the clinician could provide a prompt by sounding out the first phoneme, /s/, to stimulate the child to choose the correct item. The clinician should always use the weakest prompt possible and should be sure that the prompt focuses the client's attention on the stimulus, not on the additional prompt.

think about it

Why is it important to fade out prompts and reinforcers as quickly as possible?

Chaining Chaining is a therapy technique used to teach a skill that consists of many different components. Specifically, chaining is a sequence of behaviors, all of which must be done to be rewarded. There are three types of chaining: forward chaining, backward chaining, and total task presentation. In forward chaining, each step is taught in sequence, and the child is rewarded for completing each step as it is learned. Forward chaining is used more frequently than the other types of chaining in language and cognition tasks. For example, in teaching a child to decode, the clinician has to do a task analysis to identify the components needed to decode (i.e., recognizing the print letter, making the grapheme–phoneme association, breaking the syllable into sounds, breaking the words into syllables, etc.). Backward chaining is used to teach many self-help skills. In backward chaining, the final step of the sequence is taught first, followed by each step as the sequence regresses back to the original step. In total-task presentation, the child is required to perform all steps in the correct sequence to obtain a reward. This is used after the chain is learned using either backward or forward chaining.

Total-task presentation can be used when the child can do each individual component but does not sequence properly. Thus, it is not the learning of the discrete steps that is rewarded, but rather the proper sequencing of the steps.

Fading During the fixation stage, fading is a critical technique. Fading is the gradual removal of prompts and reinforcers so that the client responds independently to the stimulus. The key words in the definition of fading are "gradual removal." If the prompts and reinforcers are removed too quickly, the child loses the response and it is necessary to go back to the cognitive stage to relearn the skill. Another aspect of fading is bringing an already learned behavior under the control of a different stimulus. Going back to the truck-spoon-shirt example again, the clinician would substitute a different spoon to be sure the response, "spoon," is learned and generalized and is not specific to the one stimulus. Thus, in fading the antecedent stimulus may change, but the desired response remains the same (Alberto & Troutman, 1986).

TREATMENT SUGGESTIONS BASED ON ETIOLOGY

Therapy Approaches for Preschool Children with Intellectual Disabilities

Motor and/or hearing disabilities combined with cognitive, speech, and/or language deficits make a neurodevelopmental approach to therapy the most realistic and promising. In a neurodevelopmental approach, all aspects of the

Forward chaining. A series of sequenced behaviors in which the first steps of the sequence are taught first; the typical chaining approach used in teaching academic skills.

Backward chaining. A series of sequenced behaviors in which the last steps of the sequence are taught first, working backward to the beginning of the chain; frequently used to teach self-help skills.

Total-task presentation. A series of sequenced behaviors, all of which must be done completely and in sequence in order to master the skill and be reinforced.

Fading. The gradual withdrawal of prompts used to facilitate a response.

child's development are addressed, with the child achieving improved function in all modalities simultaneously. Emphasis should be placed on assisting the child through the normal stages of sensorimotor, cognitive, speech, and language development, with the use of environmental stimulation and experiential learning to facilitate the language growth. Furthermore, therapy should occur in naturalistic settings instead of contrived settings such as an isolated therapy room. Goals should be functional and chosen because they facilitate the child's ability to participate in activities that occur in his or her daily routine.

A common philosophy is that most children need to be at Piagetian sensorimotor stage late IV or early V before they are able to use symbols such as words and pictures to represent concepts. However, it is possible to use some augmentative communication systems without any presymbolic training, but these systems are limited to one icon representing one message. For example, the speech-language pathologist in a self-contained classroom for children with multiple disabilities in the severe to profound intellectual disability group placed black-and-white photographs of essential self-help items around the classroom. The teacher, classroom aides, and clinicians all provided assistance in pointing to a picture prior to the child's using the item. For example, if a child were thirsty, the teacher had the child point to a picture of a cup before receiving a cup of water. Although these children were not likely to combine photos to make early word combinations or to function at the symbolic level, they did learn to point to the picture to receive the item with prompting. Another way to encourage communication is to put something the child desires out of reach and then observe the child as he or she problem solves how to get the desired item. For example, the boy in Figure 6–4 is reaching for the cookies that are slightly out of his reach as part of a "temptation" exercise designed to have him request assistance. Another way to instigate requesting behaviors is to have a "tea party" and to serve all present except the child who is being taught to make requests. This sets up a situation to encourage the child to request the food and drink that others have received and he or she has not been given.

One major problem I have encountered in working with children and adolescents who are severely and profoundly intellectually disabled is that they do not understand the value of communication. Without the ability to understand the value of communication, the children are not motivated to develop communication. Another problem is that many of these children do not know how to imitate, which is a powerful therapy tool. Thus, efforts must be made to teach the children to imitate in order to take advantage of this technique when providing language and communication therapy. I do not have any magic solution to the question of how to instill the value of communication but, in my experience, it comes with consistent repetition of assisting the child in requesting food or drink, then providing the requested item. For example, place pudding and juice just out of reach of the child. Then assist the child in pointing to one of the items, and accompany the

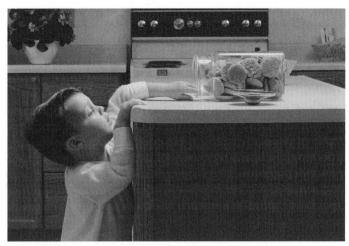

FIGURE 6–4 Temptation exercises are an excellent way to elicit communication from children who have delayed expressive language. (*Delmar/Cengage Learning*)

gesture with the verbal cue, "I want. . . .", then immediately provide that item. Of course, you must take care to only use items the child is known to like to eat and drink.

The use of generative language in augmentative communication requires that a child be at the symbolic level of functioning. It is critical that the clinician uses an integrated model that includes presymbolic skills and communication-first approaches and then moves to symbolic play schemes, followed by teaching words and symbols as a communication mode.

For children with intellectual disabilities, repetition is a key factor in achieving success in therapy. Therapy is an ongoing process that should be integrated into all daily activities. Early patterns of teaching should provide good models of communication. The adults in the child's environment must act as though they expect an answer; they should not anticipate every need. Otherwise, the child learns to be helpless instead of learning to take the initiative in communication efforts. The environment needs to be structured to facilitate learning through a variety of sensory systems, but at the cognitive level of the child. Not every child learns to communicate through speech, so a combination of speech and alternative methods such as gesturing, signing, and communication boards of all varieties must be considered.

think about it

How would you facilitate the integration of a child who uses an alternative and augmentative communication device into a traditional classroom setting?

Speech and Language for Children with Hearing Impairment

Speech and language can be taught to persons who are hearing impaired using a variety of methods of communication. Manualists support the use of sign language, including finger-spelling. American Sign Language was developed within the deaf community and is one of the most widely used signing systems. Cued speech is a supplementary system that uses a series of signals to facilitate the comprehension of spoken language. Typically, oralists do not support the use of supplementary signing systems. However, to return to one of the basic philosophies of this book, no clinician should be a purist in terms of being a manualist or oralist. Rather, whichever system works best for the child who has the hearing loss is the system that should be used. Some children may benefit from a combination of systems (total communication), and this should be analyzed carefully before assigning one communication system arbitrarily on the basis of the clinician's biases. Facilitation of speech reading should also be integrated into therapy.

A major component of therapy for children who have hearing impairment is an auditory training program. The child needs to be taught to indicate when he or she hears a sound (when the sound is on or off). The child also needs to learn to understand the sounds he or she hears (via residual hearing, hearing aids, or a cochlear implant) and to associate sounds with their sources. One way to do this is to present a sound to the child and have him or her select the item from an array of objects that makes that sound. The child could also point to a picture of the item. Other training includes recognizing and identifying volume differences of environmental sounds and speech. Eventually the child needs to discriminate between the various speech sounds.

Of course, all components of language (phonology, syntax, morphology, semantics, and pragmatics) should be incorporated into any therapy for children with hearing impairment. Particular emphasis needs to be placed on articulation and phonology. Children with hearing impairment also need instruction and guidance in voicing and natural rhythm of speech (Hegde & Maul, 2006).

Interventions for Babies Prenatally Exposed to Drugs

In addition to patting the baby at a rate of one beat per second, caregivers can use other external structuring and soothing techniques for children who are suffering the effects of maternal drug use. Swaddling the baby helps reduce the self-disrupting movements the child makes as part of his or her own distress system. Developing a consistent sucking pattern facilitates the use of a pacifier, which can also provide some soothing to the baby. The development of consistent, well-structured, predictable environments is absolutely critical, and this needs to be done primarily by providing support, structure,

TABLE 6–6 Questions for a behavioral log for drug-exposed babies

1. What is the infant's usual threshold for overstimulation?
2. What are his or her distress signals?
3. Where is the baby at this time?
4. How much stress does this activity cause?
5. What interventions were attempted?
6. What interventions worked?

Source: Compiled from information in Prenatal exposure to cocaine and other drugs: Developmental and educational prognoses, by D. R. Griffith, 1992, September, *Phi Beta Kappan*, pp. 30–34.

and guidance to the mother during high-stress tasks and situations. Finally, teaching the mother to keep a behavioral log to identify triggers and early warning signs of overstimulation can help provide a focus for intervention to facilitate the relationship between the baby, the mother, and the baby's general environment (Griffith, 1992).

In the behavioral log, questions that identify the point at which the baby becomes overstimulated should be used as guidance to provide the information needed to make environmental modifications (Table 6–6). These questions are critical in that they lead the parent through a problem-solving mode that assists the parent in helping the child. The key to helping these babies is to keep them below their threshold of tolerance. Once the level of tolerance is determined, intervention can begin. However, it is critical to respect the threshold level, because once the baby is overstimulated, it is too late. Gradually, with structured transitions, the level of tolerance can increase, and the baby's neurological systems becomes increasingly organized. This physiological organization is what could, eventually, separate children who do well in school from those who struggle academically and socially.

Children Who Are Late Talkers and Have Specific Language Impairment

In addressing therapeutic interventions with children with specific language impairment (SLI), Hadley and Schuele (1998) "argue that it is particularly important for speech-language pathologists to target socially relevant language objectives with children with SLI because these children eventually must live up to standard societal expectations in social, educational, and vocational settings" (p. 25). Teaching pragmatic skills in a contrived setting based on one-on-one interactions between the clinician and child does not adequately address socialization demands with peer groups beyond the therapy situation. Another problem that occurs in facilitating the development of social skills in children with SLI is the lack of emphasis on verbal skills needed for social competence in addition to (but separate from) nonverbal skills. Hadley and Schuele (1998) reminded us that children with SLI have language impairments in the absence of motor, sensory, emotional, or intellectual problems. Thus, the speech-language pathologist may be the only special educator who provides intervention beyond the classroom placement. Also, children with SLI are at risk academically, so enhancing their peer interaction skills may have a side effect of making the child feel more positive about school and supporting his or her adjustment to the academic setting. It is important to identify children with SLI early so that intervention in all areas of language, including social interactions with peers, can be addressed to prepare the child for the social and academic demands he or she will face when beginning school.

Children who are late talkers deserve the attention of speech-language pathologists due to the concomitant features and implications of late talking for future language and reading development. Some late talkers are considered to have a SLI because the same criteria (significant language delay in spite of normal nonverbal cognition, absence of sensory and physical deficits, and no other primary condition) is used for both deficits. However, Paul (1996), Rescorla and Lee (2000), and Whitehurst and Fischel (1994) point out that outcome data justify treating these as separate entities because late talkers have better outcomes than preschoolers with SLI (Rescorla, 2009). While there are those who argue for a categorical approach to language impairment, others follow a dimensional perspective. Rescorla (2009) cited Dollaghan (2004) in saying that a categorical approach treats SLI as a discrete disorder that specifies "a unique phenotype, etiology, base rate, and treatment regiment" (Dollaghan, p. 464, quoted in Rescorla, 2009, p. 17). On the other hand, Rescorla (2002, 2005) argued for a dimensional perspective "in which it was proposed that late talkers have below average endowment in a set of intercorrelated yet diverse language-related abilities, analogous to differential endowments for intelligence" (Rescorla, 2009, p. 17). Rescorla's use of the term *endowment* implies a constitutional basis for differences in language capabilities. Using this argument, one would say that the degree to which a late talker has language impairment depends on how severe the delay is and how prolonged it is. Some have receptive and expressive delays that are eventually (at age 4) diagnosed as SLI, while others who, for example, are late talkers with receptive language delays may resolve their delays by age 4 years. Numerous studies summarized by Rescorla indicate that while many children with early language delay score in the normal range on follow-up testing, many continue to show measurable language deficits on follow-up testing.

Rescorla (2009) conducted a study to examine "whether late talkers identified at 24–31 months continued to have weaker language and reading skills at 17 years of age than typically developing peers" (p. 16). She studied 26 toddlers who were identified as late talkers and 23 typically developing children as controls. Based on the results of previous studies and on the dimensional approach to language delay, Rescorla predicted that "the late talkers would perform close to the average range in a wide variety of language skills at age 17 years but that they would continue to manifest weaker skills than demographically matched children with typical language histories" (Rescorla, 2009, p. 20). Her predictions were upheld by the study.

EARLY INTERVENTION FOCUSING ON ACADEMIC READINESS

Most early intervention programs and therapy focus on domain-specific skills such as phoneme manipulation, letter recognition, letter sounds, counting, number knowledge, and the like, and the evidence is that these are critical skills that impact reading readiness and success in school. However, Welsh, Nix, Blair, Bierman, and Nelson (2010) suggested that it is also important to work on executive functions and cognitive skills, particularly working memory and attention control. While many studies have addressed the role of executive functions in school readiness, few have looked at their effect on emergent literacy and numeracy—that is, academics. These functions are discussed in the next section.

Facilitation of Cognitive Skills to Improve Emergent Literacy and Numeracy

Welsh and colleagues (2010) found that the development of executive function skills, particularly working memory and attention control, contributed to the development of emergent literacy and numeracy skills and predicted math and reading achievement in kindergarten. Executive functions are discussed in various contexts throughout this book, but three functions— working memory, inhibitory control, and attention set shifting—are developed mostly between ages 3–5 years. The development of these skills helps children to organize their thinking and exhibit self-control by regulating their own behaviors and reactions, and to apply rules of their environment to their own behavior.

Welsh and colleagues (2010) define working memory and attention control as follows:

> Working memory enables the retrieval of knowledge stored in long-term memory and its mental manipulation and application to foster the interpretation of novel information and the solution of problems. (p. 44)
>
> Attention control includes the capacity to focus and flexibly shift attention, as well as to ignore irrelevant stimuli and inhibit prepotent responding to stimuli, in order to respond to task demands. (p. 44)

Welsh and colleagues found that working memory and attention control help children learn more effectively by setting goals and organizing their approach to learning. They also found that executive functions are lacking or delayed in children living in poverty. Because working memory is critical to success in emergent literacy, problem solving, and math computation (all skills needed for academic success), children without developed working memory skills are at higher risk for poor school adjustment and academic underachievement due to learning problems. Furthermore, teachers report a higher incidence of inattentive behavior in students with learning difficulties, which points to the need to focus on the development of attention control during the pre-kindergarten years.

Thus, the evidence shows that it is necessary to work on domain-specific skills such as emergent literacy and numeracy in the preschool years, but it is also critical to work on domain-general skills such as working memory and attention control to facilitate learning behaviors so children can benefit from curriculum-based instruction in school.

Executive functions can be taught to preschoolers through monitoring and mediating peer interactions, providing repeated practice sessions, and providing examples of appropriate behavior and problem solving. There are also curricular programs available that focus on teaching executive functions in preschool children. One of these is Promoting Alternative Thinking Strategies (PATHS; Greenberg & Kusche, 1993), which focuses on the development of neurocognitive control. The PATHS program "targets emotion regulation, self-control, social problem-solving skills" and behavior regulation (Welsh et al., 2010, p. 50).

Another program is Tools of the Mind (ToM; Bodrova & Leong, 1996). The ToM program is based on the premise that "play provides a unique opportunity for developing critical self-regulatory skills" (Welsh et al., 2010, p, 50). Through planning make-believe play and enacting social roles, children experience opportunities for using negotiation and for interacting in reciprocal activities such as turn taking. Children are guided in using pre-planned behaviors instead of reacting impulsively. They learn reflective thinking and self-regulation. ToM is a well-researched program, with studies showing that students who have been taught using the ToM curriculum havr better vocabularies and better performance on executive function tests. They also have, according to teacher reports, fewer behavior problems.

Thence, evidence shows that the incorporation of activities designed to facilitate the development and use of working memory and attention control have positive impacts on children's academic success.

Development of Emergent Literacy in the Preschool Years

Emergent literacy is addressed in Chapters 4 and 10, so the intent here is to stress the importance of focusing on emergent literacy when providing language intervention to preschool children with language deficits. Lo, Wang, and Haskell (2009) also addressed the issue of providing intervention to at-risk children (in this case, low-income children) to facilitate the development of emergent literacy so that children are prepared to learn to read when they enter kindergarten. A child has to have phonemic awareness for alphabetic understanding, and he or she has to have alphabetic understanding to identify words in print and, therefore, to read. Lo and colleagues cited research by Schacter and Jo (2005) in noting that kindergartners from low-income urban areas "score one half of a standard deviation below the national average in reading achievement, and the gap increases to two standard deviations by the time they graduate from elementary school" (p. 12). The No Child Left Behind Act (2001) mandated that schools must close the achievement gaps between typically achieving students and disadvantaged students. In order to do this, reading achievement is a primary focus. Thus it is incumbent on speech-language pathologists and other early childhood interventionists to provide instruction in all aspects of emergent literacy. This includes teaching print concepts by exposing children to books in an interactive manner and teaching oral language skills, letter knowledge, and phonemic awareness. "Beginning reading instruction should be provided explicitly, systematically, frequently, and intensively in order to produce maximum improvement in reading" (Lo et al., 2009, p. 13).

SUMMARY

At this point, it should be clear that learning is not a random process. It is a well-orchestrated sequencing of tasks through which the language skills needed to be an effective communicator are produced. Learning is based on principles, procedures, and programs.

A therapy program encompasses fundamental principles and best practices into a comprehensive plan of action. A quality program also identifies specific activities that may be implemented to help the client achieve his or her therapy goals, including treatment variables that are used to stimulate, change, and eliminate behaviors in the therapy setting.

Regardless of the procedures selected for a child's therapy, it is critical to remember to treat the child and not the label or disability. Even though labels are sometimes necessary for financial or placement reasons, the clinician must remember to react to the child and to assess and treat the child, not the label. Also, the clinician needs to make sure the child's various systems—sensory, motor, neurological, and anatomical—are intact. This is important because a clinician should not attempt remediation of behaviors that are not responsive to behavioral interventions.

Of course, one always wonders, "Does treatment work?" ASHA has a series of functional communication measures (FCMs) designed to measure progress in as a result of treatment. FCMs are seven-point scales with level 1 being the least functional and level 7 the most functional. "According to data from ASHA'a National Outcomes Measurement System, approximately 70% of preschoolers showed gains on one or more levels on the Spoken Language Production and/or Spoken Language Comprehension FCMs" following intervention from a speech-language pathologist. (ASHA, n.d., p. 1). Clearly, speech-language pathologists have a definitive role to play in treating language disorders in preschool children and helping to prepare them for successful outcomes when they reach school age.

CASE STUDY

History

Trish is a 2-year, 5-month-old girl whose father contacted the Speech and Language Clinic because he was concerned about her language and speech development. Trish's history is positive for spastic cerebral palsy, and she has not received any speech or language therapy. The family lives on a farm about 30 miles from the clinic, but both parents work in the city. There are no other children in the family. While her parents are at work, Trish stays at home with her maternal grandparents.

Evaluation

Trish's speech and language were informally assessed using the Assessment of Language Development (see Appendix 5A) and judged to be in the 13- to 18-month age range. The Early Communication Checklist (Lombardino, Stapell, & Gerhardt, 1987) (Appendix 5D) was also used, with Trish scoring in the 14- to 16-month range. Overall, she exhibited approximately a 12-month delay receptively and expressively.

	Strengths	Weaknesses
Communicative	Excellent eye contact	Delayed receptive language
	Engages adults in play	Delayed expressive language
	Uses jargon and pointing to communicate	Oral motor weakness
		Lack of means-end and causality
		Limited symbolic play skills
Noncommunicative	Supportive family	Spastic cerebral palsy
	Attends therapy regularly	Limited language experiences beyond the home setting
	Great personality!	

Long-Term Therapy Goals

- Trish will be age appropriate in her receptive language skills.
- Trish will be age appropriate in her expressive language skills.
- Trish will enhance her oral-motor skills through a series of oral-exercises.

Language Short-Term Therapy Goals

- Trish will spontaneously use 20 words to refer to objects, events, and attributes of objects or toys presented by the clinician.
- Trish will problem solve in situations set up to tempt her by putting a toy or food item out of her reach. Trish will get the item or request help on four out of five trials for three consecutive sessions.
- Trish will engage in interactive play in schemes set up by the clinician. Interactive play schemes will be set up using a doctoring kit and a baby doll, a kitchen set, a play garage, a dollhouse, and a toy farm.
- Trish will produce multischemes spontaneously such as cooking a meal in the play kitchen, feeding it to a doll, and putting the doll to bed. Trish will complete two multischeme tasks per session.
- Trish will request help on 100 percent of the tasks that she is unable to complete independently.
- In a tea party setting, Trish will request food and drink that are used to facilitate her oral motor goals.

Oral-Motor Short-Term Therapy Goals

(Note: These were done to facilitate oral-motor skills for eating purposes, not speech.)

- With 90 percent accuracy on 10 trials, Trish will imitate tongue and lip movements made by the clinician.
- With 90 percent success on 10 trials, Trish will pucker her lips and drink through a straw.
- With 90 percent accuracy on 10 trials, Trish will lick a lollipop held by the clinician at the corners of Trish's mouth and at midline above the lips and below the lips.
- Trish will resist having the clinician pull a Lifesaver tied to a string out of Trish's mouth when the Lifesaver is held between her lips and teeth.
- Trish will use lateral and rotary chewing movements on a piece of caramel wrapped in gauze and held in Trish's mouth by the clinician, transferring the caramel from right to left and back a minimum of 10 times in 1 minute.
- Trish will bite through a sandwich cookie when it is held between her front incisors five times.

Results

Trish met all goals and was dismissed from therapy after 8 months. Her receptive language and play skills were age appropriate, and she was combining words. For example, she said "Daddy bye-bye" when her father went to get a drink of water and "baby broke"

(continues)

CASE STUDY *(continued)*

when the arm fell off a plastic doll with which she was playing. In addition, she was addressing her clinicians by name. Trish was augmenting her speech with gestures and simple signs when she was not understood. The family is to be commended for their interactive support in the therapy sessions and for following up with the goals and procedures at home. Their involvement certainly contributed to the rapid progress Trish made in therapy.

REVIEW QUESTIONS

1. The treatment stage in which the client practices, perfects, and stabilizes the new behavior is the
   a. Cognitive stage
   b. Autonomous stage
   c. Fixation stage
   d. Director's stage

2. Observable, measurable, replicable items that are based on information gleaned from careful study of the available research are
   a. Principles
   b. Procedures
   c. Theorems
   d. Of no use in therapy

3. Which of the following represent the prompting hierarchy?
   a. Stimulus → physical assist → verbal assist → visual assist → imitation/modeling
   b. Stimulus → imitation/modeling → physical assist → visual assist → verbal assist
   c. Stimulus → verbal assist → physical assist → visual assist → imitation/modeling
   d. Stimulus → verbal assist → visual assist → imitation/modeling → physical assist

4. The stage of communication development in which the child's efforts are nonverbal but intentional is the _____ stage.
   a. Perlocutionary
   b. Illocutionary
   c. Locutionary
   d. Stationary

5. An interactive framework for assessment and treatment of a child with multiple handicaps is best implemented in a transdisciplinary or inter-disciplinary setting.

    a. True

    b. False

6. IDEA funds can be used to pay for therapy for school-aged children who have a language difference.

    a. True

    b. False

7. Children must be at Piagetian stage IV before an augmentative or alternative communication system is introduced.

    a. True

    b. False

8. Sensorimotor integration is the sequence of responses that are derived through the coordination of sensory and motor systems of the body.

    a. True

    b. False

9. The use of schemes and scripts to simulate real-life settings in therapy is an excellent approach to therapy for preschool children and eventually facilitates the everyday use of skills learned in therapy.

    a. True

    b. False

10. Knowledge of the child's communicative environment is at the center of the assessment and treatment model proposed by Suzanne Morris.

    a. True

    b. False

REFERENCES

Alberto, P. A., & Troutman, A. C. (1986). *Applied behavior analysis for teachers* (2nd ed.). Columbus, OH: Merrill Publishing Company.

American Speech-Language-Hearing Association. (n.d.) *Treatment efficacy summary: Child language disorders.* Retrieved February 10, 2010 from www.asha.org/uploadedFiles/public/TESChildLanguageDisorders.pdf.

Bates, E., Camaioni, L., & Volterra, V. (1975). The acquisition of performatives prior to speech. *Merrill-Palmer Quarterly, 21,* 205–226.

Bodrova, E., & Leong, D. J. (1996). *Tools of the mind: The Vygotskian approach to early childhood* education (2nd ed.). Englewood Cliffs, NJ: Prentice-Hall.

Brady, N. (2003, March). *Communication repair strategies by young children with developmental disabilities.* Paper presented at the 36th annual Gatlinburg Conference on Research and Theory in Intellectual and Developmental Disabilities. Annapolis, MD.

Brady, N., & Halle, J. (2002). Breakdowns and repairs in conversations between beginning AAC users and their partners. In J. Reichle, D. Beukelman, and J. Light (eds.), *Exemplary practices for beginning communicators: Implications for AAC* (pp. 323–352). Baltimore, MD: Paul H. Brookes.

Cleave, P. L., & Fey, M. E. (1997, February). Two approaches to the facilitation of grammar in children with language impairments: Rationale and description. *American Journal of Speech-Language Pathology, 6*(1), 22–32.

Dunst, C. (1980). A clinical and educational manual for use with the Uzgiris and Hunt scales of infant psychological development. Austin, TX: Pro-Ed.

Fey, M. E. (1986). *Language intervention with young children.* San Diego, CA: College-Hill Press.

Greenberg, M. T., & Kusche, C. A. (1993). Promoting social and emotional development in deaf children: The PATHS Project. Seattle: University of Washington Press.

Griffith, D. R. (1992, September). Prenatal exposure to cocaine and other drugs: Developmental and educational prognoses. *Phi Delta Kappan,* 30–34.

Guralnik, D. B. (ed.). (1968). *Webster's new world dictionary of the American language.* New York: World Publishing Company.

Hadley, P. A., & Schuele, C. M. (1998, November). Facilitating peer interaction: Socially relevant objectives for preschool language intervention. *American Journal of Speech-Language Pathology, 7*(4), 25–36.

Halle, J., Brady, N. C., & Drasgow, E. (2004, February). Enhancing socially adaptive communicative repairs of beginning communicators with disabilities. *American Journal of Speech-Language Pathology, 13*(1), 43–54.

Hegde, M. N. (1995). *Clinical methods and practicum in speech-language pathology.* San Diego, CA: Singular Publishing Group.

Hegde, M. N., & Maul, C. A. (2006). *Language disorders in children: An evidence-based approach to assessment and treatment.* Boston: Allyn & Bacon.

Hodson, B. W., & Paden, E. P. (1991). *Targeting intelligible speech* (2nd ed.). Austin, TX: Pro-Ed.

Leith, W. R. (1984). *Handbook of clinical methods in communication disorders.* San Diego, CA: Singular Publishing Group.

Lo, Y., Wang, C., & Haskell, S. (2009, May). Examining the impacts of early reading intervention on the growth rates in basic literacy skills of at-risk urban kindergartners. *Journal of Special Education, 43*(1), 12–28.

Lombardino, L. J., Stapell, J. B., & Gerhardt, K. J. (1987, September-October). Evaluating communicative behaviors in infancy. *Journal of Pediatric Health Care, 1,* 5.

MacDonald, J. (1989). *Becoming partners with children: From play to conversation.* San Antonio, TX: Special Press.

Morris, S. E. (1982). *The normal acquisition of oral feeding skills: Implications for assessment and treatment.* Central Islip, NY: Therapeutic Media.

Nicolosi, L., Harryman, E., & Krescheck, J. (2004). *Terminology of communication disorders: Speech-language-hearing* (5th ed..). Boston: Lippincott Williams & Wilkins.

Owens, R. E. (1995). *Language disorders: A functional approach to assessment and intervention* (2nd ed.). Boston: Allyn and Bacon.

Owens, R. E. (1999). *Language disorders: A functional approach to assessment and intervention* (3rd ed.). Boston: Allyn and Bacon.

Paul, R. (1996). Clinical implications of the natural history of slow expressive language development. *American Journal of Speech-Language Pathology, 5,* 5–21.

Polakow, V. (1993). *Lives on the edge: Single mothers and their children in the other America.* Chicago: University of Chicago Press.

Rescorla, L. (2002). Age 9 outcomes for late-talking toddlers. *Journal of Speech, Language, and Hearing Research, 45,* 360–371.

Rescorla, L. (2005). Age 13 language and reading outcomes of late-talking toddlers. *Journal of Speech, Language, and Hearing Research, 48,* 459–472.

Rescorla, L. (2009). Age 17 language and reading outcomes in late-talking toddlers: support for a dimensional perspective on language delay. *Journal of Speech, Language, and Hearing Research, 52,* 16–30.

Rescorla, L., & Lee, E. C. (2000). Language impairment in children. In T. Layton & L. Watson (Eds.) *Early language impairment in children, Vol 1: Nature.* New York: Delmar Publishing. Company.

Schacter, J., & Jo, B. (2005, May 1). Learning when school is not in session: A reading summer day-camp intervention to improve the achievement of exiting first-grade students who are economically disadvantaged. *Journal of Research in Reading, 28*(2), 158–169.

Shulman, B. B., & Capone, N. C. (2010). *Language development: Foundations, processes, and clinical applications.* Sudbury, MA: Jones and Bartlett.

Uzgiris, I. C., & Hunt, J. M. (1975). *Assessment in infancy: Ordinal scales of psychological development.* Urbana: University of Illinois Press.

Welsh, J. A., Nix, R. L., Blair, C., Bierman, K. L., & Nelson, K. E. (2010, February). The development of cognitive skills and gains in academic school readiness for children from low-income families. *Journal of Educational Psychology, 102*(1), 43–53.

Wetherby, A. M., Alexander, D. G., & Prizant, B. M. (1998). The ontogeny and role of repair strategies. In A. M. Wetherby, S. F. Warren, and J. Reichle (vol. eds.), *Communication and language intervention series: Vol. 7, Transition in prelinguistic communication* (pp. 135–161). Baltimore, MD: Paul H. Brookes.

Provision of Speech-Language Pathology Services in the Public Schools: A Historical Perspective on the Impact of Federal Legislation on Present-Day Services

LEARNING OBJECTIVES

After completion of this chapter, the reader will be able to:

1. List and discuss the six principles that have historically guided special education law.

2. Demonstrate knowledge of federal legislation that impacts special education services in the public schools.

3. Discuss the impact of federal legislation on speech-language pathologists working in the public schools.

4. Discuss how to make an evidence-based clinical decision, particularly related to childhood language disorders.

5. Argue for or against a variety of eligibility criteria for students with special needs receiving speech-language therapy.

6. Argue the merits of center-based, mainstream, and inclusion-based placements for special education services.

7. Discuss the role of transition in special education services and how the speech-language pathologist can participate in preparing students for transitions.

8. Identify the sections of an IEP and an IFSP.

INTRODUCTION

Education of public school students who have disabilities has long been the focus of federal legislation, as well as numerous instances of case law (e.g., *Brown v. Board of Education, Pennsylvania Association for Retarded Children v. Commonwealth of Pennsylvania, Diana v. Board of Education,* The Ann Arbor case, the Rowley standard, *Lau v. Nichols, Daniel R.R. v. State Board of Education, Lisco v. Woodland Hills School District, Timothy W. v Rochester NH School District*). The purpose of this chapter is to provide an overview of federal legislation affecting public education for students with disabilities, a summary of the transitions inherent in the educational career of a student, and a discussion of the impact the laws have had on the provision of speech-language pathology services in the public schools. Traditionally education for students with severe disabilities has focused on functional content. However, the No Child Left Behind Act (NCLB) (2001) and the Individuals with Disabilities Education Improvement Act (IDEIA) (2004) have both stressed access to general education curriculum, which has led to the inclusion model as the standard of education for students with disabilities.

There is a particular focus on the provision of speech-language pathology assessment and intervention in the school setting. The Individuals with Disabilities Education Act (IDEA) and its reauthorizations and the National Joint Committee for the Communication Needs of Persons with Severe Disabilities (NJC) stress the role of communication services and supports in programming for students with disabilities. Issues such as eligibility, educational settings, access of students with disabilities to the general education curriculum, and service delivery models are discussed. In the context of this chapter, the NJC definition of *communication* is used:

> Communication is any act by which one person gives to or receives from another person information about that person's needs, desires, perceptions, knowledge, or effective states. Communication may be intentional or unintentional, may involve conventional or unconventional signals, may take linguistic or nonlinguistic form, and may occur through spoken or other modes (NJC, 1992, p. 3).

AN OVERVIEW OF KEY FEDERAL LEGISLATION AFFECTING SPECIAL EDUCATION

The Key Principles of Special Education Law

According to Moore-Brown and Montgomery (2005), there are six principles that have historically guided special education law. The first is free and appropriate public education (FAPE), which was originally set forth in the Education Amendments of 1974 (P.L. 93-380). The second principle is full education opportunity, which was promised in P.L. 93-380 but did not receive guaranteed funding until the passage of the Education for All Handicapped Children Act in 1975. A third principle is actually more of a program, called Child Find. Through educating physicians, social workers, and preschool teachers as well as through a media blitz, efforts were made to find children with handicaps who were school-aged to enroll in the public schools. A fourth principle is that all children with handicaps should receive instruction in the "east restrictive environment possible, to the extent that their handicaps permitted. Admittedly, there are some children who have handicaps so severe that they would not benefit from placement with non-impaired students, so arrangements are made for self-contained classrooms and/or special education centers for those students. Finally, children were guaranteed an individualized education through the development of annual individualized education plans (IEPs) for each child in the public schools who had an impairment.

The Elementary and Secondary Education Act of 1965 (P.L. 89-10)

The Elementary and Secondary Education Act of 1965 was the first federal legislation to address education for children with handicapping conditions, although that was not its primary purpose. P.L. 89-10 was passed to allocate funds for the education of children from low-SES backgrounds. Titles II and III of the law mandated that states develop plans to obtain materials and texts to educate the children who were considered to be of low SES. It also encouraged the provision of additional services and educational centers as part of the provisions. Although it did not consider the students with handicaps as recipients of part of the provisions, it still authorized $100 million for supplementary services and centers. In 1966, the Education and Secondary Education Act Amendments (P.L. 89-750) revised Title II of P.L. 89-10 to require that 15 percent of the Title III funding be made available for programs for students with handicaps. This requirement, Title VI, provided grants to states for "initiation, expansion, and improvement of programs and projects (including the acquisition of equipment and where necessary, the construction of school facilities) for the education of handicapped children (as defined in section 602) at the preschool, elementary, and secondary school levels" (P.L. 89-750). It also defined children with handicaps as those who are mentally retarded, deaf, hearing or speech impaired, emotionally disturbed, visually handicapped, crippled, or have other disabling health problems. States were required to submit plans to the Commissioner of Education in order to receive the federal funding. Title VI also allowed for the establishment of the National Advisory Committee on Handicapped Children and the Office of Education of the Bureau for the Education and Training of Handicapped. It was the first time in history that individuals with handicaps had representation and a federal office dedicated to their needs. It should be mentioned that the Education of the Handicapped Act of 1970 (P.L. 91-230) repealed Title VI and created a separate act. P.L. 91-230 authorized funding for centers and services, training of special personnel (including speech-language pathologists), and research in the area of education of the handicapped. It expressed a moral commitment to children with disabilities and established that "people with disabilities share the same constitutional rights as nondisabled people." In that sense, it was a civil rights statute.

> **think about it**
> Why is the Elementary and Secondary Education Act of 1965 (P.L. 89-10) of particular significance to speech-language pathologists?

Section 504 of the Rehabilitation Act of 1973 (P.L. 93-112)

Section 504 of the Rehabilitation Act of 1973 is also a civil rights statute designed to prohibit discrimination of any kind toward persons with handicaps.

Specifically, it stated that "no otherwise qualified handicapped individual in the United States . . . shall, solely by reason of his handicap, be excluded from participation in, be denied the benefits of, or be subjected to discrimination under any program receiving federal financial assistance" (School Law Register). When P.L. 94-142 was passed, funding under Section 504 would be discontinued if the state did not comply with P.L. 94-142. In other words, Section 504 did not provide funding, but it did state that it was illegal for any program receiving federal funding to discriminate on the basis of handicap. Together, Section 504 and P.L. 94-142 were the most significant pieces of legislation with regard to education of children with handicaps. Together, they set the stage for changes in the provision of educational and vocational opportunities for individuals with disabilities (Moore-Brown & Montgomery, 2005).

Education Amendments of 1974 (P.L. 93-380)

P.L. 93-380 was signed into law by President Gerald Ford on August 24, 1975 and included, among others, provisions to ensure that handicapped children were educated with non-handicapped children. States were required to formulate a plan for meeting the needs of all students with impairments. The legislators also recognized that some children have handicapping conditions that are so severe that the children cannot benefit from mainstreaming. To that end, they also authorized funds to build supplementary educational centers and to provide transportation, when needed and appropriate, for the children. P.L. 93-380 was a precursor to P.L. 94-142. It should be noted that not only did it provide full educational opportunity for children with handicaps, but it also provided opportunity for educationally deprived children, delinquent children, and migratory children.

Section 513 of P.L. 93-380 is known as the Buckley Amendment or as the Family Educational Rights and Privacy Act of 1974 (FERPA). Under FERPA, parents of students under age 18 can inspect or review official school records, files, and data relating to their child and request a hearing to challenge their child's school records. Section 438 also stated that written permission was needed to release educational records.

Another key component of P.L. 93-380 consisted of procedural safeguards. The most notable of these safeguards was the concept of due process. As stated above, parents were allowed to inspect their child's records related to the child's educational program. If the parents wanted to challenge the records, they could request a hearing before an arbitrator (due process). "For the first time, parents and handicapped children were allowed to question a school district's decision, using a systematic procedure and guaranteed rights" (Gravani, 1997, p. 17)

think about it

What are some safeguards you could put into practice to help protect yourself from being the focus of a due process hearing?

The Education for All Handicapped Children Act of 1975 (P.L. 94-142)

The Education for All Handicapped Children Act of 1975 was signed into law after congressional investigations revealed that there were more than eight million children with handicaps in the United States. However, special education needs were not being met, with at least one million not receiving services in the public schools. Congress noted that those children not being served were being prevented from taking advantage of their full and equal rights. It was also believed that many children with handicaps were currently enrolled in regular education programs, their disabilities undetected. Originally, the law presented chronological priorities, with children applying for services under P.L. 94-142 being required to be between 3 and 18 years of age. This was later amended to between 3 and 21 years of age. The priorities for placement were first those children who were not receiving any services and second, those children within each disability in relation to severity of the impairment.

P.L. 94-142 was primarily a funding statute that allocated funds needed to fully implement promises made in previous legislation, most notably FAPE, which stated that all students must be provided with an educational program designed to meet the student's individual needs at no cost to the parents. The law also clarified that children with handicaps should be educated in the least restrictive environment as much as possible (later known as mainstreaming), including participation in extracurricular and nonacademic subjects such as music, art, and physical education. A third provision of P.L. 94-142 was that only personnel who were educated and qualified in test administration could provide the necessary and appropriate testing for the evaluation and placement of students with handicaps. Furthermore, this was the first law to put into place procedural safeguards, such as the IEP, for students and their parents. Finally, the law guaranteed that students with handicaps would have the same opportunities as non-handicapped students to nonacademic services such as transportation, vocational training, counseling, and recreational activities. P.L. 94-142 recommended that services be provided for preschool children aged 3 to 5 years old, but did not mandate it.

In addition, P.L. 94-142 defined the terms *special education* and *related services*. Special education was defined as "specially designed instruction, at no cost to parents or guardians, to meet the unique needs of a handicapped child, including classroom instruction, instruction in physical education, home instruction, and instruction in hospitals and institutions." Children eligible for special education were defined as those who have educational, developmental, emotional, or physical disabilities. Related services were defined as those services needed to supplement regular classroom instruction. Specifically, related services included "transportation, and such developmental, corrective, and other supportive services," including speech-language pathology and audiology, physical therapy, occupational therapy, recreation, medical services, and counseling. Both special education and related services are geared toward allowing any child to participate fully in the educational setting. It was believed that as a result of an enriching school experience, these children would have more confidence and success in the world outside of the classroom.

Essentially, P.L. 94-142 had four primary purposes:

1. To provide assurance that all children with handicaps would receive free and appropriate public education, including special education and related services as needed

2. To protect the rights of children with handicaps and their parents through the continuation of the due process procedures set in place by P.L. 93-380

3. To evaluate the effectiveness of federal, state, and local efforts to provide special education and related services needed to educate children with handicaps

4. To provide financial support to states and local education agencies to insure that children with handicaps had full educational opportunities (Gravani, 1997)

The Individualized Education Plan (IEP)

According to the definition of the IEP written in P.L. 94-142, the speech-language pathologist is required to

1. describe the presenting problem,

2. project objectives and goals for the year,

3. determine which service delivery option will best meet the child's needs,

4. plan transitional services,

5. anticipate the length of time it will take the child to reach the goals, and

6. describe the methods by which the progress will be measured. (Taylor, 1992, p. 84)

An example of an IEP can be found in Appendix 7A. A typical IEP includes

1. The student profile

2. The current levels of performance

3. Student-centered goals

4. Teaching approaches and methodologies

5. Monitoring and evaluation techniques

6. Specialized equipment and materials set-up

7. Student-centered specific objectives

8. Special education and related services delivery plan

The IEP is an interdisciplinary document based on the evaluation of a child by all appropriate teachers and clinicians. It must be based on an evaluation of the child and updated annually. A full reevaluation must be performed every 3 years. The student profile includes information on how the student receives, processes, retains, and expresses information. It takes into account physical constraints as well as strengths and weaknesses in the cognitive and affective domains. In addition, it includes the rate at which the student learns and the conditions under which he or she best learns. The current levels of performance are based on the results of various assessments as well as data reflecting performance in therapy and in the classroom. They reflect what the child can and cannot do, as well as the student's entry level. It covers academic, self-help, language, social, prevocational, and vocational goals.

The behavioral objectives on the IEP are written for four primary reasons:

- To describe current levels of performance

- To describe the desired level of performance

- To objectify and quantify the goals

- To increase the relaying of goals to other professionals (to facilitate effective transfer of goals to other clinicians or professionals in other settings)

Behavioral objectives define the stimulus, the response, and the contingency related to each target for the child. They provide a definitive baseline (pre-intervention level of performance) and help to improve material selection. The parts of a behavioral objective are the client's name (who), the condition under which the behavior will occur (i.e., with visual assistance, with verbal prompts; see the prompting hierarchy in Chapter 6), the target behavior (short-term goal), and the criteria for mastery. Goals are long term and written in general terms. Specific objectives are the short-term goals and should include what the child will accomplish under what conditions and the criteria for mastery. Criteria for mastery should be written such that progress can be demonstrated, but not so elementary that it would be necessary to reconvene the IEP team to rewrite the IEP. Generally, providing a range of criteria (e.g., 60–85 percent) minimizes that possibility.

With the passage of P.L. 99-457, transition goals were also added to each IEP. The transition plans were originally intended to indicate how the school personnel would prepare the high school student for transition to the workforce or postgraduate education. However, they were extended down to earlier grades to help prepare students at an earlier age for activities after their school years ended and to address transition from one school level to another when appropriate.

Education for All Handicapped Children Act Amendments of 1986 (P.L. 99-457)

P.L. 99-457 was passed in 1986 and reinforced the regulations and provisions of P.L. 94-142. Essentially, it had three purposes:

1. To increase the development of handicapped infants by increasing the family's ability to serve its child;

2. To decrease educational costs by minimizing the need for special education;

3. To decease the likelihood of institutionalization.;

Congress saw a continued need for early education for all children with handicapping conditions and stressed that early identification and intervention services for children with handicapping conditions could not be ignored. To that end, it required that all children with handicaps who were 3 to 5 years of age were entitled to FAPE, thereby mandating what P.L. 94-142 had recommended. Further, it recommended public school services for families of children aged birth to 2 years. It is important to note the inclusion of the word *families* in this law. The underlying philosophy was that, by educating families on how to in teract with their children with impairments, there would be a decrease in demands for special education when the children reached school age. Students in this age group had an individual family service plan (IFSP) that addressed the needs of the family and child. The services were home based, with the clinicians' going to the homes of the students and working with the family and child. The members of Congress also stated that concerns about the federal funding of programs for children with handicaps, as well as concerns about the shortage of personnel qualified to work with children with handicaps, could not be ignored. In addition to mandating services for children with impairments aged 3 to 5 years, the law also established a new state grant program to provide early special education and related services for eligible infants and toddlers aged birth to 2 years old who had handicaps (Part H).

A variety of programs can utilize funds from P.L. 99-457, including:

*   Regional or local interagency coordination councils

*   Regional diagnostic centers

*   Models for integrated and developmental day care

*   Models to monitor progress of high-risk infants through neonatal intensive care units

- Respite care services

- Home-based services

- Transition programs

> **think about it**
>
> What are some of the difficulties you would expect to encounter when providing speech-language or aural rehabilitation services to a 3-year-old child in his or her home setting?

Children aged 3 to 5 years were guaranteed a free and appropriate education by states in order to apply for P.L. 94-142 funds. Services could be provided by local education agencies (LEAs), or the LEAs could contract with other programs, providers, or agencies. The IEP for these children is supposed to include parent instruction as desired by the parents. With regard to the birth-to-age-2 children, three categories were eligible:

Children birth to age 2 who are developmentally delayed

Children birth to age 2 who have conditions that typically result in delay

Children birth to age 2 who are at risk of substantial developmental delay (at the discretion of the state)

The Individual Family Service Plan

The IFSP is the document mandated by P.L. 99-457 for children aged birth to 2 years who receive intervention services through the auspices of the public school (either by the LEA or any agency with whom the LEA has contracted). The IFSP consists of the following components:

Statement of present level of development (cognitive, speech/language, psychosocial, motor, self-help)

Statement of the family's strengths and weaknesses

Statement of major outcomes expected for the child and his or her family

Criteria, procedures, and timeline for determining progress

Specific early intervention services necessary

Expected date of service initiation and duration

Name of case manager

Procedures for transition to a preschool program

The case manager is usually from the profession most immediately relevant to the infant, toddler, or family's needs, and who is responsible for the implementation of the program. The case manager also is responsible for coordination with other agencies and persons who can be of benefit to the child and/or his or her family.

The Individuals with Disabilities Education Act of 1990 (P.L. 101-407)

The Individuals with Disabilities Education Act (IDEA) represented an amendment of the Education for All Handicapped Children Act, including changing its name. IDEA introduced the concept of transition services, targeting students who are 15 to 16 years old who need to be prepared for transitioning from school to the community. This portion of the law resulted in the addition of social workers and rehabilitation counselors to the category of related services. Other areas that IDEA introduced into the educational platform were services were assistive technology (augmentative communication using computers and electronic communication boards), services for children with autism, and services for children with traumatic brain injury (TBI) (Gravani, 1997).

A joint committee of ASHA and the Council on the Education of the Deaf listed 12 roles of speech-language pathologists and audiologists providing services to infants and toddlers with hearing impairment through the public schools. As defined by Part H of IDEA, the roles and responsibilities are:

Participation as a member of a multidisciplinary team

Working with families

Assessment and diagnosis of hearing loss in 0- to 36-month-old children

Assessment of communication competence in 0- to 36-month-old children with hearing loss

Assessment of cognitive, motor, and social skills of 0- to 36-month-old children with hearing loss

Otologic evaluation of 0- to 36-month-old children with hearing loss

Developing and implementing the IFSP

Provision of sensory devices

Management of the sensory devices

Maximizing auditory potential (of the child)

Facilitating communication development

Facilitating cognitive development

IDEA also supported the concept of educating children with disabilities in the least restrictive environment, meaning that children with disabilities would be educated with non-disabled students to the maximum extent possible. School districts were to have a continuum of placements along with procedures to be sure that LRE was fully implemented.

Individuals with Disabilities Education Act Amendments of 1997 (P.L. 105-17)

The most significant statement in P.L. 105-17 is as follows:

> Disability is a natural part of the human experience and in no way diminishes the right of individuals to participate in or contribute to society. Improving educational results for children with disabilities is an essential element of our national policy of ensuring equality of opportunity, full participation, independent living, and economic self-sufficiency for individuals with disabilities.

No Child Left Behind Act of 2001 (PL 107-110)

President George W. Bush signed the No Child Left Behind Act of 2001 (NCLB) into law on January 8, 2002. Basically, it was a reauthorization and amendment of the Elementary and Secondary Education Act of 1965 and redefined "the role of the federal government in K–12 education" (Smith, 2003, p. 126). The major focus of NCLB was to provide all children with a fair, equal, and significant opportunity to obtain a high-quality education. The U.S. Department of Education emphasizes four pillars within the bill:

Accountability: Ensures those students who are disadvantaged achieve academic proficiency.

Flexibility: Allows school districts flexibility in how they use federal education funds to improve student achievement.

Research-based education: Emphasizes educational programs and practices that have been proven effective through scientific research.

Parent options: Increases the choices available to the parents of students attending Title I schools.

NCLB emphasized the implementation of educational programs and practices that have been demonstrated to be effective. In essence, it was a national extension of the standards-based education reform efforts undertaken in individual states (www.k12.wa.us/esea/).

Major principles of NCLB are as follows:

a. Make SCHOOLS accountable for their students' results as measured by annual statewide assessments;

b. Provide states, local education districts, and individual schools with more flexibility in how they use federal funds;

c. Provide more choices for parents of children from disadvantageous homes (i.e., parents of children attending low-achieving schools, which are frequently in low-income areas, can request a transfer to a higher achieving-school or supplemental tutoring);

   d. Emphasize proven teaching methods as indicated by results;

   e. Increase emphasis on reading instruction;

   f. Provide language instruction for students for whom English is a second language;

   g. Prepare high-quality teachers. It was determined that special education teachers have to hold a minimum of a bachelor's degree and that they pass a state special education examination or meet some alternate measure of achievement.

The writers of NCLB recommended that educators focus on the results, not the process, that they work under a model of prevention as opposed to a model of failure, and that children with disabilities be considered first as general education children, then as children with impairments (Moore-Brown & Montgomery, 2005).

Title III of NCLB addressed those students who were learning English as a second language, saying that school services for these children were developed to support educators, parents, and students who fall in this category. The issue of homeless children is addressed in Title X. The McKinney-Vento Homeless Education Assistance Act, mandated that school districts provide access to education and any other services needed by children whose families are homeless in order meet the academic standard set for all students in that district. Finally, Title IVa of NCLB provided for safe, drug-free environments in the schools, stating that this is vital for students to have success in school (www.cesa6.k12.wi.us/products_services/eseanochildleftbehind/).

> **think about it**
>
> Drawing from your knowledge of current events, the law, the rights of students with disabilities, and the opinions of educators, has the implementation of NCLB 2001 enhanced or weakened the quality of general education programs in the public schools? Has it enhanced or weakened the quality of special education programs in the public schools?

Individuals with Disabilities Education Improvement Act of 2004 (P.L. 108-446)

The Individuals with Disabilities Education Improvement Act of 2004 (IDEIA) took effect on July 1, 2005. Congress felt the urgent need for reform in special education, citing five major concerns:

1. Students with disabilities drop out of high school at twice the rate of their peers.

2. Enrollment rates of students with disabilities in higher education are still 50 percent lower than the rate of the general population.

3. Most public school educators do not feel well prepared to work with children with disabilities.

4. Of the 6 million children in special education, 50 percent are identified as having a specific learning disability.

5. Children of minority status are over-represented in some categories of special education (Moore-Brown & Montgomery, 2005).

Of significance to all special education fields, and particularly to speech-language pathologists, is the law's requirement for highly qualified special education teachers, which took effect earlier than the rest of the law (December 3, 2004). In 1998, only 21 percent of public school educators felt very well prepared to work with students with disabilities. Furthermore, 41 percent said they felt moderately well prepared for teaching this population. With regard to speech-language pathologists, some states have interpreted "highest qualified provider" to mean the highest qualified provider available. That interpretation, along with the critical shortages of special education professionals and particularly speech-language pathologists, has led to the hiring of underqualified special education professionals. This includes speech-language pathologists being hired who have only a bachelor's degree, thus not meeting what ASHA designates as the highest qualified provider (master's degree). With regard to the fourth bullet, the group of students labeled "specific learning disabled" has grown more than 300 percent since 1976. Eighty percent are in this category because they have not learned to read.It is important to note that P.L. 108-446 was not really an amendment to IDEA. Rather, as noted in the name of the law, it consisted of improvements to IDEA. Moreover, P.L. 108-446 was passed in reaction to the discrepancies between the Individuals with Disabilities Act and the No Child Left Behind Act. Its goal was "to align IDEA with the provisions of NCLB." Some of these differences are as follows:

1. NCLB mandated that all students must show progress at the same rate, and they must achieve the same outcomes. "Progress" is defined as achieving a proficiency level on statewide assessments.

2. IDEA mandated that individualized plans be made by a multidisciplinary team and an IEP team. The IEP must address the student's unique learning needs.

3. The conflict appears to be how to treat everyone individually (IDEA) and the same (NCLB) at the same time.

4. The current standard for success under NCLB is 100 percent proficiency, while the standard for IDEA is a free and appropriate education (Moore-Brown & Montgomery, 2005).

The intent and regulations of IDEIA (2004) "strengthen calls on district- and school-level personnel to ensure that students with disabilities (1) have access to the general education curriculum, (b) receive academic content that is aligned with local and statewide grade-level standards, and (c) are provided opportunities to interact with students without disabilities" (Cushing, Carter, Clark, Wallis, & Kennedy, 2009, p. 195).

The primary implications of IDEIA 2004 for speech-language pathologists are that we need to be more involved in early intervention programs, that we may be asked to provide services in private and charter schools, and that we need to be even more cognizant of functional goals that support the child's academic program. IEP development emphasizes consideration of the child's academic achievement and functional performance, so our goals must be curriculum-related and address how the child's communication disorder impacts the ability of the child to access and meet the goals of a general education classroom (Moore-Brown & Montgomery, 2005). Furthermore, children with disabilities must show adequate yearly progress, as do non-disabled children, and we need to prepare students for statewide assessments, including creating awareness of any accommodations that need to be made for a student.

Moore-Brown and Montgomery (2005) developed a table that compares and contrasts P.L. 107-110 and P.L. 108-447, reproduced here as Table 7–1.

TABLE 7–1   Compare and contrast P.L. 107-110 and P.L. 108-447

	PL 107-110	PL 108-447
Commonly Used Name	No Child Left Behind, NCLB	Individuals with Disabilities Education Improvement Act, IDEA 2004
Date Passed	January 8, 2002	December 3, 2004
Purpose	To ensure that all children have a fair, equal, and significant opportunity to obtain high-quality education and reach proficiency on challenging state achievement standards	To provide free and appropriate education for students with disabilities in public schools
Impact on Speech-Language Pathologists	Opportunities to join general education colleagues to support reading and curriculum goals for students with communication disabilities	Assessment and special education or related services or both provided for students found to have communication disabilities; responsiveness to intervention services

Source: From Making a difference in the era of accountability: Update on NCLB and IDEA 2004, by B. J. Moore-Brown and J. K. Montgomery, p. 71. Copyright 2005 by Thinking Publications.

The regulations of the Individuals with Disabilities Education Act of 2006 bring into play the role of evidence-based education by saying that when instructional plans and methods are specified on a student's IEP, the instruction must show support from scientifically based, peer-reviewed research, echoing the emphasis of NCLB (2001) on evidence-based education (Smith, 2003; Snell et al., 2003). In fact, according to the regulations of IDEA, the IEP must include "a statement of special education and related services and supplementary aids and services, based on peer-reviewed research to the extent practicable" (IDEA regulations, 300.32(a)(4), 2006).

PRACTICAL IMPLICATIONS OF THE FEDERAL LEGISLATION

Evidence-Based Practice/Evidence-Based Education

On December 18, 2001, G. J. Whitehurst presented the keynote presentation, "Evidence-Based Education," at the U.S. Department of Education's Improving America's Schools Conference. Smith (2003) quoted Whitehurst's definition of evidence-based education (EBE): "EBE is the integration of professional wisdom with the best available empirical evidence in making decisions about how to deliver instruction. 'Professional wisdom' is defined as the judgment that individuals acquire through experience" (p. 127). In addition to professional wisdom, one can make use of expert opinions and theory to guide clinical decision making when there is no evidence in the literature (Johnson, 2006).

Before moving into a discussion of the implementation of evidence-based practice in the educational setting, it is helpful to review what is meant by evidence-based practice (EBP) with regard to speech-language pathology and audiology. EBP was first addressed by the medical profession and has become a driving force in most health-related professions and, more recently, in the field of education (which is the focus of this chapter). In 2005, ASHA implemented EBP in an effort to insure that speech-language pathologists and audiologists were providing the best services possible to individuals with communication disorders. In its position statement on EBP, ASHA (2005) delineated the following actions necessary to implement EBP in the clinical practice of audiology and speech-language pathology:

- recognize the needs, abilities, values, preferences, and interests of individuals and families to whom they provide clinical services, and integrate those factors along with best current research evidence and their clinical expertise in making clinical decisions;

- acquire and maintain the knowledge and skills that are necessary to provide high quality professional services, including knowledge and skills related to evidence-based practice;

- evaluate prevention, screening, and diagnostic procedures, protocols, and measures to identify maximally informative and cost-effective diagnostic and screening tools, using recognized appraisal criteria described in the evidence-based practice literature;

- evaluate the efficacy, effectiveness, and efficiency of clinical protocols for prevention, treatment, and enhancement using criteria recognized in the evidence-based practice literature;

- evaluate the quality of evidence appearing in any source or format, including journal articles, textbooks, continuing education offerings, newsletters, advertising, and Web-based products, prior to incorporating such evidence into clinical decision making; and

- monitor and incorporate new and high quality research evidence having implications for clinical practice. (ASHA, 2005)

It is inherent upon universities to teach students how to critically evaluate research and integrate it into clinical decision making. Research should be based on a reasonable theory or hypothesis, include pre- and post-trials, compare performance variables to controls, and consist of random control trials in order to yield the most valid results. Good scientific-based research is typically published in peer-reviewed journals, so the type of journal in which the research is published can provide the clinician with some idea of the quality of the research (ASHA, 2005; Johnson, 2006; Justice & Fey, 2004).

The need to implement evidence-based practice in the schools resulted from legislation addressing education reform demanding accountability (IDEIA, 2004; NCLB, 2001). Congress was looking for efficient and effective intervention and instructional methods that would provide the best utilization of resources to create the best outcomes. To that end, Justice and Fey (2004) discuss "scaling up" in the application of the research in the school settings. They wrote that the hallmarks of science are *accumulation of evidence* (through well-designed research and systematic review of clinical practices) and *preponderance of evidence* (through careful analysis of the accumulated research). Both hallmarks are critical in the "scaling up" of EBP in the schools.

> First comes the scaling up of research, or endorsing researchers' conduct and publication of research that targets real clinical problems and, ultimately, is implemented in non-laboratory, clinical settings. Second comes the scaling up of practices, or removing barriers that affect the translation of research findings to clinical practices in schools. (Justice & Fey, 2004)

For example, there is a preponderance of research that shows a discrepancy between language abilities and cognitive abilities is not a valid criterion to determine eligibility for communication services and supports for severely disabled children. Yet it continues to be used. Thus, we must remove the barriers to the implementation of more proven criteria. (This is discussed more in the section on eligibility.)

The challenge to both the researcher and the practicing clinician is to bridge the gap between the lab and the clinic; in other words, to apply the research in the clinical setting. Johnson (2006) cited the Canadian Cochrane Network/Centre Affiliate Representatives in listing five key steps in clinical decision-making based on evidence:

1. Pose an answerable question.

2. Search for the evidence.

3. Critically appraise the evidence for its validity and relevance.

4. Make decision by integrating the evidence with clinical experience and patient and clinic values,

5. Evaluate performance after acting on the evidence. (p. 21)

Following these steps helps the clinician engage in sound, justifiable, evidence-based decision making. The first step is, of course, the most critical; one cannot answer an unasked question! So, how does one pose a question?

Posing a Question

As a guide in developing a question to study the validity of an intervention, Smith-Greenberg (2010) proposes the acronym PICO:

- P = Patient/population

- I = Intervention/treatment/exposure

- C = Comparison

- O = Outcome

The following scenario shows the application of PICO.

In keeping with the intent of IDEIA (2004) and NCLB (2001), five children with severe disabilities on your caseload are being placed in mainstream program, after 3 years in a self-contained program, to increase their access to the general education curriculum. They will spend 50 percent of their time in a resource classroom and 50 percent of their time in the regular education setting. As the speech-language pathologist for these children, you are curious as to what the evidence says about the effects placement in less restrictive environments has on communication skills of students with severe disabilities. You pose the question, "Do students with severe disabilities who spend a portion of their school day in a regular education setting with grade-level peer models demonstrate more communicative initiating behaviors than students with severe disabilities in self-contained classrooms?" In this question, (P) is the students with severe disabilities; (I) is the use of grade-level peers to model typical communicative behaviors;

(C) is the comparison of the communication behaviors of the children in each classroom setting, and (O) is the number of initiating behaviors. You then conduct a systematic review of the research, starting with studies that have addressed the issue of placement of students with severe disabilities in general education classrooms. You keep refining your search until you find the answer to your question.

In addition, you propose a question specific to your five children: "Will spending 50 percent of their time among peers with no disabilities result in an increase in the number of times the children with severe disabilities initiate interaction with their classmates compared to the number of interactions in the resource room setting?" In this question, there are five children with severe disabilities (P); (I) refers to the effect of increased exposure to peers with typical communication behaviors who could serve as models of good communication skills; (C) is a comparison of initiating behaviors in the resource room and the regular-education room; and (O) is the difference in the number of times the children initiated interactions in each setting.

You posed a question, looked for research that addressed your question, and determined if the evidence supported the decision to place these children in a less restrictive environment. You refined your search until you were determine that the evidence supported the theory that peer models would increase the communication skills of the children with severe disabilities. You then took your own data to see if the children in your group demonstrated the growth expected based on the findings in the research. All of this, combined with your knowledge of each child and your professional experience, can be used as evidence as to which placement is best for the children with whom you are working.

Evidence-Based Education

In 2003, the President's Commission on Excellence in Special Education (PCESE) was formed and charged with three primary goals. In reaction to the rising concerns about education in general and special education in particular, and in reaction to the call for evidence-based education, the commission was charged to study the existing special education system and to recommend policies that would improve the educational performance of students with disabilities and serve as a blueprint for the reauthorization of IDEA. They were also to submit a financial report to Congress for the 2004 fiscal year (Smith, 2003).

Several task forces emerged from the PCESE including the Research Agenda Task Force. This task force reviewed issues related to early childhood research, student assessment, transition services, the provision of services in the least restrictive environment (i.e., inclusion), and intervention. The task force was particularly concerned with improving the quality and quantity of research of educational practices in special education and on how to disseminate the research to the teachers in the classrooms to be put into practice (Smith, 2003). To that end, they wrote a report in July, 2002 that made recommendations with regard to the development and dissemination of research in special education. Specifically, the task force reiterated the need for introducing scientific rigor into the grant review process, for integrating and improving collaboration and coordination within the U. S. Department of Education's Office of Special Education and Rehabilitative Services (OSERS), and for defining long-term research priorities and supporting them. They also stressed the need to "support demonstration and dissemination programs in OSERS that focus on the adoption of scientifically based practices in the preparation and continuing education for teachers" (Smith, 2003, p. 131). It was believed that following through with these activities would "improve the impact of research findings" (Smith, 2003, p. 131) and facilitate evidence-based practices in the instruction of students receiving special education services.

Both IDEIA (2006) and NCLB (2001) call for the provision of education services (special and/or general) by high-quality providers using educational practices that are proven to be effective by scientifically based research (SBR):

> SBR is defined as including experimental or quasi-experimental studies, with a preference for randomized control trials (NCLB, 2001). NCLB requires accountability for all children, including student groups based on poverty, race and ethnicity, disability, and English language learners. (Smith, 2003, p. 126)

Guidelines for Providing Speech-Language Therapy Services to Students with Special Education Needs in Grades K–12

In 1984, the Council of Language, Speech, and Hearing Consultants in State Education Agencies initiated efforts to develop national guidelines for developing and implementing educational programs to meet the needs of children and youth with severe communication disabilities. These efforts culminated in a national symposium, Children and Youth with Severe Handicaps: Effective Communication, that was jointly sponsored by the US Department of Education's Office of Special Education Programs, (OSEP) and the Technical Assistance Development System (TADS) of Chapel Hill, North Carolina. (www.asha.org/NJC)

The OSEP/TADS symposium developed 33 consensus statements to address issues related to the communication needs of children with severe disabilities and how to proceed in addressing those issues. One recommendation was to increase collaboration among agencies serving this particular population, specifically ASHA and The Association for the Severely Handicapped (TASH). These two organizations met in 1986 and formed what is now known as the National Joint Committee for the Communication Needs of Persons with Severe Disabilities (NJC) (www.asha.org/NJC/history/). The stated purpose of the NJC "is to promote research, demonstration, and educational efforts, including both in-service and preservice education, directed to helping persons with severe disabilities communicate effectively" (NJC, 1992).

In 1992, the NJC published a Bill of Rights with regard to communication that all persons should expect in their daily communications:

Each person has the right to

1. request desired objects, actions, events and people

2. refuse undesired objects, actions, or events

3. express personal preferences and feelings

4. be offered choices and alternatives

5. reject offered choices

6. request and receive another person's attention and interaction

7. ask for and receive information about changes in routine and environment

8. receive intervention to improve communication skills

9. receive a response to any communication, whether or not the responder can fulfill the request

10. have access to AAC (augmentative and alternative communication) and other AT (assistive technology) services and devices at all times

11. have AAC and other AT devices that function properly at all times

12. be in environments that promote one's communication as a full partner with other people, including peers

13. be spoken to with respect and courtesy

14. be spoken to directly and not be spoken for or talked about in the third person while present

15. have clear, meaningful and culturally and linguistically appropriate communications. (NJC,1992).

> **think about it**
> How do you think the NJC's Bill of Rights will impact your approach to and justification for the provision of communication supports and services to students with severe disabilities?

In its guidelines, the NJC (1992) posited that "the specific nature of a desired functional communication system is best conceptualized in terms of its social uses" (p. 6). The NJC based its stance on addressing the communication needs of individuals with severe disabilities on empirical evidence and on the philosophical stances that (1) we need to reverse how society as a whole perceives and treats individuals with severe disabilities, and (2) we need to remember that communication is a social behavior through which one individual can influence another. The committee stressed the importance of coordinated efforts involving the family and various professionals involved in the education and development of a child with severe disabilities in assessment, diagnosis, and intervention. Therefore, the NJC developed best practices for assessment, goal setting, intervention, and service delivery. They also addressed the issue of personnel preparation. The reader is encouraged to read the guidelines at www.asha.org/NJC to become aware of the knowledge, skills, and competencies needed by the interdisciplinary team members who provide services to children with severe disabilities, particularly in the area of communication.

Impact of the Federal Legislation on Eligibility for Speech-Language Therapy in the Public Schools

In response to the NJC report, Snell and colleagues (2003) studied the application of eligibility criteria for speech-language therapy in the schools as it related to the population for severely disabled students. The NJC position statement delineated three essential characteristics of communication supports and services:

1. the determination of eligibility for services should be based on the student's "communication needs, not on reasons or criteria that are presumed or taken for granted (also called a priori criteria)" (p. 73).

2. An interdisciplinary IEP team, including the child's parents and a specialist in communication, should plan and evaluate the student's services and supports.

3. "Decisions about team members, services, settings, and how services are delivered should be based on a student's communication needs and preferences" (p. 73).

Eligibility of Students with Special Needs for Speech-Language Services in the Schools

To determine how eligibility decisions (with regard to students with severe disabilities) were being made, Snell and colleagues surveyed (by questionnaire) speech-language pathologists attending a session on eligibility at the 2001 annual conference of ASHA and the 2001 annual TASH conference. In addition, the ASHA ombudsman surveyed 796 speech-language pathologists, also in 2001. The results of their survey revealed use of the following criteria in making decisions about eligibility for speech-language therapy services:

- Student's language age equals mental age (the most frequently used criterion)

- Student too young or too old to benefit

- Student lacks prerequisite skills

- Nature or severity of student's disability

- Student's past progress not sufficient

- Caseload too large

- Restrictive interpretations of need

- Services were not educationally necessary

- Insufficient professional preparation or lack of appropriately trained staff

- Lack of funds or resources

- None: needed services always provided

Snell and colleagues (2003) maintained that all these were a priori (i.e., invalid) criteria for determining eligibility for communication services and supports, providing the reasoning discussed in the following sections.

Discrepancies Between Cognitive and Communicative Functioning and Absence of Cognitive and Other Skills Believed To Be Prerequisites

I have combined these two reasons for point of discussion and illustration. Cognitive theorists, such as Piaget, have long maintained the link between cognition and language. However, it is erroneous to make the assumption that a child cannot improve his or her ability to communicate when he or she appears to have approached capacity in terms of cognitive development or does not have the cognitive prerequisites such as object permanence, means-end, causality, or symbolic play.

An example of the ability to develop a rudimentary communication system in a student who did not have the prerequisites is a student I'll call Jason, who worked with a transdisciplinary team in a self-contained class-room. The team consisted of a special educator, an occupational therapist, a physical therapist, adult volunteers, and myself as the speech-language pathologist. Jason was 16 years old, lived in a rural area, and had never received formal education services until he was 14 years old and P.L. 94-142 was enacted. He had spastic cerebral palsy and was severely compromised orthopedically in terms of spinal deformities and contractures; he could not maintain a sitting position, and the use of his hands and fingers was very limited due to fisting. The majority of the day, Jason was positioned over a wedge because this seemed to be the most comfortable position for him (as determined by less moaning, groaning, and crying). He took nutrition through a gastric tube. Cognition was assessed using observation, developmental checklists, and parent interviews; Jason's observed and reported behaviors were those associated with a 7-month-old developmental level. With regard to communication, he was nonverbal, did not initiate, would occasionally establish eye contact, and had a few random sounds consisting of vowels only. He did not point or gesture due to the physical limitations. Technology in the late 1970s and early 1980s was not as advanced as it is today in terms of access; eye-gaze boards would not work because his communication partner would not be able to follow his eye gaze due to positioning constraints. My initial approach with this student was to engage the other adults in the room in monitoring any movements Jason made while positioned over the wedge and recording them in a log I had next to his wedge. A description of the movement, the time the movement occurred, whether or not he vocalized when making the movement, and whether or not it was a painful movement (as determined by the nature of any vocalizations accompanying the movement) were noted on the log. After two weeks of data were gathered, I analyzed the movements and determined that there were four movements he made at least five times an hour that were not accompanied by any painful vocalizations. I then assigned a "communication message" (i.e., intent) to each of those four movements as seen in Table 7–2.

All adults in the classroom, as well as his parents, were taught to respond with the appropriate phrase every time Jason made one of those four movements. Consistency in using the assigned phrases each time the movement was observed was stressed to all the staff and family. Progress was slow, but

TABLE 7–2 Jason's communication messages

Movement	Assigned Communication Message
Movement of legs side to side	"I want to go"
Turning of head to the left (when on the wedge), usually accompanied by a non-pain vocalization	"Hi"
Extension of the right arm from the shoulder	"I want to work."
Raising head straight up, usually accompanied by a non-pain vocalization	"I want to eat."

Delmar/Cengage Learning

after six months, Jason understood the message associated with the movements as evidenced by the following:

- When the school buses pulled up (you could hear them from our room) he would slide his legs side to side.

- When someone entered the room and cried out, "Hi, Jason!" he would turn his head to the left and vocalize.

- When a clinician or teacher was preparing for some one-on-one instruction, Jason would move his right arm forward when the clinician placed the materials at the base of the wedge.

- When the lunch cart arrived, Jason would raise his head straight up and vocalize.

Eventually, Jason would initiate interactions by making the movements and/or vocalizations. This, too, required some degree of vigilance on the part of the adults. It was easy to monitor the greeting response because Jason would initiate a greeting by vocalizing and turning his head when someone entered through the door that was in his line of vision. The others were harder because we had to "catch" Jason making the movement and respond, "Jason wants to go" (for example) when he was observed moving his legs even when the buses were not yet arriving. Jason also used some of the movements in response to statements and questions. For example, when it was time to go to music, the adult would say, "Jason, it's time to go to music!" and Jason would slide his legs side to side. Some would argue that this was a simple stimulus–response reaction, and, initially, it may have been. However, over time, Jason began to initiate interactions, using the movements as a rudimentary but consistent method of communication. For example, about a year into the program, Jason was having an uncomfortable day as evidenced by more pain vocalizations. When one of the aides said, "Jason, it's time to go to music!" Jason did not make his usual response of sliding legs, which we interpreted to mean he did not want to go to music that day. This indicated to us that he had, indeed, processed the comment and responded in a manner that was consistent with the fact that he probably did not want to go to music that day because he clearly was not feeling up to par.

This is an example of developing a functional communication system for an adolescent with severe disabilities who did not have the advantages that early intervention can provide due to being born in a different era. To his parents' credit, they did not institutionalize him, as so many parents were encouraged to do during the era in which he was born.

Many of the children we worked with in that classroom were not, by state criteria, eligible for communication services and supports because there was not a gap between their cognitive and communicative functioning or because they did not have the prerequisite cognitive skills. Yet we saw that even some of the most severely impaired children were able to learn a communication system. Not all were as successful as Jason, but all but one of the 22 students demonstrated some progress, even if it was limited to establishing and maintaining eye contact, vocal turn taking, and requesting attention and interaction.

> *think about it*
>
> The school district in which you work as a speech-language pathologist has strict enforcement of the language age/cognitive age gap (i.e., discrepancy model) to determine which students qualify for speech-language services. Justify why children with severe disabilities should receive your services.

Chronological Age

The "most basic argument against this criteria is that communication is essential to all persons across the lifespan" (Snell et al., 2003, p. 74). Also, augmentative and alternative communication (AAC) can be learned and beneficial at any age. Some individuals who are severely disabled will continue to grow, in terms of their ability to communicate and interact, throughout their life span.

Diagnosis

The pros and cons of diagnostic labels are discussed elsewhere in this book. However, in some cases, it can have a protective element by enabling the child to become eligible for certain services (not necessarily education services; for instance, Supplemental Security Income). However, with regard to speech and language intervention focusing on functional communication, diagnostic labels "are inadequate to predict an individual's communication potential and to decide whether services and supports are needed" (Snell et al., 2003, p. 75).

Failure to Benefit from Previous Services and Supports

Snell and colleagues (2003) point out that this essentially puts the blame for lack of progress on the student. It is much more likely that the education program is at fault. Perhaps the targeted goals are not functional, are not backed by evidence, or are inappropriately written due to inadequate testing that determined the student's strengths and weaknesses. Another factor could be lack of use of available technology to improve access to the general education curriculum.

Restrictive Interpretations of Educational, Vocational, and/or Medical Necessity

The intent and stipulations of IDEA strongly favor the provision of services and supports to students who have limitations in communication that affect their participation in and ability to benefit from educational and vocational placements. They also debunk using a diagnostic label as an eligibility criterion for communication services and supports. The NJC and IDEA stance on this is summed up by Snell and colleagues (2003), who stated, "services (including assistive technology) and placement needed by each student with a disability must be based on the student's unique needs and not on the student's categorical label" (p. 76). IDEA has, as one of its purposes, the preparation of persons with disabilities for independent living. Schools may be responsible for the procurement of AAC devices for children with communication deficits resulting from traumatic brain injury if the children do not have health insurance, because in cases of brain injury AAC support and services are considered to be medically necessary just as communication is considered to be an educational necessity.

Lack of Appropriately Trained Personnel

Based on the regulations of IDEA (and its various reauthorizations) as well as case law (such as *Timothy W. v. Rochester NH School District*, 1989), public schools and other agencies receiving federal funds for the education and training of students with disabilities are required to have appropriately trained instructional staff. Preparation of general education teachers to teach in inclusion programs is the focus of most college instruction for future teachers. However, continuing education, by law, must be provided for existing school staff (professionals and paraprofessionals) to enable them to provide access to the general education curriculum by students with disabilities.

Lack of Adequate Funds or Other Resources

There is no doubt that education, both general education and special education, is underfunded by most local and state agencies and at the national level. However, interagency agreements, a variety of public and private funding sources, and grants can be used to supplement governmental funding in order to provide the necessary resources to provide quality education.

This section has provided a listing of both established criteria (local, state, and national) and attitudes that can negatively impact the delivery of communication services and supports to children with severe disabilities. Clearly, the law is on the side of the children in stating that students' unique needs, not diagnostic labels, are the determinants in what the child needs and should receive with regard to all factors, particularly communication, in order to gain access to and benefit from his or her school years and beyond. The next area of concern is educational setting.

CENTER-BASED PLACEMENT, MAINSTREAMING, OR INCLUSION?

For every argument for inclusion, mainstreaming, and dedicated centers there is a counter-argument against them. In this section, we look at the advantages and disadvantages of each placement, moving from the least restrictive of the three (inclusion) to the most restrictive (dedicated centers).

Inclusion

Idol (1997) defined *inclusion* as being when a "student with special education needs is attending the general school program, enrolled in age-appropriate classes 100% of the day" (p. 4). Idol's study focused on the attitudes of administrators and teachers toward inclusion. Other studies have focused on variables that affected access to and performance in the general education curriculum by students in inclusion programs (Lee, Soukup, Little, & Wehmeyer, 2009; Dymond & Russell, 2004; Wehmeyer, Lattin, Lapp-Rincker, & Agran, 2003; Bender, Vail, & Scott, 1995). IDEIA (2004) stipulated that all students, including those with severe disabilities, be provided with "supplementary aids and services to ensure student involvement with and progress in the general education curriculum" (Lee et al., 2009, p. 29). Aids and services were listed as physical plant modifications, peer supports, aides or paraprofessionals, curricular adaptations, augmentation of the curriculum, and provision of alternate assessments based on grade-level standards. Of course, as Lee and colleagues pointed out, the intent of NCLB has to be considered in conjunction with IDEIA in determining how to implement the mandate that students with disabilities, even severe disabilities, have access to the general education curriculum. One of the provisions of NCLB is that *highly qualified* teachers use instructional practices and content that are evidence based (Lee et al., 2009). All the studies referenced in this discussion of inclusion have indicated that, to some degree, some general education teachers do not feel adequately prepared to work with children with special education needs.

Several factors have been identified as affecting the access children with special needs have to the general education curriculum. The MainStream Version of the Code for Instructional Structure and Student Academic Response (MS-CISSAR) (Carta, Greenwood, Schulte, Arreaga-Mayer, & Terry, 1988) is a structured observation tool used to study the impact of predetermined variables in three categories (classroom ecology, teacher behaviors, and student behaviors) that have an effect on the degree to which an inclusion program can be implemented effectively and efficiently. Specifically, they identify the following variables:

- Accommodation:
  - Paraprofessionals
  - Peer support
  - Note takers
  - Environmental adjustments

- Extended time on assignments
- Redistributed time
- Assistive technology
- Augmentation:
  - Strategies for learning
  - Strategies for test taking
  - Strategies for organization
  - Strategies for self-regulation
- Adaptation:

  - Adjusted reading demand
  - Adjusted cognitive demand (not reading)
  - Non-print content
  - Content through technology
  - Enhanced content
  - Non-traditional response(s) to instruction
  - Non-traditional instructional materials

All three categories also include "Other."

One factor is related to the curricular modifications made for the students with disabilities in the classroom activities. Dymond and Russell (2004) found that students with mild disabilities spend more time in the general education classroom than do students with severe disabilities. However, essentially no curricular modifications were made for students with mild disabilities in the classrooms Dymond and Russell observed. Some curricular modifications were made for the students with severe disabilities. Students with severe disabilities received more paraprofessional or aide support than did students with mild disabilities. Idol (2006) found that the school administrators in her study were overwhelmingly in favor of inclusion with the caveat that there be extra adults in the classroom who could assist *any* student in need of help. Yet, in practice, it appears that the students with severe disabilities may preoccupy the time of the adults in the classroom.

Another factor to be considered is how actively engaged the students with disabilities are in the general education classroom. This is directly affected by "the ways in which content is delivered to students" (Lee et al., 2009, p. 30). Lee and colleagues (2009) found that "academic engagement of students with disabilities is significantly higher during teacher-directed instruction than during seatwork in both resource room and general education settings" (p. 31). They studied the interaction of numerous student variables and teacher variables and their effect on the student's performance and engagement in the inclusion setting. One observation they made was that "teacher focus" and "student competing response" "were correlated with the degree of difficulty of tasks linked to on-grade or off-grade standards" (p. 40). (Note: The variable "teacher focus" generally referred to "the recipient of the teacher's behaviors and attention"; the "student competing responses" variable was defined as "student behaviors that are unacceptable in the context of academic instruction, academic responding, social conventions, classroom rules, and teacher direction: aggressive behavior, disruption, talking inappropriately, looking around, non-compliance, self-stimulation, and self-abusive behavior") (Lee et al., 2009, p. 35). Off-grade standard tasks related to items on the students' IEPs, while on-grade tasks related to the grade-level curricular activities and demands. When the students with special needs were engaged in less difficult tasks (i.e., off-grade standard tasks), there was more teacher focus and less student competing response; when engaged in on-grade standard tasks, there was less teacher focus and more student competing response. But there was also a tendency when the students were off-grade standard for the special education teachers to take over the instruction. Students with intellectual disabilities also did better in a general education setting when they were given "student-directed learning strategies" (i.e., self-instruction and self-evaluation). In general, the more severe the intellectual disability, the less engaged the student was in activities related to the general curriculum. (Lee et al., 2009).

Setting also played a role. Soukup, Wehmeyer, Bashinko, and Bovaird (2007) studied classroom variables affecting students with disabilities. They found that the students with disabilities did better in small instructional groups such as cooperative learning groups and one-to-one groupings. Students receiving instruction primarily in small groups had a more meaningful experience and performed better than when receiving large group (i.e., classroom) instruction. Peer support was also effective.

A concern expressed by general educators, administrators, and parents of general education students when inclusion was initially implemented was that the scores on state assessments would go down. Idol considered this fact when she evaluated the inclusion program in eight public schools. In reviewing test scores pre- and post-inclusion, it was evident that the test performance of the general education students had not been negatively affected by the inclusion of students with disabilities in the general education classrooms. Idol commented that this "finding was further substantiated by the general impressions of the teachers" (p. 85).

Idol (2006) administered a questionnaire to elementary educators to ascertain their choices on how and where to best teach students with disabilities. Their responses are summed up in Tables 7–3 and 7–4.

Among the secondary (middle and high) school educators, 77 percent thought that the best method for teaching students with special education needs was "including them with all students and having all available adults

TABLE 7–3   Responses to Idol (2006) survey, Item 7–1: "In general,
I believe students with special education needs are best educated in . . ."

Setting Description	Percent of Responses
Grade-level classes	12%
Grade-level classes with a special education teacher or assistant in the classroom with them	39%
Grade-level classes with supportive resource services	22%
Mainstreamed classes with part-time instruction in special education classes	18%
Self-contained, special education classes	2%
Separate, special education schools	0%

Source: Based on Idol (2006), p. 84.

TABLE 7–4   Responses based on Idol (2006) survey, Item 7–2: "When
students with special education needs are taught *in their grade-level classes,*
they are best taught by . . ."

Method	Percent of Responses
Including them with all students and having all available adults work with any student needing assistance	80%
Having them work with a teacher assistant	9%
Having them work with a special educator	12%

Source: Based on Idol (2006), p. 84.

work with any student needing assistance." In addition, 58 percent of this
same group of teachers indicated that other general education students are
"unaffected by the presence of the students with disabilities in their class"
(Idol, 2006, p. 88).

Cushing, Carter, Clark, Wallis, & Kennedy (2009) summed up research on
inclusion showing that students with severe disabilities benefit socially from
daily interactions with typical students in general education classrooms. Early
reports showed that students with disabilities have more friendships, improve
their communication skills, and have improved "access to social, emotional,
and instrumental supports" (p. 196). Later research indicated academic
benefits as well. The students with disabilities demonstrated "high levels of
active engagement" and "improved academic performance" (p. 196). The
students' IEPs had higher quality individualized education program goals and
reflected increased contact with the general curriculum.

Mainstreaming

Idol (1997) defined *mainstreaming* as "when students with disabilities spend a portion of their school day in the general education program, and a portion in a separate special education program" (p. 4). Some say that mainstreaming has positive effects on the child's self-concept and social adjustment and that the student feels as if he or she is more like other students than different from them (Moore-Brown & Montgomery, 2005). Others say it has a deleterious effect on self-esteem because the children realize they are different and feel inferior and/or ashamed due to these differences. Some say it helps a child with impairments to accept his or her limitations and to learn to make adjustments needed in order to be socially accepted by other students. Yet others point to the high drop-out rate of high school students with disabilities, saying that they drop out because they cannot meet the demands of regular education classrooms. One indisputable advantage of mainstreaming is that it educates non-handicapped students about individuals with disabilities. It is hoped that this awareness leads to greater understanding and acceptance of individuals with impairments. Other disadvantages include the aforementioned fact that many teachers do not feel prepared to work with special education students and the general inadequacy of regular education programs to accommodate the inherent demands of students with special needs. The regular education classrooms have a higher teacher–student ratio, making individualized instruction more difficult to achieve. Finally, that "having a label" and being placed in special education and/or related services can be stigmatizing cannot be ignored.

Dedicated Centers

Centers can be advantageous for many reasons. As outlined by Moore-Brown and Montgomery (2005), the advantages of centers over regular education settings include:

- The classes are smaller.
- There is an easing of instructional burden for regular-education teachers.
- All teachers are trained in special education.
- The facilities are built to meet the needs of students with impairments.
- The staff is committed to facilitating the educational and daily living needs of the students.
- There is generous provision of educational and therapeutic equipment and materials.
- There tends to be a greater involvement of outside agencies, volunteers, and parents in center schools as compared to regular-education schools.
- The impact of labels is minimized; all students are equal.

As with everything, there are advantages and disadvantages. Some of the disadvantages include that the students are less prepared for the "real world" when they are educated exclusively in a special education center because they have less interaction with non-handicapped peers in regular education settings. Also, the child may function well in school, but not be able to function in settings beyond the school walls. Some would argue that this is because he or she is too sheltered in a center. Since all his or her classmates are disabled in one manner or another, the student may be unaware of his or her own limitations (Moore-Brown & Montgomery, 2005).

What Do School Administrators and Teachers Think About Placement of Students with Special Education Needs?

Idol (2006) studied inclusion practices at four elementary, two middle, and two high schools to determine teachers' and administrators' principles and opinions about the practice. Out of 120 educators, "only two individuals thought that students with disabilities should be taught in self-contained special education classes, and no one thought that they should be educated in separate special education schools" (p. 84).

The primary disabilities of the students in the four elementary schools were as follows (were as shown in Table 7–5 which shows the number of students in each diagnostic category).

The types of primary disabilities of students in the four secondary schools are detailed in Table 7–6.

Clearly, learning disabilities predominate as the most frequently occurring primary disability in the middle and high schools, but speech impairments were a close second to learning disabilities in the elementary school population. The study addressed the role of the speech-language

TABLE 7–5   Number of students with various disabilities

Disability	Number of Students
Auditory	25
Autism	4
Emotional disturbances	31
Learning disabilities	103
Multiple disabilities	2
Mentally retarded (sic)	21
Orthopedic handicaps	2
Other health impairments	32
Speech impaired	91
Total	311

Delmar/Cengage Learning

TABLE 7–6 Distribution of primary disabilities among four secondary schools

Disability	Middle School	High School
Autism	3	1
Emotional disturbances	17	75
Learning disabilities	189	301
Mental retardation (sic)	9	36
Other health impairments	33	32
Speech impairments	3	2
Traumatic brain injury	2	2

Delmar/Cengage Learning

pathologists in the schools, with the general response of the educators regarding the speech and language therapy programs being that "some of this instruction—particularly language intervention—could be offered in the general education program, with the speech-language therapist serving as a consulting teacher" (p. 93). The educators also thought that having the speech-language therapist functioning as a consulting teacher would reduce the number of referrals to special education.

Idol (2006) summed up the attitudes of educational professionals as follows:

- There is a trend among educators toward inclusion.

- There is a trend among administrators toward inclusion if extra adults are available for all students who need help, not just the students with disabilities.

- Educators "had generally favorable impressions of the impact of students with disabilities on other students in their classes" (p. 91). The exception to this was students with behavior problems, but the educators noted this applied to all students regardless of whether they had disabilities.

- Regarding the resource room, many educators believe students with disabilities need tutorial assistance via resource rooms, but the curriculum in the resource room should match or support the general education curriculum.

- The educators and administrators support the use of cooperative teaching with both the general education teacher and special education teacher, but profess that this is not always financially feasible.

ROLES OF SPEECH-LANGUAGE PATHOLOGISTS IN PUBLIC SCHOOLS

As written in P.L. 94-142, speech-language pathologists in the public schools have five responsibilities. The first is identification. Through screenings and referrals, the speech-language pathologist can identify those children who are in need of a full assessment. The second responsibility is diagnosis and appraisal of specific speech and/or language disorders. Once the assessment is complete, the speech-language pathologist determines if the child meets the criteria needed to qualify for therapy, writes long- and short-term goals for the child, and convenes the IEP team. If a child does not qualify for services and/or if additional information is needed, the clinician's third responsibility is to make appropriate referrals to other professionals. The fourth responsibility is listed as "habilitation," or the provision of intervention services for each child determined to be eligible for services. Finally, the speech-language pathologist is to provide counseling and guidance about speech and language development, delays, and disorders for parents, children, and teachers. This activity can result in more appropriate referrals, thereby saving time for the clinician in the long run. The guidance can take the form of individualized work with teachers, students, and parents, as well as in-services and workshops. At faculty meetings, the speech-language pathologist can have "Two Minutes with the Speech-Language Pathologist" and provide a tidbit of information for fellow faculty members and administrators to keep in mind with regard to identification, referral, and treatment of students with speech and/or language deficits.

In the late 1980s, the collaborative approach was embraced by ASHA as the most effective means of providing intervention in the public schools. Also known as curriculum-based therapy or classroom-based strategy intervention, this method focused on collaborative team teaching, with the classroom teacher and speech-language pathologist working together to facilitate speech and language improvement in the classroom setting. Clinicians would conduct therapy in the classroom, with the clinician, classroom teacher, and aides working together to facilitate the achievement and generalization of the speech-language goals. Both the pull-out method and the collaborative method are considered to be direct therapy. The teacher and speech-language pathologist have, to some degree, to change their roles and perceptions of roles as outlined in Table 7–7.

In contrast, the consultative method is an indirect therapy approach. In the consultative model, the speech-language pathologist provides suggestions to teachers and other professionals serving the child, but does not directly intervene in the child's educational plan. These suggestions can take the form of a generalized in-service or suggestions specific to a designated classroom from which the teacher asks for ideas for facilitating language growth in his or her pupils.

TABLE 7–7 Changes in classroom members' roles

	Before Classroom-Based Strategy Intervention	After Classroom-Based Strategy Intervention
Classroom Teachers		
Self-Image:	Leader	Classroom collaborator
Strategies:	Hit-or-miss compensatory strategies	Educated guesses for language support
Language:	General discourse routines	Reflective clarification
Emotional:	Less control	More control
Motivation:	External attributions	Internal attributions
Students		
Self-Image:	Mistake maker or respondent	Language participant
Strategies:	Practice and leave	Choose and use
Language:	Predictable patterns	Risk taker
Emotional:	Follower	Leader
Motivation:	External attribution of problems	Internal attribution of problems
Speech-Language Pathologists		
Self-Image:	Resource teacher	Classroom collaborator
Strategies:	Rules and repetition	Real, usable cues
Language:	Contrived routines	Discussion and feedback
Emotional:	Therapist, frustrated	Facilitator, less frustrated
Motivation:	External attribution of problems	Internal attribution of problems

Source: Classroom-based language and literacy intervention: A programs and case studies approach, by F. C. Falk-Ross, p. 49. Copyright 2002 by Allyn and Bacon. Reprinted with permission.

Regardless of which approaches are used by a clinician, it is imperative that the goals and objectives for each student in therapy be individualized, curriculum focused, and functional. Public school therapy and, as a matter of fact, all therapy for school-aged children should be designed to facilitate academic, social, and vocational achievement by each student served by the speech-language pathologist, regardless of whether the speech-language therapy is special education or a related service.

Classifying Students as Disabled

No one will argue that it is risky to assign a label to a child because there is always the danger that the label will be assessed and treated instead of the individual child. Also, peers of the child may make fun of the child based on his or her label if they find out about it. Nonetheless, grouping by disability is the most common way of grouping children who have special needs. Even those who are grouped together as "gifted" can be the targets of ridicule. McCormick and Loeb (2003) make note of three "unfounded assumptions" that are often made as the result of grouping children by disability: "(1) that there are specific factors that have caused the disability; (2) that these factors can be identified; and (3) that all children with the same disability will benefit from the same intervention and/or instructional techniques" (p. 75).

Labeling typically occurs for two reasons: financial and placement. Thus, most educational systems continue to group children by disability regardless of the inherent dangers expressed by the above assumptions. IDEA identifies 14 areas of impairment ("labels") for which individualized instruction is mandated. These categories are listed in Table 7–7. If a child does not fall into one of these categories, he or she is at risk for having non-individualized services in the public schools. Most of the categories encompass children who have speech and/or language deficits, so there is a burden on our graduate education programs to provide instruction in as many of the 14 categories as possible. Children who are speech and/or language impaired receive special education services from the speech-language pathologist. Children in all other categories receive related services, because the categories listed in Table 7–8 are the students' primary

TABLE 7–8   Categories of disabilities listed in IDEA

Autism
Deaf-blindness
Deafness
Developmental delay
Emotional disturbance
Hearing impairment
Mental retardation
Multiple disabilities
Orthopedic impairment
Specific learning disabilities
Speech or language impairment
Traumatic brain injury
Visual impairment
Other health impairment

Delmar/Cengage Learning

placement (i.e., their special education placement) (McCormick & Loeb, 2003).

Case Load Selection

Every child who is eligible for services must be served. There cannot be waiting lists in the public schools. Yoder and Kent (1988) devised a decision-making diagram to illustrate the caseload selection process (see Figure 7–1).

One way that speech-language pathologists identify children who need to be assessed is through teacher referral. Tattershall (2002) suggested the use of a teacher observation questionnaire like one she developed to help teachers identify students who need to be seen by the speech-language pathologist. Tattershall developed her questionnaire specifically for the referral of adolescents, but it could be adapted for elementary-aged children. A copy of her Teacher Observation Questionnaire is found in Appendix 7B. Tattershall (2002) posed some excellent questions that would certainly provide some good foundation information prior to the assessment of the child. However, a criticism of Tattershall's questionnaire is that it is long and teachers may not have time to fill it out. Even though many of the questions are yes/no, there are still several questions that are time consuming to answer. This could result in the teacher not completing the questionnaire, resenting the speech-language pathologist for the demands on his or her time, or providing incomplete answers in the interest of time. None of these is a desirable outcome! It may be more beneficial and less time consuming for the speech-language pathologist to ask the questions face-to-face with the teacher. Also, interviews sometimes yield additional information that one would not necessarily get from a written questionnaire.

Selection of Assessment Tools

A reality in public schools is the lack of funds. Some school districts purchase the tests for the clinicians while others expect the clinicians at the individual schools to procure the tests themselves. Tests are very expensive, as a rule, so it behooves the clinician to choose tests that are comprehensive as well as valid and reliable. The speech-language pathologist may be better off buying a test that assesses receptive and expressive language than two separate tests. Also, many districts require that children be labeled and placed on the basis of the results on a minimum of two tests, so that should also be kept in mind when purchasing tests. It is also important to purchase and use a test for which the standardization sample reflects the characteristics of the children in the clinician's school. In addition to language tests, the clinician must have, or have access to, instruments that assess the various disorders associated with speech such as articulation deficits, phonological disorders, fluency problems, and voice disorders. Yoder and Kent (1988) developed a decision-making process to guide the clinician in evaluating tests and assessment procedures. This process can be found in Figure 7–2.

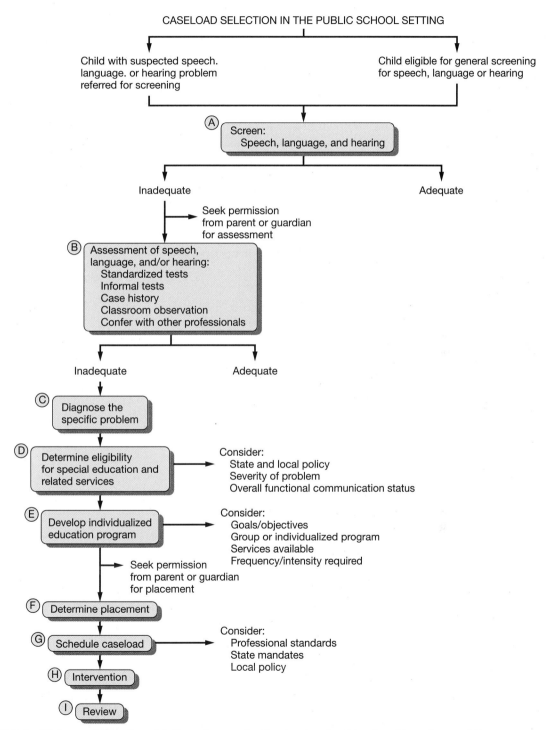

FIGURE 7–1 Yoder and Kent's guidelines for caseload selection in the school-based speech-language therapy programs. (*Source: Decision-making in speech-language pathology,* by D. E. Yoder and R. D. Kent, p. 175, 1988.)

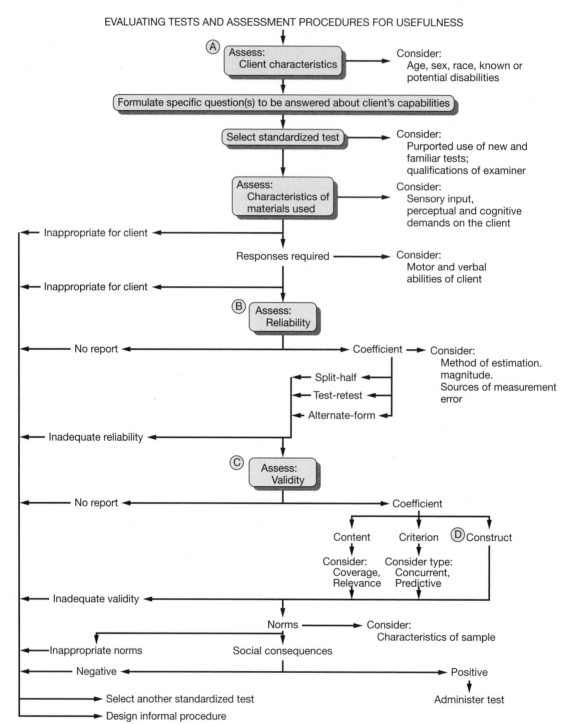

FIGURE 7–2 Yoder and Kent's process for evaluating tests and assessment procedures. (*Source: Decision-making in speech-language pathology,* by D. E. Yoder and R. D. Kent, p. 191, 1988.)

SUMMARY

This chapter has provided information on the legal requirements and implications of federal legislation focused on children with impairments. A review of the key pieces of legislation was offered, as well as an overview of the practical applications of the laws, including the roles of speech-language pathologists in the schools, approaches to therapy, and the settings in which children with handicaps are educated. It should be noted that, at the other end of the spectrum, gifted children are also considered to be receiving special education services because their education goes beyond the realm of the standard classroom. Clearly, the speech-language pathologist working with children in the public schools has an opportunity to be highly instrumental in the children's achieving their academic, social, and vocational goals.

REVIEW QUESTIONS

1. The principle of a "free and appropriate public education" was first set forth in
    a. The Education Amendments of 1974 (P.L. 93-380)
    b. The Education for All Handicapped Children Act of 1975 (P.L. 94-142)
    c. Individuals with Disabilities Education Act of 1990 (P.L. 101-407)
    d. Section 504 of the Rehabilitation act of 1973 (P.L. 93-112)

2. The Individualized Education Plan must be revised every 6 months.
    a. True
    b. False

3. The Individual Family Service Plan is written for which age group?
    a. Birth–2 years
    b. 3–5 years
    c. 6–11 years
    d. 12–18 years

4. Under FERPA, parents of students under the age of 18 can inspect or review official school records, files, and data relating to their child.
    a. True
    b. False

5. Which of the following is a civil rights statute?

   a. NCLB

   b. IDEA of 2004

   c. Section 504 of the Rehabilitation Act of 1973

   d. Education for All Handicapped Children Act

6. Speech-language pathology services can be considered special education instead of related services if the child's primary placement is a regular education classroom.

   a. True

   b. False

7. Which of the following was not a primary purpose of P.L. 94-142?

   a. Provide assurance that all children with handicaps would receive a free and appropriate public education

   b. Protect the rights of children with handicaps and their parents

   c. Ensure that all students achieve mastery on statewide achievement tests

   d. Evaluate the effectiveness of federal, state, and local efforts to provide special education and related services

   e. Provide financial support to insure that children with handicaps have full educational opportunities

8. Which of the following is not a part of an IEP?

   a. Behavioral objectives

   b. Criteria for mastery of objectives in the school setting

   c. Objectives to be taught in the family setting

   d. Baseline data

9. IDEIA 2004 mandates that all students must show progress, which is defined as achieving a predetermined proficiency level on statewide assessments.

   a. True

   b. False

10. What law introduced the concept of transition?

    a. P.L. 94-142 (Education for All Handicapped Children Act)

    b. P.L. 99-457 (Education for All Handicapped Children Act Amendments)

    c. P.L. 107-110 (No Child Left Behind)

    d. P. L. 101-407 (IDEA 1990)

REFERENCES

American Speech-Language-Hearing Association (1994, August). Service provision under Individuals with Disabilities Education Act – Part H, as amended (IDEA—Part H) to children who are deaf and hard of hearing ages birth to 36 months. Rockville, MD: Author.

American Speech-Language-Hearing Association. (2005). *Evidence-based practice in communication disorders* [position statement]. Available from www.asha.org/policy.

Bender, W. N., Vail, C. O., & Scott, K. (1995). Teacher's attitudes toward increasing mainstreaming: Implementing effective instruction for students with learning disabilities. *Journal of Learning Disabilities, 28*(2): 87–94.

Carta, J. T., Greenwood, R., Schulte, D., Arreaga-Mayer, C., & Terry, B. (1988). *Code for instructional structure and student academic response: Mainstream version (MS-CISSAR)*. Kansas City: Juniper Gardens Children's Project, Bureau of Child Research, University of Kansas.

Cushing, L. S., Carter, E. W., Clark, N., Wallis, T., & Kennedy, C. H. (2009, February). Evaluating inclusive education practices for students with severe disabilities using the Program Quality Measurement Tool. *Journal of Special Education, 42*(4): 195–208.

Dymond, S. K., & Russell, D. L. (2004). Impact of grade and disability on the instructional context of inclusive classrooms. *Education and Training in Developmental Disabilities, 39*, 127–140.

Falk-Ross, F. C. (2002). *Classroom-based language and literacy intervention: A programs and case studies approach*. Boston: Allyn & Bacon.

Gravani, E. H. (1997). Legal landmarks. In P. F. O'Connell (ed.), *Speech, language, and hearing programs in schools: A guide for students and practitioners*. Gaithersburg, MD: Aspen Publishers, Inc.

Idol, L. (1997). *Creating collaborative and inclusive schools*. Austin, TX: Pro-Ed.

Idol, L. (2006). Toward inclusion of special education students in general education: A program evaluation of eight schools. *Remedial and Special Education, 27*(2): 77–94.

Johnson, C. J. (2006, February). Getting started in evidence-based practice for childhood speech-language disorders. *American Journal of Speech-Language Pathology, 15*, 20–35.

Justice, L., & Fey, M. (2004, September 21). Evidence-based practice in schools: Integrating craft and theory with science and data. *The ASHA Leader*.

Lee, S., Soukup J., Little, T. D., & Wehmeyer, M. L. (2009, May). Student and teacher variables contributing to access to the general education curriculum for students with intellectual and developmental disabilities. *Journal of Special Education, 43*(1), 29–44.

McCormick, L., & Loeb, D. F. (2003). Characteristics of students with language and communication difficulties. In L. McCormick, D. F. Loeb, and R. L. Schiefelbusch (eds.), *Supporting children with communication difficulties in inclusive settings: School-based language intervention* (2nd ed.). Boston: Allyn & Bacon.

Moore-Brown, B. J., & Montgomery, J. K. (2005). *Making a difference in the era of account-ability: Update on NCLB and IDEA 2004.* Eau Claire, WI: Thinking Publications.

National Joint Committee for the Communicative Needs of Persons with Severe Disabilities. (1992). Guidelines for meeting the communication needs of persons with severe disabilities [guidelines]. Available from www.asha.org/policy or www.asha.org/njc.

Smith, A. (2003). Scientifically based research and evidence-based education: A federal policy context. *Research and Practice for Persons with Severe Disabilities, 28*(3), 126–132.

Smith-Greenberg, C. (2010). Moving evidence to policy and practice. www.pediatricnursing.net/conf/handouts/2010/Session_212_Greenberg.pdf

Snell, M. E., Caves, K., McLean, L., Mollica, B. M., Mirenda, P., Paul-Brown, D., Romski, M. A., Rourk, J., Sevcik, R., & Yoder D. (2003). Concerns regarding the application of restrictive "eligibility" policies to individuals who need communication services and supports: A response to the National Joint Committee for Communication Needs of Persons with Severe Disabilities. *Research and Practice for Persons with Severe Disabilities, 28*(2), 70–78.

Soukup, J. H,, Wehmeyer, M. L., Bashinsko, S. M., & Bovaird, J. (2007). Classroom variables of students with intellectual and developmental disabilities. *Exceptional Children, 74,* 101–120.

Tattershall, S. (2002). *Adolescents with language and learning needs: A shoulder to shoulder collaboration.* Clifton Park, NY: Delmar, Cengage Learning.

Taylor, J. S. (1992). *Speech-language pathology services in the schools* (2nd ed.). Boston: Allyn & Bacon.

Wehmeyer, M. L., Lattin, D., Lapp-Rincker, G., & Agran, M. (2003). Access to the general curriculum of middle-school students with mental retardation: An observational study. *Remedial and Special Education, 24,* 262–272.

Whitehurst, G. J. (2001, December 18). Evidence-based education. Keynote presentation at the U.S. Department. of Education's Improving America's Schools Conference, San Antonio, TX.

Yoder, D. E., & Kent, R. D. (1988). *Decision making in speech-language pathology.* Philadelphia, PA: B. C. Decker, Inc.

www.asha.org/NJC/history/, retrieved June 5, 2010.

www.asha.org/members/ebp/, retrieved June 6, 2010.

www.cesa6.k12.wi.us/products_services/eseanochildleftbehind/, retrieved September 20, 2009.

www.k12.wa.us/esea/, retrieved September 20, 2009.

APPENDIX 7A

Example of an IEP used in the Alachua County School District of Florida

Individual Education Plan | Front Page |

Student's Legal Name: _____ IEP Development Date: _____

Grade: _____ School: _____ Birthdate: _____ ID#: _____

Primary Exceptionality: _____

Additional Exceptionality: _____

Most Recent Evaluation Date: _____ Date of Last IEP: _____ Transition IEP *(Age 14 +)*: ☐ Yes ☐ No

---

General Factors: *Briefly describe each of the following general factors*

Student's strengths: _____

Student's interests: _____

How student input was obtained: _____

Results of the most recent individual evaluations or re-evaluations: _____
_____

Results of any state or district-wide assessments or alternate assessments: _____
_____

What concerns for their child's education have the parents expressed? _____
_____

Student's Health Needs/Concerns: _____

Special Factors: Each of the following Special Factors has been considered for this student. Check ☒ those that have been identified as needs for this student and are addressed in this IEP:

☐ Need for positive behavior intervention or strategies   ☐ Braille needs of blind/visually impaired

☐ Language needs of Limited English Proficient   ☐ Communication and language needs

☐ Need for assistive technology devices and service   ☐ Need for ESE extended school year services

☐ Need for specially designed/adaptive physical education   ☐ Need for special transportation services

---

Goal Areas: Check ☒ the areas for which present level of educational performance statements and measurable annual goals are to be included in this IEP:

☐ Instructional Domains   ☐ Transition Service Needs (age 14+)

   ☐ Curriculum and Learning Environment   ☐ Instruction   ☐ Post-school Adult Living

   ☐ Social and Emotional Behavior   ☐ Related Services   ☐ Daily Living Skills

   ☐ Independent Functioning   ☐ Community Experience ☐ Functional Vocational

   ☐ Communication   ☐ Employment   Evaluation

Transition Services *(Beginning no later than age 14 or 8th grade):* Describe the transition service needs that are to be addressed through the student's course of study, including diploma option, and in the present levels, goals, and services on the IEP.

Diploma Option: ☐ **Standard**   ☐ **Special**   [☐ **Option 1**   ☐ **Option 2**]

Does the student need instruction or assistance in self-determination or self-advocacy skills?   ☐ Yes ☐ No

If Yes, these needs are addressed in:

☐ Goals/Objectives   ☐ Accommodations   ☐ Related Services   ☐ Present Levels   ☐ Curriculum

---

Transfer of Rights:

☐ Check if the student has been informed of transfer of rights at least one year prior to reaching age of majority.

    Date of notification prior to age 17: _____   Date of 2nd notification prior to age 18: _____

Update Page # _____	Attached (Date): _____
Update Page # _____	Attached (Date): _____
Update Page # _____	Attached (Date): _____

_____ School/Cum Folder Copy

_____ Parent Copy

_____ Teacher Copy

Individual Education Plan

Student's Legal Name:		ID#:	Age:	IEP Date:

Measurable Postsecondary Goals: Beginning no later than age 16, measurable postsecondary goals are required, based on student input and transition assessments.

Transition assessments used to develop these goals included (list):

Results of transition assessments:

Postsecondary Education/Training Goal :   Following graduation from high school, the student will complete additional education/training in

Postsecondary Employment Goal: Following graduation from high school, the student will be employed in

Independent Living Goal (if needed):

Transition Services: Describe transition services for the student and a statement of interagency responsibilities or any linkages needed in order to progress toward the Measureable Postsecondary Goals.

	Services Needed		
	Yes	No	Services and/or Linkages
1. **Instruction:**	☐	☐	
2. **Related Services:**	☐	☐	
3. **Community Experience:**	☐	☐	
4. **Employment:**	☐	☐	
5. **Post-school Adult Living:**	☐	☐	
6. **Daily Living Skills:**	☐	☐	
7. **Functional Vocational Evaluation:**	☐	☐	

Responsibilities and/or Linkages for Transition Services: *A person's signature below indicates willingness to provide for the support(s), service(s), or skill(s) that relate to the Transition Plan*

Agency Represented	Responsibilities	Representative's Signature
Agency Represented	Responsibilities	Representative's Signature
Parent	Responsibilities	Parent's Signature
Student	Responsibilities	Student's Signature

_____ School/Cum Folder Copy
_____ Parent Copy
_____ Teacher Copy

Individual Education Plan

Goal Page

Student's Legal Name: _____   ID#: _____   IEP Date: _____
Date of update conference that additional annual goal(s) were added *(complete only if applicable)*: _____

Present Level of Academic, Developmental, or Functional Performance for *(Specify domain checked page1)*:

☐ Curriculum & Learning   ☐ Social & Emotional   ☐ Independent Functioning   ☐ Communication

Transition Service Need(s) addressed by this goal (age 14+):

☐ Instruction   ☐ Community Experience   ☐ Employment   ☐ Post-school Adult Living   ☐ Daily Living Skills

Based on:

Student is able to *(describe in measurable terms)*:

Student's disability affects involvement and progress in general education by (for pre-kindergarten children, participation in age-appropriate activities):

Priority educational need:

Measurable Annual Goal: *(include conditions, observable behavior, criterion, and timeline)*

Assigned Instructional Responsibilities for Goal: *(planning, implementing, documenting student performance, consulting, etc.)*
Lead Teacher/Staff: Others (s):
_____   _____
Title/Position of Person(s) Responsible   *Title/Position of Person(s) Responsible*

Benchmarks/Short-Term Objectives *(minimum of 2 steps to achieve the goal)*:

1.

2.

3.

Evaluation Plan: Describe how progress toward the annual goal will be measured _____

The student's progress toward the annual goal and the likelihood of attainment of the annual goal by the end of the year will be reported to the student's parents with each report card, at least every weeks.

Date:									
Progress toward Goal: *Report measured results in accordance with annual goal and evaluation plan*									
Likelihood of Attainment: *H - Highly Likely P - Possible U - Unlikely*									

Page 2 A B C D E F

_____ School/Cum Folder Copy
_____ Parent Copy
_____ Teacher Copy

Individual Education Plan

Service Page

Student's Legal Name: _____ ID#: _____ IEP Date: _____
Date of update conference for revision of services (*complete only if applicable*): _____

Special Education Services	Date: Initiation*	Duration*	Frequency	Location

Related Services	Date: Initiation*	Duration*	Frequency	Location

Program Modification/Instructional Accommodations	Date: Initiation*	Duration*	Frequency	Location

Supports for School Personnel	Date: Initiation*	Duration*	Frequency	Location

Supplementary Aids and Services	Date: Initiation*	Duration*	Frequency	Location

*Excluding Student Holidays/Breaks in accordance with the adopted regular school calendar, unless otherwise indicated.

Participation in state and district-wide assessment program(s):   ☐ Yes   ☐ No   ☐ N/A
If No, attach ☐ the completed Alternate Assessment Checklist **and** ☐ Notice of Non-participation to Parent
List each alternative assessment and describe why selected: ☐ Florida Alternate Assessment   ☐ Other assessments
_____
_____

Assessment Accommodations: *Describe needed accommodations for **all** testing situations.*

☐ Flexible Setting: ☐ Recording of Answers: ☐ Flexible Scheduling:
☐ Mechanical Aids: ☐ Flexible Timing: ☐ Revised Format:
☐ Other_____
For state and district-wide assessments, consult test manual to determine which of the above accommodations are permissible.

☐ Accommodations provided are allowed on state and district-wide assessments
☐ Parent has been provided an explanation for any instructional or assessment accommodations not allowed on statewide assessment
    (*letter attached*)

_____ School/Cum Folder Copy
_____ Parent Copy
_____ Teacher Copy

Individual Education Plan			Signature Page

Student's Legal Name:	ID#:	IEP Date:

Participation in Regular/Vocational/Alternative Education	**Percent of Time** *with non-disabled students*	**Purpose**

Removal from Programs with Nondisabled Students: Explain the extent, if any, to which the student will NOT participate with non-disabled students in the regular class and extracurricular and nonacademic activities:

Placement: Based on percent of time with nondisabled students

☐ **Regular Class** (80% or more with non-disabled)

☐ **Resource Room** (40% or more, but less than 80% with non-disabled)

☐ **Separate Class** (less than 40% with non-disabled)

☐ **Homebound or Hospitalized**

☐ **Separate Day School**

☐ **Residential Facility**

☐ **Juvenile Justice Facility**

☐ **Other:**

Specialized Transportation: ☐ **Not Applicable**

☐ 1. **Medical equipment required** (i.e., wheelchair, crutches, walkers, cane, tracheotomy equip, positioning or unique seating devices.)

☐ 2. **Medical condition requires a special transportation environment as per physician's prescription** (e.g. tinted windows, dust controlled atmosphere, temperature control.)   Describe: _____

☐ 3. **Aide or monitor is required due to disability and specific need of student.**   Describe:

☐ 4. **Shortened school day required due to disability and specific need of student.**   Describe:

☐ 5. **School assigned is located in an out-of-district school system.**   Describe:

Conference Notes:

Participants in Attendance at IEP Development Meeting—*have access to a copy of this IEP and have been informed of any responsibilities for the IEP implementation.*

Parent(s) _____

LEA Representative _____

ESE Teacher _____

Other IEP Team Member(s) _____

Student _____

Regular Ed Teacher _____

Evaluation Interpreter or Psychologist _____

Other Participant(s) _____

Procedural Safeguards	**Notification Attempts (Attach Invitations)**
☐ I have received a copy of *Outline of Procedural Safeguards.*	1. Date: Method:
	2. Date: Method:
☐ I have received a copy of the *Notice of Procedural Safeguards for Parents of Students with Disabilities.*	**Parents not in attendance, Procedural Safeguards sent with copy of IEP** _____
_____ _____	*Date*
Parent Signature *Date*	

Notice of Change of Placement or Services has been provided to parent: ☐ Yes   ☐ N/A, no changes

_____ School/Cum Folder Copy

_____ Parent Copy

_____ Teacher Copy

Individual Education Plan

Update Page #

Addendum to IEP Dated: _____   Addendum MUST be attached to current IEP

Student's Legal Name: _____   ID#: _____

Update Conference   Date: _____

Re-evaluation: ☐ **Planning**   ☐ **Review**   ☐ **Permanent**   ☐ **Other:**

Conference Notes:

Participants in Attendance at Update IEP Conference

Parent(s) _____   **Student** _____

LEA Representative _____   **Regular Education Teacher** _____

ESE Teacher _____   **Evaluation Interpreter or Psychologist** _____

Other IEP Team Member(s) _____   **Other Participant(s)** _____

Procedural Safeguards	**Notification Attempts (Attach Invitations)**
☐ I have received a copy of *Outline of Procedural Safeguards.*	1. Date: Method: 2. Date: Method:
☐ I have received a copy of the *Notice of Procedural Safeguards for Parents of Students with Disabilities.*	
	Parents not in attendance, Procedural Safeguards sent with copy of IEP _____
_____ _____	*Date*
Parent Signature *Date*	

Notice of Change of Placement or Services has been provided to parent: ☐ Yes   ☐ N/A, no changes

_____ School/Cum Folder Copy
_____ Parent Copy
_____ Teacher Copy

APPENDIX 7B

Teacher Observation Questionnaire

RE: John Doe

Date: _____

Permission signature: _____

Parent signature: _____

John and his parents have given permission for me to learn about his performance and participation in your class to inform our working together to improve his language and learning skills. Please complete the following checklist and add any observations we have omitted.

- How would you describe John as a student in your class?

- What do you think John needs to do to improve his work in your class?

- What is John's attention like in your class? Is he able to sustain his listening? Can he maintain his focus during individual or small group work? Does he attend well in whole group discussion?

- Does John seem to know the usual routine in your class? Is he ready when you begin your lessons? Is he ready when you give oral directions or assignments?

- Does John seem organized in your class? Does he have needed materials? Does he hand in homework on time?

- How does John participate in oral discussion? Does he make appropriate comments? Does he add to the information? How often does he comment? Are his comments appreciated by others? Does he ask questions? How often? Are they appropriate questions? Does he answer questions in a timely manner? In a clear fashion? Do you see notable differences in John's participation in whole group, small group or paired learning situations?

- What can you tell me about John's reading? Is he willing to read aloud? How well does he read orally? Does he seem to comprehend?

- What can you tell me about John's writing? Can he generate ideas for topics? Can he narrow topics to make them workable? Is he willing to write? Can he write enough? Does he express his ideas clearly? Does spelling cause him difficulty in writing? Is he avoiding challenging words because of spelling?

Source: *Adolescents with Language and Learning Needs: A Shoulder to Shoulder Collaboration.* By S. Tattershall p. 85. (2002). Clifton Park, NY: Delmar, Cengage Learning.

Chapter 8

Language Development and Impact of Language Deficits in the School Years

LEARNING OBJECTIVES

After completion of this chapter, the reader will be able to:

1. Identify predictors of a child's need for special services in adolescence.

2. List Damico and Oller's seven pragmatic referral criteria for elementary education teachers.

3. Differentiate characteristics of language development in the early and later childhood years as noted by Nippold.

4. Identify residual language problems experienced by school-age children with a history of language deficits.

5. Describe the pragmatic and form components of language in children with mental handicaps.

6. Discuss the impact of poor reading skills on one's academic and vocational life.

INTRODUCTION

Becoming school age and then entering the preadolescent and adolescent years are times of tremendous change and growth in the physical, social, academic, and personal segments of a child's life. Rosenkoetter (1995) listed some of the changes that accompany the transition from preschool to kindergarten:

1. The adult/child ratio is reduced.

2. There are an increased number of children in educational and social groups.

3. Children may be riding a school bus or participating in a carpool instead of being driven to school by the parents.

4. The family's involvement may differ between preschool and kindergarten.

5. There are increased expectations for academic performance placed on the child.

6. There is a different and more structured curricular content in kindergarten.

7. The manner of teacher instruction differs, with increased expectations for knowledge of classroom rules and routines.

Children who have a language delay or disorder frequently find these school-year transitions more difficult than typically developing children would. The transition to school creates additional demands on a child's language that are introduced by teachers and peers in the classroom setting. Children who have a language-based disorder or delay are certainly at risk of failure when they enter the academic segment of their lives. Many of the children who have transition difficulties qualify for school-based intervention, with therapy directed at reducing the impact of the language deficit on the child's academic and social progress. The involvement of the school-based speech-language pathologist in identifying children who have language deficits and in facilitating the school-year transitions is critical in establishing language competencies that play a role in the curricular changes as the child progresses through school. Nelson (1994) wrote the following:

> To succeed in the new communicative context of the early grades, children must learn to process language that is more complex and decontextualized than at home. They must recognize on their own when repairs are needed and how to make them. They must also learn new rules of communicative interaction that involve expectations for making formal requests to take communicative turns (e.g., by raising their hands) and for keeping their turns short, to the point, and responsive to topics raised by the teacher rather than initiating turns of their own. (p. 120)

think about it What impact could a preschooler's home environment have on his or her ability to adapt to school? Think about SES, parenting style, and the impact of preschool.

EFFECTS OF SPEECH AND LANGUAGE DEFICITS ON SOCIAL AND ACADEMIC ACHIEVEMENT

There have been many studies showing that speech and language deficits manifested during the preschool years have residual effects on social and academic achievement in the school years. In a 1980 study, Aram and Nation conducted a chart review of children seen at the Cleveland Hearing and Speech Center in 1973–1974 who were diagnosed with developmental speech and language disorders. A follow-up study was done 4 to 5 years after diagnosis, relying on teacher and parent ratings and the teachers' reports of the children's status based on academic achievement as measured by standardized tests. Approximately 40 percent of the children who were originally seen for developmental speech and language problems continued to have difficulties with language, articulation, or reading and spelling. In a similar study done by King, Jones, and Lasky (1982), 50 adolescents who had been seen as preschoolers at the Kent State University Speech and Hearing Clinic were assessed by parent report. Forty-two percent of the 50 adolescents still had communication problems.

There are obvious problems with retrospective studies. For one thing, the investigators must rely on whatever information is available in the child's record of his or her preschool development. Secondly, there is no control over who is in the study because severity of the problem cannot always be determined retrospectively. Children with serious motor problems and children with mild articulation problems are all included. A third problem is the subjectivity of relying on reports from parents and teachers for the follow-up study.

Longitudinal Study by Aram, Ekelman, and Nation

Aram, Ekelman, and Nation (1984) did a 10-year follow-up study of children who had been diagnosed with a language disorder and enrolled in ongoing therapy at the Cleveland Hearing and Speech Center as preschoolers. The children ranged in age from 3:5 to 6:11. Each of the 47 children was given an extensive battery of language tests in 1971. The tests measured "comprehension, formulation, and repetition of certain semantic, syntactic, and phonological features" (p. 233). Also, each child was assessed for nonverbal intelligence using the Arthur Adaptation of the Leiter International Performance Scale (Arthur, 1952). If the child failed a hearing screening, had craniofacial or neurological deficits, or had begun first grade, he or she was excluded from the study. In 1981, the researchers located 20 of the original 47 children (16 boys and four girls) and retested them. They ranged in age from 13:3 to 16:10, and the mean age was 14:10. The 1981 retesting included measures of intelligence, speech and language, academic achievement, and social adjustment. In addition, the parents of each adolescent completed a parent questionnaire (the Child Behavior Checklist; Achenbach, 1981) addressing behavior problems and social competence.

The results from the follow-up testing were summarized by the study's authors as follows:

60 percent of the verbal IQs, 80 percent of the performance IQs, and 70 percent of the full-scale IQs fell within or above the low average range. Yet, with few exceptions, most subjects continued to present deficiencies in language abilities, required special academic attention, were less socially competent, and presented more behavioral problems than their peers. Thus, it would appear that for most of this group, the language disorders recognized in the preschool years were only the beginning of long-standing language, academic, and often behavioral problems.

Five of the adolescents had not been in special education and had not repeated a grade. These students had the highest IQs, the best performance on diadochokinetic tasks (tasks requiring rapid and repetitive movements

Diadochokinetic tasks. Tasks requiring rapid, repetitive movements of the articulators; frequently elicited by having the child repeat p^t^k^ as quickly as possible.

of the articulators), and the best language abilities. The other special education services ranged from tutoring to placement in a class for children who were educable intellectually disabled. These children had the lowest IQs, the most problems with diadochokinetic tasks, and the poorest language performance. "Those with mid-range IQs and language skills required either tutoring, grade repetition, or self-contained LD class placement" (p. 240). The reader is referred to this study (Aram, Ekelman, & Nation, 1984) for a complete explanation of the test procedures used and a more extensive discussion of the results.

> **think about it**
>
> What effect does a language deficit in the preschool years have on academic adaptation?

PREDICTORS OF NEED FOR LANGUAGE INTERVENTION DURING THE SCHOOL YEARS

There are numerous factors that can be used to predict a child's need for special services at different developmental stages. For example, parental traits such as the education level of the mother "are better predictors of disabilities in adolescence than children's own behavior" (Nelson, 1998, p. 289) during the early years (birth to age 3). However, from ages 4 to 7, child-centered skills (i.e., cognitive abilities and speech, language, and communication skills) as measured by standardized tests are better predictors of a child's need for special services in adolescence (Kochanek, Kabacoff, & Lipsitt, 1990). Furthermore, teachers are the main source of referral for children in the school years. Thus, the speech-language pathologist should spend time educating the teachers about receptive and expressive language problems that can negatively impact a child's social and academic achievement. Damico and Oller (1980) noted seven pragmatic referral criteria for elementary education teachers. These criteria are outlined in Table 8–1.

Another frequent predictor for the need of special services is the age at which a child began to talk. Girolametto and colleagues (2001) studied 21 children at age 5 who had previously been diagnosed as late talkers. The children all had received previous intervention that included a parent program implemented when the children were 2 to 3 years of age and direct therapy for approximately 50 percent of the children who did not show adequate language growth in the parent program. At age 5 the children were tested on their language, with the results being compared to those of typically developing peers. Following intervention, 86 percent of the language-impaired children matched the control group in the areas of expressive grammar and vocabulary but had weaknesses on some higher-level

TABLE 8–1 Pragmatically oriented referral criteria for elementary education teachers as suggested by Damico and Oller (1980)

- *Linguistic nonfluency.* Disruption of speech production by a disproportionately high number of repetitions, unusual pauses, and excessive use of hesitation forms.
- *Revisions.* Breakup of speech production by numerous false starts or self-interruptions; multiple revisions are made as if the child keeps coming to a dead end in a maze.
- *Delays before responding.* Pauses of inordinate length following communication attempts initiated by others.
- *Nonspecific vocabulary.* The use of expressions such as *this, that, then, he,* or *over there* without making the referents clear to the listener; also, the overuse of all-purpose words such as *thing, stuff, these,* and *those.*
- *Inappropriate responses.* Utterances that appear to indicate that the child is operating on an independent discourse agenda—not attending to the prompts or probes of the adult or others.
- *Poor topic maintenance.* Rapid and inappropriate changes in the topic without providing transitional clues to the listener.
- *Need for repetition.* Requests for multiple repetitions of an utterance without any indication of improvement in comprehension.

Source: From Language, speech, and hearing services in schools, Vol. 11(2), by J. S. Damico and J. W. Oller, Jr., p. 88. Copyright 1980 by American Speech-Language-Hearing Association. Reprinted with permission.

standardized tests designed to measure the child's ability to meaningfully engage in teacher–child discourse, his or her use of pragmatic cues for resolving ambiguous sentences, and other narrative tasks. This and other studies have found that by the time the late talkers attain school age, most of them score within normal limits on norm-referenced expressive language tests. However, many of the children who achieve these normal scores "continue to have difficulties with higher level linguistic tasks that clearly distinguish them from their peers and that could place them at risk for learning and academic difficulties during the early school years" (Girolametto et al., 2001, p. 359). Girolametto and colleagues cited several studies in which the assessment of children's narrative skills revealed that the late talkers had similar mean length of utterances and content when compared to children with normally developing expressive language—the ability to convey a message through conventional means using words and symbols—but they used "significantly fewer cohesive ties and were less mature" (p. 359).

Rescorla, Hadicke-Wiley, and Escarce (1993) assessed the language of 6-year-old children who had been late talkers and found that the children scored lower than their peers on word definition tasks, verbal reasoning tasks, and auditory short-term memory tasks. When they retested the late

Expressive language. The ability to convey a message through conventional means using words and symbols; the content of what is expressed.

talkers at ages 7 and 8, the children had difficulty on sentence formulation tasks. At age 8, they also demonstrated problems in auditory processing, verbal memory, and fluency in word retrieval. Certainly, all these residual problems can affect the child's ability to succeed in school.

Even when children's early language problems appear to resolve (as documented by tests of basic communication skills), they often show evidence of difficulties when more abstract and decontextualized language is assessed or when multiple language skills must be coordinated, as when engaged in narrative retelling tasks.

The adolescent years are particularly daunting in the changes that occur not only related to academics, but also to physical, social, emotional, and vocational growth. Some of these changes are highlighted in Table 8–2.

TABLE 8–2   Characteristics of stages and tasks of normal adolescence

| Task | Stage of Adolescence | | |
	Early (10–14)	Middle (14–16)	Late (16–20)
Acceptance of the physical changes of puberty	• Physical changes occur rapidly but with wide person-to-person variability • Self-consciousness, insecurity, and worry about being different from peers	• Pubertal changes almost complete for girls; boys still undergoing physical changes • Girls more confident; boys more awkward	• Adult appearance, comfortable with physical changes • Physical strength continues to increase, especially for males
Attainment of independence	• Changes of puberty separate adolescents from children, but do not provide independence • Ambivalence (childhood dependence unattractive, but unprepared for the independence of adulthood) leads to vacillation between parents and peers for support	• Ability to work, drive, date; appear more mature; dependence lessens and peer bonds increase • Conflict with authority, limit testing, experimental and risk-taking behaviors at a maximum	• Independence a realistic social expectation • Continuing education, becoming employed, getting married—all possibilities that often lead to ambivalence about independence

(continued)

TABLE 8–2 (*continued*)

Task	Stage of Adolescence		
	Early (10–14)	Middle (14–16)	Late (16–20)
Emergence of a stable identity	• Am I OK? Am I normal? • How do I fit into my peer group? • Paradoxical loss of identity in becoming a member of a peer group	• Who am I? • How am I different from other people? • What makes me special or unique?	• Who am I in relation to other people? • What is my role with respect to education, work, sexuality, community, religion, and family?
Development of cognitive patterns	• Concrete operational thought: present more real than future, concrete more real than abstract • Egocentrism • Personal fable • Imaginary audience	• Emerging formal operations: abstractions, hypotheses, and thinking about future personal interests and emerging identity	• Formal operations: thinking about the future, things as they should be, options, consequences can be considered

Source: From Communication solutions for older students, by V. L. Larson and N. McKinley, p. 36. Eau Claire, WI, Thinking Publications. © 2003 by Thinking Publications. Reprinted with permission.

LONG-TERM OUTCOMES FOR CHILDREN WITH LANGUAGE AND SPEECH IMPAIRMENTS IN THE PRESCHOOL YEARS

Longitudinal Study by Johnson and Colleagues

Johnson, Beitchman, Young, Escobar, Atkinson, Wilson, and colleagues (1999) conducted a 14-year longitudinal study evaluating speech and language outcomes of 142 young adults; 128 had no history of speech and/or language impairment, and 14 were identified at age 5 years as having a speech and/or language impairment. The results of their study showed that children who had early language deficits continue to have deficits at age 14 in the cognitive, language, and academic domains. In addition, children who had speech deficits at age 5 demonstrated subtle, residual speech problems as teenagers. However, the children with speech deficits only did not show cognitive, language, and/or academic deficits when compared to their typically developing peers. Johnson and colleagues summarized their major findings as follows:

- High rates of continued communication difficulties in those with a history of impairments

- Considerable stability in language performance over time

- Better long-term outcomes for those with initial speech impairment than for those with language impairment

- More favorable prognoses for those with SLI than for those with impairments secondary to sensory, structural, neurological, or cognitive deficits (p. 744).

Additional information on this study can be found in Chapter 9.

Longitudinal Study of Late Talkers by Rescorla

Rescorla (2009) conducted another longitudinal study in which she followed 26 late talkers from preschool to age 17. All the children had nonverbal ability within normal limits and normal receptive language. The 26 late talkers were compared to 23 typically developing children who were matched for age, SES, and nonverbal ability. Each adolescent was given assorted standardized language tests in one 2-hour session. The results showed that the 17-year-old students who were late talkers scored "in the average range on all language and reading tasks at age 17," but they scored significantly lower on vocabulary/grammar and verbal memory factors than did their peers matched based on SES (Rescorla, 2009).

These same children were tested at age 13 years, and their scores on comparable language factors were strong predictors of the vocabulary/grammar and reading/writing factors obtained at age 17 years. The author concluded that, when compared to their typically developing peers, children who had delayed language development at age 2 to 31 months demonstrated "a weakness in language-related skills" at age 17 years. However, they scored in the expected age range on various language measures, but lower than the controls. Thus, it appears that delayed expressive language as toddlers does not cause significant language impairments at age 17. By self- and parent report, all the teenagers were making good progress in school, but still had weaker language skills than their classmates who did not have expressive language delays (Rescorla, 2009).

It is important to distinguish between late talkers and preschoolers with SLI, even though the diagnostic criteria (language difficulties with no apparent cause or primary condition) are comparable. Both groups have weak language skills when compared to their typically developing peers. Rescorla (2009) argues for a "dimensional theoretical formulation" (p. 17) that describes a child's language abilities on a spectrum. This idea was first proposed by Bishop and Edmundson in 1987 when they took exception to the idea of defining "discrete subtypes of deficits in language abilities." Rescorla (2009) also posited "that late talkers have below average *endowment* in a set of intercorrelated yet diverse language-related abilities" similar to a child's endowment for intelligence (p. 17). That is to say that, to some degree, a child's language abilities are innate, or "constitutional in origin" (p. 17).

The dimensional approach predicts that preschoolers with SLI or late talkers are very likely to continue to have weaker language skills than comparison peers who never manifested language delay because of what is presumed to be their more compromised language endowment. (Rescorla, 2009, p. 17)

Rescorla (2009) concluded that one can make the argument that children with expressive language delays as toddlers may have subclinical weaknesses in skills such as grammatical rule learning, auditory perception, verbal working memory, phonological discrimination, motor planning, and word retrieval.

> **think about it**
>
> If you were a school-based speech-language pathologist or audiologist, what would you include in an in-service for regular education teachers to educate them about the impact of speech and/or language disorders on school performance?

> **think about it**
>
> If you were a school-based speech-language pathologist or audiologist, what would you include in an in-service for regular education teachers to teach them how to make a good referral for speech, language, and/or hearing assessment?

CONTINUING DEVELOPMENT OF LANGUAGE IN THE SCHOOL YEARS

Metalinguistic skills. Skills that allow an individual to think about language in a critical manner and to make judgments with regard to the accuracy and appropriate use of language skills and functions.

Metapragmatic skills. Conscious and intentional awareness of ways in which to use language effectively in different contexts.

When considering the impact of language development on the various features of language, it is evident that children continue to acquire skills in each feature throughout childhood, but the most prevalent growth is in the areas of pragmatics and semantics. One reason for this is the expansion of the child's world beyond the home as the child enters the structured academic experience. He or she is interacting with more people in a variety of contexts that exceed the interactions focused primarily on the family and narrow preschool group. In addition, the child's metalinguistic skills and metapragmatic skills show rapid growth during this transition time.

The Development of Metalinguistic Skills

The development of metalinguistic skills is most marked at 4 to 8 years of age, but the skills continue to mature well into adolescence. Metalinguistic skills constitute a language awareness that enables the child to think and talk about language as something more than simply being a tool that enables communication (Bernstein, 1997). The development of metalinguistic skills is particularly important because some researchers believe that they appear to be critical in the child's ability to attain literacy skills (van Kleek, 1994). Other areas of change as the child progresses from childhood to adolescence include the development of metacognition, the ability to develop alternative ways to solve a problem or resolve a situation, the ability to form hypotheses and task analyze them in a constructive manner, and the capacity to make personal decisions (Larson & McKinley, 1995).

The growth accompanying the change from preschool to kindergarten, as well as from elementary school to middle school and middle school to high school, requires an increased responsibility for problem solving and for making personal decisions (Larson & McKinley, 1995), both of which are frequently problematic for children who have a language delay and/or disorder that extends beyond the preschool years.

Miller (1989) listed developmental tasks, some of which begin in childhood and extend into the preadolescent and adolescent years:

- The development of a self-identity

- Adjustment to physical and psychological changes in the body

- The development of abstract thought processes about the physical and social world, "thinking beyond the here and now," and forming opinions based on fact

- The acquisition of interpersonal skills to foster the development of peer relationships

- The development of new relationships with family members as the child increases his or her independence and lessens the emotional dependence on family

- The development of a personal system of values that impacts problem solving and the development of relationships

- The ability to consider the future and set goals

Additional milestones in the areas of language and cognition can be found in Appendix 8A. This appendix covers ages 6 to 80 years and beyond.

Another prominent change is the fact that children move from having primarily an auditory mode of learning language to also having a visual mode of learning language as they begin to read and write in the early grades in school (Bernstein, 1997).

Later Stages of Language Development

The academic, social, and vocational demands of language as the child progresses through the school years are astounding. Nelson's (1998) later stages of language development include children from third grade through

Metacognition. The ability to develop alternative ways to solve a problem or resolve a situation, the ability to form hypotheses and task analyze them in a constructive manner, and the capacity to make personal decisions.

Abstract thought processes. Thinking beyond the limits of a fact and developing opinions and expansion on a given piece of information.

adulthood; they are divided into the preadolescent age group (8 to 12 years of age) and the adolescence and transition to adulthood stage (12 to 21 years of age). During the later stages of development, children make gradual changes in their language acquisition as opposed to the rapid changes in the early and middle age periods. Nippold (1988) conducted research aimed at differentiating between the early (ages 0 to 9) and later (ages 9 to 19) stages of language development. One factor stressed by Nippold is that up to age 8, emphasis is on the acquisition of spoken language skills, whereas at age 9 and later, the emphasis is on written language skills. As children get older, they learn language from both auditory and visual input, whereas younger children learn primarily from auditory input (the speech of others). Other differences include the growth of metacognitive and metalinguistic abilities in later childhood and adolescence, as well as the processing of more abstract notions.

> **think about it**
>
> What is the impact of developing metalinguistic and metacognitive abilities on academic and pre-vocational success?

Syntactic Growth

Embedded sentences. Compound sentences in which a minimum of two independent clauses are combined to form one sentence.

Syntactic growth during the school years includes expansion of noun and verb phrases, the use of embedded sentences (also known as compound sentences; those consisting of at least two independent clauses) using words such as *unless, therefore,* and *although* (even though interpretation of these words does not occur until approximately age 7 years); the comprehension of gerunds (around age 6 years); and the use of derivational morphemes (*-er, -man, -ist*) that change verbs into nouns around 6.5 years of age. Other areas of syntactic and morphological growth include the comprehension of irregular noun–verb agreement (by the end of second grade), and the use of reflexive pronouns (Menyuk, 1969; Carrow, 1973; Bernstein, 1997).

Nippold, Mansfield, Billow, and Tomblin (2009) conducted a follow-up study of syntactic development in adolescents who had a history of language impairments. They tested 102 adolescents who had a diagnosis of SLI, 77 students with a nonspecific language impairment (NLI), and 247 typically developing children (with regard to language) (TLD). NLI children were distinguished from SLI children based on performance on nonverbal intelligence tests. Children with NLI scored below average on these tests, while children with SLI had average performance. The methodology was to gather a language sample through the use of a spoken discourse task. The discourse was elicited using a peer conflict resolution task, and the sample was then analyzed using a variety of means. The concepts and directions subtest and the recalling sentences subtest of the Clinical Evaluation of Language Fundamentals, 3rd edition (CELF-3) were also administered. The researchers found that, in terms of syntactic complexity, the typically developing children performed better than the SLI and NLI groups on the discourse analysis. On the standardized testing, the TLD adolescents again outperformed the SLI and NLI groups. The SLI students outperformed the NLI students.

Nippold and colleagues (2009) also made the point that in order to perform the daily tasks associated with a typical public high school, "adolescents must have a sufficient amount of relevant background knowledge and the ability to use and understand spoken and written language at an advanced level. Given these high expectations in schools today, it is not surprising to learn that when language impairments persist into adolescence, they frequently have a negative impact on academic performance" (p. 241). Syntactic knowledge enables individuals to generate an unlimited number of complex utterances that are required for creative expression. Most 5-year-old children are able to process and produce grammatically mature sentences consisting of subordinate clauses, and the increase in this ability through adolescence leads to an enhanced ability to express abstract ideas. Multiple studies have shown that students with language impairments use shorter, more simplistic sentence constructions than do typically developing students.

> **think about it**
>
> How does advancement in syntactic knowledge enhance a child's semantic abilities?

Growth of Lexicon in School-Age Children

There is a significant increase in lexicon, or vocabulary, in school-age children, both in terms of learning new words and being able to more clearly define them. Growth in these areas extends throughout the school years.

There is a dramatic increase in the use of words denoting temporal, spatial, logical, and familial relationships between the ages of 7 to 11 years, as well as an increase in the use of words with multiple meanings (Bernstein, 1997; Menyuk, 1971; Owens, 1996). Bernstein (1997) wrote that there is a high correlation between lexicon, "general linguistic competence, and academic aptitude" (p. 131). Throughout the school years, children increase their abilities to comprehend and use nonliteral language (abstract and symbolic language), which includes metaphors, idioms, humor, and proverbs.

An example of growth of humor is evident as children of different ages attempt to share the "Why did the chicken cross the road" joke during a conversation at dinnertime:

Lexicon. A composite list of the words and signs that comprise an individual's vocabulary.

Nonliteral language. Language that is abstract and symbolic.

7-year-old: "Why did the chicken cross the road?"
Father: "I don't know! Why did the chicken cross the road?"

7-year-old: "To get to the other side."
Family: Robust laughter.

4-year-old: "Why did chicken cross the road?"
Mother: "I don't know! Why did the chicken cross the road?

4-year-old: "Cross the road."
Family: Laughter, with the 4-year-old's laughter being the most raucous.

18-month-old: "Chicken" and laughter.
Family: Light-hearted laughter to indicate enjoyment of the attempt.

Metalinguistic devices. The ability to think about and analyze language, including the ability to understand humor, multiple meanings, inferences, and figurative language.

Clearly, the 4-year-old was beginning to implement the ability to analyze language using metalinguistic devices to convey humor in that she understood the concept of a riddle but still needed development in order to understand the punch line! The 18-month-old clued in on one word that had possibly made everyone else laugh and uttered it in order to provoke a reaction.

Another area of significant growth through the school years is pragmatics as children "learn how to become good conversational partners, how to make indirect requests, and how to process the language of the classroom" (Bernstein, 1997, p. 133). The development of social, emotional, and cognitive skills as the child progresses through school results in an expansion of the child's pragmatic capabilities. White (1975) noted communicative skills demonstrated by school-age children:

1. They can obtain and maintain adults' attention in a socially acceptable manner.

2. They can assume the roles of leader and follower among their peers.

3. They can use other individuals as a resource for help in obtaining desired information.

4. They can express appropriately emotions such as affection, hostility, and anger.

5. They can show pride in themselves and their accomplishments.

6. They can actively engage in role play.

7. They can compete with their peers in storytelling activities.

Similar growth occurs in the use of narratives, conversation, indirect requests, and topic maintenance. Children age 5 use direct requests, but by age 7 they begin to make indirect requests, an ability that grows in complexity as the child advances in age (Bernstein, 1997).

As one can see, there are many changes that children, preadolescents, and adolescents experience, and certainly all of these changes and areas of growth have the potential to be negatively impacted by the presence of a language delay or disorder.

FUNCTIONAL ILLITERACY

According to the report, State of Adult Literacy 2006, (Monten, 2007) the rate of functional illiteracy among adults 16 years and older in the United States is 21 percent. In 2003, the Organization for Economic Cooperation and Development conducted a study to compare literacy rates in six countries: the United States, Bermuda, Italy, Norway, Switzerland, and Canada. Only Italy had more citizens who are functionally illiterate than the United States; in other words, the United States came in fifth. According to the National Right to Read Foundation, "42 million Americans cannot read and 50 million can only read at the fourth or fifth grade level" (2009). Furthermore, 25 percent of America's teenagers drop out of high school. Among those who graduate from high school, 25 percent have equivalent to or less than an eighth-grade education. The prevalence of adults who are functionally illiterate is increasing at the rate of approximately 2.25 million persons each year. (McGreer, 2009). Twenty percent of high school graduates are considered to be functionally illiterate. Individuals are considered to be functionally illiterate if they cannot read and write well enough to complete everyday tasks such as filling out a job application and reading the newspaper.

The lifetime implications are numerous. The National Adult Literacy Survey (2007) found that "children who entered school without having developed some basic literacy skills are 3–4 times more likely to drop out of high school." This has vocational, societal, and financial implications. The National Institute for Literacy (2007) unveiled these disturbing facts:

1. 70 percent of prisoners in state and federal systems can be classified as illiterate.

2. 85 percent of all juvenile offenders rate as functionally or marginally illiterate.

3. 43 percent of those whose literacy skills are lowest live in poverty.

Other facts that point to the widespread impact of functional illiteracy are that 75 percent of those on welfare, 86 percent of unwed mothers, and 68 percent of those who are arrested are functionally illiterate (Washington Literacy Council, n.d.). It is estimated that 75 percent of the jobs in the United States require at least a ninth-grade reading level, yet 27 million Americans are unable to read well enough to complete a job application.

Again emphasizing the financial impact, 48.7 percent of Americans have reading and writing levels so low that they work in below-the-poverty-level-wage jobs (Clecker, 2010). Our nation spends $240 million in social service expenditures and lost tax revenues annually. Illiteracy alone costs taxpayers in America an estimated $20 billion a year (Baker, 2008).

In an effort to quantify rates of functional illiteracy based on gender, age, race, and level of education, the National Center for Education Statistics conducted the 2003 National Assessment of Adult Literacy study. They analyzed reading ability based on prose literacy, document literacy, and quantitative literacy:

> *Prose literacy* refers to knowledge and skills needed to perform prose tasks—that is, to search, comprehend, and use continuous texts. Prose examples include editorials, news stories, brochures, and instructional materials.
>
> *Document literacy* refers to knowledge and skills needed to perform document tasks—that is, to search, comprehend, and use noncontinuous texts in various formats. Document examples include job applications, payroll forms, transportation schedules, maps, tables, and drug or food labels.
>
> *Quantitative literacy* refers to knowledge and skills required to perform quantitative tasks—that is, to identify and perform computations, either alone or sequentially, using numbers embedded in printed materials. Examples include balancing a checkbook, computing a tip, completing an order form, or determining the amount of interest on a loan from an advertisement (2003 National Assessment of Adult Literacy).

On each of these tasks, scores of 0 to 500 were assigned based on the individual's performance. They defined four levels of performance: below basic, basic, intermediate, and proficient. Table 8–3 shows the scores associated with each level of performance on each of the three tasks.

In the United States, students in the fourth grade in public schools had an average score of 220 on the National Assessment of Educational Progress (NAEP). The average score of eighth graders was 261. The key findings of the 2003 study with regard to literacy levels in American adults were as follows:

1. 14 percent below basic (30 million): no more than the most simple and concrete literacy skills

2. 29 percent basic (63 million): can perform simple and everyday literacy activities

TABLE 8–3 Scores associated with each level of performance on each of the three literacy tasks

	Below Basic	Basic	Intermediate	Proficient
Prose	0–209	210–264	265–339	340–500
Document	0–204	205–249	250–334	335–500
Quantitative	0–234	235–289	290–349	350–500

Source: 2003 National Assessment of Adult Literacy.

3. 44 percent intermediate (95 million): can perform moderately challenging literacy activities; and

4. 13 percent proficient (28 million): can perform complex and challenging literacy activities.

These numbers are chilling and bring to the forefront the critical need to expose children to books, to read to them from an early age, and to provide adequate instructional activities designed to facilitate the development of reading. Two key components of this instruction are phonics and phonological awareness. Both of these components have been proven to have critical impact on a child's reading ability. It is also imperative that children be read to daily from infancy.

Appendices 8B–8D consist of a series of tables depicting literacy levels based on gender, race, age, and educational level.

TRANSITIONS EXPERIENCED BY SCHOOL-AGED CHILDREN AND ADOLESCENTS

As discussed in Chapter 7, P.L. 99-457 introduced the concept of transition into the education process. Students go through periods of transition as they move from grade to grade, school to school, and school to community, college, or the workforce. Transitions are often met with students' increased feelings of inadequacy with regard to academic competence. This feeling is most pronounced in the transition from elementary school to middle school. Middle school is the beginning of "less personal attention, more whole-class instruction, and less chance to participate in classroom decision-making" (Berk, 2004, p. 371). These factors, along with higher academic expectations, often lead to a decline in grades after the transition from elementary school. The transition from elementary to middle school has more detrimental effects on girls than boys, with boys remaining fairly stable in the transition. Overall, the timing of the shift from elementary to middle school coincides with the beginning of puberty, and one cannot help but acknowledge that the combination of the two events leads to the academic and social stress these young women feel. It should be noted that the feelings of social and academic inadequacy are not as pronounced, in fact are barely evident, in students who attend school in districts that had K–8 and 9–12 schools (no middle schools) (Berk, 2004). Berk summed up the impact of this critical transition as follows:

> School transitions often lead to environmental changes that fit poorly with adolescents' developmental needs. They disrupt close relationships with teachers at a time when adolescents need adult support. They emphasize competition during a period of heightened self-focusing. They reduce decision-making and choice as the desire for autonomy increases. And they interfere with peer networks at a time of increased concern with peer acceptance. (p. 371)

SUMMARY

The development of language has been studied heavily in the preschool population. However, it is only in the last 10 years or so that much attention has been paid to the continuing development of language in school-age children. Care should be taken to analyze the language of a child based on semantics, syntax, morphology, phonology, and pragmatics. Children who have demonstrated a delay or disorder in one or more areas of language as preschoolers should be tested and enrolled in therapy as soon as possible in order to minimize the impact of the delay or disorder on social and academic functioning. There is substantial evidence for the need to incorporate preliteracy skills into the education of all preschool children, and particularly of those preschoolers who have language delays or disorders. Literacy intervention is probably needed when the child begins and progresses through the academic curriculum.

Evidence exists in some of the recent research that indicates that even preschool-age children whose language deficits appear to have been resolved by the time they enter first grade may have some residual effects that are not noticed until the academic demands increase. Typically, there is a substantial increase in academic demands when the child enters third grade and begins to face the demands of reading textbooks for comprehension. Dealing with problem solving, abstract concepts, and increased linguistic complexity can tax a child's linguistic system, particularly if there have been previous problems. Thus, it is probably a good idea to monitor the language skills of all third graders who have a history of language delays or disorders in case there are residual elements that could impact the child's academic and social success.

CASE STUDY

Instead of the usual case study, I am including a story written by Preston Lewis who has an 18-year-old brother who is cognitively challenged, with an IQ in the 30 to 40 range. The name of the story is "A Case for Teaching Functional Skills" and I believe it captures the need to have therapy goals that are aimed at helping individuals with life-long impairments to get the most benefit out of life.

A Case for Teaching Functional Skills

By Preston Lewis

It is not uncommon to find instances of curricular content for students with moderate to severe handicaps based primarily on information from the administration of norm-referenced evaluation instruments. A dilemma often results when an attempt is made to translate test items failed at particular levels or mental ages into actual tasks to be taught. Not only were these evaluation tools never intended to be used in this manner, but the result is that students end up spending a majority of their school years being taught skills that are totally artificial or extremely age inappropriate. Given the time it takes students with moderate to severe handicaps to acquire and maintain even functional skills, there is no time or justification for devoting instruction to teaching items that are selected from a developmentally based hierarchy of supposed "prerequisite" selected skills. A scenario of the outcome for one such student is portrayed below.

My Other Brother Daryl

18 years old. TMH (30 to 40 IQ). Been in school 12 years. Never been served in any other setting than elementary school. He has had a number of years of "individual instruction." He has learned to do a lot of things!

Daryl can now do lots of things he couldn't do before!

He can put 100 pegs in a board in less than 10 minutes while in his seat with 95 percent accuracy. But he can't put quarters in vending machines.

Upon command, he can "touch nose, shoulder, food, hair, ear." He's still working on wrist, ankle, hips. But he can't blow his nose when needed.

He can now do a 12-piece Big Bird puzzle with 100 percent accuracy and color an Easter Bunny and stay in the lines! But he prefers music, but was never taught how to use a radio or record player.

He can now fold primary paper in halves and even quarters. But he can't fold his clothes.

He can sort blocks by color, up to 10 different colors! But he can't sort clothes (whites from colors) for washing.

He can roll Play Dough and make wonderful clay snakes. But he can't roll bread dough and cut out biscuits.

He can string beads in alternating colors and match it to a pattern on a DLM card. But he can't lace his shoes.

He can sing his ABCs and tell me names of all the letters of the alphabet when presented on a card in uppercase with 80 percent accuracy. But he can't tell the men's room from the ladies' room when we go to McDonald's.

He can be told it's a cloudy or rainy day and take a black felt cloud and put it on the day of the week on an enlarged calendar (with assistance). But he still goes out in the rain without a raincoat or hat.

He can identify with 100 percent accuracy 100 different Peabody Picture Cards by pointing! But he can't order a hamburger by pointing to a picture or gesturing.

He can walk a balance beam forwards, sideways, and backwards! But he can't walk up the steps or bleachers unassisted in the gym to go to a basketball game.

He can count to 100 by rote memory. But he doesn't know how many dollars to pay the waitress for a $2.59 McDonald's coupon special.

He can put the cube in the box, beside the box, and behind the box. But he can't find the trash bin in McDonald's and empty his trash into it.

He can sit in a circle with appropriate behavior and sing songs and play "Duck, Duck, Goose." But nobody else in his neighborhood his age seems to want to do that.

I guess he's just not ready yet.

Source: Reprinted with permission from *TASH Newsletter*, December 1987.

REVIEW QUESTIONS

1. There have been many studies showing that speech and language deficits manifested during the preschool years have residual effects on social and academic achievement in the school years.

   a. True

   b. False

2. Parental education is a better predictor of a child's language behaviors in adolescence than are the child's language abilities during the ages of birth to 3 years.

   a. True

   b. False

3. The development of metalinguistic skills is most marked at 3 to 6 years of age.

   a. True

   b. False

4. Skills that reflect the child's ability to develop alternative ways to solve a problem or resolve a situation, ability to form hypotheses and task analyze them in a constructive manner, and capacity to make personal decisions are _____ skills.

   a. Metalinguistic

   b. Metanarrative

   c. Metacognitive

   d. Metapragmatic

5. _____ literacy tasks are those that involve searching, comprehending, and using continuous texts.

   a. Prose

   b. Qualitative

   c. Document

   d. Narrative

   e. Quantitative

   f. Functional

6. Based on the findings of the NAEP 2008 study of literacy levels in American adults, the largest group of adults fall in the _____ performance level on literacy tasks.

   a. Below Basic

   b. Basic

   c. Intermediate

   d. Proficient

7. Metalinguistic devices enable one to think about and analyze language, comprehend humor, and understand words with double meanings.

   a. True

   b. False

8. Children who have speech impairments, but not language impairments, as preschoolers typically have residual learning problems that become apparent in grades 3 and up.

   a. True

   b. False

9. Twenty-five percent of high school graduates read at the eighth grade level or lower.

   a. True

   b. False

10. Preschoolers learn primarily through the visual mode.

   a. True

   b. False

REFERENCES

Achenbach, T. M. (1981). *Child behavior checklist*. Burlington, VT: University of Vermont.

Aram, D. M., Ekelman, B. L., & Nation, J. E. (1984, June). Preschoolers with language disorders: 10 years later. *Journal of Speech and Hearing Research, 27*, 232–244.

Aram, D. M., & Nation, J. E. (1980). Preschool language disorders and subsequent language and academic difficulties. *Journal of Communication Disorders, 13*, 159–170.

Arthur, G. (1952). *The Arthur adaptation of the Leiter international performance scale*. Washington, DC: Psychological Service Center Press.

Baker, D. (2008, July). Illiteracy in America. http://trivani.wordpress.com/2008/07/13/illiteracy-in-america.

Berk, L. (2004). Development through the lifespan. Boston, MA: Allyn & Bacon.

Bernstein, D. K. (1997). Language development: The school-age years. In D. K. Bernstein and E. Tiegerman-Farber (eds.), *Language and communication disorders in children* (pp. 127–151). Allyn and Bacon.

Bishop, D. V. M., & Edmundson, A. (1987). Language-impaired 4-year-olds: Distinguishing transient from persistent impairment. *Journal of Speech and Hearing Disorders, 52*, 156–173.

Carrow, E. (1973). *Test of auditory comprehension of language.* Austin, TX: Urban Research Group.

Clecker, B. Retrieved May 5, 2010 from http://ErzineArticles.com/?expert=Bob Clecker.

Damico, J., & Oller, J. W., Jr. (1980). Pragmatic versus morphological/syntactic criteria for language referrals. *Language, Speech, and Hearing Services in the Schools, 19,* 51–66.

Girolametto, L., Wiigs, M., Smyth, R., Weitzman, E., & Pearce, P. S. (2001, November). Children with a history of expressive vocabulary delay: Outcomes at 5 years of age. *American Journal of Speech-Language Pathology, 10*(4), 358–369.

Johnson, C. J., Beitchman, J. H., Young, A., Escobar, M., Atkinson, L., Wilson, B., et al. (1999). Fourteen year follow up of children with and without speech/language impairments: Speech/language stability and outcomes. *Journal of Speech, Language, and Hearing Research, 42*(3), 744–760.

King, R. R., Jones, C., & Laskey, E. (1982). In retrospect: A fifteen year follow-up report of speech-language disordered children. *Language, Speech, and Hearing Services in Schools, 13,* 24–32.

Kochanek, T. T., Kabacoff, R. I., & Lipsitt, L. P. (1990). Early identification of developmentally disabled and at-risk preschool children. *Exceptional Children, 56,* 528–538.

Larson, V. L., & McKinley, N. (1995). *Language disorders in older students: Preadolescents and adolescents.* Eau Claire, WI: Thinking Publications.

McGreer, M. M. (2009). House passes burden of health car costs to the illiterate, and poor. Retrieved May 5, 2010 from www.associatedcontent.com/.../house_passes_burden_of_health_care.html.

Menyuk, P. (1969). *Sentences children use.* Cambridge, MA: MIT Press.

Menyuk, P. (1971). *The acquisition and development of language.* Englewood Cliffs, NJ: Prentice Hall.

Miller, P. (1989). Theories of adolescent development. In J. Worell and F. Danner (eds.), *The adolescent as decision-maker: Applications to development and education* (pp. 13–49). San Diego, CA: Academic Press.

Monten, M. (2007, March). More than one-third of Washington, D.C. residents are functionally illiterate. *State of Adult Literacy 2006.* Retrieved May 5, 2010 from www.proliterach.org.

National Center for Education Statistics. (2003). Key concepts and features of the 2003 National Assessment of Adult Literacy. Retrieved May 5, 2010 from http://nces.ed.gov/NAAL/PDF/2006471_1.PDF.

National Center for Education Statistics. (2007). A first look at the literacy of America's adults in the 21st century. Retrieved May 5, 2010 from http://nces.ed.gov/NAAL/PDF/2006470.pdf.

National Right to Read Foundation (2009). Illiteracy: An incurable disease or education malpractice? www.nrrf.org/essay_Illiteracy.html. Retrieved May 5, 2010.

Nelson, N. W. (1994). Curriculum-based language assessment and intervention across the grades. In G. P Wallach and K. G. Butler (eds.), *Language learning disabilities in school-age children and adolescents: Some principles and applications* (pp. 104–131). New York: Merrill/Macmillan Publishing Company.

Nelson, N. W. (1998). Childhood language disorders in context: Infancy through adolescence (2nd ed.). Boston: Allyn and Bacon.

Nippold, M. A. (1988). The literate lexicon. In M. A. Nippold (ed.), *Later language development: Ages nine through nineteen* (pp. 29–47). Austin, TX: Pro-Ed.

Nippold, M. A, Mansfield, T. C., Billow, J. L., & Tomblin, J. B. (2009, August). Syntactic development in adolescents with a history of language impairments: A follow-up investigation. *American Journal of Speech-Language Pathology, 18*(3), 241–251.

Owens, R. (1996). *Language development: An introduction* (3rd ed.). Columbus, OH: Merrill/Macmillan.

Rescorla, L. (2009, February). Age 17 language and reading outcomes in late talking toddlers: Support for a dimensional perspective on language delay. *Journal of Speech, Language, and Hearing Research, 52*(1), 16–30.

Rescorla, L., Hadicke-Wiley, M., & Escarce, E. (1993). Epidemiological investigation of expressive language delay at age two. *First Language, 13*, 5–22.

Rosenkoetter, S. E. (1995) *It's a big step.* Topeka, KS: Bridging Early Services Task Force, Coordinating Council on Early Childhood Developmental Services.

van Kleek, A. (1994). Metalinguistic development. In G. P. Wallach and K. G. Butler (eds.), *Language learning disabilities in school-age children and adolescents: Some principles and applications.* New York: Merrill/Macmillan Publishing Company.

Washington Literacy Council (n.d.). Literacy statistics reference information. www.readfaster.com/education_stats.asp

White, B. (1975). Critical influences in the origins of competence. *Merrill-Palmer Quarterly, 22*, 243–266.

APPENDIX 8A

Milestones in Language and Cognitive Development Ages 6 Through Adulthood

Age	Milestone
6–8 years	Vocabulary increases rapidly, growing by approximately 20 words per day.
	Word definitions are concrete, referring to functions and appearance.
	Ability to analyze and reflect on language improves.
	Advanced understanding of infinitive phrases develops.
	Thought becomes more logical, as shown by the ability to pass.
	Piagetian conservation, class inclusion, and seriation problems.
	Understanding of spatial concepts improves, as illustrated by ability to give clear, well-organized directions and to draw and read maps.
	Attention becomes more selective, adaptable, and planful.
	Child uses memory strategies of rehearsal and organization.
	Child regards the mind as an active, constructive agent, capable of transforming information.
	Awareness of memory strategies and the impact of psychological factors (attention, motivation) on task performance improves. (p. 340)
8–10 years	Child grasps concept of double meanings.
	Child comprehends subtle metaphors and humor.
9–11 years	Word definitions emphasize synonyms and categorical relations.
	Use of complex grammatical constructions increases.
	Message is adapted to listener's needs in challenging communicative utterances.
	Conversational strategies are refined.
	Logical thought remains tied to concrete situations.
	Piagetian tasks continue to be mastered in a step-by-step fashion.
	Memory strategies of rehearsal and organization become more effective. Child begins to use elaboration.
	Child applies several memory strategies at once.
	Long-term knowledge base grows larger and becomes better organized.
	Cognitive self-regulation improves. (p. 341)
11–14 years	Child becomes capable of formal operational reasoning.
	Child becomes better at coordinating theory with evidence.
	Child can argue more effectively.
	Child becomes more self-conscious and self-focused.

Age	Milestone
	Child becomes more idealistic and critical.
	Metacognition and cognitive self-regulation continue to improve. (p. 408)
15–20 years	Individual is likely to show formal operational reasoning on familiar tasks.
	Individual masters the components of formal operational reasoning in sequential order on different types of tasks.
	Individual becomes less self-conscious and self-focused.
	Individual becomes better at everyday planning and decision-making. (p. 409)
20–30 years	If individual is college educated, dualistic thinking (dividing information, values, and authority into right and wrong) declines in favor of relativistic thinking (viewing all knowledge as embedded in a framework of thought)
	Individual narrows vocational options and settles on a specific career.
	With entry into marriage and employment situations, individual focuses less on acquiring knowledge and more on applying it to everyday life.
	Individual develops expertise (acquisition of extensive knowledge in a field of endeavor), which enhances problem solving.
	Creativity (generating useful original products) increases.
	Steady improvement occurs in mental abilities on accumulated knowledge through middle adulthood. (p. 478)
30–40 years	As family and work lives expand, the capacity to juggle many responsibilities improves.
	Creativity often peaks. (p. 479)
40–60 years	Consciousness of aging increases.
	Crystallized intelligence increases; fluid intelligence declines.
	Processing speed declines; adults compensate through practice and experience.
	On complex tasks, ability to divide and control attention declines; adults compensate through practice and experience.
	Amount of information retained in working memory declines, largely due to reduced use of memory strategies.
	Retrieving information from long-term memory becomes more difficult.
	General factual knowledge, procedural knowledge, and knowledge related to one's occupation remain unchanged or increase.
	Gains in practical problem solving and expertise occur.
	Creativity focuses on integrating ideas and becomes more altruistic.
	If individual is in an occupation offering challenge and autonomy, shows gains in cognitive flexibility. (p. 542)

(continues)

APPENDIX 8A (continued)

Age	Milestone
60–80 years	Processing speed continues to decline; crystallized abilities are largely sustained.
	Amount of information that can be retained in working memory diminishes further; memory problems are greatest on tasks requiring deliberate processing and associative memory.
	Modest forgetting of remote memories occurs.
	Use of external aids for prospective memory increases.
	Retrieving words from long-term memory and planning what to say and how to say it become more difficult.
	Information is more likely to be remembered in terms of gist than details.
	Traditional problem solving declines; everyday problem solving remains adaptive.
	Individual may hold one of the most important positions in society, such as chief executive officer, religious leader, or Supreme Court justice.
	Individual may excel in wisdom.
	Individual can improve a wide range of cognitive skills through training. (p. 616–617)
80 years and older	Cognitive changes associated with 60–80 years continue.
	Fluid abilities decline further; crystallized abilities drop as well. (p. 617)

Source: Adapted from Milestones charts in L. Berk (2004), *Development Through the Lifespan* (3rd ed.).

APPENDIX 8B

Literacy Statistics Based on the 2003 National Assessment of Adult Literacy: Percentage of Americans at Below Basic Level

Percentage of Americans Functioning at the Below Basic Level of Literacy Based on Ethnicity/Race

Race/Ethnicity	Below Basic	Total NAAL Population
White	37%	70%
Black	20%	12%
Hispanic	39%	12%
Asian/Pacific Islander	4%	4%

Percentage of Americans Functioning at the Below Basic Level of Literacy Based on Age

Age	Below Basic	Total NAAL Population
16–18 years	5%	6%
19–24 years	9%	11%
25–39 years	25%	28%
40–49 years	16%	20%
50–64 years	20%	21%
64+ years	26%	15%

Percentage of Americans Functioning at the Below Basic Level of Literacy Based on Gender

Gender	Below Basic	Total NAAL Population
Male	46%	49%
Female	54%	51%

(continues)

APPENDIX 8B *(continued)*

Percentage of Americans Functioning at the Below Basic Level of Literacy Based on Disability Status

Disability Status	Below Basic	Total NAAL Population
Vision problem only	7%	5%
Hearing problem only	4%	5%
Learning disability only	4%	3%
Other disability only	10%	8%
Multiple disabilities	21%	9%
No disabilities	54%	70%

Percentage of Americans Functioning at the Below Basic Level of Literacy Based on Educational Attainment

Educational Attainment	Below Basic	Total NAAL Population
Less than/some high school	55%	15%
GED/high school equivalency	4%	5%
High school graduate	23%	26%
Vocational/trade/business school	4%	6%
Some college	4%	11%
Associate's/2-year degree	35%	12%
College graduate	2%	12%
Graduate studies/degree	1%	11%

Source: A first look at the literacy of America's adults in the 21st century, National Center for Education Statistics, United States Department of Education, Institute of Education Sciences, NCES 2006-70.

APPENDIX 8C

Literacy Statistics Based on the 2003 National Assessment of Adult Literacy: Percentage of Americans at Each Level

Code:

- BB: Below Basic
- B: Basic
- I: Intermediate
- P: Proficient

Percentage of Americans Functioning at Each Level of Literacy per Task Based on Gender

	BB	B	I	P
Prose Literacy Level				
Men	15%	29%	43%	13%
Women	15%	29%	46%	14%
Document Literacy Level				
Men	21%	31%	33%	16%
Women	22%	35%	32%	11%
Quantitative Literacy Level				
Men	14%	23%	51%	13%
Women	11%	22%	54%	13%

Percentage of Americans Functioning at Each Level of Literacy per Task Based on Ethnicity

	BB	B	I	P
Prose Literacy Level				
White	7%	25%	51%	17%
Black	24%	43%	31%	2%
Hispanic	44%	30%	23%	4%
Asian/Pacific Islander	14%	32%	42%	12%

(continues)

APPENDIX 8C (continued)

	BB	B	I	P
Document Literacy Level				
White	8%	19%	58%	15%
Black	24%	35%	40%	2%
Hispanic	36%	26%	33%	5%
Asian/Pacific Islander	11%	22%	54%	13%
Quantitative Literacy Level				
White	13%	32%	39%	17%
Black	47%	36%	15%	2%
Hispanic	50%	29%	17%	4%
Asian/Pacific Islander	19%	34%	35%	12%

Percentage of Americans Functioning at Each Level of Literacy per Task Based on Educational Attainment

	BB	B	I	P
Prose Literacy Level				
Still in high school	14%	37%	45%	4%
Less than/some high school	50%	33%	16%	1%
GED/high school equivalency	10%	45%	43%	3%
High school graduate	13%	39%	44%	4%
Vocational/trade/business school	10%	36%	49%	5%
Some college	5%	25%	59%	11%
Associate's/2-year degree	4%	20%	56%	19%
College graduate	3%	14%	53%	31%
Grad studies/degree	1%	10%	48%	41%

	BB	B	I	P
Document Literacy Level				
Still in high school	13%	24%	54%	9%
Less than/some high school	45%	29%	25%	2%
GED/high school equivalency	13%	30%	53%	4%
High school graduate	13%	29%	52%	5%
Vocational/trade/business school	9%	26%	59%	7%
Some college	5%	19%	65%	10%
Associate's/2-year degree	3%	15%	66%	16%
College graduate	2%	11%	62%	25%
Grad studies/degree	1%	9%	59%	31%
Quantitative Literacy Level				
Still in high school	31%	38%	25%	5%
Less than/some high school	64%	25%	10%	1%
GED/high school equivalency	26%	43%	28%	3%
High school graduate	24%	42%	29%	5%
Vocational/trade/business school	18%	41%	35%	6%
Some college	10%	36%	43%	11%
Associate's/2-year degree	7%	30%	45%	18%
College graduate	4%	22%	43%	31%
Grad studies/degree	3%	18%	43%	36%

Source: "A First Look at the Literacy of America's Adults in the 21st Century", National Center for Education Statistics, United States Department of Education, Institute of Education Sciences, NCES 2006-70.

APPENDIX 8D

Averaged Score on Literacy Tasks of the National Assessment of Educational Progress (2003)

Scores Based on Educational Attainment

Educational Attainment	Prose	Document	Quantitative
Still in high school	262 (B)	265 (I)	261 (B)
Less than/some high school	207 (BB)	208	211
GED/high school equivalency	260 (B)	257 (I)	265 (B)
High school graduate	262 (B)	258 (I)	269 (B)
Vocational/trade/business school	268 (I)	267 (I)	279 (B)
Some college	287 (I)	280 (I)	294 (I)
Associate's/2-year degree	298 (I)	291 (I)	305 (I)
College graduate	314 (I)	303(I)	323 (I)
Grad studies/degree	327(I)	311 (I)	332 (I)

Source: "A First Look at the Literacy of America's Adults in the 21st Century", National Center for Education Statistics, United States Department of Education, Institute of Education Sciences, NCES 2006-70.

Chapter 9

Language-Based Learning Disabilities in the School-Age Population

LEARNING OBJECTIVES

After completion of this chapter, the reader will be able to:

1. Explain why speech-language pathologists should be part of the team that treats children with language-based learning disabilities, particularly with reading and spelling problems

2. Describe some of the problems an educational team (including the speech-language pathologist) faces in diagnosing learning disabilities in school-age children, particularly those 10 years of age and older

3. List and briefly discuss red flags for the development of a language-based learning disability.

4. Compare and contrast categories of language-based learning disabilities based on the historical approach and those based on the clinical-inferential approach.

5. Discuss the impact of a phonological deficit on reading and spelling.

6. Describe syntactic, semantic, and pragmatic disorders and delays seen in school-age children and adolescents, and discuss how they can impact academic success.

7. Discuss six problems with written language in children with learning and/or reading disabilities.

8. Define auditory processing disorder and discuss its overlap with language-based learning disabilities.

9. Discuss the impact of functional illiteracy on academic and vocational performance.

INTRODUCTION

Learning disabilities are a heterogeneous constellation of impairments that can affect various aspects of a child's abilities. For example, a child could have a graphomotor learning disability that affects his or her fine motor skills, particularly with regard to handwriting. Other children may have language learning disabilities that affect features of language such as semantics, syntax, and pragmatics and impacts oral and written language. These children frequently are at high risk for academic and social problems.

Subgroups of language-based learning disabilities include children with reading and/or spelling deficits, children with SLI, and children with general language learning impairments (sometimes referred to as nonspecific language impairment) (Gabig, 2009).

It is estimated that 8 to 10 percent of all children below 18 years of age in the United States have some type of learning disability (NINDS, 2010). The Education for All Handicapped Children Act (P.L. 94-142, 1975) included children with learning disabilities in the determination of eligibility for special education and related services in the public schools. More recently, the No Child Left Behind Act (2001), and the Individuals with Disabilities Education Improvement Act (2004) have impacted the identification, assessment, and treatment of children who have learning disabilities. Refer to Chapter 7 for a review of the legislation.

A speech-language pathologist, a critical member of the educational team, is responsible for assessing and treating language-based learning disabilities. It is important to note that not all learning disabilities are language-based. Children with non–language-based learning disabilities should be referred to professionals in occupational therapy, physical therapy, psychology, or education for remediation. However, if the learning disability is based on a language disorder, the speech-language pathologist should be involved in the child's educational process. Most language-based learning disabilities manifest as reading or spelling difficulties or both. Many of these language-based learning disabilities (LLDs) are extensions of speech and language delays and disorders occurring during the preschool years.

Some language-based learning disorders seen by clinicians serving school-age children result from traumatic brain injury and other disorders acquired in childhood. These children are discussed in Chapter 12. Children who exhibit signs of attention deficit disorder often have an accompanying LLD (see Chapter 11).

Many of the children who are diagnosed as having an LLD have very subtle deficits that may elude even the most astute clinician. Nelson (1993) described a category of children as being "ABNQ" children: They "almost but not quite" manage to keep pace with their classmates, particularly in the language-based portions of the academic curriculum. These children have relatively normal cognitive ability and remain somewhat competitive with their age-level peers. They do not have moderate to severe cognitive limitations or language delays that persist from the preschool years into older childhood. "Almost but not quite" children do not have physical or sensory impairments that interfere with acquisition of language and social interaction skills. They do have specific language and learning disabilities that interfere with their educational and social progress. Frequently, teachers refer to these children as children who "are not performing up to their potential," yet their deficits are so subtle that many times they do not perform poorly enough on tests to be easily identified as having an LLD.

In addition to the fact that many of these disorders are relatively subtle and therefore difficult to identify, another problem in identifying school-age children with LLDs is that there is no homogeneous definition of language disorders in the school-age population. At school age, delays may persist as disorders either because of the nature of the delay or because of

Learning disability. Any one of a heterogeneous set of learning problems that affect the acquisition and use of listening, speaking, writing, reading, mathematical, and reasoning skills.

Language-based learning disability. A single disorder that manifests itself in different ways at various points in development as communicative contexts and learning tasks change.

ineffective remediation during the preschool years. However, because most developmental charts stop at approximately 10 years of age, it becomes more difficult to determine if a child has a delay or a disorder in his or her language. At this point, language is less universal and more dependent on individual interests and experiences. Also, disorders due to etiologic factors, such as Down syndrome and fetal alcohol syndrome, do not disappear and need continued intervention during the school-age years.

Owing to the inherent differences among individuals, language disorders have varying effects on a child, with the impact being determined by the clinician's best judgment based on a review of the child's educational and medical records, observation, and testing. This judgment is often founded on the degree to which the language delay or disorder impacts the child's socialization and academic progress. Larson and McKinley (1995) took all of these factors into consideration and concluded that the clinician's primary job is to judge the child's abilities and disabilities based on the impact the problem or problems have on the child's social environment, academic environment, and vocational environment. It is also important to pay attention to how language delays and disorders affect reading and writing in school-age children.

> **think about it**
>
> How would a language-based learning disability impact a child academically?

DEFINITIONS OF LEARNING DISABILITIES

The legally accepted definition of learning disabilities, which was originally written in 1967 by the National Advisory Committee on Handicapped Children (NACHC), is the one provided by the United States Office of Education (USOE, 1991) in the Individuals with Disabilities Education Act. The law defines learning disabilities as a

> disorder in one or more of the basic psychological processes involved in understanding or in using language, spoken or written, which may manifest itself in an imperfect ability to listen, think, speak, read, write, spell, or to do mathematical calculations. The term includes such conditions as perceptual handicaps, brain injury, minimal brain dysfunction, dyslexia, and developmental aphasia. The term does not include children who have learning problems which are primarily the result of visual, hearing, or motor handicaps, of mental retardation, or emotional disturbance, or of environmental, cultural, or economic disadvantage. (ASHA, 1991, p. 1)

There are inherent problems in the federal definition that resulted in misinterpretations that had a direct effect on the identification, assessment, and educational programming for students with learning disabilities. In "Learning Disabilities: Issues on Definition,", ASHA (1991) delineated some of the misinterpretations:

1. The federal definition creates the impression that all people who have a learning disability have the same types of deficits and behaviors; that is, they are a homogeneous group.

2. The federal definition does not recognize that learning difficulties due to sensory, motor, emotional, economic, environmental, and cultural factors can co-exist with learning disabilities. It also fails to recognize that problems with social interaction, social perception, and self-regulation can coexist. The learning problems are not learning disabilities; however, they are problems that have been observed concomitantly with learning disabilities.

3. The federal definition leads one to believe that all individuals with learning disabilities can be assessed and educated in a uniform manner. This erroneous interpretation has had an impact on identification, assessment, and remediation of individuals with potential or confirmed learning disabilities.

4. The federal definition does not recognize that learning disabilities can be a lifelong problem; the federal definition applies only to individuals aged birth to 21 years.

5. Learning disabilities are intrinsic to the individual, presumably being associated with dysfunction in the central nervous system that results in "altered processes of acquiring and using information" (p. 2). The federal definition provides a list of terms and disorders and implies that they are causative. Indeed, some of the disorders listed in the federal definition are subtypes of learning disabilities (i.e., dyslexia), not causes of learning disabilities. An understanding of the etiology of a learning disability is essential in developing intervention.

In reaction to the federal definition, the National Joint Committee on Learning Disabilities wrote the following definition of learning disabilities in 1981:

> *Learning disabilities* is a generic term that refers to a heterogeneous group of disorders manifested by significant difficulties in the acquisition and use of listening, speaking, reading, writing, reasoning, or mathematical abilities. These disorders are intrinsic to the individual and presumed to be due to central nervous system dysfunction. Even though a learning disability may occur concomitantly with other handicapping conditions (e.g., sensory impairment, mental retardation, social and

emotional disturbance), or environmental influences (e.g., cultural differences, insufficient/inappropriate instruction, psychogenic factors), it is not the direct result of those conditions or influences. (ASHA, 1991, p. 4)

In 1991, the NJCLD rewrote its 1981 definition of learning disabilities, making the following changes:

- The word *generic* was changed to *general.*
- The term *environmental influences* was changed to *extrinsic influences.*
- The phrase *social and emotional disturbance* was changed to *serious emotional disturbance.*
- The word *direct* was deleted. (ASHA, 1991, p. 3)
- Language related to social behaviors was added.

The resulting definition is the one that has been adopted by ASHA:

Learning disabilities is a general term that refers to a heterogeneous group of disorders manifested by significant difficulties in the acquisition and use of listening, speaking, reading, writing, reasoning, or mathematical abilities. These disorders are intrinsic to the individual, presumed to be due to central nervous system dysfunction, and may occur across the life span. Problems in self-regulatory behaviors, social perception, and social interaction may exist with learning disabilities but do not by themselves constitute a learning disability. Although learning disabilities may occur concomitantly with other handicapping conditions (for example, sensory impairment, mental retardation, serious emotional disturbance), or with extrinsic influences (such as cultural differences, insufficient or inappropriate instruction), they are not the result of those conditions or influences (ASHA, 1991, p. 4).

While children with learning disabilities have certainly benefited from the enactment of the Education of All Handicapped Children Act (P.L. 94-142) (i.e., they are eligible for special education and related services in the schools), the misinterpretations of the federal definition have created problems with regard to the identification and assessment of students, as well as with the quality of services students with learning disabilities typically receive in the public schools.

However, in the Individuals with Disabilities Education Improvement Act of 2004 (IDEIA), a big step toward remediating these inadequacies in the assessment and subsequent educational programming for these students was made. Focused on student outcomes, Response to Intervention (RTI) is a systematic, problem-solving approach to measuring an individual student's response to classroom instruction, then applying that data to develop an evidence-based instructional or intervention plan for the child. RTI is discussed in more depth later in this chapter, as well as in Chapter 10.

Differentiation Between Language Disorders and Learning Disabilities

It is important to differentiate between language disorders and learning disabilities. They are separate problems, and a child can have either or both. In some children the language disorder causes the learning disability, and these children are the focus of this chapter. Language-based learning disabilities constitute a single disorder that manifests itself in different ways at various points in development as communicative contexts and learning tasks change. At the preschool level, language disorders are considered as demonstrated in a child's communicative functioning and in his or her receptive and expressive language skills. In the school-age child, it is important to look at the child's metalinguistic abilities, narrative and classroom discourse, figurative language use, and written language skills.

The Clinical-Inferential Approach to Classifying Learning Disabilities

The clinical-inferential approach to classifying learning disabilities profiles the children with language-based learning disabilities based on the review of test scores. The first profile in this approach consists of those children who have "difficulty on language and language-related tasks" (Reed, 2005, p. 135). According to Reed, this group constitutes 40 to 60 percent of the children with learning disabilities. When considering LLDs, the role that language expression and use problems and word-finding difficulties play in the child's learning problems must be considered. It is also important to pay attention to the existence of possible auditory processing problems and difficulties with speech discrimination.

A second clinical-inferential profile of learning disabilities consists of articulatory and graphomotor deficits that occur in 10 to 40 percent of individuals who have learning disabilities (Reed, 2005). Articulation, writing, and drawing difficulties characterize this group of learning disabilities. These children are often labeled as having developmental apraxia or identified as having "clumsy child syndrome."

A third, and less common, categorization is identified as a visuospatial perceptual deficit syndrome (5 to 15 percent of the population) (Reed, 2005). These children have deficits in visual discrimination and visual memory and exhibit problems with spatial orientation. They may confuse similar-looking letters, have problems orienting themselves in space, or both (Shames, Wiig, & Secord, 1994). Regardless of the type of learning disability the child exhibits, he or she typically performs within normal or near-normal limits on neuropsychological tests, although a discrepancy may occur between performance on language-based tasks and tasks that require visual-spatial and other nonlinguistic skills.

Categories of Learning Disabilities Based on Statistical Analysis

In addition to the clinical-inferential approaches to classification of LLDs, five smaller categories of learning disabilities have been proposed based on statistical analysis. As listed in Reed (2005), these categories are as follows:

1. Those with global language impairment (30% of the population)

2. Those with selective impairment of naming (16%)

3. Those with a mixed deficit of language impairment and difficulty on visual-perceptual-motor tasks (11%)

4. Those with impairment only on non-language visual-perceptual-motor tests (26%)

5. Those with normal performance on all the neuropsychological tests (13%) (pp. 135–136).

CURRICULAR DEMANDS BASED ON LANGUAGE

In the preschool years, the curricular emphasis is on language development and social-emotional growth. Activities focus on motor skills, visuospatial skills, and visual and auditory perceptual skills. Torgesen (1977) writes that preschoolers experience incidental learning that results from routine interactions with the environment. In addition, during the preschool years, children learn the value of the printed word and develop a sense of story structure as a result of exposure to books. As toddlers and preschoolers participate in book-reading routines, they learn to answer simple questions that form the basis for replying to questions in the school setting. In fact, through having the same story read and reread, many preschoolers learn to repeat the story as they flip the pages, giving the appearance of reading (Kamhi & Catts, 1989).

Incidental learning. Learning that results from routine interactions with the environment.

In kindergarten through second grade, children develop the basic skills needed for reading and writing. According to Chall (1983), children in this age bracket learn about phoneme–grapheme correspondences. That is, they begin to learn associations between the sounds they speak and hear and the printed letters (graphophonemic association). They also begin to learn about spelling, both oral and written, and begin to learn basic mathematical operations. It is through these activities that evidence of an LLD may begin to emerge. In Table 9–1, there is a list of early warning signs that a child may have an LLD.

When the child reaches the middle grades (grades 3 and 4), he or she experiences a curricular leap from decoding to reading for comprehension.

TABLE 9–1 Soft signs that may be indicative of a learning disability.

Visual-motor deficits

Letter and number reversals

Damage to supplementary motor areas of brain

Phonological deficits

History of ear infections

Higher rate of allergies and autoimmune disorders in the family

Complaints of headaches

Developmentally delayed speech onset

Source: From G. Hynd, (1991, March). Brain Morphology As It Relates to Learning Disabilities. Lecture at the 1991 G. Paul Moore Symposium. Gainesville, FL.

As expressed by Kamhi and Catts (1989), children in these grades read to learn instead of learning to read. In fact, basic skills are only reviewed; they are no longer the curricular focus. In grades 3 and 4, content areas such as English, social studies, and science are introduced. Also, mathematics includes word problems, so that even this subject area can be affected if a child has a reading disability. In addition to the shift in the curricular emphasis, around the third and fourth grades children develop "attention-demanding control processes" and learn information that must be recalled at a later time. In fact, this "controlled attentional learning" becomes a critical measure of achievement in the later school years (Torgesen, 1977). Furthermore, at this point in the education progression, executive functions begin to become a factor in a child's academic success. Executive functions are frontal lobe–based skills that enable one to set goals, organize information in working memory, manage time, attend to the task at hand, initiate tasks, self-monitor, and self-evaluate, As the child progresses through his or her educational and vocational careers, the demand on the cognitive system steadily increases, and the sophistication of the individual's executive functions plays a major role in academic, social, and vocational success.

In the upper elementary grades (grades 5 and 6), the curricular emphasis is on the acquisition of knowledge in the content areas that were introduced in grades 3 and 4. During this time, decoding skills should be fully automatic so that the child can focus his or her attention on comprehension (Kamhi & Catts, 1989). Children are exposed to more complex text and must increasingly rely on their metalinguistic and metacognitive skills to infer meaning from context, to analyze abstract language and words or phrases with multiple meanings, and to organize information in short- and long-term memory to facilitate later recall.

By the time the child reaches middle school (seventh through ninth grades), he or she should be able to read popular magazines, *Reader's Digest,* the newspaper, and popular fiction. At this point, cognitive development and its impact on reading is a bigger focus than reading development per se (Kamhi & Catts, 1989). The curriculum continues to focus on content areas, but the number of content areas expands to include more subjects. English includes literature, study skills, composition, and language arts. Social studies encompasses world geography, American and world history, and economics; science expands to biology, chemistry, and physics. In high school, foreign languages also become part of the curriculum, as do vocational education and other life-skills coursework. Students this age develop cognitive skills, including abstract reasoning, analysis, synthesis, and judgment. They learn to develop alternate hypotheses and to create strategies to test these hypotheses. They are capable of dealing with more than one point of view and glean more from their reading because they have increased ability to think abstractly.

> *think about it*
>
> What would be the impact of an LLD on academic achievement? What would be the impact of an LLD on vocational training?

IDENTIFICATION OF CHILDREN AT RISK

In Chapter 8, the persistence of deficits associated with the preschool years was discussed. The majority of affected children face some degree of struggle with academic, social, and/or vocational achievement. The following discussion targets risk factors other than those associated with specific syndromes or etiologies.

Many "almost but not quite" students are identified as academic underachievers. However, before taking this label lightly, it is important to look at the long-term impact of academic underachievement. As identified by Larson and McKinley (1995), academic underachievement can have devastating effects. Thirteen percent of high school students in the United States read below the sixth grade level, and one of every four high school students drops out of school. In addition, the impact of functional illiteracy is well documented, as outlined in Table 9–2. Recall that being functionally illiterate implies that the individual cannot read well enough to complete a job application, read directions, or read a newspaper.

Even more devastating are the findings of the Los Angeles Suicide Prevention Center, showing that 50 percent of the suicide victims between the ages of 10 and 14 years are diagnosed as being hyperactive, perceptually impaired, or dyslexic (Peck, 1982). Through suicide notes and conversations with their families and peers prior to the suicide, these children cited a lack of friends (see Figure 9–1) and having no one to talk to as contributors to their depression and low self-esteem. In addition, they cited the presence of communication problems that interfered with making and keeping friends and expressing feelings as factors affecting their decision to commit

TABLE 9–2   Demographics of functional illiteracy

85% of juvenile offenders are functionally illiterate.

70% of prisoners in state and federal systems are functionally illiterate.

85% of high school dropouts are functionally illiterate.

75% of the welfare recipients are functionally illiterate.

85% of unwed mothers are functionally illiterate.

68% of those arrested are functionally illiterate.

20% of Americans are functionally illiterate and read below a fifth-grade level.

27 million Americans are unable to read well enough to complete a job application.

90% of welfare recipients are high school dropouts.

66% of students who are not proficient readers by fourth grade will end up on welfare or in jail.

32 million adults in the United States lack basic prose literacy skills.

Source: Compiled from Washington Literacy Council; National Institute for Literacy; NCES 2007-480; Britt, 2009.

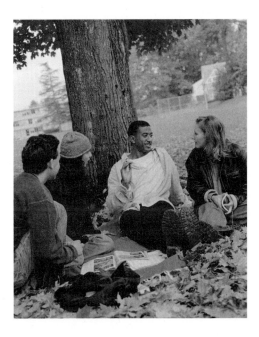

FIGURE 9–1   During the adolescent years, the value of friendship cannot be underestimated, particularly as many adolescent suicide victims claim to have no friends in whom they can confide. (*Delmar/Cengage Learning*)

suicide (Larson & McKinley, 1995). The statistics are strong enough to suggest that learning disabilities are accompanied by low self-esteem and that these children should be considered at risk for devastating academic, social, and personal problems (Peck, 1982). Even more compelling evidence that speech-language pathologists need to be involved in the assessment and treatment of LLDs is offered by Nelson (1994), who noted that 24.4 percent of youth in the general population fail to complete high school. In addition, 36.1 percent of youth with learning disabilities fail to complete high school, as do 32.5 percent of youth with speech impairments. Furthermore, 54.8 percent of youth with severe emotional disturbances fail to complete this level of schooling. Given Peck's finding that low self-esteem places children at risk for suicide, this last statistic is particularly disturbing. Table 9–3 provides more information on children who are at risk for not completing high school.

TABLE 9–3 Risk factors that precipitate dropping out of school

Many absences

Frequent tardiness

Poor grades

Low math and reading scores

Failure in one or more grades

Limited participation in extracurricular activities

Boredom with classes

Failure to see relevance of education to life goals

Disciplinary problems

Verbal and language deficiencies

Low family income or financial difficulties

Poorly educated mother

Fatherless home

Parent or sibling who dropped out

Low self-esteem

Poor social adjustment

Lack of friends

Lack of rapport with teachers

Chronic illness

Teenage pregnancy

Presence of learning disabilities

Source: Adapted from "Failure: Why Schools Must Help Children at Risk," by Sunburst Communications, 1988, *Solutions: News from Computer Educators*, 3(2), p. 1 © 1988 by Sunburst Communications.

ADHD

The presence of ADHD is another risk category that warrants attention from the speech-language pathologist. Although ADHD in and of itself is not a language-based problem or a learning disability, it can have serious consequences on students' social interactions, so pragmatic issues need to be addressed in this population. Also, many children who exhibit ADHD have reading underachievement without the phonological and linguistic deficits seen in children with reading disabilities (Lombardino et al., 1997).

Children can be at risk for poor communication (which impacts the development of social interactions and academic development) from biological and environmental deficiencies. Children who are at risk and do not get early intervention may be compromised with regard to language development and academic prowess. They may fall in the "almost but not quite" category of students, or their deficits can be more pronounced.

Academic Underachievers

Other risk factors and red flags for the development of an LLD include being a late talker, certain familial patterns, and premature and/or difficult birth. Brain studies indicate that children with an LLD possibly have a breakdown along the neural pathways that facilitate communication between the frontal cortex and the midbrain (Owens, 2004). Such a breakdown would affect the individual's executive abilities such as planning, attending, and regulating.

There is no question that a wide variety of concerns relate to identifying school-age children who are at risk for academic problems because of language-based difficulties. The question becomes how to identify these children. In most schools, observation and screening programs serve as the first line of identification. Screenings are done in a variety of ways, including paper-and-pencil tasks that are administered to whole classrooms at one sitting. In other situations, teams of volunteers give simple screening tests, which take anywhere from 5 to 15 minutes to administer. These screenings are typically done in kindergarten, in first grade, in third grade (when the curricular emphasis shifts to reading for comprehension), and in the last year in elementary school. Regardless of the type of screening or when it is done, the speech-language pathologist typically follows up with those who fail the screening by giving more complete test batteries to identify the presence or absence of a language delay or disorder that may have an effect on the child's academic, social, and vocational career. These tests are discussed more thoroughly in Chapter 13.

think about it What can you, as a speech-language pathologist or audiologist, contribute to your community in addressing the problem of high school dropouts?

Children with damage to supplementary motor areas of the brain often have characteristics similar to those who demonstrate elective mutism. They also have problems with reading silently. Approximately 60 to 70 percent of all children who have reading problems have a history of developmental articulation problems. This may be tied to a higher prevalence of otitis media and otitis media with effusion, which correlates with LLDs. It is possible that whatever puts the child at risk for ear infections may also preordain children to experience LLDs (Hynd, 1991).

A review of the family history may show a higher rate of allergies and autoimmune disorders, such as rheumatoid arthritis, lupus erythematosus, myositis, and scleroderma. In addition, children who are eventually found to have an LLD tend to have a larger number of complaints related to headaches. Parents also typically report that the child was developmentally delayed with regard to speech onset in the preschool years (Hynd, 1991).

Historically, children who are at risk for LLDs are described by their teachers as being socially adequate on entering school, but quickly showing poor performance in language-based activities and interactions in the classroom.

Other children with the same risk factors may do well in school initially, but their performance may degenerate in the late elementary or middle school years as the curricular demands rely more on reading for comprehension. Many of the children are identified in third grade when, as written earlier, they are expected to read for comprehension. This presents a problem because their struggle to decipher individual words interferes with their comprehension of text. In other cases the children are identified in grades 4 to 5 and 8 to 9 when word problems become a focus of the mathematics curriculum. Regardless of when a child's disorder is identified, early and appropriate intervention is critical to help the child keep pace with his or her peers in the academic world. Extra attention should be given to older children with learning disabilities because they tend to internalize the disorder, which can result in severe depression. In fact, serious depression and suicide among older children with a learning disability is six times the national rate (Larson & McKinley, 1995). Appendix 9A provides a list of agencies that can offer support to individuals with learning disabilities.

RISK FACTORS ASSOCIATED WITH IMPOVERISHED CONDITIONS

Families live in a state of poverty for a variety of reasons: lack of education, unavailability of jobs, lack of skills for jobs that are available, long-term effects of discrimination against minorities, and/or lack of a father in the household (Polakow, 1993). The long-term effects of poverty on language development and academic success are well documented. Specifically, there are 25 at-risk categories (see Table 9–4) that were developed by Rossetti (1996). In my opinion, 14 of the 25 categories can be directly tied to poverty. By no means do I intend to say that these 14 items are exclusive to those in impoverished situations. However, they are more frequently associated with such situations than are the non-italicized factors. The factors I associate with poverty are represented by italics in the list found in Table 9–4. (Note: This is the same as Table 1–2 but with the italics added to emphasize items relative to this discussion.)

TABLE 9–4   Factors that put a child at risk for developmental delay

1. Serious concerns expressed by a parent, primary caregiver, or professional regarding the child's development, parenting style, or parent–child interaction.
2. *Parent or primary caregiver with chronic or acute mental illness, developmental disability, or mental retardation.*
3. *Parent or primary caregiver with drug or alcohol dependence.*
4. *Parent or primary caregiver with a developmental history of loss and/or abuse.*
5. Family medical or genetic history characteristics.
6. Parent or primary caregiver with severe or chronic illness.
7. Acute family crisis.
8. *Chronically disturbed family interaction.*
9. *Parent–child or caregiver–child separation.*
10. *Adolescent mother.*
11. *Parent has four or more preschool-age children.*
12. *The presence of one or more of the following: parental education less than ninth grade; neither parent is employed; single parent.*
13. *Physical or social isolation and/or lack of adequate social support.*
14. *Lack of stable residence, homelessness, or dangerous living conditions.*
15. *Family inadequate healthcare or no health insurance.*
16. *Limited prenatal care.*
17. *Maternal prenatal substance abuse or use.*
18. Severe prenatal complications.
19. Severe perinatal complications.
20. Asphyxia.
21. Very low birth weight (<1,500 g).
22. Small for gestational age (<10th percentile).
23. Excessive irritability, crying, or tremulousness on the part of the infant.
24. *Atypical or recurrent accidents on the part of the child.*
25. Chronic otitis media.

Source: Communication intervention: Birth to three, by L. Rossetti, pp. 5–6. Copyright 1996 by Delmar, Cengage Learning.

Neuman (2008) cited numerous studies in listing consequences of poverty: "dropping out of school, low academic achievement, teenage pregnancy and childbearing, poor mental and physical health, delinquent behavior, and unemployment in adolescence and early adulthood" (p. 3). Unfortunately, poverty becomes self-perpetuating for many of these families, with subsequent generations often continuing to exist at or below the poverty level. Neuman makes the point that poverty in and of itself does not result in poor reading and academic performance. However, those who live in poverty typically have limited materials and resources that facilitate language and academic development, a lack of human capital (individuals' qualifications, education, and skills), a lack of social capital (networks, community resources, and relationships between children and adults), and fewer language supports. Research looking at the effects of poverty on language development "indicates that children who are poor hear a smaller number of words with more limited syntactic complexity and fewer conversation-eliciting questions, making it difficult for them to quickly acquire new words and to discriminate among words" (Neuman, 2008, p. 5). If the three aforementioned circumstances are addressed, children who live in poverty should have a level playing field with non-poor children with regard to language and literacy development and academic achievement (Neumann, 2008). Nonetheless, poverty's link to decreased cognitive-linguistic functioning during the preschool years foreshadows its association to diminished school achievement in primary and secondary school. On average, children who are from low-SES families perform significantly worse than non-poor and middle-class children on various indicators of academic achievement, including emergent literacy and math skills, achievement test scores, grade retention, course failures, placement in special education, high school graduation rate, high school dropout rate, and completed years of schooling (Neuman, 2008, p. 55).

Pre-Reading

Early semantic and syntactic skills are predictors of later reading success in children, but most researchers agree that the best predictor is phonological awareness. In fact, when the impact of three phonological processing skills—phonemic awareness, rapid serial naming, and phonological coding in working memory—is assessed, phonemic awareness (awareness and knowledge of distinctive features of sounds and awareness that words consist of sounds) emerged as the best predictor of later reading (Torgensen, Wagner, & Rashotte, 1994). Phonological awareness consists of three areas of understanding with regard to words: (1) words can be written or spoken; (2) spoken sounds and words have a corresponding written letter or word; and (3) words are composed of smaller segments (i.e., sounds and syllables).

A report by the National Institute for Literacy (n.d.) analyzed the pre-reading skills of children entering kindergarten in the fall. It found the following facts:

1. 67 percent had letter-recognition skills when entering kindergarten

2. 31 percent could understand the letter–sound relationship at the beginning of words

3. 18 percent could understand the letter–sound relationship at the end of words

4. 3 percent had sight-word recognition skills

5. 1 percent could understand words in context

In addition, the institute conducted the Early Childhood Longitudinal Study, in which they compared literacy skills in children who had been read to at least three times per week as opposed to children who had not been read to at least three times a week. Generally, they found that 62 percent of parents with a high SES read to their children daily, compared to 36 percent of parents with a low SES reading to their children daily. The results of this study are provided in Table 9–5.

In spring of the kindergarten year, "the children who were read to at least three times a week by a family member were almost twice as likely to score in the top 25% in reading than children who were read to less than three times a week" (National Institute for Literacy, n.d.).

The issues of reading readiness and reading success are explored in depth in Chapter 10.

TABLE 9–5   Preliteracy skills dependent upon being read to 3 times per week

Skill Mastered	Children Read to Three or More Times per Week	Children Read to Less than Three Times per Week
Letter–sound relationship at the beginning of words	76%	64%
Letter–sound relationship at the end of words	57%	43%
Sight word recognition skills	15%	8%
Can understand words in context	5%	2%

Source: National Institute for Literacy (n.d.). Literacy in the United States. www.policyalmanac.org/education/archive/literacy.shtml.

> *think about it*
>
> What can you do to facilitate the easing of children from impoverished background into the structured academic setting?

Abused and Neglected Children

Situations of impoverishment often create individuals who become isolationists to some degree; that is, they frequently avoid others, often due to mistrust. These individuals may become parents who are likely to be abusive toward or neglectful of their children. Berk (2004) wrote that these parents are "more likely to live in unstable run-down neighborhoods that provide few links between family and community, such as parks, child-care centers, preschool programs, recreation centers, and churches" (p. 268).

Risk Factors Associated with Different Cultures in American Schools

In studying language acquisition by Black children, Stockman (1996) found many similarities between the White population and those who are African American. Furthermore, he found that there are no distinctive features of African American speech and language prior to age 3 years. After that, as the child gets older, he or she has an increase in the features often associated with African American speech and language. Based on Stockman's work, van Keulen, Weddington, and DeBose (1998) summed up these characteristics as follows:

1. The phonological system of African American children changes as children grow older and varies with socioeconomic class and geographical region.

2. With few exceptions, African American children produce the same phoneme inventory as standard English-speaking children.

3. The variation of final consonant deletion is rule governed and cannot be described as "open syllables."

4. African American children use alternative ways to mark tense when the final consonant is absent, such as lengthening or nasalizing the preceding vowels.

5. Standardized articulation tests vary in items sensitive enough to reveal the presence of final consonant variations among African American speakers. Such tests are likely to show persistence in the use of deletions beyond the age when such forms are developmentally appropriate in standard English speakers (p. 85–86).

van Keulen, Weddington, and DeBose (1998) point out that while many African American children have no difficulty with understanding spoken standard English, they have difficulty with "academic English" that threatens their success in school. They write that

> In a sense, Black children who speak African American English are often limited in their knowledge of academic language and often have difficulty following directions, responding to questions, and deciphering the content of textbooks. When the textbook vocabulary is so different from the lexicon of the student and the syntax varies remarkably from the sentences heard commonly in the community, children have problems gaining the knowledge intended by the class curriculum. (p. 86)

Thus, children who speak African American English could be considered to have language deficits and differences traditionally seen in children who are limited English proficient or from non–English-speaking backgrounds. Thus, they too need instruction in standard and academic English in order to meet their potential in the standard school curriculum. When any child has difficulty learning, following directions, and generally benefiting from classroom instruction, he or she typically is referred to the speech-language pathologist for testing. Since many of African American children fail the tests due to the fact that the tests are based on standard English, it is often assumed that the child has a language disability when indeed he or she is failing due to a language difference. This has tremendous implications with regard to labeling the child and enrolling him or her in therapy (van Keulen, Weddington, & DeBose, 1998).

CLINICAL FINDINGS

The assessment and diagnosis of learning disabilities is discussed in Chapter 13; however, a few comments here are warranted. The diagnosis of a learning disability is based on "critical elements . . . elicited during psychological, educational and/or language assessments" (ASHA, 1991, p. 3). Some of these critical elements, which are based on the features of language discussed in Chapter 1, are reviewed in this section.

Phonological Deficits

Children with language-based learning disabilities frequently have trouble with phonological aspects of speech and language. Some of these children have speech that is difficult to understand due to a simplification of the manner in which sounds are produced. Children who have this type of deficit may fall into the category described above as being comprised of children with articulatory and graphomotor deficits. In other children the phonological problem is related to phonological awareness problems. That is to say, they have trouble processing the grapheme–phoneme association that helps them couple the auditory signal of the phoneme with the written letter that represents the

Segmentation. The breaking down of sentences into words, words into syllables, and syllables into phonemes.

sound. They also tend to have inferior performance on segmentation tasks. Segmentation consists of the skills needed to break words into syllables and syllables into phonemes. This includes poor letter-by-letter decoding strategies; phonological deficits contribute to this problem (Reed, 2005). In some children, poor accuracy at distinguishing sentence forms based on prosodic cues, such as pitch, stress, and pauses, is also symptomatic of LLDs.

Although these children typically perform within normal limits on neuropsychological testing, it is not uncommon for their verbal IQ to be lower than their performance IQ. This is because most of the verbal segments of IQ tests require reading, decoding, and spelling skills.

Semantic Deficits

Although morphological and phonological development are essentially complete in the early childhood years, semantics, syntax, and pragmatics continue to develop through later childhood and adolescence.

Tiegerman-Farber (1997) writes about the semantic-feature hypothesis, saying it "proposes that children establish meaning by combining features (characteristics) that are present and observable in the environment. As children continue to experience reality, their ideas and concepts about objects and events change" (p. 77). In addition, children use overextensions when learning the labels and meanings of objects. Such overextensions have broader meaning than does the adult's meaning. For example, a child may refer to all four-legged animals as dogs because the child does not use as many semantic features as the adult does when defining a word. Children normally use a variety of hypotheses and concepts to develop their lexicon. However, children with LLDs may not be able to develop these hypotheses and concepts and, hence, have an underdeveloped lexicon.

With regard to specific language features, children with LLDs show some distinctive semantic characteristics. Often these children have difficulty in organizing word meanings, particularly when multiple meanings exist for the same word. The children also have trouble in retrieving lexical items in naming tasks and spontaneous speech. This is possibly due to underdeveloped lexical systems that result in poor vocabulary and poor metalinguistic skills, such as difficulty with synonyms, antonyms, and metaphors. Children with LLDs also tend to define words in a very concrete manner. For example, they may define the word *banana* as "something you eat" and *geography* as "something you study at school."

Research shows that it can be difficult to separate semantic deficits and retrieval deficits (Leonard, 1998). In other words, it is difficult to determine whether the child has a problem with encoding the words, so that the lexicon is never stored into memory, or if the child has retrieval problems, in which case the information was encoded but cannot be retrieved from short- or long-term memory. In studying confrontational naming and spontaneous speech in these children, researchers have found several skills to be different or higher in frequency.

Confrontational naming. The naming of items as the child is confronted with the item by the clinician.

One difficulty is in retrieving the name of an item. Instead of naming an item that is shown to the child, he or she describes it. This is called circumlocution because the child evades naming an item by describing it instead.

The use of word substitutions for the target word has also been noted. In addition, a lack of specificity is seen in the language of children with LLDs, with the frequent use of low-information words such as pronouns and indefinite adverbs such as *somewhere* and *sometime* instead of more specific information. These children also may demonstrate verbal hesitancies and the use of extra verbalizations such as "um" and "uh" to cover for delays in producing target words.

It has been noted that children who have LLDs have greater difficulties in naming what has been described than do their peers. For example, if the teacher asks, "What animal has four legs and black and white stripes?" the child with a learning disability will have more difficulty providing the answer than his or her peers. These children also tend to overuse functional definitions, describing items according to their use instead of particular and distinguishing features.

The concern as to whether the issue is one of encoding or decoding may be unsolvable, so it may be more important to focus on the more immediate concern: the inability to use semantic information in a useful manner.

> **Circumlocution.** The use of an indirect manner of expression to describe an object or event when the name cannot be recalled; e.g., saying "that thing you use to unlock the door" instead of "key."

Semantic Development and Disorders in Adolescents

Nippold (1993) studied the growth of semantics, syntax, and pragmatics in adolescence. With regard to semantics, she noted that the development of literate lexicon and figurative expression are central to academic success. It is of particular importance to note that both areas are dependent on the use of metalinguistic skills in order to infer meaning from context (Nippold, 1993, p. 24).

The Literate Lexicon The literate lexicon "consists of words that commonly occur in scholarly contexts in high school and college." Nippold provided the following verbs as examples of literate lexicon: at advanced levels, "interpret, concede, predict," and at younger levels, "remember, doubt, and infer" (p. 24). Literate lexicon may not be mastered until the student is in college. A study conducted by Astington and Olson (1987) and cited by Nippold (1993) showed that a student's knowledge of literate verbs correlated with his or her reading vocabulary scores on a standardized assessment of academic achievement. This implies that comprehension and use of literate verbs are important in achieving academic success and should be a focus of intervention with adolescents who have language and/or learning disabilities (Nippold, 1993).

Figurative Expressions The understanding of figurative expressions such as proverbs, idioms, and metaphors requires the comprehension of abstract words and multiple meanings. Nippold and others found that ability to understand and use figurative expressions increases as one gets older (i.e., college students perform better on tasks involving figurative language than do young adolescents). There is evidence of a link between literacy and idiom interpretation in that performance on a task involving the interpretation of a set of idioms correlated to reading comprehension scores on a standardized measure of academic achievement (Nippold & Martin, 1989). This, too, has implications for therapy with adolescents. The learning of vocabulary requires one to infer meanings from linguistic and nonlinguistic cues, so therapy with students who have language disorders that impact academic learning should include teaching the students how to infer meaning from curricular and social contexts (Nippold, 1993).

Syntactic Deficits

Children should be combining words by 18 to 24 months of age, and failure to do so is one of the first delays observed in the syntactic development of children with specific language impairment (Paul, 1996; Rescorla, Roberts, & Dahlsgaard, 1997). Children with language-based learning disabilities typically have a lower mean length of utterance than their peers, leading to more immature and less imaginative sentence structure. They have difficulty with bound morphemes (-s, -ed), auxiliary verbs (is, be), and closed-class morphemes such as a and the (Paul, 2001). Normally, children learn syntax in short, rapid bursts of development. However, children with LLDs typically have a constant slow rate of learning syntax, and they show a poorer command of morphological items.

As a rule, children with LLDs exhibit reading deficits. Although they may have difficulties with mature syntax in their expressive language, they may not necessarily have trouble comprehending syntax in reading. However, they do have poorer sentence comprehension. This may be explained by an inadequate ability to hold a representation of the sentence in short-term memory.

Syntactic Development and Disorders in Adolescents

Nippold (1993) stated that the three areas of continued syntactic growth in the later school years and adolescence are sentence length, subordination, and cohesion devices.

Sentence Length Sentence length typically increases as youth progress through adolescence. According to Nippold (1993), increases in sentence length are due to the use of more low-frequency structures in oral and written language. Low-frequency structures used to enhance noun phrases include the use of (1) appositive constructions ("Ms Change, an art teacher, attends yoga classes on Tuesdays"); (2) post-modifications via prepositional phrases ("They guessed the magician's trick was just an illusion"); and (3) complex structures ("Before Tim could fix the car, he had to borrow a tool

TABLE 9–6 Mean length of C-units in adolescents with average language proficiency in grades 6, 9, and 12

	Grade 6	Grade 9	Grade 12
Oral Language	9.82 words	10.96 words	11.70 words
Written Language	9.04 words	10.05 words	13.27 words

Source: Based on information in Nippold (1992), p. 22.

from his neighbor, then return it when he was done"). Verb phrases are enhanced by the use of modals ("He should have gathered all the tools before starting the project"), the perfect aspect ("They had been thinking all day"), and passive voice ("The ancient stone structure was built by laborers").

Nippold (1993) noted that adolescents can have grammatically correct written and oral language but still have delays in syntax. Loban (1976) developed norms of adolescent syntax by counting C-units and T-units in the oral and written language of adolescents. "Both C-units and T-units consist of an independent clause and any modifiers, such as subordinate clauses; C-units also include incomplete sentences in answer to questions" (Nippold, 1993, p. 22). Norms related to the length of C-units are shown in Table 9–6.

The implication for speech-language pathologists who are assessing the language of an adolescent is that oral and written language samples should be collected and the mean length of C-units calculated for both. This should be compared to Loban's norms to determine if the student has a syntactic delay. In addition, the samples should be analyzed to determine what, if any, low-frequency structures are used. Nippold (1993) cautions that the clinician should bear in mind that the language samples on which the norms are based "were elicited using formal tasks, such as having students tell or write stories or converse with an adult" (p. 22). Results are likely to be different if the language sample is obtained in the student's conversation with a peer. This is confirmed by a study done by Eckert (1990) that was cited by Nippold. In an oral language sample gathered during a conversation between six adolescent girls, the most talkative girl had a mean C-unit of 7.86 words, which is average for third graders based on Loban's norms. This points out the need to obtain adolescent language samples from a variety of formal and informal contexts when determining if a student has a syntactic delay or disorder. Other signs of syntactic delays that one can ascertain from oral language samples include excessive use of false starts, hesitations, and revisions in formal conversations. (Nippold, 1993).

Subordination The use of subordinate clauses in oral and written language gradually increases in children and adolescents. Again referencing Loban (1976), norms related to the use of subordinate clauses in oral and written language are summarized in Table 9–7.

TABLE 9–7 Mean number of subordinate clauses per C-unit by students with average language proficiency in grades 6, 9, and 12

	Grade 6	Grade 9	Grade 12
Oral Language	.37	.43	.58
Written Language	.29	.47	.60

Source: Based on information in Nippold (1992), p. 22.

The use of nominal subordinate clauses predominates in oral language, while the use of adverbial subordinate clauses predominates in written language. Typically developing adolescents also show increasing use of adjectival subordinate clauses as they progress academically. There is also an increase in the types of verb phrases used. In particular, as students mature they use more participial phrases, infinitive phrases, and gerund phrases. When used in place of subordinate clauses, verb phrases "suggest even greater sophistication because of their conciseness of expression" (Nippold, 1993, p. 23). The use of concise verb phrases results in shorter sentence length, which shows that sentence length, is not necessarily an accurate indication of a student's syntactic maturity.

Cohesion Devices When conjunctions, particularly adverbial conjuncts, are used, discourse cohesion increases. Nippold (1993) maintains that "competence with adverbial conjuncts is important for literacy development and academic success" (p. 23). Adverbial conjuncts are often encountered in formal literate contexts such as textbooks and lectures. Using a writing task and a reading task, Nippold, Schwarz, and Undlin (1992) found that the use of adverbial conjuncts gradually improved with age. On the writing task, grammaticality and use of appropriate sentences improved as the students got older. They also found that "the amount of meaningful exposures" to adverbial conjuncts affected the students' competence levels.

Pragmatic Deficits

Many children with LLDs exhibit pragmatic deficits that are worse than their deficits in form and content. Indeed, some children with normal linguistic abilities may have pragmatic deficits; that is, they are unable to use language in an appropriate manner for a variety of purposes (Roth & Spekman, 1984a).

Roth and Spekman (1984b) posit that discourse organization, a segment of pragmatics, can be tested by implementing discourse within activities familiar to the child. By testing discourse in familiar activities, a scaffolding for dialogue can be set up. As part of this scaffolding, the speech-language pathologist can create opportunities for the child "to initiate conversation, to take turns, and to repair in response to self-feedback or the feedback of others in different situations" (Owens, 2004, p. 132). While playing, preschool-age children often have nonsocial dialogues, while older children engage in social monologues and in social dialogues. Thus, as the child matures, he or she becomes more aware of the use of speech and language in a social manner.

Pragmatic deficits in children with LLDs are more likely to be linguistic problems than social delays. The children exhibit poor conversational repair strategies, and they tend to be passive in groups and to ask fewer questions. The questions they do ask are simple and typically require uncomplicated answers. They also tend to have topical discontinuity, meaning that they have difficulty maintaining a topic of conversation. They may overuse meaningless starters such as, "Now, you see."

Children with LLDs also face problems with survival language, particularly when they reach middle school age. Survival language basically refers to knowing the lingo associated with peer language, but also involves knowing how to be a part of a peer group through appropriate actions. As stated earlier, many children with language disorders or LLDs have low self-esteem and do not feel as if they are part of a peer group. Thus, it is possible they may agree to participate in an inappropriate behavior if they believe it will make them an accepted member of a peer group. Thus, the survival language needed to "just say no" instead of participating in an inappropriate activity may be absent.

Nippold (1993) stated that the use of language in social contexts is a key component of an adolescent's self-identity. Pragmatic competence requires syntactic and semantic knowledge, two areas of language that are frequently deficient in school-age children with language and/or learning disabilities. Two areas of pragmatics that require special attention in adolescents are interpersonal negotiation strategies and slang expressions.

Interpersonal negotiation strategies are required in order to resolve interpersonal conflicts. As the children in Nippold's (1993) study got older, they were increasingly "aware of the wants and feelings of the participants, showed the most concern for the long-term consequences of the conflict, and were most interested in resolving the conflict through compromise and mutual agreement" (p. 26). When watching adolescent interactions, Nippold found that interpersonal negotiation strategies were used more in interactions with peers than adults and in personal situations more than work situations. Older adolescents employed the strategies more than the younger adolescents, and there were gender differences. The implications of these observations for therapy are that teaching negotiation strategies should begin with scenarios of interpersonal conflict that involve peers and personal problems.

With regard to slang expressions, Nippold (1993) stressed that this should be a focus of therapy because the use of slang expressions helps to "achieve group identity and feelings of solidarity" (p. 26). The number of slang terms used by adolescents increases at each age level and varies at each age level. The terms used also differ by gender. Nippold suggested that

Survival language. Knowing the lingo associated with peer language and knowing how to be a part of a peer group through appropriate actions and communication styles.

speech-language pathologists use peer groups of the same age and gender when identifying targets in therapy because the slang expressions are somewhat age and gender specific.

CHARACTERISTICS OF FICTIONAL AND PERSONAL NARRATIVES BY CHILDREN WITH LANGUAGE AND LEARNING IMPAIRMENTS

Fictional Narratives

There are contextual differences between oral and written (literate) language. Oral language typically is used in an environment in which the conversation partners draw information from cues in the environment such as objects and surroundings; gestures, facial expressions, and body language of conversation partners; and vocal cues, including the type of utterance and changes in pitch, loudness, and intonation. In other words, oral language is highly contextualized as a rule. On the other hand, literate language has fewer external cues and information. Therefore, it is highly decontextualized (Greenhalgh & Strong, 2001; Paul, 2001; Westby, 1984, 1991).

Greenhalgh and Strong (2001) analyzed the spoken narratives of 7- to 10-year-old students to examine differences between language impaired and typically developing children with regard to literate language use. Greenhalgh and Strong summarized the research of Paul (1995, 2001), Westby (1985, 1991), Wallach and Butler (1994), van Oers (1998), Klee (1992), Wiig and Semel (1984), and Lyon (1999) on the development of literate language. Literate language is enhanced in children who are exposed to print in many forms and who are encouraged to read and discuss their text experiences with the adults in their environment. In fact, exposure to books and other forms of print language is critical in the development of literate language. Exposure to structured oral language, such as sermons and other public speeches, also contributes to the development of literate language. "Theoretically, literate language may be linked to children's development of meaningful abstract thinking or the ability to recontextualize a previously experienced event or activity . . . so that a listener also can construct meaning" (Greenhalgh & Strong, 2001, p. 115).

A child who has deficits in literate language has problems conveying meanings, acquiring literacy, communicating effectively, and succeeding academically. Children with language impairments frequently have smaller vocabularies than their typically developing peers, use fewer complex sentences and elaborated noun phrases, and have more frequent use of nonspecific words. These deficits can also impact the development of literate language, which implies that the assessment of literate language in addition to the more traditional measures of children's language should be standard in determining a child's language abilities (Greenhalgh & Strong, 2001).

Greenhalgh and Strong (2001) cited Westby (1999), who identified four features in children's narratives that contribute to the use of literate language:

1. *Conjunctions* help clarify, organize, and provide structure to "event and object relationships in the story and make meanings explicit" (Greenhalgh & Strong, 2001, p. 116);

2. *Elaborated noun phrases* provide clarification and enhancement of the story. Their use demonstrates that a child has developed literate language.

3. *Mental and linguistic verbs* create a more literate narrative "because their occurrence indicates children's awareness of characters' mental states and their verbal abilities" (Greenhalgh & Strong, 2001, p. 116).

4. *Adverbs* indicate that the child understands the impact of time, manner, and degree on the meaning of the story.

> **Mental verbs.** Verbs that refer to different acts of thinking, such as *decided* or *thought*.
>
> **Linguistic verbs.** Verbs that refer to acts of speaking, such as *said* or *told*.

In their analyses of the narratives based on story retelling, Greenhalgh and Strong (2001) found that conjunctions and elaborated noun phrases were the most critical features in the assessment of children's literate language in their sample. They stressed that it is critical to determine the "type and grammatical role of the literate language features" (p. 121) that the child uses in his or her narratives. Analysis of the components of literate language can provide guidance in documenting the existence of a language impairment that could impact a child's academic and social success (as a communicator), as well as to guide intervention (Nippold, 1988; Gillam, Pena, & Miller, 1999; Greenhalgh & Strong, 2001).

Personal Narratives

The use of fictional narratives based on sentence and story recall is a critical part of preparing a child to be a good reader. However, with regard to teaching children how to develop a narrative, there is evidence that the use of personal narratives instead of fictional narratives is more efficacious. "Children with typical language development (TLD) are capable of producing complete and complex oral personal narratives by the time they enter first grade" (McCabe, Bliss, Barra, & Bennett, 2009, p. 195).

It is possible that elementary-aged children produce better personal narratives than fictional narratives because the content of personal narratives is more relevant to the child and easier to organize. Also, children engage in personal narratives more frequently; for example, they tell their parents, siblings, and peers about their day at school (McCabe, Bliss, Barra, & Bennett, 2008).

McCabe, Bliss, Barra, & Bennett (2008) compared personal and fictional narratives generated by 27 children aged 7:0 to 9:9 years with language impairments. The fictional narratives (elicited using a wordless picture book) were longer but less structurally complex than the personal narratives. There were also more production errors (verbal mazes) in the fictional narratives and less use of generalization. Children's personal narratives incorporated more story elements (precipitation factors, goal resolution, topic maintenance, temporal sequencing, and conclusions) than did their fictional narratives.

However, a comparison of the personal narratives of the children with language impairment to those of children with typically developing language showed that the narratives of children with language impairment were shorter and less complex. They typically did not present the sequence of events in chronological order and tended to omit key information, making it more difficult for their conversation partner to understand the intended message. Also, many of the fictional narratives of the children with language impairment were not true narratives; most of the personal narratives did meet the criteria to be true narratives. McCabe and colleagues (2008) described a non-narrative as containing no past-tense events and usually consisting "of present tense events and other picture description" (p. 199). In McCabe and colleagues' study, to be a true narrative, the narrative had to contain at least one past-tense event. This differs from the criterion established by Labov (1972) that says a narrative must contain two past-tense events in order to be a true narrative. McCabe and colleagues' scale ranged from 0 (non-narrative) to 7 (classic pattern). A classic-pattern narrative is one in which the "narrative orients the listener to who, what, when, and where something occurred, builds actions up to a high point, evaluatively dwells on it (by telling listeners the 'important part' or how the narrator felt about the events), and then resolves it" (McCabe et al., 2008, p. 198).

When the children with language impairments were using the wordless picture book to construct their fictional narratives, they tended to treat each page (picture) as a separate entity instead of recognizing the book as a story consisting of sequential events. As a result, the fictional narratives of the children with language impairment were significantly lower in quality than their personal narratives. McCabe and colleagues (2008) suggested that the characteristics of children with language impairment that possibly interfere with narrative production, particularly fictional narrative production, are:

1. Decreased working memory

2. Restricted knowledge base

3. Reduced ability to recognize the similarities between clinical and natural discourse for personal narratives

4. Limited information processing (McCabe et al., 2008, p. 201–202)

Thus, in treating children with language impairment, one should address the "infrastructure" as well as the functional production of narratives. This is discussed further in Chapter 14.

WRITING SKILLS IN CHILDREN WITH LANGUAGE-BASED LEARNING DISABILITIES

Children who have difficulties with reading, spelling, and conversational speech often have problems with writing. Children who have articulatory-graphomotor problems and children with visuospatial deficits have problems writing legibly. Children who have poor language and learning skills also exhibit difficulties with the content and form of their written language. Based on the work of several researchers (Espin et al., 1999; Parker, Tindal, & Hasbrouck, 1991; Scott, 1991; Scott & Windsor, 2000; Treiman, 1997; Watkinson & Lee, 1992), Reed (2005) listed the following problem areas with written language in individuals with learning and/or reading disabilities:

1. Productivity problems: typically fewer words used, decreased mean length of utterance, and fewer sentences used

2. Text structure: poor use of cohesion devices and poor organization of text

3. Sentence structure: lack of grammatical complexity and poor use of conjunctions

4. Spelling: use of many non-phonetic spelling errors

5. Lexicon: tendency toward repetitive use of words

6. Handwriting: poor letter formation, mixture of uppercase and lowercase, and uneven spacing

Bourassa and Treiman (2001) summarized the research on spelling difficulties in individuals with specific learning disabilities in written language. When these individuals spell, there is a high frequency of spellings that are not phonologically structured. The errors that are made can be divided into phonetic misspellings and non-phonetic errors. Bourassa and Treiman provided the examples shown in Table 9–8.

TABLE 9–8   Examples of phonetic and non-phonetic spellings

Phonetic	*plad* for *plaid*
Nonphonetic	*pad* for *plaid*
	doo for *door*
	wom for *warm*
	foz for *past*
	jry for *dry*

Source: Bourassa and Treiman, 2001.

These spellings are consistent with the phonological deficit hypothesis, which states that "these individuals compensate for their phonological weaknesses by relying heavily on visual memorization of orthographic patterns" (Bourassa & Treiman, 2001, p. 177). There are mixed reviews as to the accuracy of this hypothesis, however. Bourassa and Treiman suggested that it may be more productive to look at the misspellings in terms of how people with spelling disabilities and controls at the same spelling level differ on specific types of linguistic stimuli. Taking this approach, the authors found that students with spelling deficits were more likely to omit the internal consonants of word-initial clusters. An example they cite is *bot* for *blot*.

Another theory based on the linguistic foundations of spelling deficits is the morphological deficit hypothesis. Carlisle (1987) compared the morphologically based spelling of ninth graders with LLDs with that of non-disabled fourth graders. An example of an item was, "Warm. He chose the jacket for its ___" with the expectation that the children would write "warmth." On standard spelling tests, the ninth graders performed similarly to or worse than the fourth graders. However, on oral morphological spelling, the ninth graders performed similarly to sixth and eighth graders; that is to say, oral spelling was better than written spelling. However, the gap between oral and written spelling was greater for the ninth graders than it was for the normal children. The results "are consistent with the morphological deficit hypothesis, for they suggest that individuals with spelling difficulties have particular difficulty appreciating the way in which the English writing system reflects the morphological structure of the language" (Bourassa & Treiman, 2001, p. 178). The phonological systems of children with spelling deficits should be assessed; phonological awareness training that addresses the specific phonological deficits may help these children with their reading and spelling abilities.

SPECIFIC LANGUAGE IMPAIRMENT

Children with specific language impairment (SLI) face numerous academic and social challenges in the school transition years due to the well-documented existence of problems with peer relationships. However, it should be noted that not all children with SLI have problems with social competence (Fujiki, Brinton, & Clarke, 2002). The degree of variability of social skills in children with SLI begs for further study. Gertner, Rice, and Hadley (1994) found that many preschool children diagnosed with SLI were considered by their peers as not being a preferred playmate. In addition, Rice, Sell, and Hadley (1991) found that children with SLI preferred adults to their peers as conversational partners. In another study, Fujiki, Brinton, and Clarke (2002) studied the social behaviors of children on the school playground as opposed to the structured format of the academic classroom. They found that children with language impairment were typically more withdrawn and spent significantly less time interacting with peers than did children who did not have a language impairment. The root of these social difficulties, in part, can be traced back to the poor language abilities characteristic of children with SLI.

Fujiki and colleagues (2002) proposed that one variable affecting social development in a child with SLI is emotional regulation. They suggested that children's language impairments can influence their ability to regulate or control their emotions. These children are frequently teased because they laugh and cry more easily than their peers, with the laughter often being out of proportion when compared to that of their classmates. They may become frustrated when unable to do a task that is accomplished more readily by their peers. Additional factors that influence emotional regulation include the child's temperament, socialization practices, and cognitive functioning. Children who do not have deficits in these areas may account for those who have SLI but do not have significant social difficulties.

> **Emotional regulation.** The ability to control one's emotions and express them appropriately based on the myriad components of a setting.

Participation in Collaborative Activities

Difficulties with social interaction certainly place a child at risk in the classroom given the emphasis on group projects and other collaborative activities.

> **Collaborative activities.** Those activities that involve the joint participation and cooperation of the members of a group.

Children with SLI usually find such activities difficult. Indeed, in research on participation of children with language impairments in group activities Brinton, Fujiki, and Higbee (1998) found that these children participated significantly less often than their non–language-impaired peers, both verbally and nonverbally. This led to two primary conclusions: (1) that language-impaired children who have difficulty in group work situations do not use nonverbal methods to compensate for verbal deficits, and (2) that the success of children with SLI becoming actively involved in cooperative learning groups may depend largely on their level of social functioning. Brinton and colleagues (2000) did a pilot study to look at the functioning of children with language impairments in cooperative learning groups. Their findings verified those of Brinton, Fujiki, and Higbee (1998), particularly that the social functioning of a child with SLI significantly impacted his or her ability to integrate into a cooperative work group. However, they also found that some of the children did have more success in these small groups when compared to their performance in a full classroom activity, possibly because these groups are usually made up of children with different ability levels. This sets ups a scaffolding system in which the higher-functioning children provide models for those who do not function as well.

> **Scaffolding system.** A "stair-step" approach to problem solving in a group consisting of students at varying levels of ability, in which a high-functioning child provides a model for a lower-functioning child.

Literacy Skills and Phonological Processing in Children with SLI

A critical factor in the development of literacy skills is early exposure to books, as depicted in Figure 9–2.

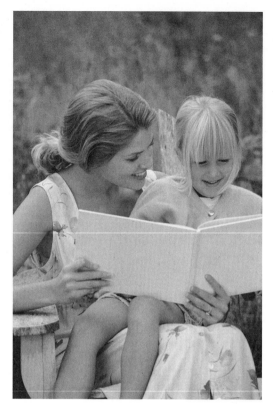

FIGURE 9–2 Exposing a child to books and reading with him or her at an early age is a crucial factor in developing literacy. (*Delmar/Cengage Learning*)

In a longitudinal study by Stothard and colleagues (1998), there was a difference in literacy skills and phonological processing, with the language-impaired children (resolved) performing worse than the controls. Those children whose language impairment had not resolved by age 5:6 and those who had general delay all exhibited "significant impairments in all aspects of spoken and written language functioning" (p. 407). Stothard and colleagues did a longitudinal follow-up study of 71 adolescents who had been diagnosed as having a speech-language impairment as preschoolers and who were in an original study by Bishop and Edmundson (1987). When the children were 4 years of age, they were divided into two groups. The general delay group had a measured nonverbal IQ that was 2 standard deviations below the mean. The SLI group had normal nonverbal intelligence. When the children were 5:6, the children in the SLI group were divided into those whose language problems had resolved and those whose SLI persisted. The general delay group was also followed. When the children with SLI were 15 to 16 years of age, they were given a test battery consisting of tests of spoken language and literacy skills, and their performance was compared to those of age-matched normal-language children. It is interesting to note that on tests of language comprehension and vocabulary, there was no difference between the children in the control group and those whose language impairments had resolved by age 5:6. In addition, it should be noted that the children whose language impairment did not resolve also had deficits on nonverbal tasks on the Weschler Intelligence Scale for Children—III. In fact, 47 percent of those children scored 1 standard deviation below the mean on nonverbal composite scores, and 20 percent fell more than 2 standard deviations below the mean. Also, with time, the children with general delay and those with unresolved SLI increasingly fell behind their peer groups in vocabulary. Based on these results, it is clear that 15-year-old-children with a longstanding history of general delay or unresolved specific language impairments have significant deficits in verbal and nonverbal language that could negatively impact academic success. Approximately 50 percent of the 15-year-old adolescents were receiving special education services, and the majority had academic problems. Even those children whose language impairments had resolved by age 5:6 exhibited "residual, but mild, processing impairments that place them at risk of later failure (e.g., in literacy skills)" (p. 417). The children in the resolved group were not diagnosed as dyslexic, and even though their "reading skills were significantly poorer than those of controls, they were not generally outside of the normal range as predicted by IQ" (p. 417).

As discussed in Chapter 8, Johnson and colleagues (1999) did a longitudinal study in which they followed children for a 14-year period. To refresh your memory, the 142 children in their study were originally diagnosed at age 5 as having language impairments and were retested at 12 and 18 to 20 years of age. Out of the 142 children, 27.5 percent had speech impairments only, 43.6 percent had language impairments only, and 28.9 percent had impairments in speech and language. There were also 142 controls selected from among the children who passed the initial screening. The results of the study indicated the following:

- Those children diagnosed at age 5 with speech impairment had only "subtle, residual speech problems as young adults but showed no long-term deficits in language, cognitive, and academic performance" (p. 755) when compared to age-level non-impaired peers.

- Children who were diagnosed as age 5 with language impairment "showed clear long-term deficits in language, cognitive, and academic domains relative to peers without early language difficulty" (p. 755).

In all these studies, it is evident that even those children whose problems appeared to be resolved in the early academic years demonstrated deficits in middle school and high school that had an impact on their social and academic success. Thus, children with SLI need to be followed by a team of specialists throughout school. This team should consist of the child's teachers, a guidance counselor, a psychologist, and a speech-language pathologist, at least. This is particularly important as the child enters the late elementary grades, middle school, and high school because this is a critical time not only in academic demands, but also in the growth of importance of peer relationships.

Questions regarding the etiology of SLI still persist. In some children, there may be a familial history of language problems and a central nervous system deficit cannot be ruled out as a causative factor. SLI is a difficult category to track in terms of causative agents due to the diversity of the problems exhibited from one child to the next and the fact that many of these children never have a causative factor identified. In fact, some researchers even question the advisability of having a label of SLI. In short, it is a heterogeneous disorder with a multiplicity of possible etiological factors.

Children who fail a screening and subsequent testing may have a specific language impairment. Leonard defines SLI as "significant limitations in language functioning that cannot be attributed to deficits in hearing, oral structure and function, or general intelligence" (Leonard, 1987, p. 1). This is an interesting diagnostic category because there is not one apparent cause and the child does not have perceptual deficits one might see in language-based learning disabilities or cognitive deficits associated with intellectual disabilities. When given a nonverbal test, the language performance scores of these children are "significantly lower than their intellectual performance scores" (Owens, 2004, p. 37). Typically, the performance IQ is above 85, but the child has a low verbal score, with the child's expressive skills being significantly below his or her receptive skills.

Rescorla (1989) estimated that 10 to 15 percent of children do not have 50 single words or combine words by 24 months of age. While many of these children develop normally, approximately 20 to 25 percent of these children with early language problems have their difficulties persist into the preschool and school age years (Paul, 1996; Rescorla, 1990; Thal, 1989). Tomblin and colleagues (1997) cited an SLI prevalence figure of 7.4 percent of all children in kindergarten. The language problems in these children frequently persist as language problems when the children become adolescents, especially as language problems related to phonological and literacy abilities (Owens, 2004). Also, usage of verbs tends to be more problematic than use of nouns. One particular deficit area in children with SLI is a limit in the use of finite verb morphemes (Goffman & Leonard, 2000). A description of semantic difficulties of children with SLI is found in Table 9–9.

In addition to the written and oral language deficits found in many children with SLI, there is documentation of difficulties with math, particularly beyond the second grade. Fazio (1999) looked at mathematical abilities in low-income children with SLI over a 5-year period. The subjects were 10 children who were 9 to 10 years of age and who had been diagnosed with SLI during the preschool years. In a 1996 study by Fazio, she found

TABLE 9–9   Several areas of semantic difficulties experienced by children with SLI

Area of Semantic Difficulty	Problems
Size of the lexicon	Smaller vocabularies
Rate of growth of the lexicon	Slower vocabulary acquisition
	Less lexical diversity
Robustness of word meaning	Less depth of knowledge about word meanings
	Less known about the meanings of individual words
	Only partial meanings of a word known
Speech of new word learning	Difficulties learning new lexical items quickly
	More exposures to a new word in context needed to abstract the meaning of the word
Word finding	Difficulties retrieving words from the cognitive store to use them in quick flow of connected speech
	The word on the "tip of the tongue"

Source: An introduction to children with language disorders, by Reed. Table 3.4, "Several areas of semantic difficulties experienced by children with SLI," p. 107. © 2005. Reproduced by permission of Pearson Education, Inc.

that children with SLI had delays in counting and basic mathematical knowledge, but they did fairly well in simple calculations in first and second grades. However, in fourth and fifth grade, these children had difficulties with math. Possible reasons for this difficulty in later elementary and subsequent years include the following:

1. The necessity of completing several steps in order to perform the calculations

2. An increase in the amount of domain-specific mathematical vocabulary

3. The need to engage in automatic retrieval of math facts instead of simply counting

4. A difficulty with rote retrieval of previously memorized material

5. A lack of active participation in group discussion of the math problems and solutions

6. Problems with underlying mechanisms such as conceptual knowledge, memory retrieval, and procedural knowledge

One of the findings of the 1999 study was that the performance of the subjects on written calculation tasks improved when they were given extra time. The children who did worst on tasks requiring working memory and language had the most difficulty with timed math tasks.

Children with SLI do not appear to have efficient problem-solving skills, in part due to the demands on working memory that hinder the automatic retrieval of math facts that results from extensive practice and the need for fewer resources. However, the children with SLI showed slow but steady growth in their math abilities over the 5-year period of the study. "Despite early delays in counting, the SLI group was not using counting as the primary means of solving calculation problems. However, learning a new set of rote material is still a formidable task for these children" (Fazio, 1999, p. 427). Children with SLI have inefficient processing of information, which places a heavier demand on verbal working memory than it does in typically developing children. This, in turn, negatively impacts working memory and interferes with the child's ability to efficiently perform on mathematical problems.

Mercer and Miller (1992) have suggested that children in third or fourth grade need automatic basic fact retrieval for increased efficiency in solving math problems. Children with SLI frequently cannot solve math problems rapidly and accurately, and counting speed is slow in children with SLI. All of these factors contribute to weak performances in math by children with SLI.

Obviously, SLI can impact multiple areas of language and academic performance in school-age children. Owens (2004) has summed up the impact of SLI on the primary features of language as seen in Table 9–10.

think about it

What would you suggest to classroom teachers to facilitate classroom participation and interactive learning by students with SLI?

TABLE 9–10 Language characteristics of children with specific language impairment

Pragmatics	May act like younger children developing typically
	Less flexibility in their language when tailoring the message to the listener or repairing communication breakdowns
	Same pragmatic functions as chronological-age–matched peers developing typically but expressed differently and less effectively
	Less effective than chronological-age–matched peers in securing a conversational turn; those with receptive difficulties most affected
	Inappropriate responses to topic
	Narratives less complete and more confusing than those of reading-ability–matched peers developing typically

Semantics	First words and subsequent vocabulary development that occurs at a slower rate, with occasional lexical errors seen in younger children developing typically
	Naming difficulties that reflect less rich and less elaborate semantic storage than actual retrieval difficulties; long-term memory storage problems probable
Syntax/Morphology	Co-occurrence of more mature and less mature forms
	Similar developmental order to that seen in children developing typically
	Fewer morphemes, especially verb endings, auxiliary verbs, and function words (articles, prepositions) than younger MLU-matched peers; learning related to grammatical function as in children developing typically
	Tendency to make pronoun errors, as with younger MLU-matched peers, but with tendency to overuse one form rather than making random errors
Phonology	Phonological processes similar to those of younger children developing typically, but in different patterns, i.e., occurring in units of varying word length rather than in one- or two-word utterances
	As toddlers, vocalize less and have less varied and less mature syllable structures than aged-matched peers developing typically
Comprehension	Poor discrimination of units of short duration (bound morphemes)
	Reading miscues often unrelated to text graphophonemically, syntactically, semantically, or pragmatically

Source: Language disorders, by Owens. Table 2.8, p. 39. © 2010 by Pearson Education, Inc. Reproduced by permission of Pearson Education, Inc.

AUDITORY PROCESSING DISORDERS

Conservative estimates are that 3 to 5 percent of the school-age population have some degree of an auditory processing disorder. Furthermore, Holston (1992) believes that a higher percentage of auditory processing disorders occurs in children with learning disabilities than in the general population. The prevalence figures may be low because many children who are perceived as having learning disabilities are not referred for auditory processing testing. In fact, auditory processing difficulties are associated with a variety of clinical populations, including children who have a history of otitis media, children in the school years who have learning difficulties, children and adults with neurological deficits, and aging individuals (DeBonis & Moncrief, 2008).

In 1996, the ASHA Task Force on Central Auditory Processing Consensus Development attempted to develop a definition of auditory processing disorders. The members of the task force believed that central auditory processes were mechanisms and processes of the auditory system and produced several behavioral patterns. The processes they identified included

- Sound localization and lateralization

- Auditory discrimination

- Auditory pattern recognition
- Temporal aspects of audition, including
  - Temporal integration
  - Temporal masking
  - Temporal resolution
  - Temporal ordering
- Auditory performance decrements with competing acoustic signals (including dichotic listening)
- Auditory performance decrements with degraded acoustic signals (ASHA, 1996; ASHA, 2005; Keith, 1999)

They defined central auditory processing disorder (CAPD) as "an observed deficiency in one or more of a group of mechanisms and processes related to a variety of auditory behaviors" (ASHA, 1996, p. 43). They went on to note that there are four issues related to the diagnosis and management of children and adults with central auditory processing disorders:

1. What does basic science tell us about the nature of central auditory processing and its role in audition?

2. What constitutes an assessment of central auditory processing and its disorders?

3. What are the developmental and acquired communication problems associated with central auditory processing disorders?

4. What is the clinical utility of a diagnosis of central auditory processing disorder?"(ASHA, 1996, p. 43)

The current terminology is auditory processing disorder (APD), as opposed to central auditory processing disorder. In 2005, the ASHA Working Group on Auditory Processing Disorders met to define the role of the audiologist in the assessment and treatment of APD. As part of their report, the working group proposed the following definition of (C)APD:

> Broadly stated, (Central) Auditory Processing refers to the efficiency and effectiveness by which the central nervous system (CNS) utilizes auditory information. Narrowly defined, (C)AP refers to the perceptual processing of auditory information in the CNS and the neurobiologic activity that underlies that processing and gives rise to electrophysiologic auditory potentials. (ASHA, 2005, p. 2)

It is important to note that the working group determined that the deficiencies in auditory processing are not caused by psychological, language, learning, communication, ADHD, or cognitive deficits, even though individuals with APD frequently have problems that coexist in these areas. In fact, individuals with auditory processing disorders have normal intelligence and hearing acuity, but they are unable to process auditory information or speech effectively. Most authorities report that auditory processing disorders cause difficulties in detection, interpretation, and categorization of sounds and that these problems may be caused by some type of dysfunction in lower- or higher-level cortical processes (Schow & Nervonne, 1996).

Children who exhibit signs of LLDs or reading and/or spelling disorders are often referred to audiologists to rule out auditory processing disorders prior to further testing. Children who have poor academic achievement, behavior problems, phonological deficits, ADHD, or problems with oral language also should be referred for auditory processing testing. It is sometimes difficult to separate an auditory processing disorder from a language deficit, owing to the underlying role of language in processing and learning. Young (1985) proposed that two types of (central) auditory processing disorders may be present in children. The first is related to attentional deficits, whereas the second includes both attentional problems and language deficits. Generally, individuals suspected of having APD frequently exhibit one or more of the following characteristics:

(a) difficulty with speech understanding in adverse listening environments,
(b) misunderstanding messages,
(c) responding inconsistently or inappropriately,
(d) frequently asking that information be repeated,
(e) difficulty attending and avoiding distraction,
(f) delay in responding to auditory directions,
(g) difficulty following complex auditory directions,
(h) difficulty with sound localization,
(i) reduced musical and singing skills, and
(j) associated reading, spelling, and learning problems. (DeBonis & Moncrief, 2008, p. 5)

Also, it is important to realize that auditory processing disorders and language processing disorders are not the same, even though they share many characteristic symptoms (ASHA, 2005). APD must include a diagnosis of deficits in the central auditory nervous system. According to the ASHA task force established in 1996, "the brain lesions associated with CAPD may be situated cortically in the left and right temporal and parietal lobes or sub cortically in the thalamus, basal ganglia, and brain stem structures"

(p. 45). However, they went on to say that some diseases and injuries lead to a broader distribution of damage. Some of these diseases and injuries include traumatic brain injury, cerebrovascular accident, tumors, multiple sclerosis, epilepsy, and Alzheimer disease.

RESPONSE TO INTERVENTION (RTI)

Response to Intervention, a systematic approach to the identification of students with learning disabilities and a means of providing early intervention for students at risk, came to prominence with the passage of IDEIA in 2004. RTI emphasizes the use of research-based interventions for students who are at risk for academic failure. The taking of data that documents students' progress in response to intensive intervention serves as a cornerstone for the identification of students who truly have a learning disability as opposed to those who may be underachieving students or students who are not performing up to standards due to inadequate instruction.

> A key element of an RTI approach is the provision of early intervention when students first experience academic difficulties, with the goal of improving the achievement of all students, including those who may have LD [learning disabilities]. In addition to the preventive and remedial services this approach may provide to at-risk students, it shows promise for contributing data useful for identifying LD. (NJCLD, 2005, p. 1)

RTI was also a response to criticisms of the long-held method of identifying children with learning disabilities—the IQ/achievement discrepancy. There are four major criticisms of using the discrepancy model:

1. Questions persist as to whether or not IQ tests really measure intelligence.

2. Some researchers' belief that IQ and academic achievement are not mutually exclusive.

3. Learning disabilities are not identified until the child had failed (wait-to-fail model).

4. "In the case of word-reading skill deficits, IQ-achievement discrepant poor readers are more alike than different from IQ-achievement consistent poor readers. (Fuchs, Fuchs, Compton, & Bryant, 2005, slide 3)

RTI uses a problem-solving approach that leads to earlier intervention and identification than the traditional IQ/achievement discrepancy model.

RTI was heralded as being a system that not only provided data based on performance that could be used to identify students with learning disabilities, but also ensured early, systematic, effective support to students who may or may not have a learning disability (Fuchs, Fuchs, Compton, & Bryant, 2005). This was the basis of the second reason for interest in RTI: overuse of special education services for students who were struggling academically but who did not have a learning disability (or any other disability). In RTI, research-based, intensive instruction was provided in general education settings, making it possible to identify students who were performing poorly due to poor instruction as opposed to performing poorly due to the presence of a learning disability (NJCLD, 2005).

Improvement in reading was a third reason for interest in RTI and is discussed in Chapter 10.

Simply put, RTI is part of a multi-tiered system of service delivery, consisting of screening, implementation of intervention in the general education setting, implementation of a supplementary diagnostic instructional trial, monitoring responsiveness to the supplementary diagnostic trial, and finally designation of disability and placement in special education programs. Most school districts assess all their students using a summative assessment annually in addition to formative assessments in the classroom throughout the year. In the RTI model, a student's performance on these tests and/or their academic growth rate is used to determine if he or she is progressing at a satisfactory rate or if he or she is at risk. Intervention is provided for children who are at risk and then the child is re-assessed. Children who do not show progress (response to intervention) are referred to a multi-disciplinary team for further evaluation and treatment, possibly in a special education setting (Fuchs, Fuchs, Compton, & Bryant, 2005).

It is important to note that, in the RTI model, assessment data based on actual response to classroom and small-group instruction can be used to partially fulfill the data needed to identify students as having a learning disability and to determine their eligibility for special education services.

> The goal of such a system is to ensure that quality instruction, good teaching practices, differential instruction, and remedial opportunities are available in general education, and that special education is provided for students with disabilities who require more specialized services than what can be provided in general education. (NJCLD, 2005, p. 5)

RTI focuses on student outcomes. It enables educators to identify students using a systematic, evidence-based problem-solving approach to assess actual student performance. Instead of relying on standardized test scores and ability/achievement discrepancies that do not reflect how a student responds to various intervention and teaching strategies, RTI measures a student's response to intervention, then uses that data to develop an appropriate instructional or intervention process based on evidence-based teaching methodologies. It is important to note that IDEIA (2004) stipulated that schools can use up to 15 percent of their Part B funds to provide "additional academic and behavioral support" to students who do not meet the qualifications to receive special education or related services but who most likely will not succeed in the general education classroom.

> *think about it*
>
> Do you agree with the use of RTI as a means of measuring academic performance? Do you think RTI results in a delay in a child's receiving special education services? If so, is the delay justified by the RTI model's systematic evaluation of the student over time with regard to the child's ability to learn in the classroom setting?

SUMMARY

An understanding of the impact of language learning disabilities on academic, social, and vocational achievement is vital to helping children and adolescents with LLD. It is also important that teachers and health professionals working in the educational setting recognize the heterogeneity of learning disabilities and the necessity to treat each child or adolescent as being unique in how his or her learning disability is manifested. LLD is often first suspected in the kindergarten years when children have difficulty with the different aspects of phonological awareness when trying to learn to read and spell(discussed in Chapter 10). The early identification of children with LLD is critical so that appropriate interventions can be developed and implemented, thereby lessening the impact the LLD has on the child's progress in school.

Neuroimaging techniques have contributed to our understanding of brain morphology as it relates to LLDs and has had an impact on the diagnostic and therapeutic process. Because LLDs can have a lifelong impact, this understanding is assuming increasing importance in educational literature. With the focus in IDEA on transition, preparing individuals with LLDs for the work place further emphasizes the importance of studying the role of language in learning disabilities.

Learning disabilities are complex and pervasive in their effects on learning and socialization of school-age children and adolescents. Speech-language pathologists need to be sensitive to the special needs of these students and willing to engage in collaborative efforts with the classroom teachers to maximize the students' abilities to experience academic success through curricular modifications and the implementation of strategies to facilitate learning.

CASE STUDY

History

Chris, a 9-year-old boy, was referred to Mercy Hospital by his third-grade teacher for a psychological evaluation because of academic problems and hyperactivity. He was referred to our clinic a year later by his teacher and the speech-language pathologist at his school to address language and academic problems possibly related to his ADHD.

Previous Testing

Chris was evaluated at Mercy Hospital in three different departments: the Pediatric Neurology Clinic, the Department of Clinical Psychology, and the Department of communication disorders.

Chris was initially seen in the Pediatric Neurology Clinic because of his parents' and teacher's concerns about his short attention span and hyperactivity. They referred Chris to the Department of Clinical Psychology, where he was tested using the Weschler Intelligence Scale for Children—Revised (WISC-R). On the WISC-R, he received a full-scale IQ of 79, a verbal IQ of 87, and a performance IQ of 73. The department also noted that he had academic weaknesses in reading, spelling, and math. Reading and spelling were at the first-grade level, and math was at the second-grade level.

Chris also was evaluated in the Communication Disorders Department. The results were that he had (1) a moderately severe language disorder for skills such as sentence formulation and repetition, (2) poor problem-solving skills, (3) difficulties with auditory processing and auditory sequencing, (4) pragmatic problems, and (5) difficulties with topic maintenance and appropriate topic switching.

Following his evaluation in the Department of Communication Disorders, Chris returned to the Pediatric Neurology Clinic for a cumulative diagnosis. They determined that Chris had ADHD and prescribed 5 mg of Ritalin to be taken each morning.

At school, Chris is repeating the third grade, and he is pulled out for supplemental instruction in reading, writing, and math. He is not receiving speech-language therapy at school.

Initial Evaluation at the Speech, Language, and Reading Clinic (SLRC)

In their initial interview, Chris' parents reported that all developmental milestones were within normal limits and that his problems did not begin until he was in kindergarten. In kindergarten, he would hug and kiss the other children, and he was teased by his classmates until he would cry. In first grade, he had surgery for a "lazy eye" and began to wear corrective glasses. His parents agreed to the referral for a speech-language evaluation at SLRC because they were concerned about his low self-esteem and his frequent temper tantrums. They were also worried about the fact that he would not establish eye contact with them and that he always "forgets what he was told to do."

On the Revised Token Test, Chris scored within an average performance range. He had difficulty with two-step commands with two modifiers ("Touch the small blue circle and pick up the small green circle."). Results of the Wide Range Achievement Test—Revised (WRAT-R) indicated that Chris' reading was at the first-grade level. He would sound out the

(continues)

CASE STUDY *(continued)*

letters and sometimes read the same word twice. However, he would read the words differently on each try. He constantly asked for feedback about his correctness. Spelling results on the WRAT-R also were at the first-grade level. He would spell quickly, using some self-corrections.

Chris was also given the Illinois Test of Psycholinguistic Abilities—3 (ITPA-3). The ITPA-3 is a relatively short multimodality test (when compared to the Woodcock-Johnson Psychoeducational Battery), so it was used to assess Chris' cognitive skills and to compare performance when the input was auditory versus visual and output was graphic versus oral versus gestural. This testing revealed strengths in grammatic closure (which addresses morphology) and sound blending. His weaknesses were auditory closure, manual expression, and auditory association (analogies). It was extremely difficult keeping him on task.

Articulation was within normal limits based on observation. No formal testing was done in this area.

Behavioral observations included the following: (1) Chris frequently perseverated on one topic, making it difficult to shift from one subtest to another in testing and from one topic to another in conversation; (2) Chris needed structure, so the session was divided into periods of work time and periods of play time that were used as breaks; (3) Chris frequently interrupted the testing with tangential comments; and (4) Chris was in constant motion.

Summary and Recommendations

Chris is a 9-year, 11-month-old boy who was referred to this clinic for language and cognition testing due to concerns about academic performance in school, low self-esteem, and frequent temper tantrums. Chris has previously been diagnosed with ADHD at Mercy Hospital. He has been tested in the pediatric neurology, clinical psychology, and communicative disorders clinics at Mercy.

At SLRC, Chris was tested using the Revised Token Test, the Wide Range Achievement Test—Revised, and the Illinois Test of Psycholinguistic Abilities—3. Performance on the Revised Token Test was in the average range. On the WRAT-R, spelling and reading were at the first-grade level. The conclusions are that Chris has a language processing disorder complicated by his ADHD. A summary of his strengths and weaknesses is as follows.

	Strengths	Weaknesses
Communicative	Average intelligence	Poor eye contact
	Interactive	Poor pragmatic skills
	Can concoct stories	Tangential conversations
	Relates events	Poor reading skills
	Likes therapy	Poor spelling skills
	Good articulation	ADHD
		Poor topic maintenance
		Poor auditory processing skills

Noncommunicative	Supportive family	Socially frustrated
	Supportive teacher	Academically frustrated
	Determined to improve	Parents functionally illiterate
	Can delay gratification	Poor reasoning skills
		Poor math skills
		Temper
		Poor affect control
		Poor focal control
		Poor visual memory
		Poor sequencing skills
		Poor handwriting

It is recommended that Chris enroll in therapy to address auditory processing skills, pragmatics, auditory and visual memory skills, grapheme–phoneme association, following directions, and topic maintenance.

Addendum to Original Report

Further Testing. One year after enrolling in therapy, at age 10 years 9 months, Chris was given the Woodcock-Johnson Psychoeducational Battery. On the test of cognition, he received the following scores:

Assessment Area	Grade Score	Age Score	Percentile Rank
Full Scale Cluster	1.8	7–4	2
Verbal Ability Cluster	5.6	10–8	50
Reasoning Ability	1.0	3–10	Below 1
Perceptual Speech Cluster	3.0	8–4	9

On the tests of achievement, which measure academic performance, he performed as follows:

Cluster	Grade Score	Age Score	Percentile Rank	Functioning Level
Reading	2.3	7–6	4	Severely deficient
Mathematics	1.7	1–7	Below 1	Severely deficient
Written Language	1.8	1–8	2	Severely deficient
Knowledge	4.7	4–7	38	Average

(continues)

CASE STUDY (continued)

The clinicians were encouraged by Chris' improvement in reading and found it not surprising that Chris' knowledge was in the low average range. As is typical with many children with ADHD and language-based learning disabilities, Chris had relatively normal intelligence, but he had trouble in specific academic areas that required concentration and adequate attending to the task.

To address the deficits in reasoning, deduction puzzles were used to help Chris chart information as a story was read to him. These deduction puzzles were eventually incorporated into his classroom activities to help him organize his school notes. Work continued on all the original goals.

Behavior management included a token economy and response-cost system. Chris earned pennies for remaining in seat and on task, and pennies were removed from the jar when off-task behaviors occurred. He could exchange the pennies for X-Men comic books and action figures. His parents were also taught this system of behavior management and they followed through with it at home.

REVIEW QUESTIONS

1. At what grades do children make the leap from decoding to read to reading for comprehension?
   a. Kindergarten–2nd grade
   b. 3rd–4th grade
   c. 5th–6th grade

2. Children who present in the clinic with difficulty in organizing word meanings, underdeveloped lexical systems, and word retrieval problems are exhibiting a _____ deficit.
   a. Semantic
   b. Syntactic
   c. Pragmatic
   d. Morphological

3. Which of the following are considered soft signs that may be indicators of a language-based learning disability?
   a. Phonological Deficits
   b. Visual-motor deficits
   c. Letter and number reversals
   d. a, b, and c
   e. a and c

  f. b and c

  g. a and b

  h. a, b, and c

4. Children with SLI frequently have difficulties with math in the later elementary years because

  a. It takes more steps to perform the calculations.

  b. They have difficulty retrieving previously memorized material.

  c. They have problems with underlying mechanisms such as conceptual knowledge.

  d. All of the above.

  e. None of the above; children with SLI don't have trouble with math.

5. Which of the following are typically indicative of children with specific language impairment?

  a. Difficulty with bound morphemes

  b. Increased mean length of utterance due to tangential conversations

  c. Failure to combine words by 18–24 months of age

  d. All of the above

  e. Both a and b

  f. Both b and c

  g. Both a and c

6. Children typically outgrow language-based learning disabilities by the time they are adolescents.

  a. True

  b. False

7. At school age, delays may persist as disorders either because of the nature of the delay or because of ineffective remediation during the preschool years.

  a. True

  b. False

8. Children who have difficulties with reading, spelling, and conversational speech rarely have difficulties with writing narratives because this taps a different part of the brain.

  a. True

  b. False

9. Children with language-based learning disabilities frequently have poor conversational repair strategies.

  a. True

  b. False

10. Children with auditory processing disorders typically have normal pure-tone hearing thresholds.

    a. True

    b. False

REFERENCES

American Speech-Language-Hearing Association. (1991). *Learning disabilities: Issues on definition* [relevant paper]. Available from www.asha.org/policy.

American Speech-Language-Hearing Association (ASHA) Task Force on Central Auditory Processing Consensus Development. (1996, July). Central auditory processing: Current status of research and implications for clinical practice. *American Journal of Audiology, 5*(2), 41–54.

American Speech-Language-Hearing Association (ASHA) Working Group on Auditory Processing Disorders. (2005, February). (Central) auditory processing disorders. *ASHA Technical Report.*

Astington, J. W., & Olson, D. R. (1987, April). Literacy and schooling: Learning to talk about thought. Paper presented at the Annual meeting of the American Educational Research Association, Washington, D. C.

Berk, L. E. (2004). *Development through the lifespan* (3rd ed.). Boston: Allyn & Bacon.

Bishop, D. V. M., & Edmundson, A. (1987). Language-impaired 4-year olds: Distinguishing transient from persistent impairment. *Journal of Speech, Langauge, and Hearing Disorders, 52,* 156–173.

Bourassa, D. C., & Treiman, R. (2001, July). Spelling development and disability: The importance of linguistic factors. *Language, Speech, and Hearing Services in the Schools, 32*(3), 172–181.

Brinton, B., Fujiki, M., & Higbee, L. (1998). Participation in cooperative learning activities by children with specific language impairment. *Journal of Speech, Language, and Hearing Research, 41,* 1193–1206.

Brinton, B., Fujiki, M., Montague, E. C., & Hanton, J. L. (2000). Children with language impairment in cooperative work groups: A pilot study. *Language, Speech, and Hearing Services in Schools, 31,* 252–264.

Britt, R. R. (2009). 14 percent of United States adults can't read. *Live Science.* Retrieved May 6, 2010 from www.livescience.com/culture/090110-illiterateadults.html. Carlisle, J. F. (1987). The use of morphological knowledge in spelling derived forms by learning-disabled and normal students. *Annals of Dyslexia, 27,* 90–108.

Chall, J. (1983). *Stages of reading development.* New York: McGraw-Hill.

DeBonis, D. E., & Moncrief, D. (2008, Feb.). Auditory processing disorders: An update for speech-language pathologists. *American Journal of Speech-Language Pathology, 17,* 4–18.

Eckert, P. (1990). Cooperative competition in adolescent "girl talk." *Discourse Processes, 13,* 91–122.

Espin, C. A., Scierka, B. J., Skare, S., & Halverson, N. (1999). Curriculum-based measures in writing for secondary students. *Reading and Writing Quarterly, 15,* 5–27.

Fazio, B. (1996). Mathematical abilities of children with specific language impairment: A 2-year follow-up. *Journal of Speech and Hearing Research, 39,* 1–10.

Fazio, B. (1999). Arithmetic calculation, short-term memory, and language performance in children with specific language impairment. *Journal of Speech, Language, and Hearing Research, 42*(2), 420–431.

Fuchs, Fuchs, Compton, & Bryan (2005). Responsiveness to intervention: A new method of identifying students with disabilities (Powerpoint presentation). Council for Exceptional Children Annual Conference, April, 2005,

Fujiki, M., Brinton, B., & Clarke, D. (2002, April). Emotional regulation in children with specific language impairment. *Language, Speech, and Hearing Services in Schools, 33,* 102–111.

Gabig, C. (2009). Understanding the nature and scope of language learning disability: Characteristics, frameworks, and connections. In D. K. Bernstein & E. Tiegerman-Farber (Eds.). Language and communication disorders in children (6th ed.), pp. 207–245. Boston, MA: Pearson.

Gertner, B. L., Rice, M. L., & Hadley, P. A. (1994). Influence of communicative competence on peer preferences in a preschool classroom. *Journal of Speech and hearing Research, 37,* 913–923.

Gillam, R. B., Pena, E. D., & Miller, L. (1999). Dynamic assessment of narrative and expository discourse. *Topics in Language Disorders, 20*(1), 33–47.

Goffman, L., & Leonard, J. (2000, May). Growth of language skills in preschool children with specific language impairment: Implications for assessment and intervention. *American Journal of Speech-Language Pathology, 9*(2), 151–161.

Greenhalgh, K. S., & Strong, C. J. (2001). Literate language features in spoken narratives of children with typical language and children with language impairments. *Language, Speech, and Hearing Services in the Schools, 32,* 114–125.

Holston, J. T. (1992, February). *Assessment and management of auditory processing problems in children.* Paper presented at the Winter Conference of the Florida Speech-Language-Hearing Association, Gainesville, FL.

Hynd, G. (1991, March). Brain morphology as it relates to learning disabilities. Lecture at the 1991 G. Paul Moore Symposium, Gainesville, FL.

Johnson, C. J., Beitchman, J. H., Young, A., Escobar, M., Atkinson, L., Wilson, B., Brownlie, E. G., Douglas, L., Taback, N., Lan, I., & Want, M. (1999). Fourteen-year follow-up of children with and without speech/language impairments: Speech/ language stability and outcomes. *Journal of Speech, Language, and Hearing Research, 42*(3), 744–760.

Kamhi, A. B., & Catts, H. W. (1989). *Reading disabilities: A developmental language perspective.* Austin, TX: Pro-Ed.

Keith, R. W. (1999). Clinical issues in central auditory processing disorders. *Language, Speech, and Hearing Services in Schools, 30*(4), 339–344.

Klee, T. (1992). Developmental and diagnostic characteristics of quantitative measures of children's language production. *Topics in Language Disorders, 12*(2), 28–41.

Labov, W. (1972). *Language in the inner city.* Philadelphia: University of Pennsylvania Press.

Larson, V. L., & McKinley, N. (1987). *Communication assessment and intervention strategies for adolescents.* Eau Claire, WI: Thinking Publications.

Larson, V. L., & McKinley, N. (1995). *Language disorders in older students: Preadolescents and adolescents.* Eau Claire, WI: Thinking Publications.

Leonard, C. M. (1998). Language. Chapter 17 in H. Cohen (ed.), *Neuroscience for rehabilitation* (2nd ed.). Philadelphia: Lippincott-Raven.

Leonard, L. B. (1987). Is specific language impairment a useful construct? In S. Rosenberg (ed.), *Advances in applied psycholinguistics,* Vol. 1 (pp. 1–39). Cambridge, UK: Cambridge University Press.

Loban, W. (1976). *Language development: Kindergarten through grade twelve* (Research report No. 18). Urbana, IL: National Council for Teachers of English.

Lombardino, L. J., Ricco, C. A., Hynd, G., & Pinheiro, S. B. (1997). Linguistic deficits in children with reading disabilities. *American Journal of Speech-Language Pathology, 6*(3), 71–78.

Lyon, R. (1995). Toward a definition of dyslexia. *Annals of Dyslexia, 45,* 3–30.

McCabe, A., Bliss, L., Barra, G., & Bennett, M. (2008, May). Comparison of personal versus fictional narratives of children with language impairment. *American Journal of Speech-Language Pathology, 17,* 194–206.

Mercer, S. P., & Miller, S. P. (1992). Teaching students with learning problems in math to acquire, understand, and apply basic math facts. *Remedial and Special Education, 13,* 19–35, 61.

National Institute for Neurological Diseases and Stroke (NINDS). (2010, May 12). *NINDS learning disabilities information page.* Retrieved Jun 12, 2010 from www.ninds.nih.gov/disorders/learningdisabilities/learningdisabilities.htm.

National Institute for Literacy (n.d.). *Literacy in the United States.* Retrieved May 6, 2010 from www.policyalmanac.org/education/archives/literacy.shtml.

National Joint Committee on Learning Disabilities (NJCLD). (1991). Learning disabilities: Issues on definition [position paper]. *ASHA, 33*(Suppl. 5), 18–20.

National Joint Committee on Learning Disabilities (NJCLD). (2005). *Responsiveness to intervention and learning disabilities.* Retrieved May 10, 2010 from www.ldonline.org/educators.

Nelson, N. W. (1993). *Childhood language disorders in context: Infancy through adolescence.* New York: Merrill/Macmillan Publishing Company.

Nelson, N. W. (1994). School-age language: Bumpy road or super-expressway to the next millennium? *American Journal of Speech-Language Pathology, 3*(3), 29–31.

Neuman, S. B. (2008*). Educating the other America: Top experts tackle poverty, literacy, and achievement in our schools.* Baltimore, MD: Paul H. Brookes Publishing Company.

Nippold, M. A. (1988). The literate lexicon. In M. A. Nippold (ed.), *Later language development* (pp. 29-47). Austin TX: Pro-Ed.

Nippold, M. A. (1993, January). Developmental markers in adolescent language: Syntax, semantics, and pragmatics. *Language, Speech, and Hearing Services in the Schools, 24,* 21–28.

Nippold, M. A., & Martin, S. T. (1989). Idiom interpretation in isolation vs. context: A developmental study with adolescents. *Journal of Speech and Hearing Research, 32,* 59–66.

Nippold, M. A., Schwarz, I. E., & Undlin, R. A. (1992). Use and understanding of adverbial conjuncts: A developmental study of adolescents and young adults. *Journal of Speech and Hearing Research, 35,* 108–118.

Owens, R. E. (2004). *Language disorders: A functional approach to assessment and intervention* (4th ed.). Boston: Allyn and Bacon.

Parker, R., Tindal, G., & Hasbrouck, J. (1991). Countable indices of writing quality: Their suitability for screening-eligibility decisions. *Exceptionality, 2,* 1–17.

Paul, R. (1995). *Language disorders from infancy through adolescence: Assessment and intervention.* St, Louis, MO: Mosby.

Paul, R. (1996). Clinical implications of the natural history of slow expressive language development. *American Journal of Speech-Language Pathology, 5*(2), 5–22.

Paul, R. (2001). *Language disorders from infancy through adolescence: Assessment and intervention* (2nd ed.). St, Louis, MO: Mosby.

Peck, M. (1982). Youth suicide. *Death Education, 6,* 29–47.

Polakow, V. (1993*). Lives on the edge: Single mothers and their children in the other America.* Chicago: University of Chicago Press.

Reed, V. A. (2005). *An introduction to children with language disorders* (3rd ed.). Boston: Allyn and Bacon.

Rescorla, L. (1989). The language development survey: A screening tool for delayed language in toddlers. *Journal of Speech and Hearing Disorders, 54,* 587–599.

Rescorla, L. (1990, June). Outcomes of expressive language delay. Paper presented at the Symposium for Research in Child Language Disorders, Madison, WI.

Rescorla, L., Roberts, J., & Dahlsgaard, K. (1997). Late talkers at 2: Outcome at age 3. *Journal of Speech and Hearing Research, 40,* 556–566.

Rice, M. L., Sell, M. A., & Hadley, P. A. (1991). Social interactions of speech- and language-impaired children. *Journal of Speech and Hearing Research, 34,* 1299–1307.

Rossetti, L.M. (1996). *Communication intervention: Birth to three.* Clifton Park, NY: Delmar, Cengage Learning.

Roth, F. & Spekman, N. (1984a, February). Assessing the pragmatic abilities of children; Part 1: Organizational framework and assessment parameters. *Journal of Speech and Hearing Disorders, 49,* 12–17.

Roth, F., & Spekman, N. (1984b, February). Assessing the pragmatic abilities of children; Part 2: Guidelines, considerations, and specific evaluation procedures. *Journal of Speech and Hearing Disorders, 49,* 12–17.

Schow, R. L., & Nervonne, M. A. (1996). *Introduction to audiologic rehabilitation.* Needham Heights, MA: Simon & Schuster.

Scott, C. M. (1991). Problem writers: Nature, assessment, and intervention. In A. G. Kamhi & H. W. Catts (eds.), *Reading disabilities: A developmental language perspective* (pp. 303–344). Boston: Allyn and Bacon.

Scott, C. M., & Windsor, J. (2000). General language performance measures in spoken and written narrative and expository discourse of school-age children with language learning disabilities. *Journal of Speech, Language, and Hearing Research, 43,* 324–339.

Shames, G. H., Wiig, E. H., & Secord, W. A. (1994). *Human communication disorders: An introduction* (4th ed.). New York: Merrill/Macmillan Publishing Company.

Stockman, I. (1996). Phonological development and disorders in African American children, In A. Kambi, K. Pollock, and J. Harris (eds.), *Communication Development and Disorders in African American Children* (pp. 117–154). Baltimore, MD: Brookes.

Stothard, S. E., Snowling, M. J., Bishop, D. V. M., Chipchase, B. B., & Kaplan, C. A. (1998). Language-impaired preschoolers: A follow-up into adolescence. *Journal of Speech, Language, and Hearing Research, 41*(2), 407–418.

Thal, D. J. (1989). *Language and gestures in late talkers*. Paper presented at the Biennial Meeting of the Society for Research in Child Development, Kansas City, MO.

Tiegerman-Farber, E. (1997). The ecology of the family: The language imperative. In D. K. Bernstein and E. Tiegerman-Farber (eds.), *Language and communication disorders in children* (pp. 60–96). Boston: Allyn and Bacon.

Tomblin, J. B., Records, N. L., Buckwalter, P., Zhang, X., Smith, E., & O'Brien, M. (1997). Prevalence of specific language impairment in kindergarten children. *Journal of Speech, Language, and Hearing Research, 40,* 1245–1260.

Torgesen, J. (1977). The role of nonspecific factors in the task performance of learning disabled children: A theoretical assessment. *Journal of Learning Disabilities, 10,* 24–34.

Torgesen, J., Wagner, R., & Rashotte, C. (1994). Longitudinal studies of phonological processing and reading. *Journal of Learning Disabilities, 27,* 276–286.

Treiman, R. (1997). Spelling in normal children and dyslexics. In B. Blachman (ed.), *Foundations of reading acquisition and dyslexia* (pp. 191–218). Mahwah, NJ: Lawrence Erlbaum.

United States Office of Education (USOE). (1991). *Thirteenth annual report to Congress on the implementation of the Individuals with Disabilities Act*. Washington, DC: Government Printing Office.

van Keulen, J. E., Weddington, G. T., & DeBose, C. E. (1998). *Speech, language, learning, and the African American child*. Boston: Allyn & Bacon.

Van Oers, B. (1998). The fallacy of decontextualization. *Mind, Culture, and Activity, 5,* 135–142.

Wallach, G. P., & Butler, K. G. (1994*). Language learning disabilities in school-age children and adolescents: Some principles and applications*. New York: Macmillan.

Watkinson, J. T., & Lee, S. W. (1992). Curriculum-based measures of written expression for learning-disabled and nondisabled students. *Psychology in the Schools, 29,* 184–191.

Westby, C. E. (1984). Development of narrative language abilities. In G. Wallach and K. Butler (Eds.), *Language learning disabilities in school-age children* (pp. 103–127). Baltimore, MD: Williams & Wilkins.

Westby, C. E. (1991). Learning to talk—talking to learn: Oral-literate language differences. In C. Simon (ed.), *Communication skills and classroom success: Assessment and therapy methodologies for language and learning disabled students,* (rev. ed., pp. 181–218). San Diego, CA: College-Hill.

Westby, C. E. (1999). Assessing and facilitating text comprehension problems. In H. Catts and A. Kahmi (Eds.), *Language and reading disabilities* (pp. 259–324). Boston, MA: Allyn & Bacon.

Wiig, E. H. & Semel, E. (1984). *Language assessment and intervention for the learning disabled* (2nd ed.). New York: Merrill.

Young, M. (1985). Central auditory processing through the looking glass: A critical look at diagnosis and management, *Journal of Childhood Communication Disorders, 9,* 31–42.

APPENDIX 9A

Organizations That Can Provide Information About and Support for Individuals with Learning Disabilities

CHADD—Children and Adults with Attention-Deficit/Hyperactivity Disorder
8181 Professional Place
Suite 150
Landover, MD 20785
www.chadd.org
Tel: 301-306-7070 800-233-4050
Fax: 301-306-7090

International Dyslexia Association
40 York Road
4th Floor
Baltimore, MD 21204
info@interdys.org
www.interdys.org
Tel: 410-296-0232 800-ABCD123
Fax: 410-321-5069

Learning Disabilities Association of America
4156 Library Road
Suite 1
Pittsburgh, PA 15234-1349
info@ldaamerica.org
http://www.ldaamerica.org
Tel: 412-341-1515
Fax: 412-344-0224

National Center for Learning Disabilities
381 Park Avenue South
Suite 1401
New York, NY 10016
ncld@ncld.org
http://www.ld.org
Tel: 212-545-7510 888-575-7373
Fax: 212-545-9665

(continues)

APPENDIX 9A *(continued)*

National Institute of Child Health and Human Development (NICHD)
National Institutes of Health, DHHS
31 Center Drive, Rm. 2A32 MSC 2425
Bethesda, MD 20892-2425
http://www.nichd.nih.gov
Tel: 301-496-5133
Fax: 301-496-7101

National Institute of Mental Health (NIMH)
National Institutes of Health, DHHS
6001 Executive Blvd. Rm. 8184, MSC 9663
Bethesda, MD 20892-9663
nimhinfo@nih.gov
http://www.nimh.nih.gov
Tel: 301-443-4513/866-415-8051 301-443-8431 (TTY)
Fax: 301-443-4279

Chapter 10

Spelling and Reading Disorders

LEARNING OBJECTIVES

After completion of this chapter, the reader will be able to:

1. Discuss acquisition and skills that determine the development of normal reading.

2. Delineate and discuss the components and importance of the emergent literacy period.

3. Discuss early indicators of reading disability and problem areas for readers identified as having a reading and/or spelling disability.

4. Discuss the roles of genetics and the central nervous system as causative factors in dyslexia.

5. Delineate the criteria for being diagnosed with a reading impairment, and discuss assessment strategies for reading disabilities.

6. Discuss how cultural diversity affects the diagnosis of a reading and/or spelling disability.

7. Differentiate between the different approaches to remediation of reading and/or spelling deficits.

INTRODUCTION

The majority of people learn to read relatively effortlessly and therefore take the skill for granted. However, 15 to 20 percent of the population of the United States has been diagnosed with a reading disorder. It is estimated that 13 to 14 percent of the school-age population nationwide needs special education services due to a handicap. Of those students, 50 percent have a learning disability. Of those students who have a learning disability, 85 percent have learning disabilities in reading and/or language processing (International Dyslexia Association, 2008). With growing understanding of the roles of phonological awareness and phonological processing in reading, the speech-language pathologist is becoming increasingly involved in the diagnosis and remediation of reading disorders. It is becoming a focus of more and more articles in the journals of the American Speech-Language-Hearing Association (ASHA), as well as the focus of many continuing education programs and conference presentations. Hence, it is fitting to include a chapter dedicated to normal and disordered reading in a book about language disorders.

NORMAL READING

Reading disability is the most prevalent learning disability, accounting for 75 to 80 percent of all learning disabilities (Livesay, 1995). Reading has phonetic, semantic, syntactic, and memory components, all of which must be integrated if a person is to be a successful reader. Therefore, to determine a child's status with regard to reading, it is necessary to assess his or her visual and auditory modalities to determine if there is a problem and, if so, where the problem lies. Using the auditory channel, an emphasis should be placed on phonics, phonetics, and linguistic information. The child must be able to decode letters to form an accurate phonological image of each word and then retrieve the definition of each word from memory. He or she must then combine syntactic and semantic information from the definitions into proper representation of a sentence. Finally, the child must combine the representations of individual sentences to comprehend the passage.

These skills are all taught in the first 3 years of elementary school, with the expectation that the child will integrate the knowledge and be a successful reader by third grade (see Figure 10–1). In kindergarten through second grade, the emphasis is on the integration of thinking and organization of sensory input and on preoperational skills. Preoperational skills typically develop between ages 2 and 7 and represent the child's emergence into conceptual development. In the third and fourth grades, the emphasis shifts to requiring a child to exercise his or her linguistic and symbolic language skills.

The content of all subject areas requires the child to abstract, analyze, and synthesize the information, with the expectation that the child can read for content and no longer needs to focus on decoding each word because word recognition and understanding have become internalized operations. Furthermore, the child is faced with a higher level of vocabulary, more complex sentence structure, and more abstract concepts.

Chall (1983) summed up this academic progression in reading by dividing the development of reading into six stages (Table 10–1). At Chall's stage 0, children learn to produce syntactically correct utterances and develop early metalinguistic skills that enable them to understand that words are made up of

> **Preoperational skills.** Skills needed to emerge into conceptual thinking and leading to prelogical thought.

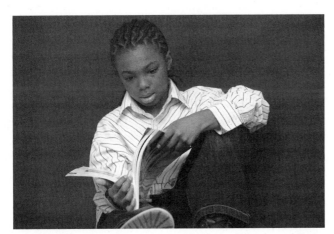

FIGURE 10–1   Children should be encouraged to engage in reading not only to gain knowledge but to enjoy reading as a daily activity. (*Delmar/Cengage Learning*)

TABLE 10–1 Stages of reading

Stage	Ages	Primary Development
0	Birth to 5–6 years	Accumulation of knowledge about letters, words, and books
1	5–7 years	Initial reading or decoding
2	7–9 years	Decoding becomes more automatic; beginning of reading for comprehension
3	9–14 years	Reading to learn; decoding skills become fully automatic
4	14–18 years	Multiple viewpoints due to increased cognitive skills, which enable abstract thinking
5	18+ years	Construction and reconstruction in critical reading; development of hypothetical-deductive reasoning

Source: Adapted from *Stages of reading development,* by J. Chall. New York: McGraw-Hill. Copyright 1983 by McGraw-Hill.

Phoneme–grapheme correspondence. The association of a printed letter with the sound it makes.

Scripts. Scenarios designed to facilitate language development and the application of language skills to reading.

letters and language is made up of words. They also learn that words go together to create phrases and sentences. At this point, the children do not understand letter order and phoneme–grapheme correspondences, meaning they cannot make the link between the printed letter and the sound it makes. However, they do show interest in initial sounds and word shapes.

In stage 1, the focus is on learning about phoneme–grapheme correspondences and learning to decode words. During stage 2, decoding becomes more automatic so children can begin to focus on meaning. They also use their knowledge of scripts and story structure to assist in reading for meaning as they develop reading fluency. Decoding skills become fully automatic by stage 3, and from that point typically developing readers advance in the complexity of the material read and focus on using reading as a means of gaining knowledge. As Chall (1983) wrote, they become critical readers.

In 1973, K. S. Goodman suggested that miscue analysis is a method typical readers use to analyze errors they make when reading aloud. Goodman suggests that nondisabled, mature readers implement three types of cues to predict the meaning of the text: semantic, syntactic, and graphophonemic. Nelson (1998) wrote the following:

> Because mature readers have considerable knowledge about language, they continually form hypotheses as they read about what they expect the texts to say. First, they use semantic cues to predict words that fit textual meaning; second, they use syntactic cues to predict words that fit syntactic contexts; and third, they use graphophonemic cues to check whether the words they have predicted fit visual perceptual information sampled from the print. (p. 409)

EARLY INDICATORS OF READING AND SPELLING DISABILITIES

In a longitudinal study by Catts and colleagues (2001), the researchers developed a model for implementation that would enhance our ability to identify kindergarten children at risk for reading difficulties. They cited several authors in writing that, "Under the most optimal conditions, at-risk children would be identified during the preschool years. Once the children are identified, home literacy programs and preschool experiences could be developed to meet these children's literacy needs" (p. 46). Furthermore, we need to identify predictive factors for reading problems other than their likely being due to other language and/or developmental disabilities or family history of reading deficits. Catts and colleagues recommended that all children with a history of speech and/or language impairments should be screened as soon as possible after starting kindergarten to determine which children have behaviors that, especially when paired with their mother's level of education, are predictive of future reading difficulties in second grade. Children who do not have a history of speech and/or language problems but who show risk factors, such as those outlined previously, should be referred by their teacher for screening. The performance of the child when screened on the factors proposed by Catts and colleagues would be analyzed to determine the probability that the child would have future reading deficits. They recommended that a 30 percent probability of having reading problems serve as the cut-off score for determining the need for further comprehensive assessment of language and phonological awareness. The factors that Catts and colleagues found to be most predictive were letter identification, sentence imitation, mother's education, deletion, and rapid automatized naming.

Shaywitz (2003) made the point that clues that may indicate a potential reading problem for a child can often be determined by listening to the child speak. Children who are late in saying their first words (i.e., after 15 months of age) and who do not combine words until after 24 months of age may be exhibiting warning signs of a potential reading problem. This does not occur in all children with reading disabilities, but it warrants attention, particularly if there is a history of reading problems in the family. Another early indicator is the persistence of difficulty pronouncing words beyond the normal period of "baby talk." As a rule, children are able to pronounce most words by age 6 years. Typically developing children may mispronounce new words as their vocabulary expands, but these mispronunciations are easily overcome as the child increases his or her awareness and understanding of the word. In addition, around ages 3 to 4 years, most children delight in rhyming verses and repetitions of sounds, but children with reading problems

> have trouble penetrating the sound structure of words and as a result are less sensitive to rhyme. Sensitivity to rhyme implies an awareness that words can be broken down into smaller segments of sound and that different words may share a sound in common; it is

a very early indicator of getting ready to read. Children's familiarity with nursery rhymes turns out to be a strong predictor of their later success in reading. (Shaywitz, 2003, p. 95)

PROBLEM AREAS FOR READERS IN TROUBLE

According to Wiig and Semel (1984), readers in trouble experience difficulty with the skills outlined in Table 10–2.

Children who experience reading difficulties frequently have trouble encoding the information, retrieving it from memory, and using phonological memory codes to decode the words (Catts & Kamhi, 2005). It is also important to analyze the child's visual and auditory skills because successful reading requires a high level of integration of both sets of skills. The integration of these skills is critical for the child to associate written language with underlying meanings and structures.

Children who exhibit deficits in reading often have difficulties with oral language and impoverished environments. Justice and colleagues (2003) have summed up relevant literature and state that preschool children who have oral language impairments "consistently show depressed performance relative to their peers on an array of emergent literacy tasks addressing both written language and phonological awareness" (p. 321). In 1990, Scarborough found that many second-grade children who were having reading problems also had significant problems in developing oral language

TABLE 10–2 Trouble areas for poor readers

Visually decoding the printed, graphic words

Integrating auditory-visual inputs

Associating printed words, phrases, concepts, and other relations with their underlying meaning

Processing the surface structure of the printed sentences and relating it to the underlying meaning

Diffculty integrating graphophonemic, syntactic, and semantic information

Generating a tentative, anticipatory hypothesis about subsequent printed messages

Verifying, rejecting, or revising the anticipatory hypothesis with reference to the actual printed, graphic representation

Trouble with developmental sensitivity to grammar in written language

Source: *Language assessment and intervention for the learning disabled*, by E. H. Wiig and E. M. Semel. Boston. Copyright © 1980 by Pearson Education. Reprinted with permission.

skills. In a 1999 study with 183 children who were classified as poor readers, Catts and colleagues found that 57 percent had receptive language difficulties as kindergartners, including problems with narrative comprehension, vocabulary, and understanding of grammar.

A major problem area for many poor readers is grammar. Children with difficulty in reading have problems correcting incorrect grammar. Regular and irregular morphemes are particularly problematic for these children. It is also known that poor readers typically have poor short-term memory for various sentence structures, which increases the problems they have because they have difficulty processing complex sentences.

Gough and Tunmer (1986) proposed a reading theory called the Simple View of Reading. There is tremendous variance in children with reading disorders, and the simple view posited that listening comprehension and word recognition can be used to explain this variance. The researchers developed a matrix that created four subgroups of reading disabilities based on listening comprehension and word recognition. This matrix is seen in Figure 10–2. The individuals who have good listening comprehension but poor word recognition are defined as being dyslexic. Those who have poor listening comprehension and poor word recognition are listed as being language-learning disabled. Poor listening comprehension and good word recognition skills define the group labeled as **hyperlexic**. Hyperlexia is frequently seen in children with autism and is often accompanied by pragmatic disorders. In an effort to define this unusual reading disorder without having it routinely associated with autism, Catts and Kamhi (2005) proposed the term *specific comprehension deficit*.

Hyperlexic. Recognizing and reading words exceeding one's cognitive and language levels, yet having little or no comprehension of what is said or read.

Finally, there is an "other" category in which word recognition and listening comprehension are good, but subtle language-based disabilities exist. The individuals in the dyslexic, hyperlexic, and language-learning disabled groups all have problems with reading comprehension, but for

Listening Comprehension	Word Recognition: Poor	Word Recognition: Good
Good	Dyslexia	Non-specified
Poor	Mixed	Specific Comprehension Deficit

FIGURE 10–2 Subtypes based on word recognition and listening comprehension. (*Source:* Catts & Kamhi, *Language and reading disabilities,* by A. G. Kamhi and H. W. Catts, Figure 4.1, "Subtypes of word recognition and listening comprehension," p. 74. © 2005. Reproduced by permission of Pearson Education, Inc.)

different reasons. The children with hyperlexia have difficulty because they have language and cognitive deficits. The children with reading and spelling difficulties have difficulty because they have poor decoding skills, often being slow and/or inaccurate in their decoding (Catts & Kamhi, 2005).

Catts and Kamhi (2005) further differentiated between subtypes of reading impairment by determining whether the individuals were rate-disabled or accuracy-disabled readers. Rate-disabled readers were defined as children who, despite having decoding skills at grade-appropriate levels, still had markedly poor reading. Accuracy-disabled readers were defined as those children who had significant deficits in decoding accuracy. In order for a child to be classified as accuracy disabled, he or she had to score at least 18 months "below grade level expectations on at least four of five different measures of word recognition" (Catts & Kamhi, 2005, p. 85). To be labeled as rate-disabled, the children "had to perform close to, at, or above grade level on four or more measures of word recognition and at least one and half years below grade-level on four of five measures of reading speed" (Catts & Kamhi, 2005, p. 85). A graphic representation of subtypes of reading disabilities is found in Figure 10–3.

In a study done to validate these subgroups, Lovett (1987) administered oral and written language tests to 96 children. There were 32 children in each of three categories: accuracy disabled, rate disabled, and typical.

Subtype	Listening Comprehension	Word Recognition
Dyslexia	Good	Phonological
		Surface
		Rate Disabled
Mixed	Poor	Phonological
		Surface
		Rate Disabled
Specific Comprehension Deficit	Poor	Good

FIGURE 10–3 Subtypes of reading disabilities. (*Source: Language and reading disabilities,* by A. G. Kamhi and H. W. Catts, Figure 4.2, "Subtypes of reading disabilities," p. 87. © 2005. Reproduced by permission of Pearson Education, Inc.)

The subjects were matched for sex, IQ, and chronological age. The results of the testing were as follows:

1. For children who were accuracy disabled, errors made while reading non-words reflected basic deficits in sound–letter correspondence rules.

2. Accuracy-disabled students had deficits in syntactic and morphological knowledge in their oral language skills.

3. In analyzing individual speech sounds, the accuracy-disabled students were significantly slower than were the rate-disabled students.

4. In naming serial-letter arrays, the accuracy-disabled students were significantly slower than were the rate-disabled students;

5. There were no differences in identifying regular and exception words (phonetic decoding and sight words) between the rate-disabled and the typical readers.

6. The rate-disabled students had significant deficits in word recognition speed, particularly in connected text.

7. The rate-disabled students were similar to the typical children with regard to oral language skills, but on tasks designed to measure rapid automatic naming, the rate-disabled students were significantly slower than the typical children.

DYSLEXIA

Originally referred to over 65 years ago as "congenital word blindness," dyslexia is a developmental reading disorder. Hynd (1991) defined dyslexia as a definable and diagnosable form of primary reading retardation with some form of central nervous system dysfunction. There is evidence that dyslexia runs in families (Leonard, 1998; Owens, 2004). Children with dyslexia have unexpected reading failures that often are accompanied by tendencies toward atypical spelling and handwriting. In addition, evidence exists to support the concept that the difficulties with phonologic awareness originate in "the phonologic component of the larger specialization for language" (Shaywitz et al., 1998).

The International Dyslexia Association (2002) defined dyslexia as follows:

> Dyslexia is a specific learning disability that is neurological in origin. It is characterized by difficulties with accurate and/or fluent word recognition and by poor spelling and decoding abilities. These difficulties typically result from a deficit in the phonological component of language that is often unexpected in relation

Dyslexia. Difficulty learning to read, often due to a neurological deficit.

to other cognitive abilities and the provision of effective classroom instruction. Secondary consequences may include problems in reading comprehension and reduced reading experience that can impede the growth of vocabulary and background knowledge.

This definition is also used by the National Institute of Child Health and Human Development (NICHD).

As outlined in Table 10–3, the American Psychiatric Association's *Diagnostic and Statistical Manual-IV* (1994) lists very specific criteria for the diagnosis of a reading disorder.

The International Classification of Diseases—10 criteria for the diagnosis of a specific reading disorder—are outlined in Table 10–4 (Lyon, 1995). With regard to the IQ discrepancy in the ICD-10 codes, questions have been raised as to whether or not IQ–reading discrepancies are a valid measure to determine the presence of dyslexia (Siegel, 1992; Stanovich, 1991). Historically, a discrepancy between IQ scores on neuropsychological tests and reading achievement scores on reading tasks has been used to determine or confirm the presence of dyslexia. However, this discrepancy is now seen as an inappropriate and invalid marker. Recent research studies do not support the use of a discrepancy-based definition of developmental dyslexia. In fact, when looking at the population of children with reading impairments minimal differences are observed between children with reading disabilities who meet discrepancy criteria and reading-disabled children who do not show a wide IQ–reading achievement gap (often referred to as "garden variety" poor readers). Measures of phonological awareness provide the most robust difference in performance between typical and impaired readers, making phonological awareness, not IQ-reading discrepancies, a better tool for diagnosing reading problems such as dyslexia.

TABLE 10–3   Characteristics of dyslexia as outlined in the *Diagnostic and Statistical Manual-IV-Revision (DSM-IV-R)*

A.   Reading achievement, as measured by individually administered standardized tests of reading accuracy or comprehension, is substantially below that expected given the person's chronological age, measured intelligence, and age-appropriate education.

B.   The disturbance in Criterion A significantly interferes with academic achievement or activities of daily living that require reading skills.

C.   If a sensory deficit is present, the reading difficulties are in excess of those usually associated with it.

Source: Reprinted from "Toward a Definition of Dyslexia," *Annals of Dyslexia,* 45 (1995) by R. Lyon with permission of the International Dyslexia Association.

TABLE 10–4   International Classification of Diseases (ICD-10; 1993) diagnostic criteria for the diagnosis of specific reading disorder

A.   Either of the following must be present:

(1)   a score on reading accuracy and/or comprehension that is at least 2 standard errors of prediction below the level expected on the basis of the child's chronological age and general intelligence, with both reading skills and IQ assessed on an individually administered test standardized for the child's culture and educational system;

(2)   a history of serious reading difficulties, or test scores that met criterion A(1) at an earlier age, plus a score on a spelling test that is at least 2 standard errors of prediction below the level expected on the basis of the child's chronological age and IQ.

B.   The disturbance described in Criterion A significantly interferes with academic achievement or with activities of daily living that require reading skills.

C.   The disorder is not the direct result of a defect in visual or hearing acuity or of a neurological disorder.

D.   School experiences are within the average expectable range (i.e., there have been no extreme inadequacies in educational experiences).

E.   Most commonly used exclusion clause: IQ is below 70 on an individual administered standardized test.

Source: Reprinted from "Toward a Definition of Dyslexia," *Annals of Dyslexia*, 45 (1995) by R. Lyon with permission of the International Dyslexia Association.

CONTRIBUTORY AND ETIOLOGICAL FACTORS IN READING DISABILITIES

Catts and Kamhi (2005) explored the causes of reading disabilities and divided the various factors into extrinsic and intrinsic causes. Extrinsic factors that contribute to reading and spelling problems included lack of exposure to the printed word, lack of instruction as to how print works, and lack of opportunity to practice reading skills. It should be noted that these extrinsic factors are not included in the definition of reading disabilities, but they deserve further attention in the literature because they may contribute to the presence of reading disabilities.

Extrinsic causes. Factors in the environment of the child that interfere with development.

Intrinsic causes. Factors within the child, such as neurological damage, that interfere with development.

Extrinsic Factors

There is increased awareness of the role of poverty as a complicating factor in reading and spelling deficits. One is always hesitant to introduce such a factor at the risk of having others overgeneralize this impact. Many families who are faced with issues related to low SES still manage to provide a stimulating environment and produce students who keep up with and/or surpass their classmates. However, there is enough evidence to recognize poverty's role in academic underachievement, and oftentimes this underachievement can be directly related to reading difficulties. Hart and Risley (1999) found that children from lower-income families do not talk about stories they have read or had read to them. They tend to focus their conversations on basic needs of daily living. Discussions that extend "beyond practical concerns" (Nelson, 2010, p. 113) are rare in children from homes of low SES. Part of this may stem from a scarcity of books in the home. Another part may be due to the decreased participation of many children from lower-SES situations in a variety of activities, both through local involvement (i.e., sports, theater, concerts) and through a variety of travels (i.e., going to Washington, D.C.). Another factor could be that the child is reflecting the focus of the discussions of the adults around him or her.

That being said, children from any home in which they are not read to in an interactive manner from an early age are at increased risk for reading and spelling disorders, regardless of SES. The acquisition of knowledge of printed words and skills such as understanding the association of words with events, developing anticipatory hypotheses, sequencing, and phonological awareness are all facilitated by being read to by one's caregivers.

Exposure to books is not the only potential difference between lower-SES homes and others. Hart and Risley (1995) studied the frequency of language-based interactions between parents and children in homes where the parents were professionals, homes that were working class, and low-income homes. The procedure was the recording of the parent–child interactions one day a month for 2 years and 5 months. The results are shown in Table 10–5.

Hart and Risley (1999) concluded with the following statement: "No matter what the family SES, the more time parents spent talking with their child from day to day, the more rapidly the child's vocabulary was likely to be growing and the higher the child's score on an IQ test was likely to be at age 3" (p. 3).

TABLE 10–5 Income level and average number of words

Income Level	Average Number of Words per Hour
Professional Homes	2,100
Working-Class Homes (Average)	1,500
Low-Income Homes	600

Source: Adapted from *The social world of children learning to talk* by B. Hart and T. R. Risley. Copyright 1999 by Paul H. Brookes.

Intrinsic Factors

There is an apparent inherited basis for reading disabilities, which are often seen in siblings and throughout generations of a family. Catts and Kamhi (2005) summed up the extensive research in this area by noting that 30 to 40 percent of parents of a child with reading disabilities also have a history of reading deficits, and that the sibling of a child with reading disabilities has about a 40 percent chance of having a reading problem as well. Twin studies have been done to solidify the argument that reading disabilities have a genetic basis. Light and DeFries (1995) studied identical and fraternal twins and documented the existence of reading disabilities in each set. Among the fraternal twins, when one twin had a reading disability, 40 percent of the other twins also had a reading disability. Among identical twins, when one twin had a reading problem, 68 percent of the twin partners also had a reading disability. It is believed that other factors contribute to the development of reading because these figures are not 100 percent. It is apparent that one can carry the gene for reading disabilities but not develop the disorder, although the chances are increased. Further research on which chromosomes carry the gene for reading disabilities is ongoing. Shaywitz (2003) expressed the belief that reading is such a complex process that no single dominant gene results in dyslexia. Early indicators show that sites on chromosomes 6 and 15 are the most likely areas associated with reading ability (Catts & Kamhi, 2005).

Three parts of the brain are instrumental in recognition of written words:

> The three areas include a left inferior frontal system (Broca's area) for analyzing words into phonologic segments for rhyming, reading, speaking, or spelling; a parieto-temporal system for analyzing the auditory components of words and connecting them to their meanings; and an occipitotemporal system that predominates 'when a reader has become skilled, and has bound together as a unit the orthographic, phonologic, and semantic features of the word' (Lyon et al., 2003, p. 5) (Nelson, 2010, p. 77)

Based on neurological studies pinpointing active areas of the brain when one reads, support is available for the role of intrinsic factors in reading disabilities. Early studies indicated that there may be an issue with hemispheric dominance for language, with individuals who have reading disabilities having mixed dominance or right-hemisphere dominance for language. This has led some to believe that left-handedness may be a marker for reading disabilities. However, there is no consistency in the literature in associating reading disabilities and handedness (Catts & Kamhi, 2005).

Much of the literature on reading supports the belief that brain abnormalities observed in people with dyslexia are an atypicality of development, just as if one extremity were larger than the other. That is to say, brain

Subcortical pathways. Interconnections in the brain that lie below the cerebral cortex.

Fissure. A deep furrow in the brain; also known as a sulcus.

Gyrus. A rounded elevation in the cerebral hemispheres.

abnormalities are structural, not physiological, anomalies. It is most likely that the central nervous system deficits are in the left temporal lobe, the right frontal lobe, and/or in the subcortical pathways that connect the left and right hemispheres (Riccio & Hynd, 1996; Owens, 2004). Leonard and colleagues (1993) used MRI studies and found that family members of individuals with dyslexia demonstrated atypical anatomical findings.

These findings included a shift of parietal tissue to the right plenum temporale, a long Sylvian fissure (a furrow within the brain) in the left hemisphere, an extra supramarginal gyrus (an elevated, rounded area in the brain), and multiple Heschl's gyri in the left and right hemispheres. Dyslexia is not part of a disease process that involves progressive weakness or deterioration of brain structures and functions. Also, some disorders that appear to be developmental may in actuality result from acquired lesions in early stages of development, with possible accompanying central nervous system dysfunction. Furthermore, significant deficits in social skills are sometimes reported in children with reading disorders. This may relate to the difficulty with increasing complexity of sentences and the general language difficulties experienced by some children who have language-based learning disabilities.

Shaywitz (2003) wrote that, in developmental dyslexia, there may not be a specific lesion that results in the reading disability. Rather, the problem is most likely in the neural pathways that develop a "glitch" during the development of the brain in the fetus. As a result, the neurons carrying the phonologic messages necessary for language do not appropriately connect to form the resonating networks that make skilled reading possible. Most likely as a result of a genetically programmed error, the neural system necessary for phonologic analysis is somehow miswired, and a child is left with a phonologic impairment that interferes with spoken and written language. Depending on the nature or severity of this fault in the wiring, we would expect to observe variations and varying degrees of reading difficulty (Shaywitz, 2003, p. 68).

Functional magnetic resonance imaging (fMRI). An MRI of the brain done while the patient performs specific tasks so the radiologist can visualize the mechanisms of the brain activated with specific tasks.

Using functional magnetic resonance imaging (fMRI), Shaywitz and colleagues (2003) progressed in efforts to map out the neural pathways for reading. They found that there are at least two neural pathways for reading. One of these pathways is activated in the early efforts associated with beginning reading, and in particular the efforts to slowly sound out words. The second pathway is faster and is more involved in skilled reading. There is a breakdown in these pathways (especially those in the back of the brain) in individuals with dyslexia.

As the field of brain pathophysiology advances, we will have better answers to the questions on the identification of structural abnormalities and neural pathway deficits in the brains of individuals with dyslexia. Galaburda (1989) reported abnormalities in brain structures and symmetries post mortem. Recent advances in the use of neuroimaging techniques such as fMRI have contributed significantly to our knowledge of the morphology of the brain (Hynd et al., 1990; Leonard, 1998).

TABLE 10–6 Tasks performed by subjects in the study by Shaywitz and colleagues (1998)

Task	Example	Adds the Demand of
Line orientation	Do [\\V] and [\\v] match?	Visual-spatial processing
Letter case	Do [bbBb] and [bbBb] match?	Orthographic processing
Single letter rhyme	Do the letters [T] and [V] rhyme?	Phonologic processing
Non-word rhyme	Do [leat] and [jete] rhyme?	Difficult phonological processing
Semantic category	Are [corn] and [rice] in the same category?	Retrieval from lexicon

Source: Based on Functional disruption in the organization of the brain for reading in dyslexia, by S. E. Shaywitz et al. 1998. *Neurobiology, 95,* 2636–2641.

Shaywitz and colleagues (1998) used fMRI techniques to study brain activation patterns in people with dyslexia. They designed a set of tasks that required their subjects to decide whether two stimuli presented simultaneously were the same or different. Their subjects included 29 readers with dyslexia and 32 unimpaired readers, all completing the tasks outlined in Table 10–6. The researchers found that the reading performance of the subjects with dyslexia was significantly impaired compared with that of the unimpaired readers. The biggest discrepancies were on the single-letter rhyme and non-word rhyme tasks, both of which require phonological processing. Using fMRI imaging, Shaywitz and colleagues (1998) found that the portions of the brain responsible for segmenting words into their phonological components functioned imperfectly in the subjects with dyslexia. Thus, the cognitive and behavioral deficits commonly associated with dyslexia were linked to problematic activation patterns in posterior and anterior language regions of the brain.

Furthermore, although magnetic resonance imaging (MRI) had been used extensively to study brain morphology in individuals with dyslexia, it had not been used to study brain morphology in children with SLI until 1997. Using the MRI scans, Gauger, Lombardino, and Leonard (1997) studied brain morphology in 11 children with SLI. They found that (1) the pars triangularis was significantly smaller in the left hemisphere of children with SLI, and (2) children with SLI were more likely to have rightward asymmetry of language structures (Gauger et al., 1997, p. 1272).

Catts and Kamhi (2005) were careful to point out that while many differences have been found in the function and structure of the brain in individuals with reading disabilities when compared to typically developing children, there is tremendous variability in these differences. Also, the differences are more diffuse in nature than those associated with acquired reading disabilities such as those found in patients with aphasia. Thus, it is probable that "individual differences in neurological development, not neurological deficits, contribute to many cases of developmental reading disabilities" (Catts & Kamhi, 2005, p. 101).

Other factors have been explored throughout the years, including the role of visual perception and processing deficits, attention deficit disorder with hyperactivity, and language problems. Language problems identified in early childhood are apparently causal factors in the development of later reading disabilities. In fact, "research indicates that 50 percent or more of children with language impairment in preschool or kindergarten go on to have reading disabilities in primary or secondary grades" (Catts & Kamhi, 2005, p. 108).

think about it Justify the position that dyslexia is a physiologically based problem.

ASSESSMENT AND DIAGNOSIS OF READING DISABILITIES

The differential diagnosis of language-based learning disabilities (LLD), dyslexia, ADHD, and auditory processing disorders can be a difficult task because there is co-morbidity among these disorders. In addition to a variety of language and cognitive tests, assessment of behavior and pragmatics should be included in a test battery for the differential diagnosis of reading disabilities and LLD. Some children are inappropriately labeled as dyslexic instead of as having LLD, especially if the language testing (lexicon, syntax, morphology, and text-level processing) reveals that the deficits in language are relatively mild. In addition, some people include a discrepancy criterion for the labeling of an individual as dyslexic. In these cases, there needs to be a discrepancy between the child's achievement and his or her expected achievement based on IQ. However, as discussed earlier, this is not viewed as a valid marker for the diagnosis of dyslexia.

Catts and Kamhi (2005) argued against the use of discrepancy criteria because a child with poor language skills will score a lower verbal IQ, which in turn lowers the overall IQ. Sometimes this lowered IQ score does not adequately reflect the difference between IQ and achievement needed in order to be diagnosed as dyslexic. It has been suggested that nonverbal IQ tests be given to children who are dyslexic; however, Stanovich (1991) found that there is little relationship between reading achievement and performance on nonverbal IQ tests. Children who do not meet the discrepancy criterion are often labeled as underachievers. Catts and Kamhi (1999) suggested that these children should be labeled as LLD because "this term focuses attention

Discrepancy criterion. The measurable difference between a child's achievement and his or her expected achievement based on IQ.

on the central role that language-learning difficulties play in these children's reading, writing, and other learning problems" (p. 66). They suggested that an extensive battery of language tests that encompass semantics, syntax, language processing, phonological processing, and reading be given.

Children who have reading disabilities and score within normal limits or high on the language-based tests would be labeled as dyslexic, whereas those children who score below age limits would be diagnosed as LLD. In other words, children who have dyslexia perform within normal limits or higher than normal on language tests; their only problem is reading. Children with LLD have a poorer performance on language tests as well as in reading, often creating a sense of frustration, as seen in Figure 10–4. Phonemic awareness is at the heart of dyslexia, so it should be tested as part of a reading battery.

Torgesen (1999) defined phonemic awareness as "a more or less explicit understanding that words are composed of segments of sound smaller than

Phonological processing. Understanding of the sound system of a language.

Phonemic awareness. Recognizing that words are made up of sounds and understanding the differences between phonemes.

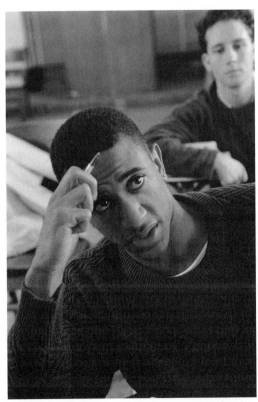

FIGURE 10–4 School-age children who have a reading and/or spelling deficit that impacts their academic progress often show signs of frustration when attempting schoolwork and homework. (*Delmar/Cengage Learning.*)

a syllable, as well as knowledge, or awareness, of the distinctive features of individual phonemes themselves" (p. 129). Phonemic awareness is embedded in the more general construct of phonological awareness and is assessed for two primary reasons: (1) to identify children at risk for reading failure prior to receiving reading instruction, and (2) to assess the level of phonological impairment in individuals who have been diagnosed with a reading disorder.

Catts and colleagues (1997) categorized assessment tasks for phonemic awareness in three categories. The first category is phonemic segmentation tasks, which include counting, pronunciation, deletion and addition of sounds to words, or reversing phonemes in words.

Phonemic synthesis is the second category. In this task, sounds are presented in isolation and the child is asked to blend them into a word. Sound comparison tasks are the third category. On sound comparison tasks, the child is asked to compare the sounds of different words. In an example of this task, the clinician presents a target word, and the child is asked to indicate which in a series of words begin with the same sound as the target word.

All these areas should be tested as part of the diagnostic process for reading impairment. A list of tests that can be used to assess phonemic awareness is found in Table 10–7.

Word recognition skills should be tested in addition to phonemic awareness. Children with reading disabilities have difficulty with orthographic processing, which enables the child to retrieve sight words from memory,

Phonemic segmentation. The act of breaking down a word into sounds.

Phonemic synthesis. The act of combining sounds presented in isolation into a single word.

TABLE 10–7 A list of tests that can be used to assess phonemic awareness

Name of Test	Author
Rosner Test of Auditory Analysis	Rosner (1975)
Lindamood Auditory Conceptualization Test	Lindamood and Lindamood (1979)
Test of Invented Spelling	Mann, Tobin, and Wilson (1987)
Test of Phonological Awareness	Torgesen and Bryant (1993)
Yopp-Singer Test of Phoneme Segmentation	Yopp (1995)
The Phonological Awareness Test	Robertson and Salter (1995)
The Comprehensive Test of Phonological Processes in Reading	Torgesen and Wagner (1997)

Source: Adapted from Assessment and instruction for phonemic awareness and word recognition skills, by J. K. Torgesen. In H. Catts and A. G. Kamhi (eds.), *Language and reading disabilities* (2nd ed.), pp. 133–135. Copyright 2005 by Allyn and Bacon (Boston).

TABLE 10–8   A list of tests that can be used to assess word recognition

Task	Name of Subtest	Name of Test
Sight Word Reading	Word Identification	Woodcock Reading Mastery Test—Revised (Woodcock, 1997)
	Reading	Wide Range Achievement Test—3 (Wilkinson, 1995)
Phonetic Decoding	Word Attack	Woodcock Reading Mastery Test—Revised (Woodcock, 1997)
Word Recognition Fluency	All 13 subtests	Gray Oral Reading Test, 3rd ed. (Wiederholt & Bryant, 1992); Word Reading Efficiency (Torgesen & Wagner, 1997); Nonword Reading Efficiency (Torgesen & Wagner, 1997)

Source: Adapted from "Assessment and Instruction for Phonemic Awareness and Word Recognition Skills" by J. K. Torgesen. In H. Catts and A. G. Kamhi, *Language and Reading Disabilities*, pp. 133–135. Copyright 1999 by Allyn and Bacon (Boston).

and with phonetic decoding, which involves applying alphabetic strategies when reading new words (Torgesen, 1999). Tests that can be used to assess word recognition skills are listed in Table 10–8.

The Assessment of Literacy and Language (ALL) is a test developed by Lombardino, Lieberman, and Brown (2005). It can be used to assess oral and written language skills for pre-kindergarten through first-grade students. The ALL consists of a caregiver questionnaire and an individually administered test with 11 norm-referenced and six criterion-referenced subtests. Examiners can screen, diagnose, and prescribe treatment for emergent literacy and language deficits for young children who are at risk for developing reading disabilities. The subtests target six areas that match Early Reading First and Reading First initiatives for development of effective reading skills, including oral language, phonological awareness, phonics knowledge, print awareness, fluency, and comprehension.

A sample battery of tests to assess the reading, writing, and spelling skills of children with suspected reading and spelling disorders is outlined in Table 10–9. It is particularly important to assess the student's knowledge of sound–letter correspondences.

In summary, comprehensive testing of language and cognition, as well as phonological awareness skills and a hearing evaluation, need to be done in order to differentially diagnose between an auditory processing disorder, a language-based learning disability, and dyslexia.

TABLE 10–9 Sample protocol for assessment of reading and spelling disorders

Test	Subtest
Comprehensive Test of Phonological Processing (Wagner, Torgesen, & Rashotte, 1999)	Phonological Awareness Composite Rapid Naming Composite Phonological Memory Composite
Woodcock-Johnson III Test of Achievement (RD book) (Woodcock, McGrew, & Mather, 2001)	Written Language (computer scored) Word Identification—Test 1 Reading Fluency—Test 2 Math Calculation—Test 5 Math Fluency—Test 6 Applied Problems—Test 10 Word Attack—Test 13 Picture Vocabulary—Test 14 Spelling—Test 7
Woodcock-Johnson Achievement Tests (SP Book)	Oral Language (computer scored) Story Recall—Test 3 Oral Comprehension—Test 15
Woodcock-Johnson III Tests of Cognition (Computer scored) (Woodcock, McGrew, & Mather, 2001)	Verbal Ability Composite Thinking Ability Composite Cognitive Efficiency General Intellectual Ability (GIA) (composite)
Gray Oral Reading Test—4 (Wiederholt & Bryant, 2001)	Fluency Comprehension Oral Reading Quotient (composite)
Test of Word Recognition Efficiency (Torgesen, Wagner, & Rashotte, 1999)	Sight Word Phonemic Decoding Total Word Reading
Brief Language Samples	Spoken, Written Language Story Re-Tell

Delmar/Cengage Learning

CULTURAL DIVERSITY ISSUES IN THE ASSESSMENT OF READING DISORDERS

Historically, there has tended to be an overdiagnosis and an underdiagnosis of literacy problems in children who are from low-SES, racially diverse, and/ or ethnically diverse backgrounds. This is problematic because there are not a wide variety of assessment tools available that are normed on these populations. It is especially problematic when taking into consideration the No Child Left Behind Act of 2001. Scarborough (2000) contended that SES is a stronger predictor of a child's literacy abilities than are assessments of emergent literacy skills, home literacy experiences, nonverbal intellect, and oral language skills. Laing and Kamhi (2003) pointed out that many standardized tests have problems with linguistic bias, content bias, and poor representation in norming samples. They wrote that linguistic bias may "be associated with the use of standardized tests and refers to a disparity between (1) the language or dialect used by the examiner, (2) the language or dialect used by the child, and (3) the language or dialect that is expected in the child's responses" (p. 45). If one adapts the test to account for these factors, the test is no longer valid in its administration and can lead to under- and/or over-referral of children who have a language difference, not a language disorder.

With regard to content validity, many tests derive their items based on the belief that most children are exposed to the same concepts and lexicon based on similar experiences in life. Laing and Kamhi (2003) also pointed out that literacy experiences such as being read to and pointing to pictures in story books may not be a traditional part of these children's experiences, and thus they are ill-prepared for tasks such as the Peabody Picture Vocabulary Test—III (Dunn & Dunn, 1997) and others that require receptively and expressively identifying pictures. Content bias occurs when the response to an item on a test could be affected by a dialectal or cultural difference.

Content bias. The effect of a dialectal or cultural difference on the responses of an individual to a test item.

Test developers need to make a conscious effort to include culturally and linguistically diverse individuals in their norming samples. Laing and Kamhi (2003) pointed out that there has been improvement in this in recent years, but there are still many tests whose norming samples do not reflect the approximate percentages of subjects that are represented in the general population. Tests that have addressed the issue of representative sampling include the Peabody Picture Vocabulary Test—III, the Test of Language Development-Primary—3 (Newcomer & Hammill, 1997), the Test of Language Development-Intermediate—2 and 3 (Newcomer & Hammill, 1988; Newcomer & Hammill, 1997), and the Test of Adolescent and Adult Language—3 (Hammill et al., 1994).

In addition to using tests with normative samples that include the background of the child being tested, the clinician can use criterion-referenced tests. These types of tools were discussed in Chapter 5, but as a reminder, criterion-referenced tests allow a clinician to test a child's language skills in a more in-depth context than does standardized testing, and the child's performance is compared to criteria developed by the clinician that permits comparison with other children who have similar cultural, ethnic, or racial backgrounds.

Other assessment devices that can be used in addition to criterion-referenced tests include obtaining and analyzing a language sample from the child and interviewing the parents of the child to develop a more complete picture of the child's form, content, and use of language, as well as a description of the child's life experiences. Laing and Kamhi (2003) also discussed two additional procedures that can be used to determine the linguistic abilities of children from culturally diverse populations. These are processing-dependent techniques and dynamic assessment techniques. Laing and Kamhi (2003) described processing-dependent tasks as being

> minimally dependent on prior knowledge or experience. Examples of processing-dependent tasks include various memory tasks (e.g., digit span, working memory, nonword repetition), certain perceptual tasks (e.g., discrimination of rapidly presented tones, sequencing tones presented in rapid sequence), and competing stimuli tasks (filtered words, auditory figure ground, competing words). (p. 46)

Dynamic Assessment

Dynamic assessment has been found to provide a more realistic picture of a child's language than do static assessments not only for children with delays or disorders, but also in the case of individuals who do not speak English as their primary language.

Dynamic assessment techniques are sometimes referred to as diagnostic therapy and are based on the work of Vygotsky (1978). Vygotsky defined a zone of proximal development as being the difference between how well a child performs on an independent task and how well the child performs when provided assistance on the same task. Thus, the clinician is able to determine the child's current level of performance as well as to determine therapy methods that can improve the child's ability on the specified task. Other dynamic assessments include test-teach-retest, graduated prompting, and task/stimulus variability. In test-teach-retest, the child is given a test and then is provided with instruction on the information he or she missed, followed by retesting on the same test. Lidz and Pena (1996) did a case study based on dynamic assessment and found that standardized tests did not provide much information on children's learning potential.

In graduated prompting, assessment and treatment occur concurrently. The child is presented with a task, then is tested for stimulability on those items missed. According to Laing and Kamhi (2003), "how well a child responds to graduated prompts can help determine which language forms and structures to target and the amount of improvement a child might be expected to make in intervention."

Graduated prompting. In diagnostic therapy, the co-occurrence of assessment and treatment, with the child being tested for stimulability on a language construct.

Stimulability. The degree to which a child can imitate a language construct presented by the clinician; the less intervention is needed, the more the child is stimulable.

In 1997, Laing, Kamhi, and Catts studied the predictive value of static versus dynamic tasks when using phonological awareness tasks to predict early reading achievement. Their study consisted of 72 typically developing children in kindergarten and first grade. During the fall and spring, each child was given a static and a dynamic measure of segmentation skills, as well as an assessment of reading performance (the Woodcock Reading Mastery Test—Revised by Woodcock, 1997). Their findings indicated that the dynamic measures of phonological awareness were better at predicting reading success than were static tests.

Task/stimulus variability can be used to modify the method by which test items are presented. For example, the clinician could present the test items in the traditional static method, or he or she could present them in a more natural method based on experiential context. Several studies were cited by Laing and Kamhi (2003) as showing that African American children tend to learn better in classrooms that are interactive and incorporate music, movement, and cooperative learning, and that these children do better on tests that are administered in their natural environment and focus on action–object orientations.

ADDRESSING READING DISORDERS IN THE SCHOOL SETTING

Individuals who have reading disabilities have trouble invoking syntactic, semantic, and graphophonemic cues into their reading, thus impeding comprehension of read material. As illustrated in Figure 10–4, students who have reading and/or spelling deficits frequently become frustrated or discouraged when attempting academic material in school. To help differentiate the academic impacts of oral and written language, see Table 10–10.

Response to Intervention

Response to Intervention, as discussed in Chapter 9, is a systematic approach to assessing a student's response to instruction. RTI asks the question, "Does instruction (i.e., strategies, methods, interventions, or curriculum) lead to increased learning and appropriate progress?" (NJCLD, 2005). As you may recall from Chapter 9, RTI was implemented for three primary reasons: (1) inadequacy of the use of the IQ–achievement discrepancy as the method for identifying children with learning disabilities; (2) overuse of special education services by students who were struggling academically but did not meet criteria for having a disability; and (3) the need for improvement in reading. The need for improvement of reading is addressed here. Research studies supported by the National Institute of Child Health and Human Development showed that the majority of students who have reading problems in the early years of school show significant improvement when participating in effective and efficient instructional programs. The report cited the work of Lyon and colleagues (2001) in saying that "early identification and prevention programs

TABLE 10–10 Differences between oral and literate language

	Oral Style	Literate Style
Function	• To regulate social interactions • To request objects and actions • To communicate face-to-face with a few people • To share information about concrete objects and events	• To regulate thinking • To reflect and request information • To communicate over time and distance • To transmit information to large numbers of people • To build abstract theories and discuss abstract ideas
Topic	• Everyday objects and events • Here and now • Topics flow according to associations of participants • Meaning is contextually based	• Abstract or unfamiliar objects and events • There and then • Discourse is centered around preselected topic • Meaning comes from inferences and conclusions drawn from text
Structure	• High-frequency words • Repetitive, predictable, redundant syntax and content • Pronouns, slang, jargon • Cohesion based on intonation	• Low-frequency words • Concise syntax and content • Specific, abstract vocabulary • Cohesion based on vocabulary and linguistic markers

Source: Adapted from Westby, C. (1991). Learning to talk- talking to learn: Oral-literate language differences. In C.S. Simon (Ed.) *Communication skills and classroom success: Assessment and therapy methodologies for language- and learning-disabled students.* Eau Claire, WI: Thinking Publications. Reprinted with permission of the author.

could reduce the number of students with reading problems by up to 70%" (NJCLD, 2005, pp. 2–3). Numerous studies looking at intervention for reading show that "instruction in small groups with high response rates, immediate feedback, and sequential mastery of topics—all typical of good teaching—are more important than the specific evidence-based program used" (NJCLD, 2005, p. 11). What this means is that, regardless of the curricular approach chosen to teach reading, small-group instruction is more effective for individuals with learning disabilities than traditional large-classroom instruction.

RTI can be used to measure the student's response to classroom strategies for teaching reading and then to determine if the student needs additional academic support in order to make appropriate progress in the area of reading. Through the provision of academic support, an instructional program that fits the child's needs and learning styles can be developed and implemented in the least restrictive environment suitable for that student.

Using the Collaborative Model to Facilitate Reading Instruction

Catts and colleagues (2001) suggested a collaborative model of classroom intervention in which the speech-language pathologist and teacher provide instruction in language and literacy to assist those children who are at risk but do not qualify for therapy in the schools, and to enhance prevention of reading difficulties by facilitating literacy in all children. These researchers suggested that the curriculum include training in phonological awareness and sound–letter correspondences and that the teachers should provide the at-risk children with extra instructional time and support in learning the skills that are foundations of literacy. They further recommended that intervention for those children who qualify for more intensive intervention with the speech-language pathologist focus on "vocabulary, grammar, pragmatics, and other language areas" (p. 46). Curriculum-based content and materials should be utilized in therapy.

Instruction in Phonological Awareness

Gillon (2000) studied the effects of training in phonological awareness on spoken language. She provided phonological awareness intervention to 61 five- to seven-year-old children who were diagnosed as having a spoken language impairment, defined as children who had a "disordered phonological system" (p. 126) and 30 children who had no speech and language deficits. The children with spoken language impairment were randomly assigned to one of three intervention programs:

1. An integrated phonological awareness program.

2. A more traditional speech-language intervention control program that focused on improving articulation and language skills.

3. A minimal intervention control program over a 4.5 month time period (p. 126).

The results were that those children who received the integrated phonological awareness intervention made significant gains in their phonological awareness and reading skills as well as in their speech articulation. In fact, the post-assessment results indicated that the children who got the integrated program matched the performance levels on phonological awareness of the typically developing children.

When a group of college students with reading disabilities was evaluated, the majority had problems with the speech production of complex phonological sequences. The authors concluded that speech processing, language processing, and speech and language production are affected by weak phonological connections (Catts, 1989). Thus, focusing on treatment methods that address phonological awareness is paramount. Catts and Kamhi (2005) made the point that children with dyslexia need therapy that targets primarily phonological processing and word recognition. Children with LLDs also need to work on phonological processing and word recognition, in addition to language comprehension. Numerous methods of reading intervention are documented in the education and speech-language pathology literature. There are several phonics computer programs that have had mixed reviews in the literature. Lombardino and colleagues (1997) stressed the need for long-term instruction in phonemic decoding for reading, spelling, and rapid word recognition. They advocated that the first step in therapy be to teach phoneme–grapheme associations using a multimodality approach. The second step should focus on irregular spelling and reading words with irregular orthographies. This should be followed by morphological manipulations in which the student learns to use sound segments to change meaning at the word level. Extensive practice is necessary to develop the rapid and automatic word recognition that is needed to have increased reading comprehension.

The Orton-Gillingham Method

The Orton-Gillingham method of teaching reading, writing, and spelling is a philosophy of teaching that incorporates an integrated curriculum of language skills. The alphabetic principle is at the core of the Orton-Gillingham method.

Alphabetic principle. The dictum governing how specific sounds in a language are represented by specific spelling patterns.

The alphabetic principle governs the orthographic structure of many languages, including English. It requires knowledge of how specific sounds are represented by specific spelling patterns. Alphabetic–phonic associations are trained from the first lesson and reinforced through phonetically controlled reading and spelling activities to form the foundation of reading and writing in alphabetic language.

The Orton-Gillingham method also focuses on the role of cognition in reading, writing, and spelling. Children are taught to think about the rules that they have learned and to apply these rules in different contexts (e.g., syllabication). Using old information to draw inferences about new information is a skill that is necessary for continued independent learning (Lombardino, 1998).

Project Read

Developed by Greene and Enfield in 1991, Project Read is a modification of the Orton-Gillingham method that also stresses input through the auditory, visual, and tactile modes. Goldsworthy (1996) described the method as a "systematic, structured, developmental approach based on the links of the language" (p. 184). It uses practice and generalization to move from the concrete to the abstract and from part to whole. The phonology component is intended for children in grades 1 to 3. It focuses on sound–symbol relationships, segmenting words into sounds, and learning syllabication patterns. The comprehension component is designed for students in grades 4 through 12. Its focus is on acquiring and organizing information using specifically designed report forms. The written expression component focuses on syntax in written language. It also includes clustering related information and editing procedures (Goldsworthy, 1996).

Lindamood Phoneme Sequencing Program (LiPS)

The Lindamood Phoneme Sequencing Program for Reading, Spelling, and Speech (LiPS) (Lindamood & Lindamood, 1998) was developed for students in pre-kindergarten to grade 12. The first three levels are specifically recommended for kindergarten students and are to be used preventively as basic building blocks toward successful reading and spelling. These levels are also recommended for students and adults with learning disabilities. Stimuli include mouth-form cards depicting the oral production plus the label and corresponding phonemes, the vowel circles, colored blocks, and letter tiles. Syllable construction and reading charts also are provided.

The LiPS program was developed to facilitate the acquisition of reading and spelling skills through a **multimodality approach** that uses auditory, visual, tactile, and kinesthetic information to teach the conceptual elements of phonemes and the corresponding graphemes. Initially, the basic auditory conceptual elements of consonant sounds are trained, followed by teaching the vowel sounds.

Objectives of ear, eye, and mouth training are dependent on the following tenets:

> **Multimodality approach.** An approach to therapy that incorporates information from all sensory systems to teach a conceptual element.

1. Sensory input is required to pair the oral motor activity with the basic auditory element.

2. Conceptualization of the distinctive features of each phoneme is required.

3. Perception of same and different number and order of speech sounds in isolation is followed by perception of minimal changes between syllable units.

4. Storage and retrieval of the agreed upon representations for phonemes and graphemes are required for reading and spelling (LeGrand, 1997).

Barton Reading and Spelling System

Developed by Susan Barton in 1999, the Barton Reading and Spelling System is also based on the Orton-Gillingham program. It can be used in individual sessions with children and adults, and a series of videotapes is available to

TABLE 10–11   Levels of the Barton System

Level 1	Phonemic Awareness
Level 2	Consonants and Short Vowels
Level 3	Closed Syllables and Units
Level 4	Syllable Division and Vowel Teams
Level 5	Prefixes and Suffixes
Level 6	Six Reasons for Silent E
Level 7	Vowel–R Syllables
Level 8	Advanced Vowel Teams
Level 9	Influences of Foreign Languages
Level 10	Greek Words and Latin Roots

Delmar/Cengage Learning

train practitioners, teachers, and parents who are interested in learning the Barton system. The Barton system also includes fully scripted lesson plans and reading materials, including color-coded letter tiles. It is divided into 10 levels, each of which contains between 10 and 15 lessons. A list of these levels is found in Table 10–11. It is anticipated that a student receiving instruction two times a week will need an average of 3 to 5 months to complete each level. According to Barton, individuals who complete all 10 levels of the program are functioning at approximately the mid–ninth-grade level of reading, spelling, and basic writing.

Wilson Reading System

The Wilson Reading System was developed by Barbara Wilson in 1988. It was originally developed to provide reading instruction to children in the upper elementary-school grades as well as adults, but it is now also available for younger children. It is a 12-step program to remediate reading and writing problems in children who have language-based learning disabilities. It, too, is based on the Orton-Gillingham approach. The phonemic awareness program emphasizes strategies that can be used for spelling and decoding. The Wilson system uses visualization techniques to help with reading comprehension and also incorporates development of oral expression. It takes approximately 1 to 3 years to complete the program, which can be used in small groups as well as one-on-one treatment sessions.

Slingerland Approach

The Slingerland Approach (Slingerland, 1977) is an example of yet another program based on the Orton-Gillingham program. An underlying philosophy of the Slingerland Approach is that individuals with dyslexia have difficulty linking the visual, auditory, and kinesthetic motor systems. According to the Learning Disabilities Association of America (2005),

> the Slingerland Approach starts with the smallest unit of sight, sound and feeling—a single letter. Expanding upon that single unit students are taught through an approach which strengthens inner-sensory association and enables the strong channel of learning to reinforce the weak. (p. 2)

The Slingerland Approach is a comprehensive language therapy system.

Laubach Method

The Laubach method was developed for the purpose of providing group instruction to high school dropouts, illiterate adults, and those for whom English is a second language. It can also be used with students in the intermediate grades in tutorial or group settings. The basic principle behind the method is the teaching of sound–symbol relationships. Consonant sounds are taught first, followed by the short vowels, and then the long vowels. Irregular spellings are then addressed, followed by reading, writing, and grammar exercises with increasing complexity. The Laubach method uses picture association cards to teach letters, sounds, and key vocabulary words. Lowercase letters are taught before uppercase letters, but both are taught in alphabetic sequence (Buchanan, Weller, & Buchanan, 1997).

Montessori Reading Instruction

The Montessori method of reading instruction uses self-paced, multisensory input to teach the letters. Visual-motor activities are designed to facilitate letter recognition and are then modified to teach writing and reading. The children participate in activities such as tracing and identifying sandpaper letters with their eyes open, then with their eyes closed. While they are tracing the sandpaper letters, they say the letter's sound. The Montessori method uses phonograms, which are alphabet cards, to construct words. A unique feature of this method is that it does not allow oral reading. Teachers check reading comprehension by writing questions on a chalkboard, then eliciting answers to the questions (Buchanan, Weller, & Buchanan, 1997).

Intervention with Stories

Prewritten narratives and the creation of novel scripts are valuable therapy tools to use with children who have language-based learning disabilities, including reading disabilities. Stories can be used to coordinate academic issues in the classroom with events happening in therapy. It is important that the stories use complete texts, events, and experiences so that children can learn the structure of stories (Naremore, Densmore, & Harman, 1995). This structure includes introducing the story, developing the components, and reaching a resolution.

By grade 2, a child should be able to get the main idea of a sentence. Thus, when reading with the child, it is helpful to point out that the first sentence in a paragraph typically reveals the general content of the entire passage. If the child can get the main idea of a sentence, he or she can move on to understanding the content of a paragraph. Reading written text from grade 3 and beyond requires the use of metalinguistic and metacognitive skills to comprehend the content of the story. Children can be taught to single out key words, then to use the repetition of those words to tie the sentences in the paragraph together (Naremore, Densmore, & Harman, 1995). Lexicon can be addressed by having the child think of synonyms for the key words. He or she can also make lists of the information words within the paragraph to help remember the key elements and sequence of events within the paragraph. Another strategy to help children remember the sequence of events is to type out the sentences of the paragraph, then cut the sentences apart into sentence strips. Then, after the child reads the paragraph, he or she can use the sentence strips to reconstruct the paragraph. This facilitates the learning of sequencing, which is critical to comprehension of a story (Naremore, Densmore, & Harman, 1995).

Stories can also be used to work on written expression. Naremore and colleagues (1995) advocate first teaching the child to state the main idea of his or her paragraph in one sentence. The child is then taught to tie each sentence back to the main idea through the use of repetition of words, pronouns, substitutions, and lists of the events. From that point, the child should be taught to make inferences and predictions using information in the paragraph and learning from past experiences. As part of this process, the child should be taught to organize his or her ideas using old and new information. This requires that the child tap into short-term and long-term memory banks.

Improving Memory

Many activities and techniques can be used to improve the memory skills needed to be successful readers and writers. One way is to tell a story to the child and have him or her repeat it back in the proper sequence. For children who have difficulty with this initially, the story can be written down on note cards that the child can read and use to reconstruct the story. Memory and concentration games are also useful tools that can be used at home and in the classroom. Playing "20 Questions" and memorizing rhymes and songs are additional helpful activities. Games that require the duplication of visual and auditory patterns are good activities for improving memory. For example, the clinician can tap out a series of knocks on the table and then have the student repeat the pattern using appropriate pauses and cadences. Alternately, the clinician could repeat a series of verbalizations (words and sounds) that the student is then required to repeat. Telling "how to" sequences likewise can be useful (Goldsworthy, 1996). An example would be to make brownies with a child and have him or her reconstruct the sequence of events that led up to eating the brownies. These are activities that can easily be implemented in the therapy room, the classroom, and at home.

Increasing Metacognitive Skills to Enhance Reading Comprehension

The development of metacognitive skills has been found to be a valid marker for later reading development. Some strategies to help students learn metacognitive skills include using advance organizers, such as having learning objectives provided prior to reading a passage, and using pretests and pre-questions.

> **Metacognitive skills.** Those skills that enable a child to solve problems, form hypotheses, analyze his or her thoughts, and make a decision.

Having advanced organizers helps the student develop strategies that enable him or her to evaluate the information read, categorize the content, and generalize the information (Nelson, 1998).

It is also important for the students to know that there is a purpose to reading. Tierney and Cunningham (1984) delineated four steps that could be utilized to increase reading comprehension:

1. Establish purpose(s) for comprehending.

2. Have students read or listen for the established purpose(s).

3. Have students perform some task that directly reflects and measures accomplishment of each established purpose for comprehending.

4. Provide direct informative feedback concerning students' comprehension based on their performance of the task(s) (p. 625).

It may be necessary to teach students to develop a self-questioning approach to reading comprehension in order to implement the four steps. Wong and Jones (1982) proposed five steps for developing self-questioning:

1. What are you studying this passage for? (So you can answer some questions you will be given later).

2. Find the main idea or ideas in the paragraph and underline it (them).

3. Think of a question about the main idea you have underlined. Remember what a good question should be like. (Look at the prompt).

4. Learn the answer to your question.

5. Always look back at the questions and answers to see how each successive question and answer provides you with more information (p. 231).

As the students learn to formulate good questions about the textual units, their reading comprehension increases.

ROLE OF THE SPEECH-LANGUAGE PATHOLOGIST IN DIAGNOSING AND TREATING DEVELOPMENTAL READING AND SPELLING DISABILITIES

In its position statement "Roles and Responsibilities of Speech-Language Pathologists with Respect to Reading and Writing in Children and Adolescents" (2001), ASHA states the following:

> Appropriate roles and responsibilities for SLPs include, but are not limited to (a) preventing written language problems by fostering language acquisition and emergent literacy; (b) identifying children at risk for reading and writing problems; (c) assessing reading and writing; (d) providing intervention and documenting outcomes for reading and writing; and (e) assuming other roles, such as providing assistance to general education teachers, parents, and students; advocating for effective literacy practices; and advancing the knowledge base (www.asha.org/policy).

Children with reading and spelling disabilities need intervention that includes speaking, listening, reading, and writing because reciprocity appears to occur in oral-written language. Dyslexia is a specific deficit in the processing of phonological information, an area about which most speech-language pathologists are well versed with regard to assessment and remediation. The primary role of the speech-language pathologist should be early identification. A test battery (see Chapter 13) that is designed to evaluate language production and processing (including phonology, semantics, and syntax) should be administered to children who are at risk for problems in reading (Lombardino et al., 1997). In addition, all children in kindergarten and first grade should be given tests of phonological awareness that predict reading disabilities. Because of the interplay between auditory and visual processing, it also makes sense for a speech-language pathologist to be involved in remediation because many children with reading disabilities also show deficits in oral language. Likewise, many of the strategies speech-language pathologists use to treat auditory processing disorders can be used to treat developmental reading and spelling disabilities. With the understanding of the phoneme–grapheme information possessed by the speech-language pathologist, it is only logical that he or she be involved in the early identification and treatment of developmental reading and spelling problems. There is no doubt that the speech-language pathologist should work collaboratively with classroom teachers and specialists in reading or learning disabilities in modifying the curriculum to facilitate optimal academic success for children with reading and spelling disabilities.

> **think about it**
>
> Many school districts do not include reading and spelling deficiencies as part of the scope of practice for their speech-language pathologists. How would you justify to a school board and other decision makers in your school district that speech-language pathologists should be actively involved in the assessment and treatment of students with reading and spelling problems?

SUMMARY

Reading and spelling disabilities are rapidly becoming one of the most referred disabilities in speech-language pathology. Over the last decade, these disabilities have received much attention in the literature, with the majority of these studies confirming that the speech-language pathologist should assume an active role in the diagnosis and treatment of individuals with reading or spelling disabilities. There have been efforts to confirm the etiology of reading and spelling disorders, with more and more evidence showing that genetics may play a role as well as specific deficits in the central nervous system. The use of functional magnetic resonance imaging has enhanced the ability of researchers to determine which areas of the brain are active in typical readers and then to compare these images to those of individuals with reading or spelling deficits. The study of reading and spelling disabilities is an exciting area in our profession, and it is paramount that speech-language pathologists make known their ability to participate in the assessment and treatment of these disorders.

CASE STUDY

Author's Note: This report greatly exceeds in length the other case studies, but the exam is very comprehensive and multifaceted.

Background Information

Wilson, a 10-year-old male, was seen at the Speech, Language, and Hearing Clinic for an assessment of his reading, spelling, and oral language skills (Diagnostic Procedure Code: 92506 Evaluation of Speech and Language).

Wilson was referred by Mrs. Samsom, a nurse practitioner at the Family Psychiatry Clinic, where Wilson had been diagnosed ADHD. His mother, Mrs. Johnson, says Wilson has difficulty focusing. He is not on medication.

Wilson is currently home-schooled by his mother, who reports that he is at the fourth-grade level. Mrs. Johnson has been concerned with Wilson's academic performance since he was in kindergarten, when he began showing

(continues)

CASE STUDY *(continued)*

signs of difficulty with writing and verbal communication skills. However, she reports that language comprehension seems to be one of Wilson's strengths, and that he does not have much trouble with memorization. Wilson has received treatment only from an occupational therapist for his difficulty with handwriting. His mother explains that Wilson uses a four-finger grasp while writing, a problem that was never successfully corrected in therapy.

Wilson's developmental history is unremarkable. He reached all his developmental milestones at the appropriate stages except for toilet training, which gave him some difficulty through kindergarten. During Wilson's delivery there was meconium staining and he had low blood sugar. Wilson has asthma, which has resulted in hospital visits on two occasions. He has a heart murmur. He has had no operations and his general health is noted to be average. There is a negative history for language learning disability in Wilson's immediate family; however, his second cousin has some language difficulties.

The purpose of this assessment was to evaluate Wilson's oral and written language abilities in conjunction with his overall cognitive abilities to determine if he has a reading disability that requires academic accommodations and/or specific intervention strategies.

Reading and Spelling Achievement Measures

The following diagnostic tools were used:

- Woodcock-Johnson Tests of Cognitive Abilities—Third Edition (WJ-COG-III) (Woodcock, McGrew, & Mather, 2001)

- Comprehensive Test of Phonological Processing (CTOPP) (Wagner, Torgesen, & Rashotte, 1999)

- Gray Oral Reading Mastery Test—4 (GORT-4) (Weiderholt & Bryant, 2001)

- Test of Word Reading Efficiency (TOWRE) (Wagner, Torgesen & Rashotte, 1999)

- Woodcock-Johnson Tests of Achievement—Third Edition (WJ-III ACH) (Woodcock, McGrew & Mather, 2001)

WJ-III Cognitive Battery

Seven subtests from the Woodcock-Johnson Tests of Cognitive Abilities—Third Edition (WJ-COG-III) were used to assess Wilson's's cognitive processing skills. These subtests were as follows: Verbal Comprehension, Visual-Auditory Learning, Spatial Relations, Sound Blending, Concept Formation, Visual Matching, and Numbers Reversed. The mean score for each subtest is 100 with a standard deviation of +/–15. Combinations of WJ-COG-III subtests are used to derive Verbal Ability, Thinking Ability, Cognitive Efficiency, and General Intelligence Ability composite scores.

Wilson's Visual Auditory Learning and Concept Formation subtest scores were in the superior range for his age. His Verbal Comprehension and Sound Blending subtest scores were in the above average range, while his Spatial Relations subtest score was in the average range for his age. He scored at the lower end of the average range on the Numbers Reversed subtest. His score on the Visual Matching subtest was depressed.

Wilson's Thinking Ability (intentional cognitive processing) was in the superior range. General Intellectual Ability and Verbal Ability composite scores were at the higher end of the average range for his age. However, his Cognitive Efficiency composite score was depressed. A discrepancy of this nature, where scores range from superior to depressed, is characteristic of a learning disability. The following table shows Wilson's standard scores and percentiles for the WJ-COG-III.

Subtests	Standard Score	Percentile
Verbal Comprehension	110	76
Visual-Auditory Learning	125	95
Spatial Relations	109	73
Sound Blending	115	84
Concept Formation	134	99
Visual Matching	71*	3
Numbers Reversed	91	28
Thinking Ability Composite	132	98
Verbal Ability Composite	110	76
Cognitive Efficiency	76*	6
General Intelligence Ability	112	80

* Score is more than one standard deviation below the mean.

Phonological Awareness

The Comprehensive Test of Phonological Processing (CTOPP) for ages 7 through 24 was used to assess Wilson's phonological awareness, phonological memory, and rapid naming skills. Six subtests of the CTOPP were given to Wilson during this evaluation: Elision, Blending Words, Memory for Digits, Rapid Digit Naming, Nonword Repetition, and Rapid Letter Naming.

The Elision subtest is a 20-item procedure that measures the extent to which an individual can say a word and then say what is left of that word after dropping out designated sounds. This test directly assesses phonemic awareness, a skill that is necessary for an individual to read and spell with accuracy. The Blending Words subtest is a 20-item procedure that measures an individual's ability to combine sounds to form words. The Memory for Digits subtest is a 21-item procedure that measures the extent to which an individual can repeat a series of numbers ranging in length from two to eight digits. The Nonword Repetition subtest measures an individual's ability to repeat nonsense words that range in length from 3 to 15 sounds. The Rapid Digit Naming subtest is a 72-item procedure that measures the speed with which an individual can name the numbers on two pages. The Rapid Letter Naming subtest measures the speed with which the examinee names letters of the alphabet. An individual's ability to rapidly name several items is often associated with reading accuracy

(continues)

CASE STUDY (continued)

and rate. The CTOPP has an average score of 10 and a standard deviation of +/–3 for each subtest. Composite scores are calculated for Phonological Awareness, Phonological Memory, and Rapid Naming. Each composite score is based on an average score of 100 and a standard deviation of +/–15.

Wilson's scores on the phonological processing subtests ranged from average to the lower end of average. All of his composite scores, Phonological Awareness (combination of Elision and Blending Words subtests), Phonological Memory (combination of Memory for Digits and Nonword Repetition subtests), and Rapid Naming (combination of Rapid Digit Naming and Rapid Letter Naming subtests) were average for his age. However, his scores indicate a slight weakness in phonological memory. His CTOPP scores are shown in the following table.

Subtest	Standard Score	Percentile
Elision	11	63
Blending Words	10	50
Memory for Digits	10	50
Nonword Repetition	8	25
Rapid Digit Naming	11	63
Rapid Letter Naming	9	37
Phonological Awareness Composite	103	58
Phonological Memory Composite	94	35
Rapid Naming	100	50

Reading, Spelling, and Mathematic Skills

The Woodcock-Johnson-III Tests of Achievement (WJ-ACH-III) were administered to measure Wilson's reading abilities for single-word reading, nonsense word decoding, and math fluency and calculation. The Story Recall subtest measured Wilson's ability to recall increasingly complex stories. The Word Attack subtest measured his ability to apply phonics skills in reading phonetically structured nonwords. The Reading Fluency subtest measured his ability to read and answer yes/no questions both quickly and accurately.

The Spelling subtest evaluated Wilson's knowledge of orthography, and the Letter-Word Identification subtest measured his sight vocabulary. The Math Fluency subtest measured his automaticity in basic arithmetic while the Calculation subtest measured Wilson's computational skills. The standard scores and percentile ranks reported for these tests are grade-based. The average score is 100 with a standard deviation of +/–15.

Wilson's scores on the Letter-Word Identification and Word Attack subtests were in the high average range for his grade. His score on the Reading Fluency and Spelling subtests fell within the average range for his grade. However, spelling was significantly lower than all other achievement test scores. On the Story Recall subtest, Wilson's score was in the superior range. An unexpected discrepancy was noted between Wilson's performance on reading tests (first three tests) and his performance on story recall, a task of spoken language.

Subtest	Standard Score	Percentile Rank
Letter-Word Identification	113	81
Word Attack	112	79
Reading Fluency	106	66
Spelling	95	37
Story Recall	130	98

Wilson's score on the Math Fluency subtest was in the average range, while his score on the Calculation subtest was in the superior range for his grade. This unexpected discrepancy in math scores was likely due to the timed constraints of the math fluency test. Wilson's scores are summarized in the following table.

Subtest	Standard Score	Percentile Rank
Math Fluency	97	41
Calculation	122	93

The Test of Word Reading Efficiency (TOWRE) was used to measure Wilson's ability to pronounce printed words accurately and fluently in timed conditions. The Sight Word Efficiency subtest was used to measure Wilson's ability to recognize familiar words as whole units (sight words). The Phonemic Decoding Efficiency subtest was used to measure Wilson's ability to decode words. Both subtests assess the number of words read in 45 seconds. The average score is 100 with a standard deviation of +/–15.

Wilson's scores on Sight Word Efficiency and Phonemic Decoding Efficiency ranged from average to above average. There was an unexpected discrepancy between sight words and phonemic decoding. The Total Word Reading score, converted from the sum standard scores, shows that Wilson's overall word reading efficiency was average for his age and grade. The results are shown in the following table.

Subtest	Standard Score	Percentile Rank
Sight Word Efficiency	96	39
Phonemic Decoding Efficiency	112	79
Total Word Reading	**105**	**64**

(continues)

CASE STUDY (continued)

On the Sight Word Efficiency subtest, Wilson read 67 words correctly and one word incorrectly in 45 seconds. On the Phonemic Decoding Efficiency subtest, Wilson read 43 words correctly and five words incorrectly in 45 seconds. For several words, Wilson initially read the word incorrectly but was able to self-correct quickly. At the end of the 45-second time frame, when the words were increasing in difficulty, Wilson was reading very few words correctly.

The Gray Oral Reading Test—4 (GORT-4) is a test used to assess reading rate and accuracy, fluency (rate + accuracy), and passage comprehension. The GORT-4 consists of a series of stories beginning with the first-grade level and progressing to advanced levels. Wilson was asked to read a story aloud as quickly and accurately as possible. He was then asked to answer five multiple-choice questions related to the story. Wilson's fluency score was computed for the story by combining his scores obtained by rate (time taken to read the passage) and accuracy (the number of errors made). The mean score for these subtests is 10 with a standard deviation of +/–3.

Wilson's score for reading accuracy was within the average range for his age. His rate, fluency (rate 1 accuracy) and passage comprehension scores were in the higher end of the average range. W's scores are shown in the table below. The Oral Reading Quotient score (fluency + comprehension) of 115, which is a measure of Wilson's overall reading ability, was high average, indicating that his reading fluency and reading comprehension are areas of strength.

Subtest	Standard Score	Percentile
Rate	12	75
Accuracy	11	63
Fluency (rate + accuracy)	12	75
Passage Comprehension	13	84
Oral Reading Quotient	115	84

Articulation

Wilson did not exhibit any articulation errors in his speech.

Hearing Screening

Wilson's hearing was not screened because his mother stated that he had been tested and his hearing was found within normal limits bilaterally. Mrs. Johnson also noted that Wilson prefers one ear over the other.

Observations

Wilson was extremely cooperative during the evaluation. He displayed excellent attention to the tasks and he worked diligently throughout several hours of testing.

Evaluation Summary

Wilson, a 10-year-old male, was seen at the Speech, Language, and Hearing Clinic for an assessment of his reading, spelling, and oral language skills (Diagnostic Procedure Code: 92506 Evaluation of Speech and Language). Wilson's test percentiles range from the 3rd to 99th. He is extremely bright and clearly demonstrates this in his Thinking Ability (98th percentile) and Verbal Ability (76th percentile) composite scores on the WJ-III Test of Cognitive Abilities. In contrast, Wilson's Cognitive Efficiency is depressed (6th percentile). This lower composite score is due mainly to his slow processing speed on the task for Visual Matching.

Wilson's reading scores, while in the normal range, were lower than expected when compared to his verbal and thinking ability scores on the WJ-III. Discrepancies between Wilson's (1) average reading and high-average language scores and (2) high thinking and verbal ability scores and low cognitive efficiency score are typical of bright children who have a developmental history of difficulty with reading, spelling, and writing.

Wilson's performance on the battery of tests suggests that his problems are consistent with a diagnosis of developmental dyslexia and dysgraphia (Developmental Dyslexia Code: 315.02 and Dysgraphia Code: 315.4) (ICD-9-CM: World Health Organization International Classification of Diseases). Wilson has compensated for these difficulties very well, due in large part to his advanced reasoning skills and his excellent home instruction. Like many very bright individuals with dyslexia, Wilson's reading scores do not fall outside the average range. The diagnosis is based on discrepancies between areas of strength and weakness that are characteristic of the individuals identified in the research literature as having "compensated dyslexia."

As reported in the *Annals of Dyslexia*, Volume 53, dyslexia is defined as

> a specific learning disability that is neurobiological in origin. It is characterized by difficulties with accurate and/or fluent word recognition and by poor spelling and decoding abilities. These difficulties typically result from a deficit in the phonological component of language that is often unexpected in relation to other cognitive abilities and the provision of effective classroom instruction. Secondary consequences may include problems in reading comprehension and reduced reading experience that can impede growth of vocabulary and background knowledge. (Lyon, Shaywitz, & Shaywitz, 2003)

As reported by the National Center for Learning Disabilities, dysgraphia is defined as "a learning disability that affects writing abilities. It can manifest itself as difficulties with spelling, poor handwriting, and trouble putting thought on paper" (www.ncld.org).

A summary of Wilson's scores for all tests administered in this evaluation are presented in the next table followed by specific recommendations. Percentile rank scores indicate the percent of individuals his age that fall below the score reported for Wilson. For example, a percentile rank of 25 on a test means that 25 percent of his peers have lower scores on this test, while 75 percent of his peers have higher scores.

(continues)

CASE STUDY (continued)

Test	Subtest	Standard Score	Percentile Rank	Descriptive Rating
CTOPP	Elision	11	63	Average
	Blending Words	10	50	Average
Composite Score	**Phonological Awareness**	103	58	Average
	Memory for Digits	10	50	Average
	Nonword Repetition	8	25	Lower end of average
Composite Score	**Phonological Memory**	94	35	Average
	Rapid Digit Naming	11	37	Average
	Rapid Letter Naming	9	63	Average
Composite Score	**Rapid Naming**	100	50	Average
WJ-III ACH	Spelling	95	37	Average
	Word Attack	112	79	Higher end of average
	Word Identification	113	81	High average
	Reading Fluency	106	66	Average
	Math Fluency	97	41	Average
	Math Calculation	122	93	Superior
TOWRE	Sight Words	96	39	Average
	Phonemic Decoding	112	79	Higher end of average
	Total Word Reading	105	64	Average
GORT-IV	Rate	12	75	Higher end of average
	Accuracy	11	63	Average
	Fluency	12	75	Higher end of average
	Comprehension	13	84	High average
	Oral Reading Quotient	115	84	High average

WJ-COG-III	Verbal Comprehension	110	76	**Average**
	Visual-Auditory Learning	125	95	**Superior**
	Spatial Relations	109	73	**Average**
	Sound Blending	115	84	**High average**
	Concept Formation	134	99	**Superior**
	Visual Matching	71	3	**Depressed**
	Numbers Reversed	91	28	**Lower end of average**
Composite Score	**Verbal Ability**	110	76	**Average**
Composite Score	**Thinking Ability**	132	98	**Superior**
Composite Score	**Cognitive Efficiency**	76	6	**Depressed**
Composite Score	**General Intelligence Ability**	112	80	**Higher end of average**

Because Wilson has a mild form of developmental dyslexia along with dysgraphia, academic accommodations and intervention will be extremely helpful in assisting him to achieve his full academic potential. Wilson will continue to advance his reading, writing, and spelling skills, despite his developmental dyslexia and dysgraphia, if his educators understand the nature of his weaknesses and if appropriate accommodations are made to provide Wilson with the optimal academic environment.

There is a high incidence of secondary emotional difficulties, such as frustration and depression, in students with learning disabilities who do not receive adequate accommodations. Wilson would benefit from alternative instructional strategies and appropriate methods of reading and writing therapy, as well as appropriate support and further instruction in the areas in which he does well and enjoys. His noticeable difficulties certainly fit the pattern of mild dyslexia and dysgraphia. Therefore, intervention may be very beneficial.

In our clinic, we have tested several gifted students with reading disabilities. We typically recommend that they (1) be given extra time to take exams and to complete in-class assignments; (2) have access to a note taker when in classes that require rapid recording of lecture material; and (3) be exempt from taking a foreign language requirement (a most difficult task for persons with dyslexia) and take, instead, a comparable number of hours in courses with cultural content.

Below are some general guidelines that might be helpful in understanding how developmental dyslexia can impact the academic performance of students who are bright yet struggling to perform comparably with their peers.

- All of these students demonstrate depressed academic performance unexpectedly given their overall intellectual abilities. Even with academic accommodations, reading fluency, spelling, and writing fluency difficulties persist.

(continues)

CASE STUDY (continued)

- These children typically do not show difficulty in listening (oral comprehension of language). Their problems are limited to processing language and other abstract symbols in the written form. Timed tests exacerbate their depressed academic performance. A much more accurate picture of their conceptual abilities is expressed when they are tested orally as opposed to having them read material and then write their responses in a limited period of time.

- Many classroom assignments that require reading and writing cannot be completed by these students in the amount of time given. We need to give these students extra time or allow them to complete their assignments at home.

- Often these children show inconsistent progress in subjects like math. Some math concepts—those that require less linguistic processing and greater visual-spatial processing—are easier. It is expected that Wilson will show stronger abilities in some math tasks than others. When gifted children are not learning a skill as quickly as expected, we need to find alternative ways to teach the concepts. They possess the conceptual ability to learn but need to have the information presented in an alternative manner.

- While they may squeeze through foreign languages with C grades, they always struggle with learning the symbols of a new language.

- Children who are gifted and insightful may internalize these difficulties and run the risk of moving away from careers in which

they have a keen interest and an ability to function unless academic subject matter is presented appropriately and/or they are afforded the accommodations that are necessary for their academic success.

Based on our findings, we recommended that

- Wilson should be allowed extra time on tests and other class work.
- Wilson could benefit from a multisensory phonics- and fluency-based instructional program.

Examples of programs are the Orton-Gillingham Program and the Barton Reading and Spelling System.

The Orton-Gillingham approach is a comprehensive phonics-based language program that utilizes a multisensory approach including auditory, visual, and kinesthetic stimuli. This type of program would be beneficial in enhancing Wilson's academic progress. This program would allow him to acquire advanced level phonics (sounds) and orthographic (spelling) skills that will improve his prognosis for academic success. Wilson should attend therapy sessions implementing this program at least two to three times per week. Components of the Orton-Gillingham program are listed below:

- Reading and spelling vowels (long and short)
- Reading and spelling of basic syllable types
- Reading and spelling with common spelling rules
- Reading and spelling rules for syllabification

- Reading and spelling regular and irregular vowel teams
- Reading and spelling word roots and suffixes
- Applying this knowledge to oral reading and written composition

The Barton Reading and Spelling System is a tutoring program that parents, volunteer tutors, resource specialists, and professional tutors can use with children, teenagers, and adults who have a learning disability. It is an adapted and simplified version of the Orton-Gillingham approach to teaching reading and spelling. It includes fully scripted lesson plans as well as all reading material, spelling lists, homework pages, and training videos.

Possible sources for these therapies include

1. A private speech-language pathologist trained in the Orton, Wilson, or Barton Reading Program in the Georgia area, Wilson's new area of residence.
2. If entered in the regular school system, Wilson should have a 504 plan developed for his academic needs.
3. Wilson should spend time using the computer. The spell-check could be especially beneficial.
4. Wilson's mother should read the information on developmental dyslexia and dysgraphia provided to her by the clinician.

Author's Note: This report was provided through the courtesy of Linda Lombardino, Ph.D.

REVIEW QUESTIONS

1. Which of the following statements characterizes learning of syntax by a child with a reading disability?
   a. They have rapid bursts of learning followed by plateaus.
   b. They have a constant slow rate of learning syntax.
   c. Neither one of the above statements is true.

2. Which of the following statements is true?
   a. The parietal bank of the planum temporale translates sound into meaningful language.
   b. The temporal bank of the planum temporale processes visual and spatial information.
   c. The temporal bank of the planum temporale translates sound into meaningful language.

3. Which of the following methods of reading instruction is a multimodality program of reading instruction that incorporates mouth-form cards, the vowel circle, syllable construction, and reading charts?
   a. Lindamood Phoneme Sequencing Program
   b. Montessori Reading Method

    c. Barton

    d. Orton-Gillingham

4. Which of the following is not based on the Orton-Gillingham program of reading instruction?

    a. Lindamood Phoneme Sequencing Program

    b. Barton Reading and Spelling System

    c. Wilson Reading System

    d. Laubach Method of Reading Instruction

5. At what age do children typically learn about phoneme–grapheme correspondences and learn to decode?

    a. 3–5 years of age

    b. 5–7 years of age

    c. 8–10 years of age

6. Children's familiarity with nursery rhymes is a strong predictor of being a successful reader.

    a. True

    b. False

7. Accuracy-disabled readers are those children who, despite having decoding skills at grade appropriate levels, still have markedly poor reading.

    a. True

    b. False

8. There apparently is a genetic basis for reading disabilities.

    a. True

    b. False

9. Based on fMRI studies, cognitive and behavioral deficits commonly associated with dyslexia have not been linked to problematic activation patterns in posterior and anterior language regions of the brain.

    a. True

    b. False

10. In graduated prompting, assessment and treatment of reading disabilities occur concurrently.

    a. True

    b. False

REFERENCES

American Psychiatric Association. (1994). *Diagnostic and statistical manual of mental disorders-IV* (4th ed.). Washington, DC: Author.

American Speech-Language-Hearing Association. (2001). Role and responsibilities of speech-language pathologists with respect to reading and writing in children and adolescents [position statement]. www.asha.org/policy.

Barton, S. (2000). *Barton reading and spelling system.* San Jose, CA: Bright Solutions for Dyslexia, LLC.

Buchanan, M., Weller, C., & Buchanan, M. (1997). *Special education desk reference.* San Diego, CA: Singular Publishing Group.

Catts, H. W. (1989). Speech production deficits and reading disabilities. *Journal of Speech and Hearing Disorders, 54,* 422–428.

Catts, H. W., Fey, M. D., Zhang, X., & Tomblin, J. B. (1999). Language bases of reading and reading disabilities: Evidence from a longitudinal investigation. *Scientific Studies of Reading, 3,* 331–362.

Catts, H. W., Fey, M. D., Zhang, X., & Tomblin, J. B. (2001). Eliminating the risk of future reading difficulties in kindergarten children: A research-based model and its clinical implemenation. *Language, Speech, and Hearing Services in the Schools, 32,* 38–50.

Catts, H. W., & Kamhi, A. G. (1999). *Language and reading disabilities.* Boston: Allyn and Bacon.

Catts, H. W., and Kamhi, A. G. (2005). *Language and reading disabilities* (2nd ed.). Boston: Allyn and Bacon.

Catts, H. W., Wilcox, K. A., Wood-Jackson, C., Larrivee, L. S., & Scott, V. G. (1997). Toward an understanding of phonological awareness. In C. K. Leong and R. M. Joshi (eds.), *Cross-language studies of learning to read and spell: Phonologic and orthographic processing.* Dordrecht, The Netherlands: Kluwer Academic Press.

Chall, J. (1983). *Stages of reading development.* New York: McGraw-Hill.

Dunn, L., & Dunn, L. (1997). *Peabody picture vocabulary test—III.* Circle Pines, MN: American Guidance Service.

Galaburda, A. M. (1989). Ordinary and extraordinary brain development: Anatomical variations in developmental dyslexia. *Annals of Dyslexia, 39,* 67–79.

Gauger, L. M., Lombardino, L. J., & Leonard, C. M. (1997, December). Brain morphology in children with specific language impairment. *Journal of Speech, Language, and Hearing Research, 40,* 1272–1284.

Gillon, G. T. (2000). The efficacy of phonological awareness intervention for children with spoken language impairment. *Language, Speech, and Hearing Services in the Schools, 31,* 126–141.

Goldsworthy, C. L. (1996). *Developmental reading disabilities: A language-based treatment approach.* San Diego, CA: Singular Publishing Group.

Goodman, K. S. (1973). Analysis of oral reading miscues: Applied psycholinguistics. In F. Smith (ed.), *Psycholinguistics and reading* (pp. 158–176). New York: Holt, Rinehart and Winston.

Gough, P., & Tunmer, W. (1986). Decoding, reading, and reading disability. *Remedial and Special Education, 7,* 6–10.

Greene, V. E., & Enfield, M. L. (1991). *Project Read*. Bloomington, MN: Language Circle Enterprise.

Hammill, D., Brown, V., Larsen, S., & Wiederholt. J. (1994). *Test of adolescent and adult language–3*. Austin, TX: Pro-Ed.

Hammill, D., & Newcomer, P. (1997). *Test of language development-intermediate—3*. Austin, TX: Pro-Ed.

Hart, B., & Risley, T. R. (1995). *Meaningful differences in the everyday experience of young American children*. Baltimore: Paul H. Brookes.

Hart, B., & Risley, T. R. (1999). *The social world of children learning to talk*. Baltimore: Paul H. Brookes.

Hynd, G. (1991, March). Brain morphology as it is related to learning disabilities. Lecture at the 1991 G. Paul Moore Symposium, Gainesville, FL.

Hynd, G., Semrud-Clikeman, M., Lorys, A., Novey, E., & Eliopulos, D. (1990). Brain morphology in developmental dyslexia and attention deficit disorder/hyperactivity. *Archives of Neurology, 47*, 919–926.

International Dyslexia Association (2002, November). A definition of dyslexia. Retrieved March 10, 2010 from www.interdys.org.

International Dyslexia Association. (2008). Retrieved March 10, 2010 from www.interdys.org.

Justice, L. M., Chow, S., Capellini, C., Flanigan, K., Colton, S. (2003, August). Emergent literacy intervention for vulnerable preschoolers: Relative effects of two approaches. *American Journal of Speech-Language Pathology, 12*(3), 320–332.

Laing, S. P., & Kamhi, A. (2003, January). Alternative assessment of language and literacy in culturally and linguistically diverse populations. *Language, Speech, and Hearing Services in the Schools, 34*(1), 44–66.

Laing, S., Kamhi, A. G., & Catts, H. W. (1997, November). Dynamic assessment of phonological awareness in school-age children. Paper presented at the annual convention of the American Speech-Language-Hearing Association, Boston.

Learning Disabilities Association of America (2005). *Adult literacy reading programs for literacy providers: LDA fact sheet*. Retrieved April 20, 2010 from http://www.ldaamerica.org/aboutld/professionals/adult_literacy.asp.

LeGrand, H. (1997). Unpublished manuscript. Gainesville, FL.

Leonard, C. M. (1998). Language. Chapter 17 in H. Cohen (ed.), *Neuroscience for rehabilitation* (2nd ed.). Philadelphia: Lippincott-Raven.

Leonard, C. M., Voeller, K. K. S., Lombardino, L. J., Morris, M. K., Hynd, G. W., Alexander, A. W., Andersen, H. G., Garofalakis, M., Honeyman, J. C., Mao, J., Agee, F., & Staab, E. V. (1993). Anomalous cerebral structure in dyslexia revealed with magnetic resonance imaging. *Archives of Neurology, 50*, 461–469.

Lidz, C. S., & Pena, E. D. (1996). Dynamic assessment: The model, its relevance as a nonbiased approach, and its application in Latino-American preschool children. *Language, Speech, and Hearing Services in the Schools, 27*, 367–377.

Light, J. G., & DeFries, J. G. (1995). Comorbidity of reading and mathematical disabilities: Genetic and environmental etiologies. *Journal of Learning Disabilities, 28*, 96–106.

Lindamood, C. H. & Lindamood, P. C. (1979). *Lindamood auditory conceptualization test*. Allen, TX: DLM Teaching Resources.

Lindamood, P., & Lindamood, P. (1998). *Lindamood phoneme sequencing program for reading, spelling, and speech.* Circle Pines, MN: American Guidance Service Publishing.

Livesay, Y. (1995). Dyslexia and reading instruction: Presented to California educators, legislators, and advocates. Answers, *1*, 1–8.

Lombardino, L. J. (1998). Unpublished manuscript. Gainesville, FL.

Lombardino, L. J., Lieberman, R. J., & Brown, J. C. (2005). *Assessment of literacy and language.* San Antonio, TX: Harcourt Assessment.

Lombardino, L. J., Ricco, C. A., Hynd, G., & Pinheiro, S. B. (1997). Linguistic deficits in children with reading disabilities. *American Journal of Speech-Language Pathology, 6*(3), 71–78.

Lovett, M. W. (1987). A development approach to reading disability: Accuracy and speed criteria of normal and deficient reading skill. *Child Development, 58*, 234–260.

Lyon, R. (1995). Toward a definition of dyslexia. *Annals of Dyslexia, 45*, 3–30.

Lyon, G. R., Shaywitz, S. E., & Shaywitz, B. A. (2003). A definition of dyslexia. *Annals of Dyslexia, 53*, 1–14.

Lyon, G. R., Fletcher, J. M., Shaywitz, S. E., Shaywitz, B. A., Torgesen, J. K., Wood, F., et al. (2001). Rethinking learning disabilities. In C. E. Finn Jr., A. J. Rotherham, and C. R. Hokanson Jr. (eds.), *Rethinking special education for a new century* (pp. 259–287). Washington, DC: Thomas B. Fordham Foundation. Retrieved from www.excellence.net/library/special ed/index.html.

Mann, V. A., Tobin, P., & Wilson, R. (1987). Measuring phonological awareness through the invented spellings of kindergarten children. *Merrill-Palmer Quarterly, 33*, 365–389.

Naremore, R. C., Densmore, A. E., & Harman, D. R. (1995). *Language intervention with school-age children: Conversation, narrative, and text.* San Diego, CA: Singular Publishing Group.

National Joint Committee on Learning Disabilities. (2005). *Responsiveness to intervention and learning disabilities.* Available from http://www.ldonline.org

Nelson, N. W. (1998). *Childhood language disorders in context: Infancy through adolescence.* New York: Merrill/Macmillan Publishing Company.

Nelson, N. W. (2010). *Language and literacy disorders: Infancy through adolescence.* Boston: Allyn & Bacon.

Newcomer, & Hammill (1988). *Test of language development-intermediate—2.* Austin, TX: Pro-Ed.

Newcomer, & Hammill (1997). *Test of language development-primary—3.* Austin, TX: Pro-Ed.

Owens, R. E. (2004). *Language disorders: A functional approach to assessment and intervention* (4th ed.). Boston: Allyn and Bacon.

Riccio, C. A., & Hynd, G. W. (1996). Neuroanatomical and neurophysiological aspects of dyslexia. *Topics in Language Disorders, 16*(2), 1–13.

Rosner, J. (1975). Rosner test of auditory analysis. In *Helping Children Overcome Learning Disabilities.* New York: Walker and Company.

Robertson, C., & Salter, W. (1995). *The phonological awareness test.* East Moline, IL: LinguiSystems.

Scarborough, H. S. (1990). Very early language deficits in dyslexic children. *Child Development, 61*, 1728–1743.

Scarborough, H. S. (2000, September). *Predictive and causal links between language and literacy development: Current knowledge and future directions.* Paper presented at the Workshop on Emergent and Early Literacy: Current Status and Research Directions, Rockville, MD.

Shaywitz, S. E. (2003). *Overcoming dyslexia: A new and complete science-based program of reading problems at any* level. New York: Alfred A. Knopf.

Shaywitz, S. E., Shaywitz, B. A., Pugh, I. R., Fulbright, R. K., Constable, R. T., Mencel. W. E., et al. (1998). Functional disruption in the organization of the brain for reading in dyslexia. *Neurobiology, 95,* 2636–2641.

Siegel, L. S. (1992). An evaluation of the discrepancy definition of dyslexia. *Journal of Learning Disabilities, 25,* 618–629.

Slingerland, B. (1977). *A multi-sensory approach to language arts for specific language disability children.* Cambridge, MA: Educators Publishing Service.

Stanovich, K. E. (1991). Discrepancy definitions of reading disability: Has intelligence led us astray? *Reading Research Quarterly, 26,* 1–29.

Tierney, R. J., & Cunningham, J. W. (1984). Research on teaching reading comprehension. In P. D. Pearson (ed.), *Handbook of reading research* (pp. 609–655). New York: Longman.

Torgesen, J. K. (1999). Assessment and instruction for phonemic awareness and word recognition skills. In H. W. Catts and A. G. Kamhi (eds.), *Language and reading disabilities.* Boston: Allyn and Bacon.

Torgesen, J. K., & Bryant, B. (1997). *The comprehensive test of phonological processes in reading.* Austin, TX: Pro-Ed.

Torgesen, J. K., & Wagner, R. K. (1997). *Test of word and nonword reading efficiency.* Austin, TX: Pro-Ed.

Vygotsky, L. (1978). *Mind in society: The development of higher psychological processes.* Cambridge, MA: Harvard University Press.

Wagner, R., Torgesen, J., & Rashotte, C. (1999). *Comprehensive test of phonological processing.* San Antonio, TX: The Psychological Corporation.

Wiederholt, J. L., & Bryant, B. R. (2001). *Gray oral reading tests* (4th ed.). Austin, TX: Pro-Ed.

Wiig, E. H., & Semel, E. (1984). *Language assessment and intervention for the learning disabled* (2nd ed.). New York: Merrill.

Wilkinson, J. S. (1995). *The wide range achievement test—3.* Wilmington, DE: Jastak Associates.

Wilson, B. (1988). *Wilson language training.* Millbury, MA: Author.

Wong, B. Y., & Jones, W. (1982). Increasing metacomprehension in learning disabled and normally achieving students through self-questioning training. *Learning Disability Quarterly, 5,* 228–240.

Woodcock, R. W. (1997). *Woodcock reading mastery test—rev.* Circle Pines, MN: American Guidance Service.

Woodcock, R. W., McGrew, K. S., & Mather, N. (2001). *Woodcock-Johnson tests of cognitive abilities—third edition.* Itasca, IL: Riverside Publishing.

Yopp, H. K. (1999). A test for assessing phonemic awareness in young children. *The Reading Teacher, 49,* 20–29.

Chapter 11

Attention Deficit Hyperactivity Disorder

LEARNING OBJECTIVES

After completion of this chapter, the reader will be able to:

1. Explain the relationship between attention deficit with hyperactivity disorder (ADHD) and language-based learning disabilities.

2. Explain some of the brain activities typically associated with the areas believed to be damaged in children with ADHD.

3. Explain the statement, "ADHD is not about paying attention; rather, it is about controlling attention."

4. Explain the role of cognition and processing in the assessment and treatment of ADHD.

5. Explain why achievement testing is considered part of the assessment process in children with ADHD.

6. Discuss how problems with focal and associative control can impact problem solving.

7. Describe the typical language skills of children with ADHD.

8. Explain the behaviors and symptoms associated with each of the seven types of control systems.

INTRODUCTION

Co-morbidity. The coexistence of one or more disorders.

Up until 1980, attention deficit hyperactivity disorder (ADHD) was known by a variety of terms such as Still's syndrome, Strauss syndrome, hyperkinetic syndrome, and hyperkinetic impulse syndrome. Grossly underdefined and overdiagnosed in the 1970s and 1980s, ADHD became a catch-all term used to describe children who had unruly and/or disruptive behaviors at home and in the classroom. In 1994, the *Diagnostic and Statistical Manual-IV* (American Psychiatric Association) described types of ADHD and a standard was set for definitive diagnosis. Since ADHD is not a language disorder, the reader may wonder why it is included in a book dedicated to language disorders. As is discussed later in this chapter, there is frequently co-morbidity of auditory processing disorders, reading and spelling disorders, and language and learning disabilities with ADHD. For that reason, it is important for speech-language pathologists and audiologists to understand the impact of ADHD on children and adolescents and how it can affect their academic and social performances.

WHAT IS ADHD?

ADHD is best defined in terms of what it is and what it is not. ADHD is not just a behavior management problem. It is not a learning disability, nor is it an auditory processing disorder. Most importantly, it is not a label to be randomly applied to any child who has trouble sitting still or paying attention. ADHD is a neurobehavioral disorder that typically begins in childhood and continues into adulthood. There are instances in which it has not been diagnosed until adolescence or even adulthood. Inattention, hyperactivity, and impulsivity are the elemental behaviors of ADHD. The National Institute of Mental Health (NIMH) (2009) pointed out that just about all children display these behaviors and attributes at some time. In order to be diagnosed with ADHD, the child must exhibit the symptoms in more than one setting for 6 or more months. According to NIMH and the American Psychiatric Association (1994), ADHD has three subtypes:

1. **Predominantly hyperactive-impulsive:** At least six symptoms are in the hyperactivity-impulsivity categories. No more than six symptoms of inattention are present, although some symptoms of inattention may be present.

2. **Predominantly inattentive:** At least six symptoms are in the inattention category and there are fewer than six symptoms of hyperactivity-impulsivity.

3. **Combined hyperactive-impulsive and inattentive:** The patient has six or more symptoms of inattention and six or more symptoms of hyperactivity-impulsivity. (www.nimh.nih.gov/health/publications/attention-deficit-hyperactivity-disorder/complete-index.shtml).

Most children who have ADHD have the combined hyperactive-impulsive and inattentive type. Children who have the predominantly inattentive type typically do not have problems getting along with their peers and are not as likely to act out, and for those reasons are often overlooked. Even though they are quiet and not a problem in the classroom, they are not focusing their attention and not attending to the tasks at hand (www.nimh.nih.gov/health/publications/attention-deficit-hyperactivity-disorder/complete-index.shtml). Problems with social status and peer acceptance are critical areas of concern about children with ADHD. Socialization is hindered by "intrusiveness and sometimes aggression resulting from hyperactivity and impulsiveness, coupled with inattentiveness to social cues" (Arnold, 2002, p. 18).

While attending to the task at hand and overactivity are the most frequently assigned symptoms of various forms of ADHD, Arnold (2002) wrote that impulsivity is the unifying symptom of all types of ADHD. He further notes that "patients with the disorder act before they think, react before they think, speak before they think, and even think before they think, jumping to conclusions prematurely" (p. 8). Arnold further stated that there is some preliminary evidence that ordinary activities are not as inherently rewarding for the child with ADHD as they are for the patient's peers. Thus, is appears that the symptom of impulsivity is the one that has the most impact on the individual's social status and acceptance by his or her peers.

> **think about it**
>
> Why should speech-language pathologists be knowledgeable about ADHD although it is not a language disorder?

INCIDENCE AND PREVALENCE OF ADHD

Prevalence estimates for ADHD range from 2 to 18 percent in various community samples of school-aged children. In 2003, the Centers for Disease Control and Prevention (CDC) conducted the National Survey of Children's Health, in which they concluded that approximately 8.8 percent of children aged 6 to 17 years in the United States had a diagnosis of ADHD (Pinborough-Zimmerman et al., 2007). The CDC (2007) also cited statistics from Pastor and Reuben's 2008 National Health Interview Survey in noting the following prevalence figures:

- Number of children 3–17 years of age ever diagnosed with ADHD: 4.5 million

- Percent of children 3–17 years of age ever diagnosed with ADHD: 7.2 percent

- Percent of boys 3–17 years of age ever diagnosed with ADHD: 10 percent

- Percent of girls 3–17 years of age ever diagnosed with ADHD: 4.3% (p. 7)

ADHD is twice as common in boys as in girls. However, it should be noted that between 1997 and 2006, there was a 4 percent increase in the number of girls diagnosed with ADHD, compared to a 2 percent increase in boys (Pastor & Reuben, 2008). The prevalence in adults is unknown. although in adults the sex ratio of identified ADHD is almost equal (Nelson, 1993; Arnold, 2002).

THREE CATEGORIES OF SYMPTOMS OF ADHD

There are three categories of symptoms of ADHD: control and regulation of attention, impulsivity, and activity (American Psychiatric Association, 1994). Following is a discussion of each of these categories.

Control and Regulation of Attention

In ADHD, controlling attention, rather than paying attention, is the problem. Paying attention implies the presence or absence of attention, or both; controlling attention refers to the ability to stay on task by focusing selectively on the appropriate stimuli. Everything is equally important to the child with ADHD, and he or she cannot isolate and focus on the important issues.

According to the National Institute of Mental Health (2009), children who have symptoms of inattention may:

- Be easily distracted, miss details, forget things, and frequently switch from one activity to another

- Have difficulty focusing on one thing

- Become bored with a task after only a few minutes, unless they are doing something enjoyable

- Have difficulty focusing attention on organizing and completing a task or learning something new

- Have trouble completing or turning in homework assignments, often losing things (e.g., pencils, toys, assignments) needed to complete tasks or activities

- Not seem to listen when spoken to

- Daydream, become easily confused, and move slowly

- Have difficulty processing information as quickly and accurately as others

- Struggle to follow instructions (NIMH, 2009)

The academic impact of being unable to focus attention is that the child cannot determine what the important facts and activities are and channel his or her attention accordingly. This also leads to free-flight associations and the answering of questions in an unexpected manner. Lack of focus also can be problematic for these children because when they know the answer, they are likely to burst out with the reply without following the traditional rules of raising their hands and waiting to be called on. In the time children with ADHD spend waiting to be called on, they will probably forget the answer. Therefore, in an attempt to answer correctly, they blurt out the answer without waiting.

With regard to social impact, the child who is labeled as having ADHD is often perceived as rude and uncaring by his or her peers. Because of the problems with associative control, he or she is likely to have pragmatic problems that interfere with being a good communication partner. These pragmatic problems include speaking out of turn, failing to maintain a topic, and switching topics inappropriately.

> *think about it*
>
> Explain the following statement: "ADHD is not about paying attention; it is about controlling attention."

Impulsivity

Impulsivity. Acting without premeditation, thought, or concern about consequences.

Impulsivity is defined as the neurological inability to sustain inhibition. Impulsivity, then, has no premeditation or malicious intent. The child does not think before acting. Behaviors "just happen" and the child usually is unable to explain why they occurred or demonstrate understanding of the consequences of the action.

Children who have symptoms of impulsivity may:

- Be very impatient

- Blurt out inappropriate comments, show their emotions without restraint, and act without regard for consequences

- Have difficulty waiting for things they want or waiting their turns in games

- Often interrupt conversations or others' activities (NIMH, 2009)

Academically, impulsivity results in the child's being disorganized in his or her overt academic activities and in his or her thought processes. Socially, impulsivity makes the child always want to be first—to always be the winner. Because of affective control problems, this child is likely to act out inappropriately when he or she loses, which, as with so many aspects of this disorder, affects the child's interaction with his or her peers. In fact, many children with ADHD are described by their parents as having no friends. Impulsivity also impacts negatively on the child's ability to delay gratification.

Activity

NIMH identified the following symptoms of ADHD in children who have symptoms of hyperactivity. These children may:

- Fidget and squirm in their seats

- Talk nonstop

- Dash around, touching or playing with anything and everything in sight

- Have trouble sitting still during dinner, school, and story time

- Be constantly in motion

- Have difficulty doing quiet tasks or activities (NIMH, 2009)

Some children with symptoms primarily in the inattentive category are underactive, and the ADHD may go undetected until fourth or fifth grade. At that time, their academic and social frustrations are likely to be expressed through behavior problems and failure to succeed in school. These children benefit from having teachers who are aware of possible warning signs of inattentive ADHD and who can monitor them as soon as any soft signs indicative of ADHD are noticed. These soft signs include not finishing school work, crying excessively, laughing excessively, not living up to their academic potential, and not having many friends.

In contrast, the child who is overactive may be labeled a "motor mouth" and described as fidgety and being unable to sit still. The child with the hyperactive and impulsivity components of ADHD is often identified much earlier than the child with just the inattentive signs because of the hyperactive component. However, it is important for the child to be tested carefully before the label of ADHD is applied. As stated previously, ADHD is not a label to be applied automatically to all children who have difficulty sitting still in school.

SEVEN FRAGILE CONTROL SYSTEMS

For a child to attend to a task, he or she must develop internal control and organization, much as was discussed in Chapter 2 in the section on babies born to mothers who are drug abusers. Twelve control systems have been documented, but this discussion is limited to seven systems.

A major problem for children with ADHD is focal control. Focal control is the ability to select what is important and attend to that over all other distractions and information (Heyer, n.d.). For example, in a traditional classroom, noises include paper shuffling, pencils tapping, and students moving around. Children with ADHD cannot focus their attention on what is important (i.e., the teacher's talking) and tune out the insignificant noises. Also, when they do pay attention to the correct stimulus, it is likely that, as the teacher is talking, they do not attend to what the teacher is saying even though it may be important. That is to say, everything is of equal importance to the child with ADHD.

As a result of poor focal control, the child has to work hard at concentrating on what is being said in the classroom. This effort is called mental effort control. Because it takes so much mental effort to focus on what is important, many children with ADHD experience mental fatigue. Then the tiredness, coupled with the lack of focal control, compounds the child's difficulties in learning in the classroom (Heyer, n.d.).

A third control system that poses problems for the child with ADHD is associative control. Associative control is what enables people to maintain a conversation by stating issues that are relevant to the conversation (Heyer, n.d.). A child with ADHD has free-flight ideas during conversational exchanges, with these free-flight ideas being tangential to the content and intent of the conversation.

Focal control. The ability to select what is important and attend to that over all other distractions and information.

Mental effort control. Work at concentrating, resulting in mental fatigue when excess energy is expended on focal control.

Associative control. Control that enables a person to maintain a conversation by stating issues that are relevant to the conversation.

TABLE 11–1 Conversation with a child with deficits in associative control*

T: I really like your red fingernail polish. Who painted them for you?

C: Mom

T: Your mom fixed your fingernails. Were you playing dress up?

C: We had pizza for supper.

T: You had pizza for supper. Was it good?

C: My grandmother has a garden with tomatoes in it.

T: Did your grandmother eat pizza with you?

C: No, she has a garden with tomatoes and she waters the garden. She lives at the river.

T: Your grandmother lives on the river. That must be fun.

C: My grandpa has a boat and we took swim lessons.

*T, therapist; C, child.
Source: Delmar/Cengage Learning

Table 11–1 contains a transcript of a conversation with a child with ADHD. The conversation started with the clinician asking the child about her red fingernail polish. As can be seen from the transcript, most of what the child said was somewhat related to the color red, but each contribution to the conversation was a tangential thought. We can see the tangential relationships with the red possibly reminding her of the tomato sauce on the pizza and the sauce reminding her of the tomatoes in her grandmother's garden. Similarly, watering the garden reminded her of the river, and the river is associated with the boat and swimming lessons. However, the original conversation, which was to be about the fingernail polish, never developed.

Children who have problems with associative control are also likely to answer questions correctly, but not as expected. For example, if the child is asked, "What is your name?" the child is likely to say, "The same as my mother's," which may be correct but is not what is expected in the way of an answer.

The fourth type of control is called appetite control, but it does not have anything to do with eating! Rather, appetite control is the ability to delay gratification, which is difficult for individuals with ADHD.

Delayed gratification refers to the ability to continue providing the correct and expected behaviors even when a delay exists between the response and the provision of reinforcement. Children with ADHD expect immediate reinforcement, which can be problematic in the classroom. Many times, children with appetite control problems are considered noncompliant because they have difficulty following rules when gratification is not offered immediately (Heyer, n.d.). Problems with peers also may develop because the child with ADHD may not be able to meet behavioral criteria that have been set for the class to receive positive reinforcement. For example, a

Appetite control. The ability to delay gratification, which is typically problematic for children with ADHD.

Delayed gratification. The ability to continue providing the correct and expected behaviors even when a delay exists between the response and the provision of reinforcement.

teacher may say that the class will have a party on Friday if all the students complete their work in a timely manner on Wednesday and Thursday. The child with ADHD may not be able to complete the work, and furthermore, he or she may not be able to delay the gratification for 2 days if the work is complete. Thus, the party is at risk for his or her classmates, with the child with ADHD becoming a culprit if he or she does not complete the work in the specified time period.

Behavior control is another control system that creates difficulty for children with ADHD. A child with ADHD may be totally impulsive (Cantwell & Baker, 1992; Heyer, n.d.; Lahey et al., 1987). This, again, is due to a lack of organization of the central nervous system, particularly the parts of the nervous system that control impulsivity.

Behavior control. Impulsive behavior due to a poorly organized central nervous system.

Complicating the issue is the fact that many children with ADHD cannot predict the consequences of their actions (Heyer, n.d.). Thus, telling a child he or she should not perform a certain behavior because of the resultant negative reactions may be futile, which makes implementing behavior management techniques very difficult. ADHD is not diagnosed solely on the basis of behavior management problems. Due to the other symptoms of ADHD, such as impulsivity, poor quality control, and poor internal control systems, the use of traditional behavior management techniques often is ineffective with these individuals.

A sixth type of control issue for children with ADHD is affective control. Many of these children have inappropriate affect; they laugh too much and cry too much (Heyer, n.d.; Weintraub & Mesulam, 1983).

Affective control. Inappropriate affect and expression of emotions.

When a joke is told or something funny happens in class, the child is likely to laugh out of proportion to the silliness or to laugh inappropriately at incidental behaviors. Likewise, when something sad or disappointing occurs, the child is likely to cry uncontrollably. A fifth-grade boy who was in therapy at the University of Florida Speech and Hearing Clinic had particular difficulty with uncontrollable crying when he became frustrated with the task. Compounding the problem for him was his embarrassment at crying in front of the student clinician. Therefore, a system was worked out whereby he would put his head down on the table when he was going to cry, the student clinician would excuse herself, and the supervisor would help the child work through his frustration. Eventually, the crying subsided and he was able to deal with his frustrations in a positive manner with the student clinician.

The final control system to be discussed in the context of ADHD is quality control, which refers to a person's ability to provide an explanation for his or her own actions.

Quality control. A person's ability to provide an explanation for his or her own actions.

Many children with ADHD cannot explain their actions, particularly those that occur impulsively. Frequently reminding a child of the potential consequences of his or her behavior is ineffective because the child cannot predict the consequences of that behavior. Also, children with ADHD often cannot control their behavior, so it becomes difficult for them to explain why they behaved in a particular way (Heyer, n.d.). For example, the child with ADHD typically likes to be first at everything, including lining up. If another child gets in front of him or her, he or she is likely to push the other child. When asked why he or she pushed the other child, the child with ADHD most likely responds with, "I don't know—I just did it." These kinds of responses are very frustrating for parents and teachers to hear, but the truth is that the child truly does not know why he or she pushed the other child because it was an impulsive, not a planned, action.

It is easy to see how problems with these seven control systems can interfere significantly with the academic and social progression of a child with ADHD. They also lead to labeling and mislabeling.

WHAT CAUSES ADHD?

Although it is difficult to pinpoint one cause of ADHD, there are several factors under consideration as being causative. For example, there is some evidence to suggest that a mother who smokes or drinks during her pregnancy will have a child with increased risk of inattention and hyperactivity. Some children who suffer from a traumatic brain injury or other neurological events may also show signs of ADHD (Barkley, 2000). This is particularly true in instances in which the brain injury occurs in the frontal lobe, which regulates many of the behaviors and executive functions that are typically problematic for individuals with ADHD.

Although most children who have signs of ADHD do not have a history of significant brain injuries, one cannot help but be struck by the fact that for many children with ADHD there is a history of pregnancy and/or birth complications. However, not all children who have a history of pregnancy and/or birth complications develop ADHD. In fact, less than 10 percent of children with ADHD have any history of brain injury; disruptions in the development of the brain, particularly the frontal cortex, seem to be a more likely explanation (Barkley, 2000). According to Arnold (2002), there is a high incidence of genetic predisposition in most cases of ADHD. Problems associated with two dopamine genes (the DAT1 dopamine transporter gene and the D4 dopamine receptor gene) have been noted in many cases of ADHD. Clinical evidence of the involvement of these genes is supported by the fact that individuals who have ADHD and are treated with drugs to enhance the neurotransmission of dopamine typically show some resolution or lessening of the symptoms (Arnold, 2002).

ADHD is an inability to maintain focused, selected attention. It is thought to be related to disruptions in transmission and metabolism along subcortical pathways connecting the midbrain to the prefrontal cortex. These are the areas of the brain that play roles in executive functioning tasks such as directing attention, self-regulation, organizing information, making and executing an action plan, and inhibiting inappropriate actions. These skills are problematic in children with ADHD and frequently lead to a misdiagnosis of the child as being lazy, unmotivated, and/or disruptive.

THE RELATIONSHIP OF ADHD TO LANGUAGE AND LEARNING DISABILITIES

The relationship of ADHD to language disorders and learning disabilities in children is receiving much attention in the literature. While any clear-cut relationship between the two disorders is disputable, one cannot ignore that some children have a co-morbidity of language-based learning disabilities, auditory processing disorders, reading disorders, and ADHD. In fact, it is estimated that 20 to 30 percent of children with confirmed ADHD "have at least one type of learning disability in math, reading, or spelling" (Barkley, 2000, p. 98). Mayes, Calhoun, and Crowell (2000) reported a higher percentage of co-morbidity between ADHD and learning disabilities, finding that 70 percent of those with ADHD also had a learning disability, with learning disabilities in written expression language (65%) being twice as common as a learning disability in reading, writing, or spelling. Conversely, they also found that, in a population of 73 children with a learning disability, 82.2 percent also had ADHD. In comparing groups of children with ADHD only, learning disability (LD) only, and ADHD and LD, they made the following observations:

- Those with LD and ADHD have more severe learning problems than those children with LD without ADHD.

- Those with LD and ADHD have more severe attention problems than those children with ADHD without LD.

- Children with ADHD without LD still have learning problems.

- Children with LD without ADHD still have "some degree of attention problems" (p. 417)

Mayes, Calhoun, and Crowell (2000) suggested, based on these observations, that "learning and attention problems are on a continuum, are interrelated, and usually coexist" (p. 417). They were particularly interested in studying the coexistence of written expression language disorders. Using scores for 86 children diagnosed with ADHD on the written expression subtest of the Weschler Individual Achievement Test (WIAT), which assesses compositional writing (ideas and development, organization, vocabulary, sentence structure, grammar, capitalization, and punctuation). Mayes and colleagues found that 65.1 percent of the children with ADHD had a learning disability in written expression. Compare this to the other types of learning disabilities found in the 86 children:

- 26.7 percent had a learning disability in basic reading (19.8%) or reading comprehension (19.8%).

- 31.4 percent had a learning disability in numerical operations.

- 30.2 percent had a learning disability in spelling.

- 68.9 percent had a learning disability in one or more areas.

With regard to reading disorders and ADHD co-occurrence, it should be noted that ADHD does not cause the reading problem; rather, they are two separate problems, each with their own causative agents (Catts & Kamhi, 1999). ADHD may impact reading, particularly silent reading comprehension, but, again, the ADHD is not the cause of the reading problem (Shaywitz et al., 1995). Shaywitz, Shaywitz, Fletcher, and colleagues (1996) found that learning disability and ADHD are separate disorders, but both are symptomatic for executive impairments and processing impairments. They went on to say that reading disabilities and ADHD have a combination of symptoms that are seen in each separate disorder, so that there may be an association between the two diagnoses through a combination of factors.

Pastor and Reuben's (2008) survey yielded the following prevalence figures (2004–2006) on ADHD and LD:

- Approximately 4.7 percent of children 6 to 17 years of age had ADHD without LD, 4.9 percent had LD without ADHD, and 3.7 percent had both conditions.

- Older children, 12 to 17 years of age, were more likely than younger children, 6 to 11 years of age, to have each of the diagnoses (ADHD without LD, LD without ADHD, and both conditions).

- Among children 6 to 11 years of age, no significant change was found in the percentage of children with ADHD. However, among children 12 to 17 years of age, an average annual increase of 4 percent occurred in the number of children with ADHD.

- Boys were more likely to have each of the diagnoses (ADHD without LD, LD without ADHD, and both conditions).

- Boys (6.7%) were more than twice as likely as girls (2.5%) to have ADHD without LD.

- Boys (5.1%) were about twice as likely as girls (2.3%) to have both conditions.

- Boys (5.6%) were about one-third more likely than girls (4.3%) to have LD without ADHD (p. 3).

It is unclear why boys are diagnosed with ADHD, LD, or both conditions more frequently than girls. One possible explanation for the disparity between boys and girls is that boys have disruptive behaviors, especially in school, more frequently than girls (Pastor & Reuben, 2008).

Rutter, Tizard, and Whitmore (1970) studied the presence of learning, neurological, and psychiatric disorders in a group of children on the Isle of Wight and found that children who had "overt behavior disorders" had significant learning problems, particularly in the area of reading. Twenty-five percent of the children in their study who had reading disabilities also had a psychiatric behavioral disorder such as ADHD or oppositional disorders. The effects of ADHD on language and learning can clearly make an impact on a child's academic and social success in school.

Learning differences also exist between the two groups (the ADHD group and the learning- and/or language-disabled group). According to Arnold (2002), 20 to 25 percent of children who have ADHD also have learning disorders. Children with ADHD show higher co-morbidity of learning disabilities and more underachievement, particularly in mathematics. They are also slower on rapid naming tasks than are children with ADHD only (Cantwell & Baker, 1992; Edelbrock, Costello, & Kessler, 1984; Hynd et al., 1991; Lahey et al., 1984; Lahey et al., 1987). In a study reported by Barkley (2000), it was found that children with ADHD "performed much worse on tests involving perceptual-motor speed or eye-hand coordination and speed. They also made more mistakes on a memory test. In particular, they had more trouble consistently recalling information they had learned as time passed" (pp. 137–138). Lazar and Frank (1998) compared the performance of three different groups (ADHD plus LD, LD only, and ADHD only) on tasks of problem solving, working memory, and attention-inhibition cueing. They found that the ADHD plus LD group and the LD-only group both did worse than the ADHD-only group.

Thus, while the exact relationship between ADHD and various types of learning disabilities remains unclear, there is indisputable evidence that they frequently co-occur, often sharing many of the same signs and symptoms yet maintaining enough unique characteristics that they are more likely being seen as co-morbid disorders than a single disorder. Grizenko, Bhat, Schwartz, Ter-Stepanian, and Joober (2006) maintained that, based on a review of the literature, the underlying neurocognitive mechanisms of learning disabilities and ADHD are different, but "it has been suggested that children with ADHD and learning disabilities may have a common frontal lobe dysfunction" (p. 47).

---

think about it

As a speech-language pathologist, you provide therapy for a 14-year-old boy who has reading and spelling deficits. He also has ADHD, and he comes for therapy for a 1-hour session at 3:30 three days a week (he gets out of school at 3:00). You believe he is not progressing because of the complications of ADHD and seeing him after a long day at school. What would you tell him and his parents?

ADHD AND OTHER LABELS

Hyperkinetic. Having persistent and exaggerated motor movements.

Children with ADHD historically were labeled as having hyperactive child syndrome, as being hyperkinetic, or as having minimal brain dysfunction. As explained previously, children with ADHD have many features in common with children who are learning disabled; in fact, in many children with ADHD, learning disabilities coexist (Hynd et al., 1991). Regardless of whether a child is learning disabled or has ADHD, multiple professions are involved in diagnosing and treating the child. The participation of more than one professional in diagnosis is often due to the fact that the child with ADHD typically presents a multiplicity of problems. The child's impulsivity may be misinterpreted as a behavior management problem. Problems with affective control and delayed gratification can be mislabeled as immaturity and/or noncompliance. Therefore, many negative labels can be applied to a child who is not properly diagnosed as having ADHD and can lead to disruption in the child's home and academic life.

In addition, as with learning disabilities, ADHD has complex effects on families. The parents are frequently called to the school because the child is not living up to the expectations of the academic system. It should be pointed out that some children with ADHD can be so retiring that they "blend into the wallpaper" and are mislabeled as overly shy (Edelbrock, Costello, and Kessler, 1984; Hynd et al., 1991). However, these children also suffer socially and academically because of the same types of problems demonstrated in children in whom the ADHD is more overt. The "wallpaper children" are often found to have only a few friends and to be at risk academically even though they are not "troublemakers," which is how many children with ADHD are labeled. Parents are confused as to why the child does not try harder or why the child continues to misbehave in the presence of negative consequences of the misbehaviors. Some parents feel embarrassed because their child causes a problem in the classroom, and others are ashamed because their child is not living up to the expectations of the teacher or performing at a level appropriate to his or her age, education, and family background. Thus, the time prior to the diagnosis of ADHD can be more frustrating for families than knowing the child's diagnosis. As upsetting as the diagnosis of ADHD can be, the definitive diagnosis at least offers an explanation for the child's academic and/or social difficulties. The diagnosis also opens the door to the implementation of appropriate treatment protocols.

Uncertainties regarding the cause and prognosis of ADHD can also have a debilitating effect on families. The parents tend to blame themselves or each other, which can produce tension in a home that is, most likely, already experiencing a high level of stress because of the child's difficulties. Fear about the future can also create emotional turmoil in the families. It is absolutely critical that families receive adequate counseling regarding ADHD so that they have an understanding of the symptoms of the disorder and learn methods of managing the ADHD.

Parent support groups can be helpful. In one parent support group meeting, several parents complained that the worst part of the day was the time between when the child woke up and when he or she walked out the door to go to school. Frequently, there were delays in getting dressed and the child forgot to brush his or her teeth, getting halfway to school only to realize that something (lunch, homework, and coat) had been left at home. The parents shared strategies that they had found helpful, and they all benefited from this type of sharing. One parent recorded morning instructions for her child on a digital recorder. The child was able to listen to the recorder with its constant reminders regarding what he should be doing guiding him through the morning activities. Both parents found it much easier to provide the constant reminders via the recorder than it was to keep going to the child's room to remind him of what he was supposed to be doing. Another mother made a checklist that hung in the child's room. Once everything was checked off, the child went to the kitchen for breakfast and then checked another list by the front door to be sure he had done all he was supposed to do and that he had everything he was supposed to take to school.

It is important to keep the lines of communication open between the families, the school personnel, and any other professionals who may be providing therapy for the child. When a strategy is found that is effective with a child, everyone involved should share in its implementation to ensure consistency in how the child's problems are handled in different settings. This consistency is essential in developing the internal control that many children with ADHD lack.

ADOLESCENTS WITH ADHD

Children and adolescents who have ADHD need guidance in understanding how they process information and how they should participate in social and academic settings. Impulsivity is a frustrating component of ADHD, and students with impulsivity should work closely with an adult (teacher, counselor, parent, etc.) who can help them understand the nature of their impulsivity and how it interferes with learning and social interactions.

These students should receive instruction in problem solving, working with others, and understanding themselves as participants in academic situations (Tattershall, 2002). Rutter, Tizard, and Whitmore (1970) did a study to document co-morbidity of psychiatric, neurological, and learning disorders. They found that 25 percent of the children who had reading problems also had either ADHD or oppositional disorders.

Students who do not have hyperactivity need some of the same direction that is provided for students with hyperactivity, particularly in the areas of problem solving and understanding themselves and the nature of ADHD. They should receive counseling about how to self-monitor their attention and what to do when attentional problems interfere with their social and academic progress. Teachers, counselors, and parents should be sure the adolescent understands the nature of ADHD and its impact on learning.

Adolescents with ADHD are likely to have problems with pragmatics. Heyer (1995) found that the use of language for social purposes (i.e., pragmatics) is the most significant language deficit found in children with ADHD. Children with ADHD have difficulty with "self-talk," a critical need in learning to self-mediate one's social behaviors. They also have difficulty responding to questions, with their responses often not related to the question (although possibly in some tangential way). The children with ADHD often have difficulty following the rules of a conversation with regard to turn taking, not interrupting, maintaining a topic, and switching a topic.

Children and adolescents with ADHD need instruction in the rules that govern how to be a communication partner. Tattershall (2002) suggested that the adolescents collect and report anecdotes about communication exchanges in which they believed they were successful and in which they felt unsuccessful. Sharing these anecdotes with an adult can help the student analyze his or her strengths and weaknesses in social conversations and academic settings. Likewise, the adolescents can observe communication exchanges among their peers, analyze them (including via role play), and adopt strategies that were effective in the conversations. Larson and McKinley (1987) made the point that language therapy for adolescents (with or without ADHD) should focus primarily on pragmatics, with semantics, syntax, and phonology being addressed under the umbrella of pragmatics. Teenagers need to learn survival language and be able to relate to their peers in order to succeed socially and academically.

DIAGNOSING ADHD

The diagnosis of ADHD in a child requires the input of a diagnostic team made up of psychiatrists, psychologists, educators, audiologists, and speech-language pathologists. Newhoff (1986, 1990) supported the participation of speech-language pathologists on the team due to the co-morbidity previously mentioned. Psychiatrists should be involved in the diagnosis of ADHD because many of these children receive medications to help control the symptoms, and as many as 45 percent of children who are diagnosed with ADHD also have another psychiatric problem such as depression, anxiety, and/or low self-esteem. Psychologists are involved in the diagnosis through the administration of tests such as the Weschler Intelligence Scale for Children—Revised (Weschler, 1974). Reasearchers have found that while children with ADHD earn scaled scores of 10 to 13 on most subtests, they typically score 6 or 7 on those subtests that relied on selective attention (digit span, arithmetic, coding, and mazes) (Newhoff, 1986). Educators and parents can provide information on the child's behavior and attitudes that may result from ADHD and are observed in the child's natural settings.

Objectives of the Evaluation

The child who comes to the speech-language pathologist is probably being seen to determine if a language-based learning disability is present. Therefore, the evaluation of the child by the speech-language pathologist is exclusionary. That is, the speech-language pathologist is trying to determine whether the child's academic and social problems are due to the presence of a language-based learning disability. If no language-based learning disability is present, the clinician can make observations based on the child's performance in the evaluation session that can help to confirm or reject a possible diagnosis of ADHD.

As with all other evaluations, the first question to be asked of the referral source is, "What do you want me to answer as a result of this evaluation?" If the answer is, "I want to know if this child has ADHD," it is necessary to explain to the parent or referral source that you, as the speech-language pathologist, are not able to make the definitive diagnosis of ADHD. What you can do is determine if the child has a language-based learning disability and analyze the child's learning style and behaviors to see if signs and symptoms of ADHD are present. If necessary, appropriate referrals can then be made to other professionals, such as educators, psychologists, and psychiatrists, who should be involved in the treatment of ADHD. Similarly, an audiologist can be consulted to provide testing to rule out or prove the existence of an auditory processing disorder.

A second objective is to provide a baseline from which to monitor progress and judge the effectiveness of treatment. This also involves identifying the child's strengths that can be utilized to enhance his or her performance in academic and social settings.

A third objective is to determine the child's eligibility for school services. As stated in Chapter 8, to qualify for special education services in the schools, the child's condition frequently must be labeled. Therefore, the question of whether the child's disorder should be labeled needs to be studied from a fiscal, an emotional, and an academic perspective. Fiscally, if the child qualifies for a special education service, the funding is different than it would be for a regular education student who is not receiving any special education services. Emotionally, it can be devastating to a parent, and to the child, to have the condition labeled as ADHD. After a staffing conference in which her child was identified as having ADHD and placed into some special education services, a mother said, "You know, I have been trying to convince his teachers! But, to sit here and hear three professionals from different disciplines say that my child has ADHD was very hard. I wanted to stop the labeling, even though I know he needs this extra help to succeed in school."

Similar to describing the strengths the child has, the evaluation process should also describe deficits needing management. To minimize the stigmatization of the student, careful consideration needs to be given to determine what management strategies can be incorporated into the classroom to help the child be more successful academically and socially. Also, if the child is to be removed from class ("pulled out"), this needs to be scheduled carefully so that the child does not miss the same academic subjects every time he or she goes to a therapy session outside of the classroom.

Eight Diagnostic Focus Areas

When evaluating a child to determine whether he or she has ADHD, it is important to address eight diagnostic categories to have a complete picture of the child's status with regard to possible ADHD, academic achievement, and social aptitude.

Cognition

The first category is cognition. As discussed in Chapter 13 cognition is assessed using multimodality testing. This means that the subtests are varied in terms of stimulus input (auditory or visual) and response modality (oral, written, or gestural). What is critical is to determine the modalities through which the child best responds to the provision of information, then to capitalize on that information to design the child's academic program. For example, the same young man who had problems with affective control had tremendous difficulty on spelling tests. He was punished at home for poor spelling grades, and his classmates made fun of him for his low grades on spelling tests (the students graded each other's papers). In therapy, it was determined that he spelled much better orally than he did when he had to write his answers. Therefore, the clinician approached the teacher and asked whether the child could take his spelling tests orally in the future. The teacher agreed to a trial run, and over the next 4 weeks the child's spelling grade improved from an F to a B. More important than the grade was the change in the child's self-esteem. Further explanation of this child's spelling difficulties can be found in the case history at the end of this chapter.

Processing

Processing. How the child handles information that is presented to him or her visually and aurally.

Processing is the second category that needs to be assessed. Processing determines how the child handles information that is presented to him or her visually and aurally.

Children can have normal vision and hearing but have a breakdown in the neurological connections that permit them to process and understand the information that is presented. Just as with cognition, it is important to determine whether the child processes better when information is presented visually or aurally. Then, if necessary, teaching strategies can be modified to accommodate the child's best learning modalities, which may in turn assist him or her in using focal control. Audiologists should provide an assessment of auditory processing abilities in any child who is being evaluated for ADHD. It could be that some of the child's behaviors (such as poor academic performance and not following directions) are due to an auditory processing disorder, not ADHD. It could be that the child has both.

Achievement

The assessment of achievement is particularly important when the child has already completed 2 or more years of school. Achievement testing enables the clinician to determine what the child has learned, or achieved, during his or her academic career. Achievement testing is often done annually in schools but is also frequently done by school psychologists when a child's academic performance is a cause for concern.

Language

Language testing should include a variety of skills, such as those outlined in Table 11–2. Problem-solving skills require higher-level cognitive skills that are frequently associated with the development of metalinguistic, metacognitive, and metapragmatic skills. In other words, the child needs to know how to analyze language and develop sequenced plans of action to solve problems. Because of problems with focal and associative control, problem solving is usually a source of difficulty for children with ADHD.

Socially, children with ADHD usually have poor pragmatic skills. They typically do not respond to environmental cues that serve as regulators for pragmatic interactions with other individuals. They frequently ignore social rules, which further impedes their social adaptations and can result in lowered self-esteem owing to the lack of friends. Therefore, it is important to assess the child's pragmatic skills, looking at subareas such as topic maintenance and topic switching.

Involving the child in a story-telling scheme is a critical part of the diagnosis of language problems that may be contributing to academic problems associated with ADHD. Metanarrative skills are of particular concern.

> **Metanarrative skills.** The ability to analyze stories, extract appropriate details from a story, and comprehend a story.

TABLE 11–2 Areas of focus in language testing for children suspected of having ADHD

Problem-solving skills

Auditory skills

Visual skills

Sequencing

Pragmatic skills

Extracting detail

Story schema

Associative responses

Topic maintenance

Topic switching

Source: Delmar/Cengage Learning

Special attention should be paid to how well the child extracts detail from a story, primarily because of the problems children with ADHD have with focal control. It is also important to help the child stay focused on the story and to minimize the tangential remarks that may occur owing to problems with associative control. Finally, the clinician should look at the child's ability to hypothesize about what is going to happen as the story progresses.

Attention

Many people believe that having ADHD means that the child cannot pay attention. However, it is controlling attention, not paying attention, that is problematic for children with ADHD. Therefore, the child's abilities with regard to focal and associative control need to be assessed carefully to determine if the child can control his or her attention sufficiently to benefit from traditional academic instruction (Heyer, n.d.).

Behavior

As mentioned earlier, ADHD is not a behavior management problem *per se*. It does, however, present challenges to traditional methods of behavior management that are employed to address some of the child's behaviors. Classroom observations, teacher feedback, and parental reports are critical in assessing the behavior of children with ADHD. All must work together to develop a plan of action that enables the child to succeed academically and socially without frustrating the child in his or her efforts to participate in classroom lessons and social interactions.

Medical Factors

Psychostimulants. Medications that have antidepressant effects and stimulate the production of dopamine, which acts on the frontal lobe to improve executive functions.

Children who have a hyperactive component frequently benefit from the use of psychostimulants. In fact, one way it is known that ADHD is related to central nervous system dysfunction is the fact that the children with this disorder typically respond positively to the use of psychostimulants to help control their ability to maintain appropriate attending skills. Therefore, it is mandatory for teachers, parents, and any specialists working with the child to make careful, controlled observations of the child's behavior to determine whether the medicine is having a positive effect on the child. The child also needs to be monitored to be sure the levels of medication are not so high that the child is too sedated to respond appropriately in the academic setting.

Social and Environmental Interaction

As with the medical aspects of the evaluation, it is important to have multidisciplinary and parental reports on the child's social interactions. Many children with ADHD are considered class clowns or viewed as loners. Either way, it is likely that the child has negative social interactions with most of his or her peers. This can lead to lowered self-esteem and elevated levels of depression in the child with ADHD. The social and environmental interactions of the child need ongoing monitoring, with appropriate intervention to prevent additional problems related to poor self-esteem and/or depression.

TREATMENT OF ADHD

Arnold (2002) delineated three goals that should be addressed when developing the initial treatment plan for an individual with ADHD.

1. Give the patient and family the necessary information. Explain the nature of the disorder and expected effects of the prescribed medication, including "side effects, the expected duration of treatment, possible alternatives, and the targets of treatment" (pp. 107–108).

2. Facilitate acceptance of the plan and future compliance. Debunk misinformation the family may have, and cite scientific evidence.

3. Optimize the placebo effect (for some patients, just knowing the prescription is available can lead to improvement of symptoms).

Placebo effect. An inactive treatment that has a suggestive effect on the individual's symptomology.

In addition, the speech-language pathologist should bear in mind the role of language in a cognitive-behavioral treatment paradigm, which is frequently employed when providing intervention for children with ADHD. According to Vail (1987), children need a combination of four factors in order to focus their attention: arousal, a filter, language, and appropriate work. The child's attention is alerted and made ready through arousal of the cognitive system. Then a filter that eliminates internal and external distractions is activated in order to focus his or her attention. The child's thought processes are focused on and organized using language. Language enables the child to task analyze, categorize, and sort ideas, to prioritize, and to acknowledge cause and effect. The child's work level must be monitored for difficulty in order to be sure that lack of attention is the problem instead of tasks that are too difficult or inappropriate (Nelson, 2010).

Four Areas of Management of ADHD

Academic

In the classroom, teachers rely on students being able to attend to what is being taught. Therefore, teaching students to pay attention, sustain attention, and process information as it is presented is critical to learning. For most children, this is learned through incidental teaching as teachers make comments like, "I like the way you are listening." However, for many children with learning disabilities and/or ADHD, learning to control attention becomes almost a subject in and of itself. This is particularly true for the children who have ADHD.

If a child is unable to attend in class, his or her schoolwork will fall behind and the child may face adverse ramifications in terms of academic and social progress. As stated in Chapter 8, poor academic and social adjustment often lead to low self-esteem in school-age children, particularly in the late elementary and middle school years. Therefore, it is even more critical that these children be afforded instruction that focuses on developing their ability to learn internal control and organization so that they can attend to the task at hand in academic and social settings.

Academically, it is important to provide structure for the child both in the classroom and at home when doing homework. Likewise, the teacher and homework helpers should individualize the interaction, working through the modalities that are the most successful for individual children. Also, structuring the environment so that the child can complete his or her assignments is critical. Fifty percent of children with ADHD fail their courses due to productivity problems. That is to say, they fail because they do not complete their work. One strategy that has been employed successfully by some teachers is to break the assignments into smaller units. For example, if the students are to complete 20 mathematics problems, the assignment could be divided into four sets of five problems for the child with ADHD. After completing the first set, the child could turn them into the teacher and pick up the next set. The same types of strategies should be employed across the academic spectrum because most children with ADHD have decreased achievement in reading, spelling, and written language.

Cantwell and Baker (1985) studied the cognitive styles of children with ADHD and noted that these children demonstrate a cognitive impulsivity in addition to the behavioral impulsivity commonly associated with ADHD. These children make decisions quickly without filtering through all the relevant information. Children with ADHD are often gifted, which makes one question the idea that children with ADHD may be cognitively impaired. Rather, they do not manage their knowledge in an appropriate and systematic manner. They are nonreflective about the information at hand, which leads to quick decisions that are sometimes incorrect or inappropriate (Nelson, 1993).

Memory Deficits It is also important to focus on memory deficits when working with children with ADHD. Table 11–3 delineates the different areas of attention that are usually deficient in children with ADHD and that contribute to memory problems.

Selective attention and its effects on memory are similar to focal control. When presented with a myriad of stimuli, the child cannot attend to what is important (Heyer, n.d.).

Focused attention requires that the child complete an activity, usually under a time constraint (Heyer, n.d.). This is important because the child may have difficulty accessing his or her memory bank to "call up" the information needed to complete a task. For example, a child who is taking a test on a story that has been read to the class may have trouble remembering the important information in the story in time to complete the test. Teachers often report that a child with ADHD seems to daydream at times when attention should be focused on a specific classroom task. The student in Figure 11–1 demonstrates this behavior.

Selective attention. The attention needed to focus on what is important among myriad stimuli.

Focused attention. The requirement that a child complete an activity, usually under a time constraint.

TABLE 11–3   Memory deficits in children with ADHD

Selective attention	Focusing on what is important amid myriad stimuli
Focused attention	Having a specific activity that must be done, usually under a time constraint
Sustained attention	Similar to focused attention but a little less time restricted
Divided attention	Determining how much attention should be given to each activity
Vigilance	Completing the whole task without falling behind; needed to develop a memory bank

Source: Adapted from *Programming for children with attention deficit disorders,* by J. L. Heyer, n.d. West Lafayette, IN: Purdue Research Foundation.

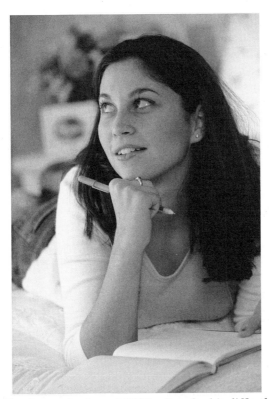

FIGURE 11–1   Students who have ADHD often find it difficult to remain focused on the task at hand, tending to daydream or be distracted by other events in the environment. (*Source: Delmar/Cengage Learning*)

Sustained attention. The ability to remain on task, but without the time constraints of focused attention.

Divided attention. Determining how much attention to give to each activity.

Vigilance. The attention skills needed to develop and use a memory bank.

Sustained attention is somewhat similar to focused attention, but in this case the child does not complete the task because he or she cannot stay focused on the task, rather than having difficulty recalling the important information.

Divided attention is a problem for the child with ADHD because he or she cannot decide how much attention to give to each activity (Heyer, n.d.). Problems with divided attention interfere with the ability to multitask. For example, most children in third grade have homework in two or three subject areas per night. The child with ADHD has difficulty determining how much time to allot to each subject so that all of the assignments are completed.

Vigilance is important because it underlies the development of a memory bank. The child has a poor memory bank because he or she cannot stay focused enough on the information at hand in order to store it (Heyer, n.d.).

For example, the young man who had difficulty with written spelling tests had trouble with vigilance. In fact, being unable to complete written spelling tests is a classic example of difficulty with vigilance. An example would be if a child is busy writing word number three when the teacher calls out word number four. By the time the teacher gets to word number five, the child has fallen behind and cannot remember the words that have been called out. Consequently, these children fail to complete the spelling test because they have trouble refocusing and recalling the words that have been called out by the teacher.

As a rule, vigilance, divided attention, and sustained attention are the attention factors that create the biggest memory deficits in children with ADHD (Heyer, n.d.). Therefore, many children with these disorders do better on self-paced tasks cut into small units than they do on timed tasks. Other treatment strategies are suggested in Table 11–4.

TABLE 11–4 Treatment strategies to use with children who have ADHD

Provide a consistent routine across all environments.

Break assignments down into smaller groups (e.g., five mathematic problems at one time instead of 20).

Give simple, single instructions or directions.

Prepare for changes.

Strengthen the strengths as much as address the weaknesses.

Maximize function and circumvent or minimize the weaknesses.

Source: Delmar/Cengage Learning

Behavioral

As stated previously, ADHD is not just a behavior management problem. However, the behavior of the affected children is problematic. The first step in remediation of some of the behavioral issues is to make sure the child knows that he or she is responsible for his or her own behavior. This is a time-consuming task, but it is nonetheless absolutely critical. It requires addressing each of the control and attention areas and developing strategies that can be used to foster their development.

Behavioral treatment can be direct, via behavior modification using a cognitive-behavioral approach, or indirect, via training through parent and teacher education. Promoting communication between school and home is critical and can be accomplished through daily checklists. Setting clearly defined rules and procedures can be of benefit to the child as well, as long as the rules are consistently enforced at home and at school, as well as in any other settings in which the child is a participant. Typical behavior management strategies can be adopted, including a token economy system, time out, and response cost systems (Arnold, 2002).

> **Behavior modification.** The implementation of an intervention plan to change, modify, or correct an individual's behavior.

Medical

Drugs make the central nervous system more accessible to learning. They help with the activity level, the impulsivity, and the attention, but they do not increase knowledge. They do increase the parent–child and teacher–child interaction time and quality, so an increase in positive responses to learning becomes a benefit of the medication.

Frequently some confusion occurs when a physician says he or she is going to treat hyperactivity by prescribing a psychostimulant. The stimulants do not stimulate behavior directly. Rather, they stimulate neurotransmitters to increase the production of dopamine, which in turn improves the control and attention devices the child has at his or her disposal. The fact that children with ADHD respond to the psychostimulants lends support to the belief that biological factors underlie the disorder (Nelson, 1993). It is also important to note that the drugs are psychologically, not physiologically, addictive. In other words, the child may think he or she needs the drugs when they no longer are needed, but this is not a physiological craving in the way that drugs such as nicotine are.

The most common medication used for treating the hyperactivity component of ADHD is Ritalin (methylphenidate), which has been used since 1956. Side effects of Ritalin and other stimulants are difficult to document owing to the fact that children taking it suffer from a wide variety of conditions and treatments. Side effects are limited primarily to loss of appetite and some trouble sleeping. These side effects frequently are dosage related, meaning they can be alleviated by adjusting the dosage. Grizenko, Bhat, Schwartz, Ter-Stepanian, & Joober (2006) studied the response to methylphenidate of 95 children (aged 6–12 years) diagnosed with ADHD only and children with both ADHD and learning disabilities (LD). They looked at both of these groups because, even though the neurocognitive mechanisms of LD and ADHD are different, a review of the research indicates that both groups may have "a common frontal lobe dysfunction" (Grizenko et al, 2006, p. 47). Grizenko and colleagues found that 75 percent of the students who had ADHD only (i.e., no LD) had a positive response (i.e., reduction in symptoms) to the methylphenidate, while only 55 percent of those with ADHD and LD responded to the drug. They conducted further analyses and found differences depending on the type of learning disabilities (math disability and/or reading disability).

Methylphenidate appears to have an effect on executive functions in children with ADHD only. Several studies have shown that children with ADHD and math disabilities are particularly vulnerable because both of these deficits involve problems in the areas of the brain that manage executive function (i.e., the frontal lobe) (Grizenko et al., 2006). This could be one explanation as to why there is less response to treatment by methylphenidate in children with ADHD and a math disability than in the other groups (ADHD only or ADHD with a reading deficit only).

Adderall, Concerta (also a commercial name for methylphenidate), and Dexedrine Spansule are also used to treat symptoms of ADHD. The advantage to these drugs is that they do not have to be given during school hours (Arnold, 2002). In recent years even more drugs have become available including Vyvanse, Focalin, Focalin XR, and Daytrana. All of the drugs mentioned so far are stimulants that stimulate the production of the neurotransmitter dopamine. Strattera (atomoxetine) is a nonstimulant that boosts the levels of norepinephrin, which is also a neurotransmitter. It is the only nonstimulant approved for the treatment of ADHD (www.rxlist.com/script/main/art.asp?articlekey=104501&page=6#some). Regardless of whether or not the physician chooses to use pharmacological agents to control hyperactivity in children with ADHD, it is important to remember that it is parents, not pills, that make children mind.

Social

The fourth area of management is the social aspect of dealing with ADHD. As stated previously, many children with ADHD are perceived as rude and uncaring, so these issues need to be addressed. The children also need to be taught how to deal with their emotions appropriately. The psychologist is the most likely person to work with these particular aspects. In addition, the teacher might explain ADHD to the whole class in an effort to ease some of the confusion regarding the disorder. It is also critical to monitor the social status of the child with ADHD because of the inclination to poor self-esteem and depression, particularly among older children. Behavior therapy should be provided to help children analyze the situations in which they find themselves and to practice problem solving as it relates to personal and academic problems. The use of positive reinforcement is critical, and timing is important. Remember that delayed gratification is difficult for children with ADHD, so frequent use of positive reinforcement is essential. The use of behavior management, particularly positive reinforcement, is admittedly difficult because children with ADHD tend to elicit primarily punitive responses from teachers, parents, and peers. This often results in inconsistent attempts at behavior management, with increases in depression and delinquency.

SUMMARY

ADHD is a multifaceted disorder that can have profound effects on the academic and social growth of school-age children. The speech-language pathologist plays a key role in the diagnosis of ADHD by providing language and cognitive testing that can either rule out a learning disability or establish the possibility that the learning disability may coexist with the diagnosis of ADHD. Family members and all professionals who are involved in the education and therapy process should work together to develop a consistent plan of interaction to maximize the opportunity for the child with ADHD to find success in his or her academic and social growth.

CASE STUDY

History

Paul is an 11-year-old boy who was referred to the speech and hearing clinic for evaluation due to poor performance in school. He lives at home with his parents, both of whom are in their late 40s. He has an older brother who is attending a technical school in another state. Paul is in the process of repeating fourth grade due to poor performance on a statewide assessment test and general academic difficulties. He is receiving speech-language therapy at his school for 1 hour a week in a group of five children. According to his parents, Paul has always been an active child who frequently gets in trouble at home and at school. He does not have any friends at school or at home. He cries with frustration almost every night when working on homework and has difficulty organizing his assignments and remaining focused enough to be able to complete the assignments. His father is functionally illiterate.

(continues)

CASE STUDY *(continued)*

Evaluation

On the Peabody Picture Vocabulary Test, Paul scored in the 83rd percentile. The Test of Language Development–Intermediate was administered with the following results:

Subtest	Raw Score	Percentile	Standard Score
Sentence Combining	11	9	6
Characteristics	38	37	9
Word Ordering	9	5	5
Generals	7	2	4
Grammatic Comprehension	6	9	6

Composite scores were as follows:

	SC	CH	WO	G	GC	Sum of Std. Scores	Quotients
Spoken Language (SLQ)	6	9	5	4	6	30	73
Listening (LiQ)		9			6	15	85
Speaking (SpQ)	6		5	4		15	68
Semantics (SeQ)		9		4		13	79
Syntax (SyQ)	6		5		6	17	72

Paul's profile is a jagged line, which is often indicative of learning disabilities. He showed relative strengths in characteristics, and his biggest weaknesses were generals and word ordering.

	Strengths	Weaknesses
Communicative	Lexicon	Written spelling
	Decoding skills	Syntax and morphology
	General knowledge	Pragmatics
		Reading comprehension
		Poor attending skills
		Narrative writing and story development
		Short-term memory

	Strengths	Weaknesses
Non-communicative	Cooperates in therapy	ADHD
	Responds to behavior management techniques	Home environment not intellectually stimulating
	Relative strength in mathematics	Poor handwriting
		Frustrated by school work

Therapy

When Paul began therapy, we initially focused on his reading comprehension and spelling skills, as well as attending skills and short-term memory. We also addressed writing narratives. His decoding skills were within normal limits, but apparently this did not translate into his spelling when taking a spelling test. His comprehension of short paragraphs was good, but broke down with longer readings.

Paul is in a class in school where they have a spelling test every Friday, and he typically fails these tests. It does not appear so much a matter of not being able to spell as it is not being able to keep up as the teacher goes through the spelling list. This is a source of embarrassment for him. When therapy started, Paul did not like to write and his handwriting was at times illegible. He did not understand punctuation and thus omitted it entirely in his written assignments. He had a relative strength in mathematics, making low Bs to high Cs on most math assignments.

Paul did not have vigilance, which is frequently a problem area for children who have ADHD when it comes to spelling tests. Paul would hear the first spelling word spoken by the teacher, but by the time she had

gotten to the third word he was just finishing up writing the first word and was hopelessly lost and behind. Over the course of therapy, it was discovered that Paul could spell words more accurately when he could spell them orally than when he had to write them. We contacted his teacher to see if he could take his tests orally before or after school and she agreed. His scores went from an F to a B on the spelling tests. We also worked on handwriting skills and referred him to an occupational therapist for help in this area.

Paul loved to concoct stories, some fictional and some fabricated. For example, he frequently spoke of letters he had received from his brother. When the clinician remarked to Paul's mother that the letters from his brother meant a lot to Paul, Paul's mom said his brother had not written any letters to Paul and rarely interacted with him when he was home.

Paul was a sports enthusiast, and this was usually the focus of his stories. An example of his written stories before intervention is depicted on the next page. Notice the fact that there is no punctuation, several words are illegible (hence a translation is printed below the story), and there is no true introduction, elaboration, or conclusion to the story:

(continues)

CASE STUDY *(continued)*

> *my trip to ther footBall Game oF*
> *me anD may pan wint to a fuotBall Gam*
> *It wiss tan somach fan tf it tuck*
> *we Juse goi ter in time so we*
> *watch it wase fun*
> *and it wass so mach*
> *fun it wane and I sod a fuot*
> *Ball gqiv skor a 100 AD*
> *tougireaper shan wathuse*
> *he hes hand oo hurt so he*
> *luft the Game*
> *theny*
>
> *I wint to ney Bas Bali Plan*
> *and about Bull aier and astonote*
> *I wio Ba cacact anD ILmt to Bee on*
> *the Araves tim*

Writing Sample from an 11-Year-Old Boy with ADHD and Language-Based Learning Disabilities

Translation (punctuation added): My Trip to the Football Game.

Me and my dad went to a football game. It was fun so much fun it took we just got there in time so we watch it was fun and it was so much fun it won and I saw a football player score a 100 touchdown. Shane Matthews his hand got hurt so he left the game. The end.

I want to be a baseball player and a football player and astronaut. I want be a catcher and I want to be on the Braves team.

After four months of intervention, Paul wrote the following story.

> once up a time ther woss a mane
> namD Bill ray he haD a moter-
> sikle anD He hao amoxer sikle
> anD it cuas namD ak
> Harley DaribSon anD he coDe
> Go so fast it couD Go 295 MHP.
> qnD so he Bou a noue moteni
> sikle haDe Harler pariDson
> anD he Gao me a riDe on heis
> noe motnsikre he wint nell
> fast he rick 300 MAP anD
> I wase "skarD'] cha
> aente AnD I sull a sqyrei
> and lust of tree's
> Becuse he tockme on q riDe
> on a moter Citle rov rov
>
> the EnD

Writing Sample from an 11-Year-Old Boy with ADHD and Language-Based Learning Disabilities After 4 Months of Intervention.

Notice the addition of periods at the end of each line (he defined a sentence as a line of words) and more cohesion within the story. There is a distinct beginning, development, and conclusion to the story, in comparison to his previous stories.

Translation (punctuation added): Once upon a time there was a man named Bill Ray. He had a motorcycle and he had a motorcycle and it was named a Harley Davidson and he could go so fast. It could go 295 miles hour per and so he bought a new motorcycle named Harley Davidson and he gave me a ride on his new motorcycle. He went real fast. He reached 300 mhp and I was "scared"! And I saw a squirrel and lots of trees. Because he took me on a ride on a motorcycle. Rev Rev. The End

Notice that this story has an introduction, an elaboration, and a conclusion. There is more elaboration and cohesion within the story. It is more legible and has fewer spelling

(continues)

errors. He still has not mastered the science of punctuation. When asked what a sentence is, Paul said it was a line of words with a dot at the end. He took this quite literally as indicated by the column of dots down the right side of the page (after each line of words).

It should also be noted that we referred Paul to a local psychiatrist for evaluation of possible ADHD and consideration of medication. The psychiatrist confirmed our suspicions and prescribed Ritalin, which Paul took each morning before school and each afternoon after school. It has been reported that sometimes the handwriting of children with ADHD improves when they are placed on Ritalin. This is because these drugs act on the frontal lobe, and this may account for the improvement in handwriting we saw in the second story above.

Conclusion

Paul was dismissed from therapy when the family moved out of state. He was able to move on to the fifth grade, and while he was not an academic star, he consistently made Bs and Cs. His written assignments were more organized and legible. His short-term memory improved and he made some friends, which is critical for an early adolescent.

REVIEW QUESTIONS

1. Which of the following groups represents behaviors and skills that are typically problematic language behaviors for children diagnosed as having ADHD?
   a. Poor problem-solving skills, good auditory skills, good sequencing skills, poor pragmatic skills
   b. Fair problem-solving skills, poor auditory skills, poor sequencing skills, poor pragmatic skills
   c. Good problem-solving skills, poor auditory skills, poor sequencing skills, fair pragmatic skills
   d. Poor problem-solving skills, poor auditory skills, poor sequencing skills, poor pragmatic skills

2. Which of the following represent the areas of management of children with ADHD?
   a. Academic, behavioral, medical
   b. Academic, behavioral, medical, social
   c. Academic, medical, social
   d. Behavioral, medical, social

3. ADHD is just a learning disability.
   a. True
   b. False

4. Medications for ADHD are physiologically addictive.
    a. True
    b. False

5. Attention needed to complete a specific activity, usually under a time constraint, is
    a. Selective attention
    b. Sustained attention
    c. Focused attention
    d. Vigilance

6. Memory needed to sufficiently focus on information to develop a memory bank is
    a. Selective attention
    b. Focused attention
    c. Divided attention
    d. Vigilance

7. Difficulty with the _____ control system results in the child with ADHD having difficulty with delaying gratification.
    a. Appetite
    b. Affective
    c. Associative
    d. Mental effort

8. Inability to select what is important is due to problems with which control system?
    a. Quality
    b. Associative
    c. Focal
    d. Mental effort

9. ADHD is one of several causes of reading disabilities.
    a. True
    b. False

10. Which of the following statements is not true?
    a. There appears to be no genetic basis for ADHD.
    b. Problems with dopamine receptors are common in ADHD.
    c. Disruptions in the development of the frontal cortex seem to occur in many children with ADHD.
    d. Both a and b.
    e. Both b and c.
    f. Both a and c.

REFERENCES

American Psychiatric Association. (1994). *Diagnostic and statistical manual of mental disorders.* Washington, DC: American Psychiatric Association.

Arnold, L. E. (2002). *Contemporary diagnosis and management of attention-deficit/hyperactivity disorder* (2nd ed.). Newtown, PA: Handbooks in Health Care Co.

Barkley, R. A. (2000). *Taking charge of ADHD—revised edition.* New York: The Guilford Press.

Cantwell, D. P., & Baker, L. (1985). Interrelationships of communication, learning, and psychiatric disorders in children. In C. S. Simon (ed.), *Communication skills and classroom success: Assessment of language-learning disabled students* (pp. 43–61). Austin, TX: Pro-Ed.

Cantwell, D. P. & Baker, L. (1992). Issues in the classification of child and adolescent psychopathology. *Journal of the American Academy of Child Adolescence, 27,* 532–533.

Catts, H. W., & Kamhi, A. G. (1999). *Language and reading disabilities.* Boston: Allyn & Bacon.

Centers for Disease Control. (2007). *Attention deficit hyperactivity disorder (ADHD).* Retrieved July 9, 2009 from www.cdc.gov/nchs/fastats/adhd.htm.

Edelbrook, C., Costello, A. J., & Kessler, M. D. (1984). Empirical collaboration of attention deficit disorder. *Journal of the American Academy of Child Psychiatry, 23,* 285–290.

Grizenko, N., Bhat, M., Schwartz, G., Ter-Stepanian, M., & Joober, R. (2006). Efficacy of methylphenidate in children with attention-deficit hyperactivity disorder and learning disabilities: A randomized crossover trial. *Journal of Psychiatry and Neuroscience, 31*(1), 46–51.

Heyer, J. L. (n.d.). *Programming for children with attention deficit disorders.* Purdue University Continuing Education. West Lafayette, IN: Purdue Research Foundation.

Heyer, J. L. (1995). The responsibilities of speech-language pathologists toward children with ADHD. *Seminars in Speech and Language, 16,* 275–288.

Hynd, G. W., Lorys, A. R., Semrud-Clikeman, M., Nieves, N., Huettner, M. I. S., & Lahey, B. B. (1991). Attention deficit disorder without hyperactivity (ADD/WO): A distinct behavioral and neurocognitive syndrome. *Journal of Child Neurology, 6,* 37–43.

Lahey, B. B., Schaughency, E. A., Hynd, G. W., Carlson, C. L., & Nieves, N. (1987). Attention deficit disorder with and without hyperactivity: Comparison of behavioral characteristics of clinic-referred children. *Journal of the American Academy of Child and Adolescent Psychiatry, 26,* 718–723.

Lahey, B. B., Schaughency, E. A., Strauss, C. C., & Frame, C. L. (1984). Are attention deficit disorders with and without hyperactivity similar or dissimilar disorders? *Journal of the American Academy of Child Psychiatry, 23,* 302–309.

Larson, V. L., & McKinley, N. (1987). *Communication assessment and intervention strategies for adolescents.* Eau Claire, WI: Thinking Publications.

Lazar, J. W., & Frank, Y. (1998). Frontal systems dysfunction in children with attention-deficit hyperactivity disorder and learning disabilities. *Journal of Neuropsychiatry and Clinical Neuroscience, 10,* 160–167.

Mayes, S. D., Calhoun, S., & Crowell, E. W. (2000, September). Learning disabilities and ADHD: Overlapping spectrum disorders. *Journal of Learning Disabilities, 33*(5), 417–424.

National Institute of Mental Health. (2009). Retrieved March 10, 2010 from www.nimh.nih.gov/health/publications/attention-deficit-hyperactivity-disorder/complete-index.shtml.

Nelson, N. W. (1993). *Childhood language disorders in context: Infancy through adolescence.* New York: Macmillan Publishing Company.

Nelson, N. W. (2010). Childhood language disorders in context: Infancy through adolescence. New York: Macmillan Publishing Company.

Newhoff, M. (1986). Attentional deficit—What it is, what it is not. *The Clinical Connection* (Fall), 10–11.

Newhoff, M. (1990). Attention deficit hyperactivity disorder: Defining our role. *The Clinical Connection* (1st Quarter), 10–12.

Pastor, P. N., & Reuben, C. A. (2008, July). Diagnosed attention deficit hyperactivity disorder and learning disability: United States 2004–2006. National Center for Health Statistics. *Vital Health Statistics, 10*(237). Retrieved February 13, 2010 from www.cdc.gov/nchs/data/series/sr_10/Sr10-237.pdf.

Pinborough-Zimmerman, J., Satterfield, R., Miller, J., Bilder, D., Hossain, S., & McMahon, W. (2007, November). Communication disorders: Prevalence and comorbid intellectual disability, autism, and emotional/behavioral disorders. *American Journal of Speech-Language Pathology, 16*(4), 359–367.

Rutter, M., Tizard, J., & Whitmore, K. (eds.). (1970). *Education, health, and behavior.* London: Longmans Green.

Shaywitz, B. A., Fletcher, J. M., Holahan, J. M., Shneider, A. E., Marchione, K. E., Stuebing, K. K., et al. (1995). Interrelationships between reading disability and attention-deficit/hyperactivity disorder. *Cognitive Neuropsychology, 1,* 170–186.

Shaywitz, S. E., Shaywitz, B. A., Fletcher, J. M., et al. (2006). Prevalence of reading disability in boys and girls: Results of the Connecticut longitudinal study. *Journal of the American Medical Association, 264,* 98–1001.

Tattarshall, S. (2002). *Adolescents with language and learning needs: A shoulder to shoulder collaboration.* Clifton Park, NY: Delmar, Cengage Learning.

Vail, P. L. (1987). *Smart kids with school problems: Things to know and ways to help.* New York: E. P. Dutton.

Weintraub, S., & Mesulam, M. M. (1983). Developmental learning disabilities of the right hemisphere: Emotional, interpersonal, and cognitive components. *Archives of Neurology, 40,* 463–468.

Weschler, D. (1974). *Weschler intelligence scale for children—revised.* San Antonio, TX: Psychological Corporation.

www.rxlist.com/script/main/art.asp?articlekey=104501&page=6#some, retrieved Februay 13, 2010.

Chapter 12

Language and Communication Deficits Associated with Acquired Brain Injury in Children

LEARNING OBJECTIVES

After completion of this chapter, the reader will be able to:

1. Define *acquired brain injury* and *traumatic brain injury* (TBI).

2. Discuss problems a clinician would expect to see in individuals who have sustained a mild TBI, a moderate TBI, and a severe TBI.

3. Discuss the causes and characteristics of head injuries associated with different age groups (pediatric and adult).

4. Discuss, list, and briefly describe the three categories of symptoms associated with TBI.

5. Discuss a minimum of five language functions within the umbrella term *executive functions*.

6. Define *impairment, disability,* and *handicap* as explained by the World Health Organization.

7. Describe the language differences in diagnosis and treatment between children with TBI and adults with TBI.

8. Discuss what professionals should be involved in the multidisciplinary assessment and treatment of children with TBI and describe the roles of each.

INTRODUCTION

This chapter focuses on acquired brain injury, with an emphasis on traumatic brain injury. According to the Brain Injury Association of America,

> an acquired brain injury commonly results in a change in neuronal activity, which effects [sic] the physical integrity, the metabolic activity, or the functional ability of the cell. An acquired brain injury may result in mild, moderate, or severe impairments in one or more areas, including cognition, speech-language communication; memory; attention and concentration; reasoning; abstract thinking; physical functions; psychosocial behavior; and information processing. (1997) (www.biausa.org/education. htm#anoxic).

They define traumatic brain injury as

> an insult to the brain, not of a degenerative or congenital nature but caused by an external physical force, that may produce

a diminished or altered state of consciousness, which results in an impairment of cognitive abilities or physical functioning. It can also result in the disturbance of behavioral or emotional functioning. These impairments may be either temporary or permanent and cause partial or total functional disability or psychosocial maladjustment. (1986) (www.biausa.org/education.htm#anoxic).

An average of 66 to 82 percent of all head injuries are classified as mild. It is estimated that there are 1.4 million instances of head injury annually in the United States. Of those 1.4 million, 50,000 die, 235,000 are hospitalized, and 1.1 million are treated and released from an emergency department. There is no way to estimate the number of unreported and untreated head injuries. Among children aged birth to 14 years, there are 2,685 deaths, 37,000 hospitalizations, and 435,000 visits to an emergency department annually (Langolis, Rutland-Brown, & Thomas, 2004). Appendix 12A list ways in which head injuries can be reduced in the home environment.

Males are twice as likely to sustain a head injury as are females. The age ranges with the highest risks are the birth-to-4-years-old population and teenagers aged 15 to 19 years. Adults aged 75 years and older have the highest rate of hospitalization and death due to traumatic brain injury, and African Americans have the highest death rate (Langolis, Rutland-Brown, & Thomas, 2004). African Americans and Native Alaskans have the highest rate of hospitalization due to TBI (Langolis, Kegler, Butler, et al., 2003).

Researchers at the Centers for Disease Control and Prevention estimated that a little more than 2 percent of the population of the United States, or 5.3 million Americans, have a lifelong or long-term need for assistance in performing activities of daily living as a result of a TBI (Thurman, Alverson, Dunn, Guerrero, & Sniezek, 1999). Individuals who sustain a TBI and survive can have a variety of speech and language disorders, including (but not limited to) voice, motor speech, articulation, cognitive, word-retrieval, executive function, and pragmatic deficits. In addition, they may have neurological or physical damage resulting in dysphagia, which is another area in which the speech-language pathologists can assist these individuals.

The next section presents the definition of traumatic brain injury.

DEFINING TRAUMATIC BRAIN INJURY (TBI)

Kay and the Mild Traumatic Brain Injury Committee of the Head Injury Special Interest Group of the American Congress of Rehabilitation Medicine (1993) have defined traumatic brain injury as follows:

Traumatically induced physiological disruption of brain function, as manifested by *at least one* of the following:

1. any period of loss of consciousness

2. any loss of memory for events immediately before or after the accident

3. any alteration in mental state at the time of the accidents (e.g., feeling dazed, disoriented, or confused)

4. focal neurological deficit(s) that may or may not be transient; but where [sic] the severity of the injury does not exceed the following:

    • loss of consciousness for approximately 30 minutes or less;

    • after 30 minutes, an initial Glasgow Coma Scale (GCS) of 11–15; and

    • post-traumatic amnesia (PTA) no greater than 24 hours.

The definition by Kay and colleagues incorporates diagnostic criteria, thereby making it more functional than the definition by the Brain Injury Association of America.

The Individuals with Disabilities Education Act (IDEA), which is the federal law that defines the rights of children with disabilities in the public schools, defines TBI as follows:

An acquired injury to the brain caused by an external physical force, resulting in total or partial functional disability or psychosocial impairment, or both, that adversely affect a child's educational performance. The term applies to open and closed head injuries resulting in impairments in one or more areas, such as: cognition; language; memory; attention; reasoning; abstract thinking; judgment; problem-solving; sensory, perceptual, and motor abilities; psychosocial behavior; physical functions; information processing; and speech. The term does not apply to brain injuries that are congenital or degenerative, or brain injuries induced by birth trauma. (*U.S. Federal Register, 57*[189], p. 44802, 1992)

It is important that IDEA designates TBI as a diagnostic category because it makes children with head injury eligible for services in the public schools. IDEA calls for the reintegration of children with traumatic brain injury into the classroom. Teachers of students with TBI report that language disabilities are the factors that cause the greatest interference with success in school, so the designation of TBI as a diagnostic category in IDEA has significant implications for speech-language pathologists in the schools. According to ASHA, 5,775,722 children aged 6 to 21 years with disabilities were served in the schools under IDEA Part B in the 2000–2001 school year. Of those children, 14,884 received therapy for communication and learning problems resulting from TBI (Castrogiovanni, 2010).

UNDERLYING COMPLICATIONS

Cognitive and language deficits due to TBI are rarely related to a single factor. Many secondary mechanisms exist that can create complications after the immediate injury. For example, the child may have seizure activity. In fact, many children with head injuries are placed on seizure medications as a prophylactic measure to minimize or prevent the occurrence of seizures. Swelling of the brain tissues also may be present. In closed-head injuries, in which tissue swells, a tight cavity is created between the brain and the cranium, leaving no place for the excess fluid. Therefore, the intracranial pressure increases and results in a decline in the child's status. Hypoxia (lack of oxygen), hemorrhage, and the development of blood clots can also contribute to increased damage following the actual accident.

Secondary damage may occur after a TBI and may also affect the degree of impairment experienced by the child. One example of secondary damage is cerebral edema, which can contribute to increased intracranial pressure. Cerebral edema is the "accumulation of fluid between the brain and skull, within the ventricles, or within the brain lesion" (Ylvisaker, Szekeres, & Feeney, 2001, p. 748). The edema may be limited to the area of the brain around the injury site or be present throughout the brain. Intracranial pressure is due to accumulation of cerebrospinal fluid, water, or blood within the skull. The fluid accumulation can compress or displace brain tissue.

Another type of secondary damage is hemorrhage. There are two types of hemorrhage: intracerebral, in which blood in the brain tissue causes diffuse axonal injury, and extracerebral, in which there is bleeding into the meninges.

Seizures, yet another type of secondary damage, may occur within 1 week post injury (early onset), or after the first week (late onset). Finally, hypoxic-ischemic damage may occur as a result of reduced oxygen and blood supply to the brain. This can be due to cardiopulmonary deficits, an increase in intracranial pressure, or cerebral vasospasms. In addition, critical areas of the brain such as the hippocampus may suffer further damage from pathological neurotransmitter surges (Ylvisaker, Szekeres, & Feeney, 2001).

A summary of the primary and secondary mechanisms associated with the different types of brain trauma is found in Figures 12–1 and 12–2.

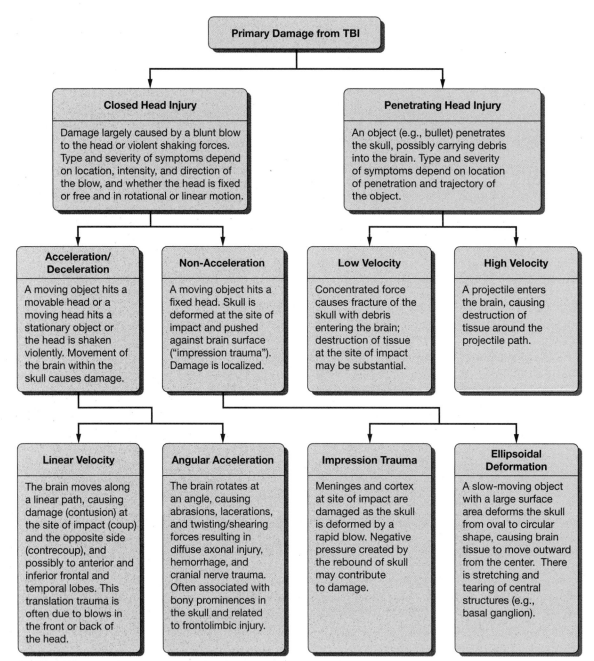

FIGURE 12–1 Mechanisms of immediate injury in closed and open traumatic brain injury.

(*Source:* Communication disorders associated with traumatic brain injury, by Mark Ylvisaker, Shirley F. Szekeres, and Timothy Feeney. In *Language intervention strategies in aphasia and related neurogenic communication disorders* (5th ed.), edited by R. Chapey. Philadelphia: Lippincott Williams & Wilkins. Copyright 2009 by Lippincott Williams & Wilkins. Reprinted with permission. http://lww.com.)

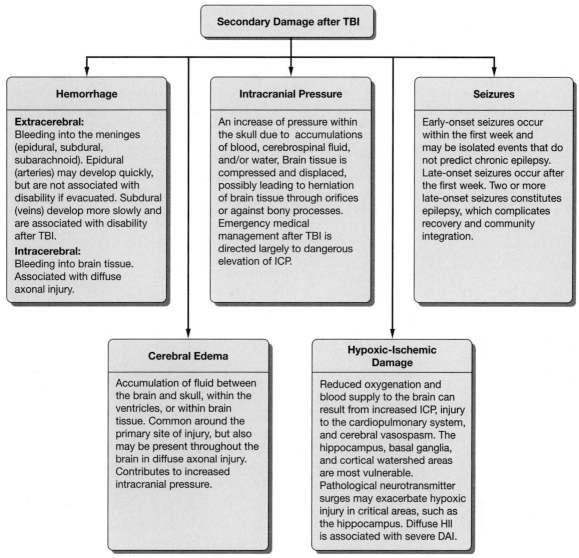

FIGURE 12–2   Pathologic events that often follow severe TBI and contribute to impairment.
(*Source:* Communication disorders associated with traumatic brain injury, by M. Ylvisaker, S. Szkeres, and T. Feeney. In *Language intervention strategies in aphasia and related neurogenic communication disorders* (4th ed.), edited by R. Chapey. Philadelphia: Lippincott Williams & Wilkins. Copyright 2001 by Lippincott Williams & Wilkins. Reprinted with permission. http://lww.com.)

INITIAL EFFECTS OF TBI

A frequent initial effect of TBI is coma. Confusion and posttraumatic amnesia (PTA) are also frequently observed immediately after the injury. In mild injuries commonly associated with a concussion, a loss of consciousness occurs that lasts less than 30 minutes and PTA lasts less than 1 hour. An injury is regarded as moderate if a loss of consciousness or PTA is present for more than 30 minutes but less than 24 hours. In severe cases, the coma lasts for more than 6 hours and the PTA lasts for 1 to 7 days. In very severe cases, the PTA lasts for more than 7 days (Russell, 1993). The status of the child on the Glasgow Coma Scale (see Table 12–1) and the length of the PTA can be predictors of how the child will do with regard to recovering language and cognitive functions. However, in the pediatric population, this needs to be interpreted with much caution as the Glasgow Coma Scale was developed for use with adults.

The child may also have retrograde amnesia, which is difficulty remembering events leading up to the accident. Abnormal behaviors such

> **Retrograde amnesia.** A common sequela of traumatic brain injury that creates difficulty in remembering events that led up to the accident.

TABLE 12–1   Glasgow Coma Scale

Eye opening (E)	
spontaneous	4
to speech	3
to pain	2
nil	1
Best motor response (M)	
obeys	6
localizes	5
withdraws	4
abnormal flexion	3
extensor response	2
nil	1
Verbal response (V)	
oriented	5
confused conversation	4
inappropriate words	3
incomprehensible sounds	2
nil	1

Coma Score (E + M + V) = 3–15

11–15: Mild brain injury

9–12: Moderate brain injury

3–8: Severe brain injury

Source: From *Management of head injuries,* by B. Jennett and G. Teasdale, 1981, p. 78. By permission of Oxford University Press.

as irritability, aggression, anxiety, hyperactivity, lethargy, and withdrawal may also be observed in the period immediately after the injury. Motor dysfunctions such as rigidity, tremor, spasticity, ataxia, and apraxia may also be observed.

Apraxia. A neurological deficit in the cortex that hinders one's ability to make voluntary motor movements even when the muscles function normally.

CAUSES OF BRAIN INJURY IN CHILDREN

According to the Brain Injury Association of America, acquired brain injury can occur as a result of

- Airway obstruction;

- Near-drowning, throat swelling, choking, strangulation, crush injuries to the chest;

- Electrical shock or lightening strike;

- Trauma to the head and/or neck;

- Traumatic brain injury with or without skull fracture, blood loss from open wounds, artery impingement from forceful impact, shock;

- Vascular Disruption;

- Heart attack, stroke, arteriovenous malformation (AVM), aneurysm, intracranial surgery;

- Infectious disease, intracranial tumors, metabolic disorders;

- Meningitis, certain venereal diseases, AIDS, insect-carried diseases, brain tumors, hypo/hyperglycemia, hepatic encephalopathy, uremic encephalopathy, seizure disorders;

- Toxic exposure-poisonous chemicals and gases, such as carbon monoxide poisoning. (www.biausa.org/education.htm#anoxic).

Traumatic brain injury is the result of an external force, such as a direct blow to the head, impacting "the head hard enough to cause the brain to move within the skull or if the force causes the skull to break and directly hurts the brain" (www.biausa.org/education.htm#anoxic). The most common causes of direct force injuries are motor vehicle accidents, firearms, falls, and being struck with an object. Sports injuries also fall in this last category.

A rapid acceleration and deceleration of the head can force the brain to move back and forth across the inside of the skull. The stress from the rapid movements pulls apart nerve fibers and causes damage to brain tissue (www.biausa.org/education.htm#anoxic). Vehicle accidents, particularly rollovers, and physical violence can result in these types of injuries. This is also the type of injury associated with shaken baby syndrome, which is discussed in the following section. In the infant and toddler age range, most head injuries are due to falls or abuse. In the older preschool population, the most common cause of injuries is falling. Elementary school–age children are most likely to acquire head injuries as a result of sports, bike accidents, skateboarding accidents, pedestrian accidents, or accidents in which they are passengers in a car. Adolescents are more likely to suffer head injuries as a result of car crashes, usually at high speeds (Reed, 2005).

Shaken Baby Syndrome

The American Academy of Pediatrics (AAP) prefers use of the term abusive head trauma (AHT) to describe head (and brain) injuries in children due to inflicted injuries, which includes shaken baby syndrome (SBS), injuries due to blunt impact, and injuries due to a combination of blunt impact and shaking. Their reasoning for expanding the term (from *shaken baby syndrome* to *abusive head trauma*) was to "broaden the terminology to account for the multitude of primary and secondary injuries that result from abusive head trauma, some of which contribute to the often-permanent and significant brain damage sustained by abused infants and children" (Christian, Block, & the Committee on Child Abuse and Neglect, 2009). Christian and colleagues (2009) state that shaking is the most frequent cause of abusive head trauma. In 2001, the American Academy of Pediatrics reported "95% of serious intracranial injuries and 64% of all head injuries in infants younger than 1 year were attributable to child abuse." (p. 206) There is usually evidence of prior episodes of abuse, and "specific evidence of previous cranial injuries (e.g., old intracranial hemorrhages) from shaking episodes is found in about 33%–40% of all cases" (AAP, 2001, p. 207).

Who Is Abused?

SBS is seen primarily in children under the age of 2 years, with the majority of cases occurring before 12 months of age. The average child with SBS, also known as shaken impact syndrome, is between 3 and 8 months old (Neurosurgery Today, 2005). While it can be seen in children up to age 5 years, most cases are seen under age 2 years (www.nim.nih/gov/medlineplusency/article/0004.htm).

When one combines the categories of abuse and neglect, 772,000 children were reported as abused or neglected in 2008. Of these, the age group with the highest incidence of abuse and neglect were children below 1 year of age, with 21.7 out of 1000 children being abused or neglected. Other incidence statistics include:

- 51.3 percent of abused or neglected children are female and 48.3 percent are male.

- 45.1 percent are White.

- 16.6 percent are African American.

- 20.8 percent are Hispanic.

Children with disabilities are often abused, with 15 percent of the children who were reported as being abused in 2008 having a disability ("mental retardation, emotional disturbance, visual or hearing impairment, learning disability, physical disability, behavioral problems, or another medical problem") (U.S. Department of Health and Human Services, 2010). Of those 15 percent, 5.3 percent had behavior problems, 6.2 percent had some other medical condition, and 3.7 percent were emotionally disturbed.

Who Are the Perpetrators of Child Abuse?

The American Academy of Pediatrics (AAP) characterized the parents of children who are shaken as having emotional factors, having unrealistic expectations of their child, being stressed, or being victims of domestic violence and/or substance abuse. Those who react out of emotion typically are tense and frustrated. They usually report that their actions were due to their baby's crying or irritability and their own inability to calm the infant. Many times these parents also report that they are under much stress. The AAP found that parents who reported being under financial, social, environmental, or biological stress were more prone to engage in "impulsive or aggressive behavior" (2001, p. 206). They also found that some parents who are prone to being abusive have unrealistic expectations for their child, even having "role reversal" in which they expect the child to fulfill or meet the parent's needs (2001).

In 81.2 percent of the cases of child abuse reported in 2008, the perpetrator was a parent (38.3% mother alone, 18.1% father alone, 17.9% both parents). In another 6.5 percent of the cases, the perpetrator was a relative (nonparent). With regard to parentage, 90.9 percent of the abusive parents were the biological parent, 4.4 percent were step-parents, and 0.7 percent were adoptive parents.

Signs and Symptoms of Shaken Baby Syndrome

Disabling effects from being shaken can occur as a result of being shaken for as little as 5 seconds (www.nim.nih/gov/medlineplusency/article/0004.htm). The damage is caused by "extreme rotational cranial acceleration induced by violent shaking or shaking/impact" (AAP, 2001, p. 206). Symptoms that an infant has been shaken may be evident immediately, but they usually reach a peak within 4 to 6 hours following the incident. Thus, some infants who are shaken and then put to bed may have their death attributed initially to sudden infant death syndrome (SIDS). Babies who have been shaken typically present with any combination of the following physical findings upon medical examination:

- Retinal hemorrhage
- Closed head injury (subdural, epidural, subarachnoid, subgaleal injury)
- Lacerations
- Contusions
- Concussions
- Bruises to face, scalp, arms, abdomen, or back
- Soft tissue swelling which may indicate a fracture to the skull or other bones
- Abdominal injuries
- Chest injuries
- Abnormally low blood pressure
- Tense fontanel (soft spot)

If the child has anoxia during the shaking, he or she can suffer from irreversible brain damage. The child can have additional brain damage if "the injured nerve cells release chemicals that add to the oxygen deprivation to the brain" (*Neurosurgery Today*, 2005).

The diagnostic constellation is retinal hemorrhage (present in 75–90% of cases), subdural and/or subarachnoid hemorrhage, and little or no evidence of external cranial trauma (AAP, 2001).

Other symptoms that a child has been shaken include:

- Altered level of consciousness
- Drowsiness accompanied by irritability
- Coma
- Convulsions or seizures
- Dilated pupils that do not respond to light
- Decreased appetite
- Vomiting
- Posturing in which the head is bent back and the back arched
- Breathing problems and irregularities
- Abnormally slow or shallow respiration
- Cardiac arrest
- Death (*Neurosurgery Today*, 2005)

Outcomes and Disabilities Resulting from SBS

The mortality rate in SBS is 15 to 38 percent of all cases (AAP, 2001). Infants who were comatose when they were first evaluated medically have the worst outcomes, with 60 percent either dying or having severe motor dysfunction, spastic quadriplegia, or profound intellectual disabilities. Infants with permanent neurological disability from being shaken may have seizure disorders, visual disturbances including cortical blindness or other blindness, cerebral palsy, static encephalopathy, paralysis (possibly due to cervical spinal injury), epilepsy, learning disabilities, and/or intellectual disabilities (AAP, 2001; *Neurosurgery Today*, 2005; Christian, Block, & the Committee on Child Abuse and Neglect, 2009).

Speech-language pathologists (and all persons who work with children) should be aware of the signs and symptoms of abuse; we are ethically and legally responsible for reporting any suspicion that a child is being abused or neglected. It is also important to maintain a healthy relationship with parents of the children we serve; having a child with an impairment can be stressful. The parents need to know they have our support and can trust us to help them seek assistance if the stresses and challenges of having a child with a communication disorder of any type become overwhelming.

Some children who have a history of being shaken but who never received medical attention may demonstrate behavior problems, learning disabilities, or motor deficits that become evident later in their childhood years (AAP, 2001).

Acquired Aphasia Secondary to Convulsive Disorders and Cerebrovascular Disease

Acquired aphasia secondary to convulsive disorders often includes unknown etiological factors. The problems can be either sudden or gradual in onset. According to Nelson (1993), Landau-Kleffner syndrome is a convulsive disorder characterized by epileptic discharges and severe language comprehension deficits. Nelson also referred to encephalopathies that are secondary to infection or irradiation. These include disorders due to tumors, encephalitis, meningitis, and cancer treatments. The extent of the damage in the last two categories varies with the extent and location of tissues involved, the age of the child, and the general health of the child.

> **Aphasia.** Impairment of the abilities to comprehend and express language resulting from acquired neurological damage.

In 1989, the death rate for children under 15 years of age from cerebrovascular disease (which contributes to stroke) was 4 per 100,000, compared to 2296 per 100,000 in adults. Over one-third of strokes in children occur in the first 2 years of life. Usual etiological factors are sickle cell anemia, cardiac disease, vascular occlusions or malformations, and hemorrhage (Reed, 1994). Reed summarized much of the research in this area as outlined in Table 12–2.

TABLE 12–2 Associated physical, cognitive, perceptual, motor, behavioral, and social problems in children with acquired aphasia due to traumatic brain injury

Area	Effect of Traumatic Brain Injury
Gross and fine motor	Severe TBI: spasticity, delayed motor milestones Mild TBI: fine motor and visuomotor deficits, reduction in age-appropriate play and physical activity
Cognitive	Problems with long- and short-term memory, conceptual skills, and problem solving Reduced speed of information processing Reduced attending skills
Perceptual motor	Visual neglect, visual field cuts Motor apraxia, reduced motor speed, poor motor sequencing
Behavioral	Impulsivity, poor judgment, disinhibition, dependency, anger outbursts, denial, depression, emotional lability, apathy, lethargy, poor motivation
Social	Does not learn from peers, does not generalize from social situations Behaves like a much younger child, withdraws Becomes distracted in noisy surroundings, becomes lost even in familiar surroundings

Source: Adapted from *An introduction to children with language disorders* (2nd ed.), by V. A. Reed, p. 368. Copyright 1994, Macmillan College Publishing Company.

Sports Injuries

Approximately 60 percent of high school students participate in organized sports. In addition, organized sports such as tee ball and soccer are available through community recreation programs for children at a young age (Duff, 2009). Sports injuries are a cause of brain injury receiving much attention. The most common head injury is a concussion. According to the American Academy of Neurology, a concussion is "any alteration of mental status due to a biochemical force affecting the brain with or without loss of consciousness" (Duff, 2009). Most concussions are characterized by the symptoms associated with mild brain injury. Athletes who have sustained a concussion typically complain of being off balance, having headaches, and feeling mentally sluggish. The athlete typically recovers with no residual effects. However, the issue of repetitive concussions and their cumulative toll is receiving much attention.

A National Collegiate Athletic Association (NCAA) football study (Guskiewicz et al.) found an association between the number of reported prior concussions in NCAA football players and the likelihood of sustaining another concussion. The study found that players reporting more than 3 prior concussions were three times more likely to sustain another concussion than players who reported no prior concussions. Among players reporting 2 prior concussions they were 2.5 times more likely to sustain another concussion. Players that reported only 1 prior concussion were 1.4 times more likely to sustain another concussion. (www.dvbic.org/TBI—The-Military/Cumulative-Concussions.aspx)

At this time, the research is inconclusive regarding the cumulative pathologic effects of multiple concussions or regarding how many concussions one can safely sustain, even when there is apparent recovery. The U.S. Department of Defense is keeping abreast of the studies being conducted on NCAA athletes in an effort to obtain guidance as to when injured military troops can safely return to active duty (www.dvbic.org/TBI—The-Military/Cumulative-Concussions.aspx).

The February 23, 2010 edition of the NCAA News contained an article by Jack Copeland, who reported the following data:

- Concussion is the second most frequent injury in fall football and women's soccer, and the fourth most frequent injury in field hockey, men's soccer, and women's volleyball.

- Concussion accounts for 7.2 percent of game injuries across the five fall sports and 4.7 percent of injuries suffered during practice.

- Of every 1000 student-athletes who take the field in any given competition, 2.7 suffer a concussion in football, compared to 2.1 in women's soccer and 1.1 in men's soccer.

- Concussions during competition accounted for about 11 percent of injuries in women's soccer, 9 percent of injuries in field hockey, 6 percent of injuries in football and men's soccer, and 4 percent of injuries in women's volleyball.

"The common injury mechanisms in the sports are blocking and tackling in football and direct player contact while heading the ball in men's and women's soccer, while more than half of competition injuries in field hockey are due to contact with apparatus (primarily the stick or ball)" (Copeland, 2010). New rules regarding contact to and with the head or helmet in collegiate football were implemented in 2005 and, along with stricter enforcement of contact rules, have led to a decrease in the number of concussions sustained by college football players. (Copeland, 2010). An adjunct focus to the NCAA studies on concussion is research on long-term effects of repeated concussions on the brain. In particular, the rates of occurrence of Alzheimer's and other dementias in professional football players is being studied.

The speech-language pathologist has a responsibility to promote awareness of activities that can result in head injury and how to safely participate in those activities in order to minimize the possibility of sustaining a head injury. Students who do sustain a head injury need the support of the speech-language pathologist in making the transition from the rehabilitation program (if one was necessary) back into the school setting. This includes educating teachers about accommodations such as providing note takers and copies of instructional materials, placing the student in a seat where there are minimal distractions, making alternative testing arrangements, and other such accommodations.

> **think about it**
>
> Do you believe the current guidelines regarding the return of athletes to competition following a concussion are stringent enough? Who should have the final word as to when an athlete resumes playing following a concussion? What would be other roles and responsibilities with regard to sports of a speech-language pathologist in a high school?

TYPES OF INJURIES

The World Health Organization (WHO) (1980) classified injuries such as TBI in three ways: impairment, disability, and handicap. They defined *impairment* as a disruption or abnormality in mental or physical functioning. When an impairment limits participation in life activities, the result is a disability. In 2001, the WHO revised their terminology, substituting *activity reduction* for *disability*. This terminology refers to a reduction in the individual's ability to effectively and successfully participate in activities that are important to a quality life, such as comprehending reading material, conversing with others, and remaining organized and focused in work and social settings. A handicap historically referred to the social deficits that occur as sequelae to an injury or illness. In 1998, the word *participation* was substituted for *handicap*. This refers to the individual's decreased ability to participate in work, school, social situations, community activities, and so on.

Closed Head Injuries and Penetrating Head Injuries

Closed head injury. A non-penetrating brain injury in which the skull may be intact or fractured, but the meninges are intact.

It is important to differentiate among the various terms frequently used to describe head injury. A closed head injury is a nonpenetrating brain injury in which the skull may be intact or fractured, but the meninges are intact (Hegde, 1996). It is possible in these cases to have a minor head injury without brain injury. Nonpenetrating brain injuries typically result in diffuse pathological changes in the brain and are more frequent in civilian life than are penetrating head injuries (Murdoch & Theodoros, 2001). A blunt blow to the head usually causes the damage to the brain. Shaking of the head (such as in shaken baby syndrome) is also a frequent cause of closed head injury. Closed head injuries can be due to a moving object hitting a moving head or due to a moving head colliding with a fixed object. Both scenarios result in the brain moving within the skull, resulting in damage to the brain. These mechanisms of injury are known as acceleration/deceleration injuries, as compared to nonacceleration injuries, in which a moving object collides with a stationary head and results in localized damage at the point of impact (Ylvisaker, Szekeres, & Feeney, 2001). A penetrating head injury, which is also known as an open head injury, results in a fracturing or perforation of the skull with the meninges becoming torn or lacerated (Hegde, 1996). An example of a penetrating head injury is a gunshot wound.

Coup and Contrecoup Injuries

Two other terms that are frequently encountered when studying traumatic brain injury are *coup injury* and *contrecoup injury*. In a coup injury, the injury is at the point of impact. This type of injury occurs when a blow to the head results in the brain moving and slamming against the point of impact. A contrecoup injury is a brain injury opposite from the impact. In these cases, a second injury occurs as the brain "bounces from the point of impact to the opposite side of the skull" (Blosser & DePompei, 2003, p. 17). Coup and contrecoup injuries are associated with a linear velocity mechanism that frequently is the result of trauma in the front or the back of the head (Ylvisaker, Szekeres, & Feeney, 2001).

Diffuse and Focal Injuries

It is also important to know whether the child has a focal lesion or a diffuse lesion. In a focal lesion, the damage is limited to a small area of the brain. This is in contrast to a diffuse lesion, which causes widespread damage. In diffuse lesions a twisting movement of the brain frequently occurs, which can force tissues together, pull tissues apart, or create a tearing of axonal fibers as the injury occurs (Blosser & DePompei, 2003). Depending on the site of the damage, a diffuse lesion can be expected to be much more devastating to the child's cognition and language than a focal lesion. The majority of injuries are consistent with frontolimbic damage, and the deficits can be grouped into three categories: cognitive, executive functions, and psychosocial and behavioral (Ylvisaker, Szekeres, & Feeney, 2001).

Nelson (1993) advocated dividing brain injury into four etiological categories: "(1) focal acquired lesions, (2) diffuse lesions associated with traumatic brain injury, (3) acquired childhood aphasia secondary to convulsive disorder, and (4) other kinds of brain injury or encephalopathy" (p. 116). Focal acquired lesions are frequently caused by strokes in children (and adults). These strokes are commonly the result of emboli associated with

Penetrating head injury. An open head injury resulting in a fracturing or perforation of the skull with the meninges becoming torn or lacerated.

Coup injury. Injury at the point of impact, occurring when a blow to the head results in the brain moving and slamming against the point of impact.

Contrecoup injury. A brain injury opposite from the impact as the brain bounces from the point of impact to the opposite side of the skull.

Focal lesion. A lesion in which the impact is concentrated in one small area of the brain.

Diffuse lesion. A lesion in which the damage is spread throughout a large area of the brain or over several small areas, resulting in comprehensive deficits.

congenital heart disease. They may also be associated with vascular disorders due to sickle cell anemia. The strokes often result in left hemisphere lesions, from which recovery usually is fairly complete.

SYMPTOMS AND EFFECTS OF TBI

Individuals with mild TBI may have a functional disability due to physical, cognitive, behavioral, or emotional symptoms that may persist after the injury. As a result of a mild head injury, the individual may have problems with memory, attention, and executive functioning. The child may be anxious, depressed, or irritable. Language effects include mild word-retrieval deficits (Levin, Eisenberg, & Benton, 1989; Sohlberg & Mateer, 1989).

TBI can result in various functional changes affecting language, sensation (including hearing), thinking, cognitive-communication deficits, physical well-being, and/or emotions. TBI can also result in increased risk for conditions such as epilepsy, Parkinson's disease, and Alzheimer's disease. Other brain disorders that normally occur with higher prevalence in the aging population are also more likely to occur in an individual who has sustained a TBI (National Institute of Neurological Disorders and Stroke, 2002). The degree to which an individual is affected by a TBI is quite diverse, with various combinations of effects creating varying degrees of handicap and disability.

Physical Symptoms

The first category consists of physical symptoms including dizziness, headaches, insomnia and other sleep disturbances, nausea, and vomiting. Blurred vision and sleep disturbances also may occur. Unexplained lethargy, quickness to fatigue, and other sensory losses may also occur in individuals with TBI (Green, Stevens, & Wolf, 1997; Bogaert-Martinez, 2007).

TBI and Auditory Disorders

According to Dennis (n.d.), audiologists should expect to see a variety of auditory and vestibular symptoms in individuals who have sustained a head injury. These symptoms include "ear aches, aural fullness, tinnitus and hyperacusis, dizziness and vertigo, distorted hearing, and hearing impairment" (Dennis, n.d.). They also may complain of sensitivity to loud noises. As a personal aside, my daughter took a blow to the side of the head from a kicked soccer ball in a high school match; the force of the impact gave her a mild concussion and ruptured her tympanic membrane.

It is important that audiologists be sensitive to the fact that the memory loss, deficits in executive functions, attention deficits, and emotional and behavioral disturbances "can have a significant impact on auditory and vestibular evaluation and rehabilitation" (Dennis, n.d.).

Central auditory deficits are another possible manifestation of TBI (Dennis, n.d.).

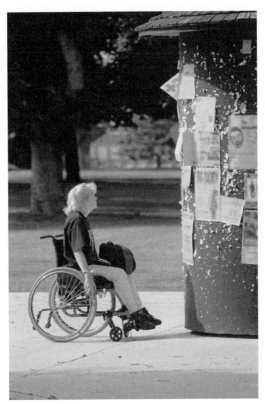

FIGURE 12–3   TBI can affect an individual's mental, social, emotional, and physical states. (*Delmar/Cengage Learning*)

Cognitive Deficits

The second category of symptoms relates to cognitive deficits. Traumatic brain injury can significantly impact cognitive and communication abilities. When examining and determining the cognitive deficits that have occurred as the result of a TBI, the clinician must be careful to ascertain that the cognitive deficits are not due to emotional or other causes besides the traumatic brain injury. Cognitive deficits frequently observed include poor attention skills, difficulty in concentrating, memory deficits, difficulty thinking, problem-solving deficits, perceptual deficits, problems with speech or language or both, and difficulty with executive functions (Green, Stevens, & Wolfe, 1997; Bogaert-Martinez, 2007). "Cognitive-communicative impairments are those impairments of communication related to impairments of linguistic (e.g., syntax, semantics, metalinguistic skills) as well as nonlinguistic cognitive functions (e.g., attention, perception, and memory" (Coelho, DeRuyter, & Stein, 1996, p. S6; American Speech-Language-Hearing Association, 1987, 1990). Executive functions include goal setting, self-awareness, initiating tasks, self-directing and self-monitoring, self-evaluation, self-inhibiting, and planning (Coelho, DeRuyter, & Stein, 1996). All of these cognitive factors combine and interact with receptive and expressive language skills. Nelson (1993) warned of possible enduring effects on language development and learning, however. Diffuse lesions associated with TBI resulting from falls, vehicular accidents, or abuse are the primary focus of this chapter. In these cases, it is not unusual to see relatively good language recovery in young children; however, long-term sequelae in terms of linguistic processing and cognition are common (Ewing-Cobbs, Fletcher, & Levin, 1985; Satz & Bullard-Bates, 1981).

In the pediatric population, lesions causing language deficits initially may be limited to the surface structure of the brain. However, as the learning demands increase, as they do in grades 3 and 4, the deficits become more apparent. Clinicians must understand the relationship between cognition and language because impaired cognitive processes (i.e., perception, memory, reasoning, and problem solving) interfere with language processes (Russell, 1993).

Behavioral Changes

Behavioral changes with or without alterations in the degree of emotional responsivity constitute the third category of symptoms. Again, these symptoms must exist in the absence of other psychological, physical, or emotional stresses. Behavioral changes include emotional lability, disinhibition, irritability, and quickness to anger (Green, Stevens, & Wolf, 1997). Other behavioral and emotional deficits include frustration, depression, anxiety, mood swings, impulsivity, agitation, apathy, paranoia, confusion and aggression (Bogaert-Martinez, 2007; Dennis, n.d.).

Effects of TBI on Personality

According to National Institutes of Health (1984) criteria, three types of personality changes exist following a TBI. The first is apathy, in which the child does not care about what happens. He or she has reduced interest in the usual activities and challenges, which is often misinterpreted as compliance or absence of a behavior problem. However, that misinterpretation often reinforces the apathy. In other words, the caregivers treat the child as if he or she has a behavior problem, and, because the child may have trouble making them understand otherwise, the apathy is reinforced. The second personality change occurs when the child is overly optimistic regarding the extent of the disability. Although positive thinking can be a good trait, caution should be taken to ensure that the child has realistic expectations regarding the rate and degree of recovery. The third change entails a loss of social restraint and judgment. In these cases, the child often becomes tactless and talkative. He or she can become hurtful, which frequently damages his or her relationships with family members. He or she may also have rage outbursts of abnormal intensity in response to trivial frustration.

COMMUNICATION DISORDERS FREQUENTLY SEEN IN CHILDREN WITH TBI

Castrogiovanni (2010) summarized the communication disorders (and disorders impacting communication) frequently seen in children with TBI:

- Understanding and producing written language

- Understanding and producing spoken language

- Pragmatics (particularly "the more subtle aspects of communication, such as body language, and emotional and nonverbal signals")

- Sensory (hearing, smell, touch, taste)

- Spoken language deficits including intonation and inflection

- Dysarthria

- Aprosodia

- Attention disorders

- Cognitive disorders

- Behavior problems

Any or all of these problems can be present in pediatric and adult patients who are living with the effects of TBI.

> **Dysarthria.** A motor speech disorder resulting from generalized weakness of the oral musculature.
>
> **Aprosodia.** The inability to either produce or comprehend the affective components of speech or gesture.

Communication Deficits in the Acute Recovery Period

During the acute recovery period, speech production deficits may occur, such as difficulty with the production of consonants and possible mutism. The child also may have speech comprehension problems and word retrieval deficits during the acute recovery stages. When shown common objects, the child may have difficulty describing them. Syntactic problems including a limited mean length of utterance, difficulty in constructing sentences, and fewer utterances may be observed. In children old enough to write, deficits in this area may be noted.

Long-Term (Residual) Effects Of TBI On Communication

Possible long-term effects include persistent word retrieval problems and a reduction in spontaneous speech. When speech does occur, it may be characterized by reduced fluency, in part due to the word retrieval difficulties. Pragmatic problems are common. Subtle comprehension problems that result in reading problems, poor mathematic reasoning skills, and general poor academic performance may be present. Memory problems may persist. Behaviorally, hyperactivity and impulsivity are frequently observed in children who are post-TBI. An additional problem may involve residual confusion, in which the child is unable to recognize his or her own deficits.

Language and Communication Deficits Seen in Children with TBI

Language characteristics occurring after closed head injury are outlined in Table 12–3. In addition to the language characteristics, psychological difficulties, which include depression, anger, and behaviors inappropriate for the situation, are frequently noted.

The child who sustains a TBI may have deficits in specific language areas as well as in metacognitive and metalinguistic skills. These deficits also impact the child's ability to organize narratives (Reed, 2005).

It is helpful for intervention purposes to work with the child in his or her natural settings to facilitate the development of language skills that can be used to combat these problem areas.

Impact of TBI on Academics

Ylvisaker and Szekeres (1989) identified seven problem areas in the academic arena for children who have sustained a TBI:

1. Limited self-awareness with regard to their communication problems

2. Poor planning, impacting the quality and organization of narratives

3. Difficulty initiating conversation with teachers and peers

4. Problems with inhibition, leading to the use of inappropriate statements

TABLE 12–3 Language deficits in children with TBI

Concentration
Sustained attention
Memory
Nonverbal problem solving
Part or whole analysis and synthesis
Conceptual organization and abstraction
Processing
Reasoning
Executive functioning (formulating goals, planning to achieve goals, carrying out plans)

Source: Adapted from *Mild traumatic brain injury: A therapy and resource manual,* by B. S. Green, K. M. Stevens, and T. D. W. Wolfe. Copyright 1997 by Delmar, Cengage Learning.

5. Failure to self-monitor, affecting behavior and comprehension

6. General self-evaluations that do not lead to constructive responses

7. Lack of flexibility in problem solving

> **think about it**
>
> A 16-year-old high school student sustains a head injury in a head-on car collision. After 4 months of rehabilitation, he has returned to school and rejoined his old classes. His teachers report that he is not keeping up with the workload and has trouble sustaining focus on a task. They think he needs to be in a resource room where special strategies can be implemented and more individualized instruction can take place. However, the student does not want to leave his regular classroom and classmates. As a member of the school's special education services faculty, how would you address this situation?

COMPARISON OF PEDIATRIC AND ADULT APHASIA

Pediatric children usually exhibit nonfluent aphasia with mutism, effortful speech, and impaired repetition skills. Syntactic problems, auditory comprehension deficits, anomia, and reading and writing difficulties also may be present. Children are less likely than adults to show paraphasia, jargon, and fluent aphasia.

In fluent aphasia, the child does not have difficulty initiating speech, but he or she typically uses few, if any, content words. Syntax and prosody frequently remain intact, so the person appears to be speaking in sentences, but the sentences cannot be understood with regard to content.

Associated deficits in pediatric acquired aphasia include attentional disturbances and language impairments. As already mentioned, these language impairments include anomia. Also included are trouble with figurative and abstract language, difficulty in organizing the production of language, and problems in comprehending language. Cognitive and communication deficits result in academic underachievement. In her examination of the long-term residual effects of pediatric aphasia, Lees (1997) observed that, with adequate treatment, some children may achieve a relatively normal language profile based on testing used to measure progress after intensive therapy. However, Lees cautioned that, for some children, these normal language profiles masked persistent high-level difficulties, such as those involving auditory verbal processing and lexical recall, which interfered with successful progress in school. Organically based behavioral and emotional deficits interfere with social interactions and impede the social-emotional growth that normally occurs during the school-age years. The child also may have perceptual-motor deficits that result in visual-field cuts, motor apraxia, or both.

Nonfluent aphasia. Slow, labored, effortful speech, word retrieval deficits, and motor planning deficits due to a lesion or lesions in the anterior language area and left premotor cortex (Broca's area).

Paraphasia. The unintentional substitution of an incorrect word for an intended word.

Anomia. Lack of the ability to recall names of people, common objects, and places.

The individual who has sustained a TBI initially may demonstrate an aphasia-like set of symptoms. However, much of the research indicates that the traditional aphasic syndromes are uncommon following TBI in children and adults. A child who has a diffuse injury is more likely to demonstrate impairment in receptive and expressive language accompanied by persistent cognitive deficits. Ylvisaker and colleagues (2001) wrote that "communication challenges following TBI are most often 'nonaphasic' in nature, that is, they co-exist with intelligible speech, reasonably fluent and grammatical language, and comprehension adequate to support everyday interaction" (p. 754).

Children who do not present with aphasia in its classical terms still are likely to have language deficits that are not evident in routine interactions. Specifically, these deficits include problems with following complex oral directions, confrontational naming, and word fluency (Sarno, 1984). Ylvisaker and colleagues (2001) reflected the findings of many clinicians and caregivers in noting that children with TBI often have deficits in interactive competence as cognitive and social demands increase. Taken together, the array of communication deficits exhibited by children with TBI are labeled by ASHA as cognitive-communicative impairment (Ylvisaker, Hanks, & Johnson-Green, 2003). A listing of impairments associated with frontolimbic damage can be found in Table 12–4.

TABLE 12–4 Vulnerable frontolimbic structures and frequently associated impairments

---

Frontolimbic Injury and Executive System Impairment

Reduced awareness of personal strengths and weaknesses

Difficulty setting realistic goals

Difficulty planning and organizing behavior to achieve the goals

Impaired ability to initiate action needed to achieve the goals

Difficulty inhibiting behavior incompatible with achieving the goals

Difficulty self-monitoring and self-evaluating

Difficulty thinking and acting strategically and solving real-world problems in a flexible and efficient manner

General inflexibility and concreteness in thinking, talking, and acting

Frontolimbic Injury and Cognitive-Communication Impairment

Disorganized, poorly controlled discourse or paucity of discourse (spoken and written)

Inefficient comprehension of language related to increasing amounts of information to be processed (spoken or written) and to rate of speech

Imprecise language and word-retrieval problems

Difficulty understanding and expressing abstract and indirect language

TABLE 12–4   (*continued*)

Difficulty reading social cues, interpreting speaker intent, and flexibly adjusting interactive styles to meet situational demands in varied social contexts

Awkward or inappropriate communication in stressful social contexts

Impaired verbal learning

Frontolimbic Injury and Cognitive Impairment

Reduced internal control over all cognitive functions (e.g., attentional, perceptual, memory, organizational, and reasoning processes)

Impaired working memory

Impaired declarative and explicit memory (encoding and retrieval)

Disorganized behavior related to impaired organizing schemes (managerial knowledge frames, such as scripts, themes, schemas, mental models)

Impaired reasoning

Concrete thinking

Difficulty generalizing

Frontolimbic Injury and Psychosocial and Behavioral Impairment

Disinhibited, socially inappropriate, and possibly aggressive behavior

Impaired initiation or paucity of behavior

Inefficient learning from consequences

Perseverative behavior; rigid, inflexible behavior

Impaired social perception and interpretation

Source: From Communication disorders associated with traumatic brain injury, by M. Ylviskar, S. Szkeres, and T. Feeney. In *Language intervention strategies in adult aphasia and related communication disorders* (4th ed.) by R. Chapey (ed.), pp. 745–808. Philadelphia: Lippincott, Williams, & Wilkins. © 2001 by Lippincott, Williams & Wilkins. http://lww.com.

As a rule, recovery from mild TBI in children is usually excellent, while recovery from severe TBI is less certain. However, generally speaking, recovery in children is more complete than in adults regardless of the severity of the TBI (Bijur, Haslum, & Gloning, 1990). Murdoch and Theodoros (2001) suggested three reasons why recovery is more complete in children than in adults. First, it may be due to the different nature of the impacts causing TBI in children versus adults, childhood TBI generally being associated with lower-speed impacts. Second, it may be related to differences in the basic mechanisms of brain damage following head injury in the two groups, which in turn are related to differences in the physical characteristics of children's heads and adult's heads. Third, it may be the result of greater plasticity in the child's brain (p. 248).

Even though their recovery is more complete, children with severe TBI frequently have residual and persistent language deficits as one would find in aphasia. These deficits include word-finding and naming problems, difficulty with expressive language (verbal, gestural, and written output) (Alajouanine & Lhermitte, 1965), and deficient repetition of words and sentences (Murdoch & Theodoros, 2001). In a study by Levin and Eisenberg (1979), the Neurosensory Center Comprehensive Examination for Aphasia (NCCEA) (Spreen & Benton, 1969) was administered to a group of children and teenagers who had sustained a closed head injury. Eleven percent of their subjects had deficits in auditory comprehension; 4 percent had impaired verbal repetition; 12 percent had dysnomia. The same test and a similar age grouping was used in a study by Ewing-Cobbs and colleagues (1985) who found linguistic impairments (especially naming problems, dysgraphia, and reduced verbal production) in a significant portion of their subjects when they were less than 6 months post event. Ewing-Cobbs and colleagues concluded that their subjects demonstrated a subclinical aphasia due to the stages of language acquisition their subjects were in when they incurred their injury. In a later study by Ewing-Cobbs and colleagues (1987), they administered the NCCEA to 23 children and 33 adolescents who had TBI. In this study, they found significant language impairment in most of their subjects, with graphic and expressive functions being the most affected.

In a series of studies by Jordan and colleagues (Jordan, Ozanne, & Murdoch, 1988), 20 children between the ages of 8 and 16 years who had sustained a TBI were tested using the Test of Language Development series and the NCCEA. When compared to a control group matched for age and sex, the children with TBI were mildly language impaired 12 months after the injury. The language impairment was similar to that found in adults, creating the impression of a subclinical aphasia with dysnomia. At 24 months post injury, Jordan and Murdoch (1990) found that the naming deficit had persisted and verbal fluency had declined. This further solidifies the argument that children who sustain a moderate to severe TBI have residual language deficits (Murdoch & Theodoros, 2001).

Dysnomia. Loss of ability to name people, places, or things; may also be referred to as anomia.

RIGHT HEMISPHERE DAMAGE

Historically, the right hemisphere has been attributed with three primary responsibilities:

1. A site of speech in left-handers

2. The hemisphere that could take over functions after damage to the left hemisphere in children and in some adults

3. The hemisphere most likely to be implicated in denial or neglect in hemiparesis (Payne, 1997, p. 300)

Interest in right hemisphere damage (RHD) did not emerge until the 1960s and 1970s, when it was found that the right hemisphere plays a critical role in linguistics, prosody and affect, lower-order perceptual skills such as visual tracking, and higher cognitive skills (Payne, 1997).

A right hemisphere deficit is "an acquired disorder of linguistic, non-linguistic and extralinguistic processes resulting from damage to the right hemisphere" (Payne, 1997, p. 345). Linguistic processes affected include auditory comprehension, word fluency, naming body parts, grapheme omissions and substitutions in writing, and reading sentences aloud (Payne, 1997). Although there is clear evidence of some linguistic deficits being associated with right hemisphere deficits, Myers and Blake (2008) made the point that linguistic deficits are usually mild and not typical of aphasias associated with left hemisphere damage. More typically, individuals with right hemisphere deficits have difficulty with pragmatics, particularly general problems with language use and discourse. In fact, pragmatic deficits are the primary communication disorder in right hemisphere deficits (Blake, 2007).

With regard to language functioning in individuals with RHD, Myers and Blake (2008) pointed out that "their command over basic linguistic structures is usually adequate, and they may do well in superficial or straight-forward conversation. Their communication problems typically become apparent in more complex communicative events in which verbal and non-verbal contextual cues must be used to assess and convey communicative intent" (p. 963). Thus, those individuals who have RHD and also communication impairments (not all do) typically are not believed to be aphasic.

Nonlinguistic deficits include deficits in those skills that are associated with attention and perception and their roles in "normal recognition, integration, and interpretation of important cues" (Payne, 1997, p. 301). Nonlinguistic deficits also encompass orientation in time and space. Nonlinguistic deficits include unilateral or hemispatial neglect, in which the individual has the motor and sensory capabilities to respond, yet he or she does not orient or respond to stimulation on the side of the body that is opposite the hemisphere of the lesion. Numerous researchers cited by Myers and Blake (2008) reported that neglect is most often associated with damage in the frontal, temporal, or parietal cortex. However, they acknowledge that subcortical lesions, particularly in the thalamus, can also lead to unilateral neglect.

It was mentioned previously that people with RHD have difficulties with attention. This includes problems with arousal (decreased attentiveness and alertness) and orientation. Thus, it may take more intense sensory input to gain the attention of the child, and he or she may need more time than normal to attend to the stimulation and react. Individuals with RHD also have problems with some of the same attention systems discussed in Chapter 11 regarding ADHD, including vigilance, sustained attention, and selective attention.

Attention deficits may impair the appreciation of the verbal and visual cues that specify the context within which communication takes pace. Children may be less able to shift attention, actively or covertly, during conversations. They may be less able to sustain attention to stimuli anywhere in the environment and to filter out distracters Thus, they may not be able to attend selectively to important information during communicative events. (Myers & Blake, 2008, p. 967)

Furthermore, increased complexity of conversations and/or directions proves problematic due to the attention deficits exhibited by children with RHD.

Another nonlinguistic deficit, visual disturbance, is frequently associated with right hemisphere damage. A description of visual disorders can be found in Table 12–5.

Extralinguistic deficits are those that play a role in prosodic and pragmatic interpretation and use and information organization (such as abstraction), thereby affecting the ability to communicate (Payne, 1997). Myers and Blake (2008) listed macrostructure deficits, selection and integration deficits, producing informative content, and generation of alternative meanings as examples of extralinguistic deficits. A macrostructure is an "overall theme, central message, or main point of narratives, pictured scenes, situations, or discourse" (Myers & Blake, 2008, p. 969). When faced with complex communications, individuals with RHD have difficulty developing macrostructures. As written by Myers and Blake, one must be able to interpret information and draw inferences in able to develop macrostructures. These abilities are compromised by RHD. This includes extracting detail from both

TABLE 12–5 Classification of selected right hemisphere visual syndromes that impair language functions

Disorders of Visual Processing	Relationship to Language	Site of Lesion
Disorders of gaze instability	Causes problems in reading	Frontal lobe eye fields
Disorders of visuoverbal processing	Alexia	Hemialexia: Splenium of the corpus callosum. Visuospatial alexia: Right occipital cortex or subcortical disconnections.
	Agraphia	Frontoparietal or temporoparieto-occipital areas
Disorders of visuosymbolic processing	Acalculia	Left or right hemispheres, anywhere

Source: Adult neurogenic language disorders, by Joan C. Payne, p. 308. Copyright 1997 by Delmar, Cengage Learning.

conversation and a picture or photograph and integrating the information into the generalized context of the current discussion (written or verbal).

With regard to producing informative content, individuals with RHD can be taciturn or verbose. Those who are taciturn do not contribute sufficiently to an exchange of information. Those who are verbose are hyperverbal but contribute little substantive information to the conversation. This may partially be attributed to the pragmatic deficits previously noted (Myers & Blake, 2008).

People with RHD have difficulty generating alternative meanings. As explained by Myers and Blake (2008), "it often happens that we must generate different, less familiar, or alternative meanings during discourse. Sometimes this occurs because we need to accommodate new information that alters our original interpretation" or use a word or phrase meaning that is less familiar to us (p. 972). This includes skills such as revising our initial interpretation of information, or using connotative and metaphoric meanings to convey our thoughts (Myers & Blake, 2008).

Individuals with RHD also have difficulty processing emotional content, showing difficulties in interpreting and expressing emotional content when interacting with others. Current research is inconclusive as to the origin of this problem. The problem could be "the result of an altered internal experience of emotion, reduced levels of arousal, cognitive interference or some combination thereof" (Myers & Blake, 2008, p. 975). Deficits related to this type of difficulty for children with RHD include poor comprehension of facial expressions of conversation partners, reduced facial expression by the child, and difficulty comprehending and expressing emotional information.

Haynes and Pindzola (2008) summed up the sequelae of RHD as shown in Table 12–6.

TABLE 12–6   Sequelae of Right Hemisphere Damage

General Symptoms

Neglect of the left half of space

Denial of illness

Impaired judgment

Impaired self-monitoring

Poor motivation

Visuospatial Deficits

Visual memory and imagery problems

Facial recognition difficulties (disorientation to person)

Geographic and spatial disorientation (to place)

Visual field deficits (especially left)

Visual hallucinations

Visuoconstructive deficits (constructional apraxia)

(continues)

TABLE 12–6 (*continued*)

Deficits in Affect and Prosody

Indifference reaction

Reduced sensitivity to emotional tone

Impaired prosodic production and comprehension

Linguistic Deficits

Problems with figurative language (interprets literally)

Impaired sense of humor

Comprehension of complex auditory material

Word fluency

Word recognition and word–picture matching

Paragraph comprehension

Higher order communication deficits

Difficulty organizing information

Tendency to produce impulsive answers with unnecessary detail

Insensitive to contextual cues and pragmatic aspects of communication

Source: Haynes & Pindzola, DIAGNOSIS AND EVALUATION IN SPEECH PATHOLOGY, Table 8.7 "Sequelae of Right Hemisphere Damage" p. 245, © 2008. Reproduced by permission of Pearson Education, Inc.

ASSESSMENT

Neuropsychological testing of an individual who has sustained a TBI should be completed by a multidisciplinary team that includes professionals from medicine, nursing, social work, psychology, physical therapy, occupational therapy, psychiatry, audiology, and speech-language pathology.

Mood and behavior changes can be due to the injury or an emotional reaction to the injuries. Testing of cognitive abilities includes assessment of auditory and visual processing skills and a determination of attention abilities, similar to those assessed in ADHD. Of particular interest are the child's abilities to sustain attention and to use selective attention, divided attention, and alternating attention (Mateer & Moore-Sohlberg, 1992).

Testing of language abilities should concentrate on the comprehension of single words and sentences, auditory discrimination skills, and expressive language abilities. Assessment of memory and learning should be done in conjunction with language testing and should focus on auditory and visual memory, immediate and delayed recall, and the ability to learn new information. Intelligence testing should analyze verbal intelligence, nonverbal intelligence, and general knowledge.

Alternating attention. The ability to shift attention between tasks that have different cognitive demands.

Communication should be assessed and analyzed in a variety of contexts. This involves observing the child with TBI interacting in a multiplicity of settings with different individuals. It is necessary to evaluate how they interact with each other and to eventually modify the communication behavior of the injured individual as well as his or her communication partners. Blosser and DePompei (2003) presented a diagram, shown in Figure 12–4, that illustrates the interrelated aspects of communication.

Executive functioning refers to setting and executing goals and the ability to self-evaluate. Many individuals who have suffered a TBI have trouble with motivation and personal drive. Accident-induced lethargy contributes to this problem, which may occur even in individuals who were highly motivated and self-directed prior to the accident. Tests of dissimulation that assess the child's effort and motivation also should be completed (Green, Stevens, & Wolf, 1997). Problems with executive functioning may be manifested as reduced deficit awareness, poor goal-setting skills, lack of initiation of tasks, poor self-monitoring, difficulty in making and keeping a schedule, and poor time efficiency.

Testing of academic skills and achievement should include subject-specific testing. This includes mathematics, vocabulary, reading, and spelling. Abstract reasoning and concept formation testing should address problem-solving skills and the ability to make appropriate judgments. Motor strength, coordination, and manual dexterity should be part of the assessment of fine

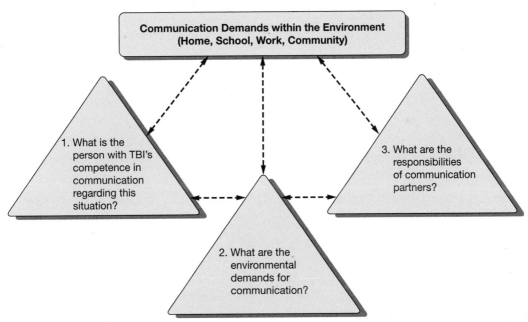

FIGURE 12–4   Interrelated aspects of communication. (*Source: Pediatric traumatic brain injury: Proactive intervention*, by J. Blosser and R. DePompei. Clifton Park, NY: Delmar, Cengage Learning, 2003.)

motor control and speed. Orientation in space and time, visual and tactile perceptual abilities, and responses to varying sensations may have a negative effect on the testing of sensory and perceptual skills.

Finally, a complete personality inventory and psychosocial examination should be done. Children who have suffered a TBI are reported to undergo personality changes after the accident, so this should be assessed by a competent psychologist, psychiatrist, or both (Green, Stevens, & Wolf, 1997).

When assessing the strengths and weaknesses of an individual who has suffered a TBI, the professionals involved must communicate frequently and regularly in order to follow the changes that occur as the child's physical injuries resolve. It is important to remember that the child may fatigue easily, so testing should be done in several short sessions, as opposed to one long session. Sensitivity to the child's emotional state is also important so that the individual does not become overly frustrated or depressed by his or her performance on the varying tasks that are presented.

A list of assessment tools that are appropriate for use with children who have sustained a TBI is found in Table 12–7.

There are many tests and scales that can be used to determine the severity of a brain injury and to measure associated disability. These tests are listed in Table 12–8.

TABLE 12–7 Language tests suitable for use with children with TBI

Test	Authors
Preschool Language Scale—3 (PLS-3)	Zimmerman et al. (1992)
Receptive-Expressive Emergent Language Test—Second Edition (REEL-2)	Bzoch and League (1991)
Clinical Evaluation of Language Fundamentals—Third Edition (CELF-3)	Semel, Wiig, and Secord (1995)
Clinical Evaluation of Language Fundamentals—Preschool (CELF-P)	Wiig, Secord, and Semel (1992)
Peabody Picture Vocabulary Test—Third Edition (PPVT-III)	Dunn and Dunn (1997)
Hundred Pictures Naming Test (HPNT)	Fisher and Glenister (1992)
Boston Naming Test (BNT)	Kaplan et al. (1983)
Test of Language Competence—Expanded Edition (TLC)	Wiig and Secord (1989)
Test of Word Knowledge (TOWK)	Wiig and Secord (1992)
Test of Problem Solving—Elementary (TOPS-Elementary)	Bowers et al. (1994)
Test of Problem Solving—Adolescent (TOPS-Adolescent)	Bowers et al. (1991)
Queensland University Inventory of Literacy (QUIL)	Dodd et al. (1996)
Test of Phonological Awareness (TOPA)	Torgesen and Bryant (1994)
School Age Oral Language Assessment (SAOLA)	Allen et al. (1993)

TABLE 12–8   Assessments commonly used to measure injury severity and associated disability

Assessment Procedure	Description
Glasgow Coma Scale (Teasdale and Jennett, 1974)	A three-category (eye opening, motor response, verbal response), 15-point scale commonly used to measure the initial severity of TBI. Scores of 8 or lower within the first several hours after injury are typically classified as severe injuries, 11–12 as moderate, and 13–15 as mild.
Duration of Coma	Generally based on time from injury to eye opening and resumption of normal sleep-wake cycles. Measured in minutes or hours for mild to moderate injuries and in days, weeks, or months for severe injuries. Sometimes used more informally to refer to the period of significantly altered consciousness.
Duration of Posttraumatic Amnesia	Based on time from injury to resumption of orientation and integration of day-to-day memories. Very hard to establish with precision in severe cases.
Galveston Orientation and Amnesia Test (GOAT) (Levin et al., 1979)	A 11-question test of orientation to person, place, and time and of memory for recent, post-injury events as well as for most recent preinjury events.
Glasgow Outcome Scale (Jennett & Bond, 1975)	A five-category global outcome scale: death, persistent vegetative state, severe disability (conscious, but disabled and dependent), moderate disability (disabled but independent), and good recovery (relatively normal life, but possibly with ongoing minor impairment).
Rancho Los Amigos Levels of Cognitive Functioning (Hagen, 1981)	An eight-level scale of cognitive recovery, based on observations of responsiveness, purposeful activity, orientation, memory, self-regulation, spontaneity, independence. Levels: no response, generalized response, localized response, confused-agitated, confused-nonagitated, confused-appropriate, automatic-appropriate, and purposeful-appropriate.
Disability Rating Scale (Rappaport et al., 1982)	A rating scale developed to track improvement of people with TBI from coma to community. Includes subscales for impairment (similar to GCS), disability (cognitive ability for feeding, toileting, and grooming), and handicap (level of community functioning and employability).
Functional Assessment Measure (FIM + FAM) (Hall, 1992)	A rating scale that adds 12 domains for disability to the 12 domains of the older Functional Independence Measure (FIM). The additional items, added specifically for individuals with brain injury, include swallowing, reading, writing, orientation, attention, safety judgment, emotional status, and adjustment to limitations.
ASHA-FACS (Frattali et al., 1995)	A rating scale designed to assess functional communication with greater precision than is possible with most general disability rating tools.
Communication Effectiveness Survey (Beukelman, 1998)	A survey designed to assess functional communication in natural contexts.
Community Integration Questionnaire (Willer et al., 1994)	A 15-item questionnaire designed to assess home and social integration and productivity in the following domains: household activities, shopping, errands, and leisure activities.

Source: From "Communication disorders associated with traumatic brain injury," by M. Ylvisaker, S. F. Szekeres, and T. Feeney. In *Language intervention strategies in aphasia and related neurogenic disorders* (4th ed.), by R. Chapey (ed.), pp. 745–808. Copyright 2001 by Lippincott Williams & Wilkins.

STAGES OF RECOVERY OR IMPROVEMENT

Szekeres, Ylvisaker, and Holland (1985) defined three stages of improvement based on the Rancho Los Amigos Levels of Cognitive Functioning (Hagen, 1981). As described by Szekeres and colleagues, the early stage is compatible with the Ranchos Los Amigos (RLA) levels 2 to 3. The behaviors at this stage range from the initial generalized responses to environmental stimuli to external stimulus-specific responses. These stimulus-specific responses include localizing to sound, visual tracking, appropriately using common objects, and following simple commands. This stage is frequently referred to as the sensory or coma stimulation stage of treatment, with the child needing intensive support from others.

During the middle stage (RLA levels 4–6), the child may initially be disoriented, confused, and agitated but is more active and alert than in the early stage. Typically, these children experience improvement slowly. They may become more goal-directed but still have difficulty in planning a course of action to achieve the goals. Memory continues to be impaired, although some improvement in episodic memory and focused attention may occur. The children continue to need support from others in their environment, although simplifying and structuring the environment may facilitate eventual independence.

The last stage is equivalent to RLA levels 7 and beyond. The goal at this stage is to help the child achieve his or her ultimate level of independence through the fading of environmental supports. The child may have residual communication and cognitive deficits, with therapy focusing on the development of compensatory strategies and functional skills that can be used in the child's natural settings (Ylvisaker, Szekeres, & Feeney, 2001).

TREATMENT

Interdisciplinary Teams

Interdisciplinary teams (IDT) for the treatment of acquired brain injury (via shaken or blunt trauma, tumor, progressive neurological diseases, or vascular problems such as stroke) should be the norm regardless of setting. In some instances, the team may consist of members across several settings, such as the team for a school-age child. Regardless, the team needs to hold structured meetings (via conference call, teleconferencing, or other electronic means if all are at different settings) in order to monitor the child's progress and modify the treatment plan to accommodate any progress the child has made as well as any changes that may need to be made due to changes in the child's environment, caregiver network, health, and the like.

In keeping with the recommendations of the Commission on Accreditation of Rehabilitation Facilities (e.g., CARF, 2007) and Individuals with

Disabilities Education Improvement Act of 2004 (IDEIA), ASHA recommended that an IDT for individuals with acquired brain injury consist of the following individuals:

- The child with the acquired brain injury
- Members of the child's family and/or caregiver network
- A coordinator
- Professionals from varied disciplines needed to have a "comprehensive assessment process, treatment plan, and discharge plan" (Joint Committee on Interprofessional Relations Between the American Speech-Language-Hearing Association and Division 40 (Clinical Neuropsychology) of the American Psychological Association, 2007, p. 3)

These professionals may include any of the following, depending on the needs of the child and his or her family:

- Speech-language pathologist
- Clinical neuropsychologist
- Audiologist
- Rehabilitation psychologist
- Behavioral specialist
- Dietitian
- Educator
- Occupational therapist
- Physical therapist
- Primary care physician
- Psychiatrist
- Physiatrist
- Rehabilitation nurse
- Social worker
- Case manager
- Therapeutic recreation specialist
- Vocational rehabilitation counselor
- Paraprofessionals (such as speech-language pathologist assistants, teacher aides, or nursing aides) (Joint Committee, 2007, pp. 3–4).

Treatment should focus on the functional knowledge and skills needed for the individual to participate at his or her optimal level in his or her everyday settings and activities.

Each child should have an evidence-based treatment plan with goals that focus on functional outcomes. The goals should reflect those needed within each discipline, but also overall therapy goals that reflect the team's treatment plan. It is also critical that a discharge plan be developed that reflects a "description of functional ability and level of independence/dependence" anticipated at the time the child is discharged from his or her rehabilitation program (Joint Committee, 2007, p. 6).

Factors Affecting Treatment

Factors affecting treatment include the stage of recovery, etiological factors, and age at the time of injury. Age is important because the younger the child, the greater the plasticity of the brain. Plasticity refers to the ability of the undamaged areas of the brain to compensate for the damaged areas of the brain. It is believed that the more plasticity the brain has, the better the chances for natural recovery of some function. Regardless, therapy is needed to help manipulate the plasticity to ensure that the child recovers his or her maximum abilities (Rose, Johnson, & Attree, 1997). The type of treatment pursued varies based on the severity of the injury, the amount of time elapsed since the injury, and the constellation of impairments (Bogaert-Martinez, 2007).

Environmental enrichment is a key to recovery. A common consequence of traumatic brain injury in humans is a reduction in cerebral arousal-activation. In combination with other common neuropsychological impairments such as those involving inattention, memory, and motivation, this can result in significantly reduced levels of interaction between the child and his or her environment. Coexisting sensory and motor impairments can restrict interaction still further. Clinicians agree that to increase levels of interaction between children who have brain damage and their environments is a vital part of any rehabilitation process.

Because children suffering from residual effects of TBI fatigue easily, it is usually recommended that initial therapy sessions be brief and frequent. In other words, four 15-minute sessions per day may be more productive than a single 1-hour session. Functional communication goals should be targeted in individual and group therapy. Determining readiness to return to school or work should be a prime consideration. Thus, it is important to focus not only on functional goals but also compensatory strategies that can be used to minimize the deficits. The rehabilitation team, including family members, also needs to work closely with the child's school or work personnel to facilitate the transition back into the child's natural settings. Initially, an appropriate classroom setting may be a class specifically designed for children recovering from TBI or a classroom for students with learning disabilities (Iskowitz, 1997).

Focus Areas in Therapy

During the acute phase, therapy is likely of focus on sensory stimulation and working closely with the family to encourage responses from the child. Although speech and language abilities are a concern, during this stage issues related to self-care, swallowing, and feeding may be paramount. However, as the child progresses, more attention can be focused on speech and language goals and preparing the child to return to his or her home and school environment. This includes focusing on prospective memory, which is the ability to remember to do things at the appropriate time (such as taking prescribed medications), and functional memory. Functional memory includes the skills needed to learn new information, recall old information, remember situational details, and function independently (Green, Stevens, & Wolf, 1997). It is also important to address pragmatic issues with the client, with an emphasis on social skills such as carrying on a conversation, sharing, greeting, and cooperating, in order to facilitate interaction with others in the client's natural environments (Ylvisaker et al., 1992).

> **Prospective Memory.** Memory involved in remembering to do daily activities at the appropriate time.
>
> **Functional Memory.** Memory needed to recall previously learned information, to learn new information, to remember situational details, and to function independently.

Cognition is an additional focus in therapy. This includes addressing memory, attention, reasoning ability, organization, efficient information processing, perceptual skills, and learning. However, there are impediments inherent in TBI that make therapy more challenging. For example, people with TBI frequently have difficulty taking previous consequences into consideration when making decisions. They also frequently have reduced initiation, which can also impede executive functions such as decision making. Deficits in working and strategic memory, poor organizational skills, and impaired memory of previous consequences to decisions impede improvement in cognition. There is also difficulty with maintenance and generalization of skills beyond the therapy setting to the child's natural environments. Children with TBI frequently exhibit oppositional behavior and this, combined with poor ability to learn from previous consequences, impedes behavior management in children with TBI (Ylvisaker, Szekeres, & Feeney, 2001).

Compensatory and Restorative Training

Ylvisaker, Hanks, and Johnson-Greene (ASHA, 2003) discussed cognitive and behavioral rehabilitation of children and adults after brain injury. They differentiated between two approaches: compensatory and restorative. Compensatory training addresses the development of skills to adapt to and compensate for the deficits the child is experiencing as a result of his or her brain injury. For example, for a child who has lost much of his or her ability to communicate through speech, therapy could focus on learning how to use an augmentative or alternative communication device or system. Restorative training, on the other hand, addresses the specific deficits in an effort to improve the functions related to those deficits. Again using the example of a child having difficulty communicating through speech, restorative training would focus on assisting the child in regaining functional speech. Regardless, both approaches are based on goals developed "to enhance the person's capacity to process and interpret information and to improve the person's ability to function in all aspects of family and community life" (ASHA, 2003, p, 1).

Section 504 of the Rehabilitation Act

Students who have a head injury and receive special education and related services can be covered by Section 504 of the Rehabilitation Act, which "protects individuals with disabilities from discrimination and ensures that children with disabilities have equal access to an education" (Duff, 2009, p. 4) (see Chapter 7). However, in order to qualify for coverage, the student must have a substantial limitation (due to a physical or mental impairment) in one or more major life activities. These include ambulatory issues (not being able to walk), sensory issues (impaired vision or hearing), difficulty breathing, difficulty speaking, difficulty with self-care, difficulty performing manual tasks and/or working, and difficulties related to classroom performance (i.e., writing, learning, reading, and doing math calculations). Even if the student only needs accommodations made and not direct therapy, he or she is still covered under Section 504.

Response to Intervention Model

Many therapists use the Response to Intervention model. The RTI model is discussed in depth in Chapter 9. Basically, it is an approach that allows a thorough assessment of a student's ability to perform when provided with appropriate and adequate instruction. The assessment is based on structured observation of the student in the classroom in order to get real-time functional measures. It can help identify children who may have learning disabilities or other problems that interfere with academic progress, and can be used to develop and implement intervention strategies to assist the student in meeting his or her educational goals within the least restrictive environment. This model is often used with students who have sustained a brain injury to assess their ability to function adequately in the classroom and identify supports to help them get the maximum benefit from their educational activities (Duff, 2009).

Why Do Some Individuals with Head Injury Succeed Post Injury When Others Do Not?

(Author's note: The information discussed in this section is based on narratives from adults with head injury who have had successful recoveries. However, the information can have significant effects on how we, as speech-language pathologists and audiologists, approach rehabilitation with individuals, whether adult or child, who have sustained a head injury.)

Despite the best efforts of a treatment team (including the child), some individuals just do not make the adjustment to post-injury life. Ylvisaker and Feeney (2000) wondered why and found two major themes to establishing new identities, which seemed to be the key to having successful recoveries: "engagement in meaningful life activities" and "reconstruction of a satisfying sense of self" (quoted inFraas and Calvert, 2009, p. 315). Fraas and Calvert (2009) followed up on the findings of Ylvsaker and Feeney through the analysis of narratives obtained from 31 adults who had sustained a head injury. Fraas and Calvert attempted to determine what characteristics were common to a group of survivors of head injury who had successful recoveries and were leading productive lives. The 31 survivors included 21 males (average age 43:10 years) and 10 females (average age 44:40 years). Their etiologies were as follows:

- Males: 11 TBI; 8 cardiovascular accident; 2 tumor or seizure disorder

- Females: 5 TBI; 3 cardiovascular accident; 2 tumor or seizure disorder

Several subthemes emerged from the narratives. Fraas and Calvert organized these subthemes into four main themes:

1. Development of social support networks

2. Grief and coping

3. Acceptance of injury and redefinition of self

4. Empowerment

In regard to development of social support networks, 87 percent of the survivors indicated that "strong support (e.g., family and friends) was a key to their successful recovery" (Fraas & Calvert, 2009, p. 320). Other factors were having a strong marriage and the importance of having supports for the family to help them cope with their own needs, emotions, and responsibilities. With regard to grief and coping, 87 percent said they had feelings of denial, 84 percent experienced anger, and 84 percent experienced depression. Some attributed their faith to getting them through the grief stages, and several indicated they had to make "adaptations in their coping styles" before they were able to experience success after sustaining their head injury.

Eighty-four percent of the survivors in the Fraas and Calvert (2009) study indicated they achieved acceptance of the injury and redefinition of self, which was (according to Fraas and Calvert) consistent with the findings of Ylvisaker and Feeney (2000), who found that relinquishing the former selves and developing new identities (i.e., redefining themselves) was key to having a successful recovery. Sixty-eight percent of Fraas and Calvert's subjects said the "emotional and psychological changes necessary to finally accept their injuries took a long period of time to fully emerge" (p. 321). Components of redefining themselves included focusing on aspects of their lives that they wanted to improve from their preinjury personas, such as becoming a better husband, spending more time with their children, or generally being a nicer person. Eighty-one percent of the survivors were successful in accepting their "new selves" and 68 percent found they had new roles to play and achieve.

Empowerment was vital in successful recovery. The individuals who felt successful in postinjury life were those who made "accomplishments that have empowered them to become independent, resourceful, and eager to give back to their communities" (Fraas & Calvert, 2009, p. 322). Driving was a big factor in feeling independent, as was procuring employment. However, 92 percent of the individuals were employed preinjury; 19 percent remained employed in a part-time capacity postinjury. 42 percent were involved in volunteer work or had returned to school to learn new skills. Finally, acquired brain injury advocacy was important to many of the survivors. "The desire to contribute, advocate (48%), and give back (52%) has empowered many of the participants" (p. 322). These findings are consistent with Ylvisaker and Feeney's (2000) second major theme of engaging in meaningful activities. The characteristics of the individuals who felt empowered fell into three main categories:

1. "Self-esteem or self-efficacy (e.g., developing independence)

2. Actual power (e.g., being assertive and learning new skills)

3. Community activism (e.g., giving back to the community and ABI advocacy)" (Fraas & Calvert, 2009, p. 324)

Fraas and Calvert strongly encouraged the use of narratives in order to have a "holistic look at the needs of their patients," (p. 325) thereby enhancing the recovery process. They assessed the attitudes and beliefs of speech-language pathologists who had employed narratives in their interactions with children with head injury and found that the clinician's own attitudes and beliefs "with regard to the psycho-social and vocational challenges of the survivors" were improved. This is one reason I encourage students to read biographies, autobiographies (in particular), and memoirs of individuals who have experienced head injury, either as the individuals themselves or as part of the injured individual's support network. Several books related to head injury are listed in Appendix E in this book. The use of narratives could be a key strategy in defining an appropriate treatment plan and certainly could be used with adolescents who have sustained a head injury and are likely to have periods of denial and anger, perhaps even more so than adults.

Treatment Summary

Regardless of the age of the individual with TBI, the setting, or the approach, treatment needs to be focused on having the child be an active participant in the therapy process. Therapy should address the development of skills that enable the child to succeed in school, independent living, working environments, and social activities. Blosser and DePompei (2003) delineated the skills needed to effectively communicate in each of these settings. These skills are outlined in Table 12–9. I have included the skills needed

TABLE 12–9   Individual skills necessary for effective communication in various environments

School	Employment
Maintain adequate vocabulary	Attend regularly
Request information	Communicate effectively
Respond to questions	Follow directions
Follow directions	Organize day and job routines
Comprehend lectures	Adapt to changes
Read for functional comprehension	Recognize mistakes
Write for functional expression	Correct mistakes
Organize for planning and sequencing	Care for work area
Store and recall information for later use	Ask for help
	Use socially acceptable manners
Social	Use nonaggressive socially correct language
Monitor actions	Demonstrate initiative
Manage time	Cope with constructive criticism
Understand cultural diversity	**Independent Living**
Respect others	Plan daily routine
Use correct pragmatics	Carry out daily routine
Demonstrate socially acceptable manners and language	Use public transportation
	Know community resources and how to access them
	Advocate for self without offending others
	Manage finances

for employment for two reasons: (1) some adolescents over age 18 may seek employment instead of continuing in school, and (2) it is helpful for the child's rehabilitation team to know the skills that the child will need when he or she begins to work. These skills should be incorporated into the rehabilitation plan.

SUMMARY

Based on studies conducted over the last 20 years, Murdoch and Theodoros (2001) concluded that while children who suffer a mild TBI usually fully recover, those who have moderate to severe TBI events do not fully recover. Receptive language is not as impaired as expressive language, and the children have compromised "expressive oral language skills, including verbal fluency and naming to confrontation" (p. 251). In the initial stages, the child typically has reduced verbal output, even to the point of mutism in some cases. In the long term, they have subtle high-language deficits characterized by poor verbal fluency, word-finding difficulties, and dysnomia. Generally speaking, the language impairments following moderate to severe TBI in children are similar to those found in adults. Speech-language pathologists see these children in therapy as they are integrated back into their home and school setting following the TBI.

Over the last several years, speech-language pathologists have held discussions regarding the need to establish medical tracks and school-based tracks in speech-language pathology coursework. However, the population of students with TBI helps point out the need to have both types of education, regardless of the professional's primary employment site. Those who work with a child in the medical setting need to understand the educational setting to which the child will return as soon as possible. Likewise, those in the educational setting need to be familiar with the long-term sequelae of TBI and to understand the nature of the injury and recovery process. These children also need to be followed closely throughout their academic careers to monitor possible residual deficits that may play a role in a child's educational and social progress.

Children returning to their school settings following a TBI need to be monitored to gauge the effect the TBI and its residual deficits have on the individual. Careful attention needs to be paid to his or her ability to adapt to the old surroundings and to be sure the child does not become depressed and/or frustrated to the point that it is not possible for him or her to continue in that setting. This may involve providing therapy in community-based settings, with the clinician going to the client instead of having the client come to a therapy setting. Functional goals should be established that relate to the needs and interests of the child and his or her family (Blosser & DePompei, 1989; DePompei & Blosser, 1987, Coehlo et al., 1996).

CASE STUDY

History

Luke, a 18-year old, left-handed male was seen on July 23, 2010 for an initial speech and language evaluation. He had suffered a gunshot wound to the left frontal lobe in a drive-by shooting when he was 17 years old and, consequently, had aphasia. During the first 6 months following the trauma, Luke received speech-language therapy, physical therapy, and occupational therapy five times a week in a residential rehabilitation center. During this time, he also worked with a homebound teacher on his schooling. He has continued with outpatient speech-language therapy two times a week since he was discharged from the residential rehabilitation center. Luke and his family recently moved to Centerville and have been referred to the Rehabilitation Clinic for continued therapy. Luke had difficulty with the subject matter at the ninth-grade level and did not return to school following discharge from the rehabilitation center. He did continue to work with a homebound teacher for 3 months until he was 18 but did not graduate.

Luke wears glasses, has a brace on his right leg, and has a moderate (40 dB) hearing loss in his right ear. Luke has taken 100 mg of Dilantin three times a day since the shooting to control seizures.

Assessment

Luke's speech, language, and cognitive functions were assessed using the Western Aphasia Battery during his initial visit to the Rehabilitation Center. The results of the subtests were as follows.

Spontaneous Speech	Information content	9/11
	Fluency, grammatical competence, paraphasias	5/11
	Total	14/20
Auditory Comprehension	Yes/No questions	60/60
	Auditory word recognition	51/60
	Sequential commands	47/80
	Total	158/200
Repetition		84/110
Naming	Object naming	44/60
	Word fluency	11/20
	Sentence completion	11/11
	Responsive speech	8/11
	Total	72/110

(continues)

Reading	Comprehension of sentences	34/40
	Reading commands	14/20
	Written word stimulus—object–choice matching	6/6
	Written word stimulus—picture–word matching	6/6
	Written word stimulus—written word–choice matching	6/6
	Spoken word stimulus—written word–choice matching	3/4
	Letter discrimination	4/6
	Spelled word recognition	1/6
	Spelling	2/6
	Total	76/110
Writing Apraxia	Not assessed due to Luke's fatigue	60/60
Constructional, Visuospatial, and Calculation Tasks	Drawing	26/30
	Block design	9/9
	Calculation	18/24
	Raven's Progressive Matrixes	31/37
	Total	84/110
Aphasia Quotient		75

In the spontaneous speech test, Luke's speech was characterized as often being telegraphic; however, some grammatical organization was evident. Certain paraphasias were noted. On the auditory comprehension subtest, Luke answered yes/no questions with 100 percent accuracy. On the auditory word recognition section, he achieved 85 percent accuracy and did not demonstrate difficulty with any particular category. Luke scored 59 percent on sequential commands, which demonstrated his difficulty when commands were increased in length and complexity (two or more steps).

On the repetition subtest, Luke performed with 84 percent accuracy. The longer sentences and phrases proved to be the most difficult for Luke to repeat.

Luke was able to name objects with 73 percent accuracy. On the word fluency section, he was able to name 10 animals in 1 minute, indicating decreased word fluency. One paraphasia was noted (*cantaloupe* for *antelope*). He was 100 percent accurate on the sentence completion section, and his responsive speech was 80 percent accurate.

On reading comprehension of sentences, Luke was 85 percent accurate. It took him a long time (average 3 to 5 minutes) to complete the task. The additional time appeared to help him answer items correctly.

On the reading commands section, Luke was 70 percent accurate. He had difficulty reading each command aloud and received only partial points on the more complex commands. On choice matching of written and spoken words, Luke was 75 to 100 percent accurate. He had more difficulty identifying the written word from an orally presented target, as opposed to pointing to a picture or object that matched the written word or pointing to the written word that matched the picture.

On the letter discrimination section, Luke was 67 percent accurate. He performed with 17 percent accuracy on spelled word recognition and 33 percent accuracy on spelling words. It was noted that Luke finger spelled the letters on the table, but he was unable to process what individual letters together would spell.

The client was able to perform upper limb, facial, instrumental, and complex gestures upon command with 100 percent accuracy. His responses were quick and appropriate.

Luke showed little difficulty with constructional tasks. He was able to freehandedly draw the figures required with 87 percent accuracy. All but one of his drawings were appropriate; he drew a square when asked to draw a circle. On the Block Design subtest, which tests visuospatial skills, he was able to quickly put four blocks together in the desired pattern with 100 percent accuracy.

Calculation tasks were 75 percent accurate. He showed no difficulty with addition and multiplication but had some errors in subtraction and division. This may have been partially due to the examiner's presentation of the cards; combined oral and visual stimulation was not provided.

The Cinderella story was used to assess Luke's expressive narrative speech and language ability. His speech was characterized as nonfluent with an abundance of fillers such as "ya know," "and all this," and "and everything," and contained many pauses. He had much difficulty initiating sentences and produced false starts throughout the story.

Summary

Luke presents with mild auditory and reading comprehension problems, even though his scores were relatively high for these subtests. This was evidenced by his frequent delay of response and/or requests for repetition. His speech is nonfluent and is characterized by a short mean length of utterance, frequent pauses, false starts, and fillers. His speech at times was also telegraphic. Luke demonstrated letter-processing problems visually and auditorily. He also showed problems spontaneously naming functional objects and performing sequential commands.

Impression

Luke presents with Broca's aphasia, characterized by his nonfluent speech, a greater production of nouns and verbs compared to other grammatical forms, agrammatic speech, and an abundance of pauses and fillers.

Recommendations

It was recommended that Luke receive individual therapy two times a week for 1-hour sessions. Therapy concentrated on sentence production of Wh- interrogatives and object relatives. It was also recommended that he receive a full audiological evaluation.

REVIEW QUESTIONS

1. A contrecoup injury is one in which the injury to the brain is at the point of impact only.

   a. True

   b. False

2. Severe TBIs are characterized by a loss of consciousness lasting 1 to 24 hours.

   a. True

   b. False

3. Individuals who have sustained a closed head injury are likely to demonstrate attention disorders, impulsivity, and fluctuating moods.

   a. True

   b. False

4. Falls are the leading cause of TBIs in the age 5 to 64 population.

   a. True

   b. False

5. According to IDEA, TBI includes brain injuries that are congenital.

   a. True

   b. False

6. As defined by WHO, which of the following defines an impairment?

   a. A decreased ability to participate in work, school, social situations, and so on

   b. A reduction in the individual's ability to effectively and successfully participate in activities of life

   c. A disruption or abnormality in mental or physical functioning

7. Cerebral edema is an example of primary damage resulting from a TBI.

   a. True

   b. False

8. Children who have sustained a TBI usually exhibit nonfluent aphasia as opposed to fluent aphasia.

   a. True

   b. False

9. Which of the following should be included in an assessment battery for children with a TBI?

   a. Tests of academic skills and achievement

   b. Tests of executive functioning

    c. Language tests

    d. Personality inventory and psychosocial examination

    e. All of the above

    f. a, b, and c

    g. a, c, and d

10. Usually receptive language is not as impaired as expressive language in individuals who have sustained a moderate to severe TBI.

    a. True

    b. False

REFERENCES

Alajouanine, T. & Lhermitte, F. (1965). Acquired aphasia in children. *Brain, 88,* 653–662.

Allen, L., Leitao, S., & Donovan, M. (1993). *School age oral language assessment.* South Fremantle, Western Australia: Language-Learning Materials, Research and Development.

American Academy of Pediatrics. (2001, July). Shaken baby syndrome: Rotational cranial injuries—technical report. *Pediatrics, 108*(1), 206–210.

American Speech-Language-Hearing Association (ASHA). (1987). The role of speech-language pathologists in the rehabilitation of cognitively impaired individuals: A report of the subcommittee on language and cognition, *ASHA, 29,* 53–55.

American Speech-Language-Hearing Association (ASHA). (1990). Guidelines for speech-language pathologists serving persons with language, socio-communicative, and/or cognitive communicative impairments. *ASHA, 32,* 85–92.

American Speech-Language-Hearing Association (ASHA). (2003). Rehabilitation of children and adults with cognitive-communication disorders after brain injury [technical report]. Available from www.asha.org/policy.

Beukelman, D. R. (1998). Communication effectiveness survey. In C. M. Frattali (ed.), *Measuring outcomes in speech-language pathology* (pp. 334–353). New York: Thieme.

Bijur, P. E., Haslum, M., & Gloning, J. (1990). Cognitive and behavioral sequelae of mild head injury in children. *Pediatrics, 86,* 337–344.

Blake, M. L. (2007, November). Perspectives on treatment for communication deficits associated with right hemisphere brain damage. *American Journal of Speech Language Pathology, 16,* 331–342.

Blosser, J. L., & DePompei, R. (1989). The head injured student returns to school: Recognizing and treating deficits. *Topics in Language Disorders, 9,* 19–32.

Blosser, J. L., & DePompei, R. (2003). *Pediatric traumatic brain injury: Proactive Intervention* (2nd ed.). Clifton Park, NY: Delmar, Cengage Learning.

Bogaert-Martinez, E. (2007*). Assessment and treatment of traumatic brain injury within the ECHCS polytrauma system of care.* Retrieved July 5, 2009 from www.dol.gov/vets/grants/07conference/TBI_AUG9.PPT.

Bowers, L., Huisingh, R., Barrett, M., Orman, J., & LoGuidice, C. (1991). *Test of problem solving—elementary.* Nerang East, Queensland, Australia: Pro-Ed.

Bowers, L., Huisingh, R., Barrett, M., Orman, J., & LoGuidice, C. (1994). *Test of problem solving—elementary.* Nerang East, Queensland, Australia: Pro-Ed.

Bzoch, K. R., & League, R. (1991). *Receptive-expressive emergent language test, second edition.* Austin, TX: Pro-Ed.

Castrogiovanni, A. (2010). Communication facts: Special populations: Traumatic brain injury 2010 edition. http://www.asha.org/research/reports/tbi.htm.

Christian, C. W., Block, R., & the Committee on Child Abuse and Neglect. (2009). Abusive head trauma in infants and children. *Pediatrics, 123*(5), 1409–1411.

Coelho, C. A., DeRuyter, F., & Stein, M. (1996, October). Treatment efficacy: Cognitive-communicative disorders resulting from traumatic brain injury in adults. *Journal of Speech and Hearing Research, 39*(5), S5–S17.

Commission on Accreditation of Rehabilitation Facilities. (2007). *Medical rehabilitation accreditation and standards.* Retrieved August 2, 2007, from www.carf.org/Providers.aspx?content=content/Accreditation/Opportunities/MED/AccreditationStandards.htm.

Copeland, J. (2010, February). New data suggest shift in college football concussions rate. www.ncaa.org/wps/portal/ncaahome?WCM_GLOBAL_CONTEXT=/ncaa/ncaa/ncaa+news/ncaa+news+online/2010/associationwide/new+data+suggest+shift+in+college+football+concussions+rate_02_23_10_ncaa_news.

Defense and Military Veteran's Brain Injury Website. Retrieved March 11, 2010 from www.dvbic.org/Service-Members—Veterans/TBI-Awareness.aspx.

Dennis, K. (n.d.). Current perspectives on traumatic brain injury. Retrieved June 10, 2010 from www.asha.org/aud/articles/CurrentTBI.htm.

DePompei, R., & Blosser, J. (1987). Strategies for helping head-injured children successfully return to school. *Language, Speech, and Hearing Services in the Schools, 18,* 292–300.

Dodd, B., Holm, A., Qerlemans, M., & McCormack, M. (1996). *Queensland University inventory of literacy.* Nerang East, Queensland, Australia: The University of Queensland.

Duff, M. (2009, July 14). Management of sports-related concussion in children and adolescents. *The ASHA Leader.*

Dunn, L. M., & Dunn, L. M. (1997). *Peabody picture vocabulary test—third edition.* Circle Pines, MN: American Guidance Service.

Ewing-Cobbs, L., Fletcher, J. M., & Levin, H. S. (1985). In M. Ylvisaker (ed.), *Head injury rehabilitation: Children and adolescents* (pp. 71–89). Austin, TX: Pro-Ed.

Ewing-Cobbs, L., Levin, H. S., Eisenberg, H. M., & Fletcher, J. M. (1987). Language functions following closed head injury in children and adolescents. *Journal of Clinical and Experimental Neuropsychology, 9,* 575–592.

Fisher, J. P., & Glenister, J. M. (1992). *The hundred pictures naming test.* Victoria, Australia: ACER.

Fraas, M. R., & Calvert, M. (2009, November) The use of narratives to identify characteristics leading to a productive life following acquired brain injury. *American Journal of Speech-Language Pathology, 18,* 315–328.

Frattali, C. M., Thompson, C. K., Holland, A. L., Wohl, C. B., & Ferketic, M. M. (1995). *The American Speech-Language-Hearing Association functional assessment of communication skills for adults (ASHA FACS).* Rockville, MD: ASHA.

Green, B. S., Stevens, K. M., & Wolfe, T. D. W. (1997). *Mild traumatic brain injury: A therapy and resource manual.* San Diego, CA: Singular Publishing Group.

Hagen, C. (1981). Language disorders secondary to closed head injury. *Topics in Language Disorders, 1,* 73–87.

Hall, K. M. (1992). Overview of functional assessment scales in brain injury rehabilitation. *NeuroRehabilitation, 2,* 98–111.

Haynes, W. O., & Pindzola, R. H. (2007). Diagnosis and evaluation in speech pathology (7th ed.). Boston, MA: Allyn & Bacon.

Hegde, M. N. (1996). *Pocket guide to assessment in speech-language pathology.* Clifton Park, NY: Delmar, Cengage Learning.

Iskowitz, M. (1997, June 16). Overcoming obstacles of pediatric TBI. *Advance for Speech Language Pathologists, 7*(24), 5.

Jennett, B., & Bond, M. (1975). Assessment of outcome after severe brain damage: A practical scale. *Lancet, 1,* 480–484.

Joint Committee on Interprofessional Relations Between the American Speech-Language-Hearing Association and Division 40 (Clinical Neuropsychology) of the American Psychological Association. (2007). Structure and function of an interdisciplinary team for persons with acquired brain injury. Available from www.asha.org/policy.

Jordan, F. M., & Murdoch, B. E. (1990). Linguistic status following closed head injury: A follow-up study. *Brain Injury, 4,* 147–154.

Jordan, F. M., Ozanne, A. E., & Murdoch, B. E. (1988). Long-term speech and language disorders subsequent to closed head injury in children. *Brain Injury, 2,* 179–185.

Kaplan, E., Goodglass, H., & Weintraub, S. (1983). *Boston naming test.* Philadelphia: Lea & Febiger.

Kay, T., & the Mild Traumatic Brain Injury Committee of the Head Injury Special Interest Group of the American Congress of Rehabilitation Medicine. (1993). Definition of mild traumatic brain injury. *Journal of Head Trauma Rehabilitation, 8*(3), 86–87.

Langolis, J. A., Kegler, S. R., Butler, J. A., et al. (2003). Traumatic brain injury-related hospital discharges: Results from a fourteen state surveillance system, 1997. *Morbidity and Mortality Weekly Reports, 52*(55-04), 1–18.

Langolis, J. A., Rutland-Brown, W., & Thomas, K. E. (2004). *Traumatic brain injury in the United States: Emergency department visits, hospitalizations, and deaths.* Atlanta, GA: Centers for Disease Control and Prevention, National Center for Injury Prevention and Control.

Lees, J. (1997). Long-term effects of acquired aphasias in childhood. *Pediatric Rehabilitation, 1*(1), 45–49.

Levin, H. S., & Eisenberg, H. M. (1979). Neuropsychological impairment after closed head injury in children and adolescents. *Journal of Pediatric Psychology, 4,* 389–402.

Levin, H. S., Eisenberg, H. M., & Benton, A. L. (1989). *Mild head injury.* New York: Oxford University Press.

Levin, H. S., O'Donnell, V. M., & Grossman, R. G. (1979). The Galveston orientation and amnesia test: A practical scale to assess cognition after head injury. *Journal of Nervous and Mental Diseases, 167,* 675–684.

Mateer, C., & Moore-Sohlberg, M. (1992, September). Current perspectives in cognitive rehabilitation. Presented at a conference entitled Speaking of Cognition . . . Assessment and Intervention Strategies. Sponsored by Rehabilitation Services Midwest Medical Center, Indianapolis, IN.

Murdoch, B. E., & Theodoros, D. G. (2001). *Traumatic brain injury: Associated speech, language, and swallowing disorders.* Clifton Park, NY: Delmar, Cengage Learning.

Myers, P. S., & Blake, M. L. (2008). Communication disorders associated with right hemisphere damage. In R. Chapey (Ed.), *Language intervention strategies in aphasia and related neurogenic communication disorders* (pp. 963–987). Philadephia, PA: Lippincott Williams & Wilkins.

National Head Injury Foundation. (1985). *An educator's manual: What educators need to know about students with traumatic brain injury.* Framingham, MA: Author.

National Institute of Neurological Disorders and Stroke. (2002, February). *Traumatic brain injury: Hope through research.* NIH Publ. #902-158. Bethesda, MD: National Institutes of Health.

National Institutes of Health. (1984). *Head injury: Hope through research.* NIH Publication No. 84–2478, pp. 1–37. Bethesda, MD: Author.

Nelson, N. W. (1993). *Childhood language disorders in context: Infancy through adolescence.* New York: Macmillan Publishing Company.

Neurosurgery Today. (2005, November). Shaken baby syndrome. Retrieved June 6, 2010 from www.neurosurgerytoday.com.

Payne, J. C. (1997). *Adult Neurogenic Language Disorders: Assessment and treatment. An ethnobiological approach* (pp. 157–158). San Diego, CA: Singular Publishing Group, Inc.

Rappaport, M., Hall, K. M., Hopkins, H. K., Belleza, T., & Cope, D. N. (1982). Disability rating scale for severe head trauma: Coma to community. *Archives of Physical Medicine and Rehabilitation, 63,* 118–123.

Reed, V. A. (1994). *An introduction to children with language disorders* (2nd ed.). New York: Macmillan Publishing Company.

Reed, V. A. (2005). *An introduction to children with language disorders* (3rd ed.). New York: Macmillan Publishing Company.

Rose, F. D., Johnson, D. A., & Attree, E. A. (1997). Rehabilitation of the head-injured child: Basic research and new technology. *Pediatric Rehabilitation, 1*(1), 3–7.

Russell, N. K. (1993, April). Educational considerations in traumatic brain injury: The role of the speech-language pathologist. *Language, Speech, and Hearing Services in the Schools, 24,* 67–75.

Sarno, M. T. (1984). Verbal impairment after closed head injury: Report of a replication study. *Journal of Nervous and Mental Disease, 172,* 475–479.

Satz, P., & Bullard-Bates, C. (1981). Acquired aphasia in children. In M. T. Sarno (ed.), *Acquired aphasia* (pp. 399–426). New York: Academic Press.

Semel, E., Wiig, E. H., & Secord, W. A. (1995). *Clinical evaluation of language fundamentals—third edition.* San Antonio, TX: Pro-Ed.

Sohlberg, M. M., & Mateer, C. A. (1989). *Introduction to cognitive rehabilitation theory and practice.* New York: Guilford Press.

Spreen, O., & Benton, A. L. (1969). *Neurosensory centre comprehensive examination for aphasia.* Victoria, British Columbia, Canada: University of Victoria.

Szekeres, S., Ylvisaker, M., & Holland, A. (1985). Cognitive rehabilitation therapy: A framework for intervention. In M. Ylvisaker (ed.), *Head injury rehabilitation: Children and adolescents.* Boston: College-Hill Press/Little, Brown.

Teasdale, G. M., & Jennett, B. (1974). Assessment of coma and impaired consciousness: A practical scale. *Lancet, 2,* 81–84.

Thurman, D., Alverson, C., Dunn, K., Guerrero, J., & Sniezek, J. (1999). Traumatic brain injury in the United States: A public health perspective. *Journal of Head Trauma and Rehabilitation, 14*(6), 602–615.

Torgensen, J. K., & Bryant, B. R. (1994). *Test of phonological awareness.* Nerang East, Queensland, Australia: Pro-Ed.

U. S. Department of Health and Human Services, Administration for Children and Families, Administration on Children, Youth and Families, Children's Bureau. (2010). *Child maltreatment 2008.* Available from www.acf.hhs.gov/programs/cs/stats_research/index.htm#can.

Wiig, E. H., & Secord, W. A. (1989). *Test of language competence—expanded edition.* San Antonio, TX: The Psychological Corporation.

Wiig, E. H., & Secord, W. A. (1992). *Test of word knowledge.* San Antonio, TX: The Psychological Corporation.

Wiig, E. H., Secord, W. A., & Semel, E. (1992). *Clinical evaluation of language fundamentals—preschool.* San Antonio, TX: The Psychological Corporation.

Willer, B., Ottenbacher, K. J., & Coad, M. L. (1994). The community integration questionnaire. *American Journal of Physical and Medical Rehabilitation, 73,* 113–117.

World Health Organization (1980). *International classification of impairments, disabilities, and handicaps: A manual for classification relating to the consequences of disease.* Geneva, Switzerland: Author.

World Health Organization (2001). *International classification of function, disability, and health.* Geneva, Switzerland: Author.

Ylvisaker, M., & Feeney, T. (2000). Reconstruction of identity after brain injury. *Brain Impairment, 1*(1), 12–28.

Ylvisaker, M., Hanks, R., & Johnson-Green, D. (2003). Rehabilitation of children and adults with cognitive-communication disorders after brain injury. *ASHA Supplement, 23,* 59–72.

Ylvisaker, M., & Szekeres, S. (1989). Metacognitive and executive impairments in head-injured children and adults. *Topics in Language Disorders, 9,* 34–49.

Ylvisaker, M., Szekeres, S., & Feeney, T. (2001). Communication disorders associated with traumatic brain injury. In R. Chapey (ed.), *Language intervention strategies in aphasia and related neurogenic communication disorders* (4th ed.). Philadelphia: Lippincott Williams & Wilkins.

Ylvisaker, M., Szekeres, S., Haarbauer-Krupa, J., Urbanczyk, B., & Feeney, T. (1992). Speech and language intervention. In G. Wolcott and R. Savage (eds.), *Educational programming for children and young adults with acquired brain injury.* Austin, TX: Pro-Ed.

Zimmerman, I. L., Steiner, V. G., & Pond, R. E. (1992). *Preschool language scale—3.* San Antonio, TX: The Psychological Corporation. www.biausa.org/education. htm#anoxic, retrieved June 9, 2010. www.dvbic.org/Service-Members---Veterans/TBI-Awareness.aspx, retrieved February 11, 2010. www.nim.nih/gov/medlineplusency/article/0004.htm, retrieved June 4, 2010.

APPENDIX 12A

Prevention of Head Injury at Home

The Defense and Veteran's Brain Injury Center offers the following suggestions to prevent head injuries at home:

1. Wear a seat belt every time you drive or ride in a motor vehicle.

2. Never drive while under the influence of alcohol or drugs.

3. Always buckle your child into a child safety seat, booster seat, or seat belt (depending on the child's height, weight, and age) in the car.

4. Wear a helmet and make sure your children wear helmets when:

   • Riding a bike, motorcycle, snow mobile, or all-terrain vehicle.

   • Playing a contact sport, such as football, ice hockey, or boxing.

   • Using in-line skates or riding a skateboard.

   • Batting and running bases in baseball or softball.

   • Riding a horse.

   • Skiing or snowboarding.

5. Avoid falls in the home by:

   • Using a step stool with a grab bar to reach objects on high shelves.

   • Installing handrails on stairways.

   • Installing window guards to keep young children from falling out of open windows.

   • Using safety gates at the top and bottom of stairs when young children are around.

   • Maintaining a regular exercise program to improve strength, balance, and coordination.

   • Removing tripping hazards, using non-slip mats in the bathtub and on shower floors, and putting grab bars next to the toilet and in the tub or shower.

6. Make sure the surface on your child's playground is made of shock-absorbing material (e.g., hardwood mulch, sand).

7. Keep firearms stored unloaded in a locked cabinet or safe. Store bullets in a separate secure location.

Source: www.dvbic.org/Service-Members—Veterans/TBI-Awareness.aspx, retrieved March 11, 2010.

Chapter 13

Assessment of Language Disorders in School-Age Children

LEARNING OBJECTIVES

After completion of this chapter, the reader will be able to:

1. Describe three goals that guide the evaluation process.

2. Cite four key questions that should be asked when analyzing a language sample of a school-age child.

3. Explain why an IQ–achievement discrepancy is not a good tool for diagnosing a child as dyslexic.

4. Discuss three constructs that should be noted through the analysis of a language sample.

5. Discuss why it is better to assess narrative discourse and expository discourse than straightforward discourse analysis when testing adolescents.

6. Discuss why it is difficult to differentially diagnose auditory processing disorders, language problems associated with ADHD, and language-based learning disabilities.

INTRODUCTION

When discussing the assessment of language disorders in preschool children, consideration must be given to lexicon, semantics, syntax, morphology, and pragmatics and to analyzing these areas of language within the context of normal development. In the school-age population, however, the clinician needs to be concerned about the impact of the features of language on learning, and particularly the impact of language deficits on reading, spelling, writing, and socialization. The population of school-age children with language impairments and disorders is quite diverse. One faction of this population is made up of children whose preschool delays evolve into disorders during the school years as greater language demands are placed on the child. These children are discussed in Chapter 5. However, the bulk of the children seen for assessment and treatment during the school years have problems that affect their reading, spelling, and writing. These children have a language-based learning disability that has a negative impact on their academic, social, and vocational progress. These children are the focus of Chapters 13 and 14.

COMPONENTS OF THE EVALUATION

The evaluation process is guided by three goals. The first objective is to determine the reality of the problem. The child's communication behavior needs to be described, with particular emphasis on the areas of greatest deviation from expected behaviors. Is the child's language within normal limits, delayed, or disordered? Because few norms are available against which to compare diagnostic data in the school-age population, it is important to compare the information gained through the diagnostic process with acceptable criteria for the mental and chronological ages of the student. It is also necessary to make a severity statement, including a notation as to how much of a problem the disorder is for the child. This includes evaluating the impact that the language or learning disability has on the child's academic and social progress.

A second goal of the diagnostic process is to determine the etiology of the problem. What causal factors may be related to the presenting problem? Emerick and Haynes (1986) differentiated predisposing, precipitating, and perpetuating etiologic factors, and this distinction is particularly important when talking about the school-age population. Predisposing factors are defined as "agents that dispose or incline an individual toward communication impairment" (Emerick & Haynes, 1986, p. 9).

In children with language delays in the preschool years, a persistence of the delay may occur as a disorder. Thus, the language delay could be a predisposing factor in the child's language disorder. Precipitating factors "actually bring about the onset of the problem" (Emerick & Haynes, 1986, p. 9) and may not always be identifiable.

Perpetuating factors are "responsible for the persistence of the abnormality" (Emerick & Haynes, 1986, p. 9). These may include such factors as lack of early identification and treatment, unreasonable demands in the classroom when the disorder is taken into account, and the student's own lack of understanding about his or her language deficits.

> **think about it**
>
> How would you proceed with identifying and modifying or eliminating perpetuating factors in a child's classroom?

Predisposing factors. Factors that dispose or incline an individual toward an impairment related to his or her language and communication skills.

Precipitating factors. Factors that result in the onset of the language and/or communication problem.

Perpetuating factors. Factors that result in the persistence of the language and/or communication problem.

The third goal of the evaluative process with school-age children is to provide a clinical focus. When all of the information is gathered, what can be done to help the child improve with regard to language, academic progress, and social goals? Effectively obtained diagnostic information is the basis for clinician accountability when determining therapy goals. To this end, when evaluating adolescents, it is particularly important to make sure they understand the importance of what the clinician is doing. The clinician should be straightforward with the child and acknowledge the pressure the child may feel in the evaluation process. Alternatives could be discussed, as well as the socio-economic repercussions of language disorders that affect the child's learning in school and carry over into adulthood. Adolescents need to feel that they have some control, so it is a good idea to let the adolescent be the focus during the interviews. Questions should be directed to the adolescent during the history-gathering process, and the results should be discussed directly with the adolescent.

Observation

Observation as a component of a complete assessment battery was discussed in Chapter 5. Just as it is important to evaluate how a child uses (or does not use) language in his or her natural settings, it is critical to observe school-age children and adolescents in a variety of settings. For example, they should be observed in the classroom, noting the following in particular:

- What strategies (e.g., use of a planner, recording lectures, using a note taker) does the student employ to be able to maintain compliance with the classroom demands?

- Does the student interact with his or her peers?

- Does the student interact with the teacher?

- Where in the classroom does the student sit?

- Does the student volunteer to ask or answer questions?

- Does the student answer questions when directly called on?

- Does the student request that the teacher repeat the question?

- Is the student organized?

- Does the student ask for clarification when needed (i.e., when he or she does not understand the assignment of instructions)?

- Does the student remain attentive?

- Does the student daydream?

- Is the student disruptive?

- Does the student appear frustrated?

- Does the student appear to have given up?

- Does the student appear angry?

In addition to the classroom, students should be observed during unstructured times such as lunchtime, during interactive classes such as physical education, art, or music classes, and on the school grounds interacting with peers before and after school. Finding the answers to questions like those above across a variety of settings can help determine the direction the speech-language pathologist, audiologist, and other school personnel take in designing the assessment and intervention process for the student.

The information from the observation could also be helpful in gathering documentation needed to make appropriate referrals.

Screening

In most school settings, a child's speech and language skills can be screened without getting permission from the parents. A screening serves to identify children who are not using speech and language as expected based on the child's chronological age and academic abilities. A screening simply provides information that, based on the test used to provide a preliminary evaluation of the child's speech and language skills, there is or is not reason to suspect a possible speech or language deficit. Screenings can be administered individually using instruments that take 5 to 15 minutes to determine if a child is at risk. Some screening tools can be administered as paper-and-pencil tasks to an entire classroom at one time. Regardless of the type of screening done, the only conclusion that can be drawn is that the child apparently is within normal limits with regard to speech and language skills or that the child is at risk for speech and language problems and should be evaluated further. A screening does not result in a diagnosis.

Case History

As with any evaluation, the history is a critical component in the assessment of an individual with a language-based learning disability. It may be gathered through a written history form and through a preassessment interview with the student and his or her family. When evaluating the effect of language on a child's academic and social development, it is critical to analyze carefully the child's daily environment and the impact that his or her family and peers have on the child's language. It is also important to look at the child's educational history. What academic subjects are particularly challenging for the child? What are his or her grades? Does the child actively participate in the educational process? The answers to these questions can provide important guidance to the clinician in planning the assessment and treatment processes. The passage of the Individuals with Disabilities Education Act (IDEA) reinforced the educational expectations outlined in Public Laws 94-142 and 99-457 but added an educational focus on the child's transition from school to work. Transition is a required focus for all children receiving special education services who are 16 years old and older. However, for children with severe deficits or multiple problems, educators are encouraged to introduce vocational training prior to age 16 years. Thus, the case history of a school-age child should also reflect information related to previous, current, and future vocational education.

A detailed medical history also should be taken. The presence of seizure disorders should be carefully noted, as well as any medications that the child takes on a regular basis. The presence of allergies or autoimmune disorders in the child or family members should be documented carefully because some studies show a history of these types of disorders in the families of children with language-based learning disabilities. Also, any history of drug abuse by the child should be documented.

Previous testing should be reviewed carefully, although usually there is no need to go back to developmental milestones for children with language-based learning disabilities. For children who have severe delays that have carried over into the school-age years, the milestones may be of interest, particularly those relating to the development of the features of language.

Student Interview

An interview is a directed conversation that proceeds in an orderly fashion to obtain data, to convey certain information, and to provide release and support for the sharing of information. For older elementary, middle school, and high school students, it is particularly important to make the student feel that he or she has some control over what happens in the assessment process. Time should be given to the student to vent any concerns, problems, or feelings with regard to the disorder and its diagnosis and treatment. When assessing a student who has a language-based learning disability, it is important to get the student's perspective on the problem (Larson & McKinley, 1995). This is particularly important when assessing students who are in middle or high school. Larson and McKinley (1995) suggested that the clinician determine the student's feelings and attitudes about thinking, listening, and speaking. Negative attitudes can adversely affect the logical thought processes needed to survive in academic and social situations. As stated earlier, many students with language-based learning disabilities develop a sense of learned helplessness in which they come to believe that outcomes cannot be controlled. They become passive participants in the academic world and develop an inability to be persistent in their approach to learning. These students are likely to become ineffective problem solvers; they believe they cannot think, so they do not think. They believe that educators, family members, and clinicians have low expectations, and this influences their desire to set and achieve higher goals. All of these factors are compounded into a negative self-image and an increased prevalence of depression in the learning-disabled population when compared to their nondisabled classmates.

Larson and McKinley (1995) also pointed out the importance of knowing the student's feelings and attitudes toward listening. Many students with language-based learning disabilities express listening barriers that are excuses for their poor academic achievement. For example, comments frequently include statements such as, "The teacher is boring" and "The teacher does not like me." The students may criticize the speaker's looks, actions, and speaking style. They may also listen for isolated facts without taking in the whole picture. Some students may get overly stimulated or emotionally involved with the topic, sometimes allowing their own personal prejudices to interfere with listening to the speaker and with their comprehension of the subject. They may listen as long as the topic is easy, but shut down when the content becomes more complicated.

Feelings and attitudes toward speaking also are important to ascertain (Larson & McKinley, 1995). The first step is to determine if poor communication is due to a poor attitude about speaking, to a disordered communication system, or to both. Does the student believe he or she has nothing to say, in which case the root of the problem may be language-based, or does he or she have a speech disorder (voice, fluency, articulation) that interferes with his or her desire to communicate with others? Does his or her attitude vary from setting to setting or speaker to speaker? Many adolescents will not admit to a communication disorder unless it affects communication with their peers.

Assessing the student's learning environment also is important. What is the child's learning style? Does he or she do better on oral or written examinations? Are there environmental factors or social-emotional factors that affect the student's ability to learn?

All of the above information should be obtained prior to proceeding with the testing portion of the diagnostic process.

> **think about it** What are some other questions that you would ask a high school student that you would not ask a middle school child when you conducting a preassessment interview with him or her? Justify the questions.

Language Sample

A predominant part of any evaluation of a school-age child is the language sample, in which the clinician gathers approximately 50 to 100 utterances (depending on the analysis system to be used) and carefully analyzes the child's spontaneous language use. In younger elementary school–age children, a language sample should be obtained in the assessment situation. Usually, toys and books can be presented to encourage the child to engage in dialogue with the assessing clinician. To thoroughly assess the speech and language of adolescents (middle and high school students), it is beneficial to get one language sample of the child talking with a peer, one talking to a teacher, and one talking with a family member (Hegde, 1996).

A conversational language sample is a critical part of the evaluation of any individual with communication impairment. As shown in Table 13–1, Weiss, Tomlin, and Robin (2000) listed activities that can be used to elicit a language sample for different age groups as well as ideas of what to look for when analyzing the language sample. The sample should be analyzed from several perspectives and can be one of the most valuable pieces of

TABLE 13–1   Language sampling across the life span

Age Range	Suggested Sampling Activities	Items to Look for:	Helpful References
Infants and Toddlers (preverbal to emerging language: approximately birth to 2 years of age)	• Observation of the child with the primary caregiver(s). • Use a variety of familiar and unfamiliar toys; place some just out of reach or make them otherwise inaccessible without assistance from an adult. • Coggins and Carpenter (1981) suggested a sample of 45 minutes duration.	• Evidence of responsiveness on the part of the caregiver(s) to the child's initiated bids. Compare styles of interactions: Does the infant provide clear signals of interest in interaction? • Evidence of developing communicative interactions, e.g., protoimperatives and protodeclaratives. • Evidence of nonlinguistic comprehension strategies, e.g., imitation of ongoing actions versus evidence of true word comprehension. • Evidence of the child's repertoire of volitional vocalizations and speech sounds; these areprecursors to word use. • Evidence of real word use: (1) resemblance to an adult word, (2) consistent phonetic form, (3) used in consistent context. • Analysis of early words in terms of pragmatic function and semantic categorization.	Rossetti (1990); Coggins and Carpenter (1981); Bates (1976); Chapman (1978); Proctor (1989); Owens (1996); Dore (1974); Bloom (1973); Nelson (1973)
Preschoolers (approximately 2 to 5 years of age)	• Collect several language samples with different conversationalists in different settings and with different degrees of structure. 50–200 utterances are usually recommended. • Use materials that lend themselves to the creation of scenarios, e.g., dollhouse, toy farm.	• Evidence of assertiveness and responsiveness in conversations and their different proportions relative to the different samples collected. • Evidence of age-appropriate syntactic structure and use of grammatical morphemes as per mean length of utterance and developmental sentence scoring, for example.	Fey (1986); Brown (1973) and Miller (1981) for mean length of utterance analysis; Lee (1974) for developmental sentence scoring; Retherford (1993)

Preschoolers	• Use open-ended requests for information that does not constrain response length and complexity, e.g., "Tell me about. . . ." • Use a variety of familiar and unfamiliar materials and follow the child's lead. • Although conversation samples are most often used, you can also use prompts for personal narratives, scripts, and story retelling. Be sure to use a lot of visual support materials.	• Evidence of a variety of vocabulary words in the sample, e.g., type–token ratio, as per Templin (1957). • Evidence that the child is accommodating language to his or her listeners via responses, requests for clarification, or presuppositional skills; question comprehension is evident by appropriate responses made to questions asked. • Evidence of observation of turn-taking rules; little if any "simultalk" occurs. • Child can maintain a topic for several turns.	Brinton and Fujiki (1989)
School-Age Children (approximately 6 to 12 years of age)	• Provide prompts for personal narratives, fictional stories, and scripts with visual support, e.g., "Make up a story about something that's not real." • Use of interview questions as per Evans and Craig (1992): (1) What can you tell me about your family? (2) Tell me about school. (3) Tell me about what you like to do when you are not in school. • For older children, collect both written and oral samples. Collect samples of classroom discourse from both ends of the formal–informal continuum.	• Evidence of a cohesive discourse structure: What is the overall structure of the discourse and how adequate is it? • Use of later-developing syntax forms: postmodification of nouns, coordinate conjunctions, adverbial clauses, infinitives, complements, and subjunctive modals. • Evidence of more sophisticated sentence repair strategies or use of alternation rules when faced with communication breakdowns.	Hughes, McGillvray, and Schmidek (1997); Roth and Spekman (1986); Scott (1988); Nippold (1998); Weiss and Johnson (1993); Damico (1991); Westby (1994)

(continues)

TABLE 13–1 *(continued)*

Age Range	Suggested Sampling Activities	Items to Look for:	Helpful References
Adolescents (junior high school and high school age)	• Use activities that require story creation or retelling either with or without visual support. • Collect a sample of expository discourse. • Elicit samples of both oral and written discourse. • Use written materials to prompt conversations, e.g., a provocative newspaper article.	• Evidence of perspective taking and acknowledgment of others' perspectives and opinions. • Greater finesse should be expected in terms of discourse cohesion and structure. • Comparison of cohesion in samples in which information is shared versus not shared with the audience.	Hughes, McGillvray, & Schmidek (1997)
Adults	• Story generation and story retelling without visual stimuli; context not shared. • Fable retelling, proverb interpretation, picture descriptions; use of picture sequences, orcartoon stimuli.	• Sentence complexity, completeness of episode structure, proportion of core information presented (in recall), proportion of revisions, and words per minute.	Nicholas and Brookshire (1993); Chapman (1997); Chapman, Ulatowska, Franklin, Shobe, Thompson, and McIntire (1997); Chapman, Levin, and Culhane (1995); Ulatowska, Chapman, Highley, and Prince (1998)

Source: Language disorders, by A. L. Weiss, J. B. Tomlin, and D. A. Robin. In J. B. Tomlin, H. L. Morris, and D. C. Spriesterbach (eds.), *Diagnosis in speech-language pathology* (2nd ed.), pp. 153–155. Copyright 2000 Delmar, Cengage Learning.

diagnostic data that the clinician has. First, just as with preschoolers and younger school-age children, the sample should be analyzed in terms of the features of language. Does the child have appropriate semantics, syntax, and prosody? The presence of word-retrieval problems should also be documented. Differentiation between speech dysfluencies and dysfluency due to language-based problems should be noted. Does the student use false starts, verbal mazes, circumlocution, imprecise language, excessive pauses, repetitions, and other devices that interfere with his or her expressive language skills? The mean length of utterance also should be determined.

Second, the conversational language sample should be analyzed with regard to the child's use of language for various functions. For example, using the Damico (1985) analyses of conversational language, it can be determined whether a student is an assertive or passive communicator by comparing the number of times the student initiates conversation with the number of times he or she responds to the initiations of his or her conversation partner. It can also be used to determine whether a child uses language for a variety of functions, such as sharing information, receiving information, greeting, and negotiating.

The conversational language sample should be analyzed in terms of the quality and the quantity of information. Is the student able to generate a sample of 50 to 100 semantically and syntactically acceptable utterances? It not, what factors interfered with the student's production of an adequate sample? With regard to the quality of information, the clinician should look at the accuracy of the message. Are the topics discussed relevant and coherent? Is the message full of verbal mazes, or is it fluent with appropriate pragmatics? These issues should be considered carefully when analyzing the quality of a language sample (Larson & McKinley, 1995).

Metalinguistics

Children must make a transition from acquiring functional use of language during the preschool years to developing the ability to think and talk about language as a tool during the school-age years. They learn that language can be used to think, learn, problem solve, and communicate. As a child's language matures, he or she becomes more able to attend not only to the context of a message, but also to how the message is transmitted (Brown, 1978; Flavell, 1977; Flavell & Wellman, 1977). This is due, in part, to an increase in metalinguistic skills. Metalinguistic skills allow a child to think about language in a critical manner and to make judgments with regard to the accuracy and appropriate use of language skills and functions. These skills appear to be related to environmental stimulation, play, cognitive development, academic achievement, and reading ability (Shaywitz & Cherry-Wilkinson, 1982).

The development of metalinguistic skills also leads to the formation of metacognitive skills. *Metacognitive skills* refer to an increasing ability to think about and analyze how a problem can be solved. In other words, metacognition is a skill that underlies a child's ability to become a logical thinker and problem solver.

Discourse Parameters

The child's language should be analyzed in terms of his or her use of cohesion devices to maintain conversational continuity. These devices include repetitions of key words in the conversation and following a logical progression of thought as the dialogue progresses. Critical listening is a primary component of comprehension of a conversation. To be a critical listener, one must be a critical thinker. This implies that, to be a mature conversationalist, a child must have well-developed metalinguistic and metapragmatic skills. Critical listening includes the ability to engage in inductive and deductive thinking, to distinguish between facts and opinions, and to make inferences (Larson & McKinley, 1995).

Narratives

The role of narratives in the assessment of language in school-age children must not be overlooked. At age 5 to 7 years, children can produce true narratives. This is a good age to begin narrative journals to track the child's development in writing as he or she progresses through the elementary years. Children aged 7 to 11 years can summarize and categorize stories. By age 11 to 12 years, they can produce more complex stories; between the ages of 13 to 15 years, children learn to analyze stories. By the time a child is 16 years old, he or she should be able to formulate abstract statements about the themes and messages of books (Larson & McKinley, 1995).

In addition to knowing what kind of information a child can glean from a story, it is important to assess the child's knowledge of story structure. Can he or she identify the common elements of a story? Does the child understand the rules that dictate the construction of a story (Mandler & Johnson, 1977; Rumelhart, 1975; Stein & Glenn, 1979; Thorndyke, 1977)? One way to evaluate the extent of a child's knowledge of story structure elements is to elicit oral and written fictional narratives (McCabe, Bliss, Barra, & Bennett, 2008).

The speech-language pathologist should obtain fictional narrative samples, both oral and written, from students. In a school-age child, a fictional narrative can be elicited by giving the child a wordless picture or story book and asking him or her to tell or write you a story about that book. Another way to elicit a fictional narrative is to have the child retell or write a story told by the examiner (McCabe, Bliss, Barra, and Bennett, 2008).

An adolescent could be encouraged to produce a fictional narrative based on recalled memories of certain events, experiences, or people. He or she also could produce a fictional narrative based on an article he or she read in a magazine or newspaper.

Personal narratives in both age groups (elementary aged children and adolescents) can be elicited by asking the student, "Tell me about your . . . (day, classes, participation in sports and/or other activities, family, goals, etc.)" (McCabe, Bliss, Barra, and Bennett, 2008). It is important to obtain personal narratives because they provide different information regarding a child's language use and complexity than that gleaned from fictional narratives. As discussed in Chapter 9, children and adolescents with language impairment do significantly better with regard to cohesion, use of story elements, and semantic and syntactic complexity on personal narratives than they do on fictional narratives (McCabe, Bliss, Barra, & Bennett, 2008).

Oral narratives should be analyzed in much the same manner as the conversational speech sample. In addition, when the oral and written narratives are evaluated, the clinician should document the number of different words (NDW; a measure of semantic diversity), the accuracy of the information, the presentation of the information, the cohesion, and the incorporation of story elements (such as a beginning, an elaboration, a logical sequence, and a resolution into the narrative) (McCabe, Bliss, Barra, and Bennett, 2008). Information obtained from the analysis of all types of narratives (conversational, personal, fictional, oral, and written) should be compared and integrated into a summary of the child's developmental level with regard to the features of language. This information should then be considered, along with information from other diagnostic sources and activities, in developing a functional plan for language remediation for the student.

Thus, with regard to language in school-age children and adolescents, it is important to assess their ability to comprehend and produce different types of narratives. A child's abilities with regard to narration can provide a window of observation into how well he or she integrates information conveyed through language (Larson & McKinley, 1995).

The use of narratives to determine the types of components and the features of literate (written) language a student uses can provide guidance in intervention. It also helps document the existence of a language impairment that could impact a student's academic and social success (Greenhalgh & Strong, 2001).

> **think about it**
> Many teenagers, when asked to write a narrative, are likely to respond with, "What do you want me to write about?" What suggestions for topics could you provide that would challenge the child yet yield a narrative of sufficient length?

General Testing

Clinicians who provide services for school-age children must be adept at analyzing the language skills of students from kindergarten through twelfth grade. Language-based learning disabilities are multifaceted disorders that need specialized assessment using modality-specific testing instruments. The assessment battery should consist of standardized tests that assess language and cognition using instruments such as the Woodcock-Johnson III Psycho-educational Battery (Woodcock & Johnson, 1977, Woodcock et al. 2001a, 2001b) and the Detroit Test of Learning Aptitude (Hammill, 1998). Tests should be used that enable the clinician to compare the child's overall verbal skills with his or her nonverbal (frequently referred to as performance) skills. Many schools use a discrepancy score between verbal and nonverbal IQ as an eligibility criterion for placement in special education or related services in the schools.

Standardized testing is a critical component of any assessment battery for children who are school aged. Standardized testing allows the student's performance to be compared to that of peers in a normative sample and can provide a more complete picture of a child's specific strengths and weaknesses. However, one needs to remember that standardized testing typically provides a snapshot of a specific construct. That is to say, items are often tested out of context or a language construct is tested with only two or three items. Therefore, it is critical that the clinician analyze each incorrect item to determine what skills or knowledge are necessary to answer the question correctly. In doing so, it is probable that a pattern will emerge that answers a question more important than "What did the student miss?"; the question "Why did the child miss these items?" yields information that can be used as a foundation for generating goals in therapy and recommendations to facilitate classroom participation and performance.

Another component of an assessment battery is criterion-referenced tests, discussed in Chapter 5. The reader is encouraged to review that information because it applies to the school-aged population as much, if not more, than to the preschool population.

TESTING CHILDREN WITH AUDITORY PROCESSING DISORDERS

It is estimated that some degree of auditory processing difficulty is present in 3 to 5 percent of the school-age population. In addition, a much higher percentage of auditory processing disorders occur in children with learning disabilities than in the general population (Holston, 1992). These prevalence figures may be low because many children with learning disabilities are not referred for auditory processing assessment.

Hearing starts at the outer ear and ends at the auditory nerve, which transports the auditory information to the brain. The auditory signal is then separated from nonessential background sound and translated into a meaningful, clarified message. The skills needed for this translation develop mostly in the first 5 years of a child's life.

Although *auditory perception* and *auditory processing* frequently are used interchangeably, there are distinct differences in the meanings of this terminology. Auditory acuity refers to the sharpness and clarity with which sound is perceived by the ear. Auditory perception is the identification, interpretation, or organization of sensory data received through the ear (Holston, 1992). Auditory processing refers to the processing of auditory information throughout the auditory system, including the outer and middle ear. Young (1985) defined processing as the neuropsychological transmission of the stimuli from one point in the brain to another. He referred to the comprehension of the stimuli as perception. A central auditory processing disorder refers to "auditory processing that begins at the level of the cochlear nuclei in the brain stem, ascending ultimately to the cortex" (Wallach & Butler, 1994, p. 383). Sometimes, *auditory processing* and *central auditory processing* are used interchangeably, although ASHA now recommends the use of *auditory processing* as the correct designation for these disorders.

> **Auditory acuity.** The sharpness and clarity with which sound is perceived by the ear.

Individuals with auditory processing problems have normal hearing acuity and intelligence but are unable to process auditory information effectively. Most authorities report that auditory processing disorders cause difficulties in detection, interpretation, and categorization of sounds and that these problems may be due to some type of dysfunction in lower- or higher-level cortical processes (Schow & Nerbonne, 1996).

On the basis of several different profiles, children are frequently referred for assessment of their auditory processing. Young (1985) proposed that two types of auditory processing disorders may be present in children. The first is related to attentional deficits, whereas the second includes both attentional problems and language deficits.

Children who are believed to have reading problems or language-based learning disabilities are often referred to an audiologist for testing to rule out auditory processing as a causative factor in their learning problems. Children who have poor academic achievement, ADHD, behavior problems, phonological deficits, and problems with oral language also should be referred for further evaluation of their auditory processing abilities (Wallach & Butler, 1994).

At times, it is difficult not only to separate language disorders from auditory processing disorders but also to differentiate between children with ADHD and children with auditory processing disorders. This is because many of the symptoms of ADHD are also reported as symptoms for auditory processing problems. These symptoms include hyperactivity, impulsivity, distractibility, and difficulty in staying on task (Holston, 1992).

Table 13–2 presents a list of typical behaviors associated with auditory processing disorders in childhood. This list can be used by classroom teachers as a guide in making referrals of children who are struggling academically to audiologists and speech-language pathologists.

Over the years, there traditionally have been at least two methods of identifying children who need further evaluation for a possible auditory

9. Difficulty understanding rapid speech or persons with an unfamiliar dialect

10. Frequent requests for information to be repeated

Other indications of a possible APD include problems with reading, spelling, and handwriting, as well as articulation and language disorders. Children who demonstrate any of these behaviors in the classroom or demonstrate academic performance that is below what one would expect should be referred to an audiologist for a complete audiological evaluation and to a speech-language pathologist for an assessment of language problems (which are often displayed by individuals with auditory processing disorders).

One way in which clinicians can differentially diagnose a language-based learning disability and an auditory processing disorder is to test the child using non–language-based auditory input (see the APD testing battery pages 594–595) and language-based auditory input (as found in most language assessments). Knowing how the child performs on language-based tasks versus non–language-based tasks can help provide a differential analysis that helps answer the question, "Why did this student miss this item?" This is an instance in which differential diagnosis clearly is critical in order to know the cause of the student's deficits and its impact on his or her academic performance. The input of the speech-language pathologist and audiologist is necessary to help determine whether the primary deficit is auditory processing difficulties, language or learning deficits, or cognitive deficits before proceeding with the development of an intervention plan. The role of the audiologist and classroom teacher in the assessment and diagnosis of a school-age child with a suspected auditory processing disorder are expanded in the next section.

Assessment Procedures for Auditory Processing Disorders

Testing for auditory processing disorders is based on three important assumptions. The first is that testing auditory processing requires a series of tests that assess auditory memory, auditory closure, auditory discrimination, and auditory figure-ground perception (Keith, 1988). A second assumption is that the auditory system is redundant; therefore, it is necessary to reduce and manipulate the redundancies by filtering, alternating between the right and left ears, compressing the message, lowering the signal-to-noise ratio, and presenting competing noise in the opposite or same ear. The neuroanatomical and language redundancies challenge the mechanism, so the testing should also address the redundancies (Keith, 1988).

The third assumption had to do with cause and effect. If a child tests positive for auditory processing disorders, it is difficult to determine whether the auditory processing problems are the cause or the result of the language problem (Northern & Downs, 1991). It is almost certain that, because language has a strong auditory component, the auditory processing disorder contributes to the language difficulties. However, until a definitive relationship can be forged between language disorders and auditory processing disorders, the reader should take care when considering the diagnostic information for purposes of labeling a child's disorder and determining eligibility for services. It is possible that some children do not perform well on auditory processing tests owing to metalinguistic and metacognitive disorders that affect the outcome of the testing (van Kleeck, 1984).

In its 2005 *Technical Report on (Central) Auditory Processing Disorders*, ASHA stated that APD "is best viewed as a deficit in the neural processing of auditory stimuli that may coexist with, but is not the result of, dysfunction in other modalities" (p. 3). As with many other language disorders, assessment of auditory processing disorders should involve a team consisting of audiologists, speech-language pathologists, teachers, psychologists, and neurologists in the testing of an individual with difficulty processing auditory information. In fact, the 1996 ASHA Task Force on CAP Consensus Development implicitly stated that auditory processing disorders should be addressed using a multidisciplinary approach. The multidisciplinary team should take the following into account when diagnosing an auditory processing disorder:

- The physical structure of the acoustic stimulus

- The neural mechanism that encodes the stimulus

- The perceptual dimensions that arise from the encoding

- The interactions that occur between perceptual processes and the activation of the higher level resources

- The nature of the pathological process (ASHA, 1996, pp. 41–42)

Each team member has a unique set of tests that can be used to help define the patient's ability to process information using the auditory channel. For example, the speech-language pathologist should employ tests of language across modalities, paying particular attention to performance of skills that are tested using the auditory channel only, then performance of the same skills using the visual modality only. It should be noted here that due to the neurological organization of language processing, the child may demonstrate problems with visual processing as well, but the deficits are more pronounced in the auditory modality (ASHA, 2005). Receptive and expressive abilities also should be analyzed, as well as standardized and functional assessment of form, content, and use of language. DeBonis and Moncrieff (2008) recommended that speech-language pathologists administer the following tests of auditory perceptual skills:

- Lindamood Auditory Conceptualization Test (Lindamood & Lindamood, 1979)

- Test of Auditory-Perceptual Skills—Revised (Gardner, 1996)

- Comprehensive Assessment of Spoken Language (Carrow-Woolfolk, 1999)

- Language Processing Test (Richard & Hanner, 1995)

- Comprehensive Test of Phonological Processing (Wagner, Torgesen, & Rashotte, 1999)

- The Listening Test (Zachman, Huisingh, & Barrett, 1992)

- Auditory Processing Abilities Test (Swain & Long, 2004)

The educator should provide information as to how the child functions in the classroom setting and a description of the environment. For example, do the teacher and student use a variety of assistive listening devices, and are there visual and acoustic distractions in the classroom? The teacher can also provide insight regarding the child's personality and performance in groups, his or her ability to follow directions, and how the child is performing academically. Some behaviors that teachers (and family members) can provide insight into include the following:

> difficulty understanding spoken language in competing messages, noisy backgrounds, or in reverberant environments; misunderstanding messages; inconsistent or inappropriate responding; frequent requests for repetitions, saying "what" or "huh" frequently; taking longer to respond in oral communication situations; difficulty paying attention; being easily distracted; difficulty following complex auditory directions or commands; difficulty localizing sound; difficulty learning songs or nursery rhymes; poor musical and signing skills; and associated reading, spelling, and learning problems. (ASHA, 2005, p. 5)

The audiologist should use assessment procedures designed to demonstrate the integrity of the central auditory nervous system and central auditory processes. These procedures include evaluation of the integrity of the peripheral auditory system, clinical observation, and electrophysiological measures (Friel-Patti, 1999; Keith, 1999). In addition to a thorough case history (addressing medical, social, and educational considerations), and observation of the student in a variety of sound environments, the task force specifically recommended the following auditory tests:

- Thorough basic auditory battery, including pure tones, speech recognition, and immitance

- Analysis of temporal processes

- Ability to localize and lateralize to sound

- Monaural low redundancy speech tests

- Dichotic stimuli

- Binaural interaction procedures (ASHA, 1996; Keith, 1999)

TABLE 13–3 Sample auditory processing battery

Test	Author
Synthetic Sentence Identification (SSI)	Jerger and Jerger (1974)
Dichotic Digits	Musiek (1983)
Staggered Spondaic Words (SSW)	Katz (1962)
Pitch Pattern Sequence (PPS)	Pinheiro (1977)
Duration Pattern Sequence (DPS)	Baran, Musiek, Gollegly, et al. (1987)
Random Gap Detection Test (RGDT)	Keith (2000)
Test for Auditory Processing Disorders in Children (SCAN-C) or Adults (SCAN-A)	Keith (1986)

Delmar/Cengage Learning

Other professionals can also contribute to the differential diagnosis of these children. The psychologist can provide invaluable information on the status of the patient's cognitive and learning skills, and the neurologist can provide information regarding the integrity of the neurological system with regard to auditory signal and language processing through the use of MRI and CT scans and neurochemical analysis.

A sample battery of tests for auditory processing disorders is found in Table 13–3.

> *think about it*
>
> What would you do if the testing is inconclusive or, based on test results, a student does not meet the criteria for therapy?

TESTING LANGUAGE SKILLS IN CHILDREN WITH SPECIFIC LANGUAGE IMPAIRMENT (SLI)

Early identification of children with SLI is particularly important because communication functions and academic development are frequently at risk in this population. Children with SLI frequently have reading disorders in addition to more global impairment in academic subjects (Aram, Ekelman, & Nation, 1984; Catts, 1991, 1993; Stark et al., 1984). Not only is early identification important, but also it is advantageous to reassess the children over time (even if they are receiving intervention) in order to monitor linguistic variables that are typically associated with long-term deficits in children with SLI.

The child's use of morphosyntactic structures should be followed, as well as more general measures such as mean length of utterance and quantitative and qualitative growth in lexicon. The best way to measure these constructs is through a spontaneous language sample (in addition to more formalized measures) (Goffman & Leonard, 2000). The assessment of language in children who have SLI should include comparisons both across and within language domains. This involves comparing the child's performance on tasks assessing form (phonology, morphology, and syntax), content (semantics), and use (pragmatics). Bliss (2002) wrote, "At more specific levels, comparisons should be made within grammatical categories for noun and verb phrase expansion (e.g., articles versus demonstrative pronouns or auxiliaries versus copulas) and between grammatical categories and grammatical structures (e.g., auxiliaries versus simple and complex sentence use)" (p. 35).

It is also important to assess the child's usage of verbs because this is a language form that is typically problematic for children with SLI (Goffman & Leonard, 2000; Grela & Leonard, 2000; Bliss, 2002).

In addition, adolescents who have language-based learning disabilities should be assessed and provided with intervention as early as is feasible. This is due to the impact that language-based learning disabilities have, not only on language, but also on academic, social, and subsequent vocational activities. Bliss (2002) advocated the use of discourse analysis but cautioned the reader that basic conversation is not necessarily problematic for these adolescents, so it may not reflect the extent of the language and/or learning deficits. Narrative discourse is useful for the assessment of topic maintenance, referencing, and event sequencing. Likewise, expository discourse, which is commonly encountered in the classroom, can provide insight into the child's ability to describe and explain different phenomena, to persuade, and to argue (Larson & McKinley, 1995; Nelson, 1998; Paul, 2001). Metalinguistic skills, metapragmatic skills, and metacognitive skills should also be assessed in adolescents with language-based learning disabilities, as well as social skills and word-retrieval skills (Bliss, 2002).

> **think about it**
>
> What would you expect to learn from a written narrative that may indicate a language and/or learning disability that you would not learn from a conversation? Why is this information critical?

Ultimately, the best test of the abilities of a child with SLI is to assess his or her functional communication ability in a wide variety of settings. How well does he or she exchange information with others? Are his or her pragmatics appropriate? Damico (1993) noted that effective communication is based on three criteria: "the effectiveness of meaning transmission, the fluency of meaning transmission, and the appropriateness of meaning transmission" (p. 29). Larson and McKinley (1995) advocated that a descriptive assessment including a descriptive analysis and an explanatory analysis be done.

A descriptive analysis focuses on directly observing and recording behaviors that (1) have been found to be necessary for successful communication in selected contexts in which the student is likely to communicate and in selected modalities that the student is likely to use, and (2) are believed to be valid indices of communicative difficulty. An explanatory analysis determines the causal factors for the communication disorder that was observed during the descriptive analysis (p. 83).

It is important when assessing a school-age child or adolescent with SLI that an evaluation of the student's environment, including curriculum variables, teachers' attitudes and philosophies, and social demands be conducted (Larson & McKinley, 1995). All of these factors can greatly affect the student's ability to learn and use language and to succeed socially and academically.

TESTING LANGUAGE SKILLS IN SCHOOL-AGE CHILDREN WITH INTELLECTUAL DISABILITIES OR MULTIPLE DISABILITIES

Testing the school-age child with intellectual disabilities or multiple disabilities (e.g., motor, sensory, and/or intellectual disabilities) poses a different set of problems than testing most school-age children. These children are likely to have attention and motivation problems, lack of conventional verbal output, poor motor skills, and cognitive skill deficits. It may be necessary to divide the testing into several short periods of time instead of one long session. In addition, it may be helpful to increase the amount of reinforcement that is offered to the child in order to help keep him or her motivated to complete the tasks. If the child is nonverbal and/or has physical problems that negate pointing as a response mode, it may be necessary to use an alternative response mode such as eye gaze or head wands for pointing. It also may be necessary to give the child extended time in which to respond. Children with multiple handicaps may need time not only to formulate the correct response but also to motor plan how to make that response.

Other test adaptations may be necessary, such as modifying the test items; however, this would result in an invalid administration. At times, one may have to use a standardized test to gain specific information about the child's language. However, if the test does not include children with handicaps in its normative sample, the test is not valid for the children with handicaps. It could be used to gain information about some of the child's language constructs, but the test could not be scored. A clinician can employ "out-of-level testing" (Berk, 1984), which involves using a test for a child whose age is not included in the normative sample. Again, this enables the clinician to gain information about the child, but no score can be obtained. For lower-functioning school-age children, it may be beneficial to use developmental checklists and tests such as the Communication and Symbolic Behavior Scales—Developmental Profile (CSBS-DP) (Wetherby & Prizant, 2002). The CSBS is normed for developmental ages 8 to 24 months and chronological age 9 months to 6 years. The results of the CSBS and similar tests (see Chapter 5) can be used to guide further assessment, plan intervention, and document change over time.

In 1988, Sattler proposed *testing of limits* as a method of adaptations for following up on standardized test administrations. These modifications include providing extra time to respond, providing supplemental cues to the child, changing the response modality (for example, using gestural output instead of verbal output), and asking questions that can help the child clarify and prepare his or her response. Testing of limits can provide information as to how the child approaches a task and the impact of his or her disabilities on test performance (McCauley, 2001).

Another type of testing that can be done is discrepancy testing. McCauley (2001) defined discrepancy testing as "the comparison of performances in two different behavioral or skill areas (e.g., between ability and achievement) to determine whether a discrepancy exists" (p. 158). Some school districts use discrepancy testing as a means of justifying educational assistance for a child.

Generally speaking, the child with cognitive challenges should be tested in a variety of settings in order to get a true picture of his or her communicative abilities. Behavioral observations and language samples can be helpful in providing an adequate assessment of their functional communication skills (Bliss, 2002).

> **think about it**
> Based on test scores, many children with intellectual disabilities and/or multiple disabilities may not qualify for therapy. Do you believe a child who does not have a discrepancy between his or her mental age and language age should receive therapy? Justify your answer.

TESTING LANGUAGE SKILLS IN CHILDREN WITH ADHD

Children with ADHD frequently are restless and fidgety, unable to sit still for the duration of a test, and excessively talkative. All of these behavioral manifestations of ADHD can contribute to making it difficult to assess a child with ADHD. According to Barkley (2000), lack of behavioral inhibition is at the root of the impulsivity, inattention, and hyperactivity seen in children who have ADHD. Behavioral inhibition is a cognitive deficit that significantly interferes with executive functioning skills. This, in turn, has the potential to affect assessment results in these children. This is particularly important when one considers that there may be overlap of language impairments and ADHD, with estimates that co-morbidity of these two problems ranges from 20 to 60 percent (Oram et al., 1999).

Oram and colleagues (1999) proposed three hypotheses related to language assessment of children who have ADHD. The first hypothesis is that the children's behavioral manifestations of ADHD do not interfere with formal testing. This may be due in part to the nondistracting environment and one-on-one interaction that typically characterize language assessments. Contrary to this first hypothesis, the second hypothesis is that the ADHD does interfere with testing, which may lead to an underestimation of the child's true ability on language tasks. The third hypothesis is that the ADHD interferes with the child's performance on specific tasks, namely those "that require a greater degree of sustained attention, inhibition, and/or organization" (p. 73). Oram and colleagues designed a study to test the third hypothesis through the language testing of three groups of children: controls (24 private-school children), children with ADHD and language impairment (LI), and children with ADHD only. Fifty-three children aged 7 to 11 years old who were diagnosed with ADHD were tested using three language tests. These tests were the Test of Word Finding (TWF) (German, 1986), the Clinical Evaluation of Language Fundamentals—Revised (CELF-R) (Semel, Wiig, & Secord, 1987), and the Auditory Analysis Test (Rosner & Simon, 1971). "Language impairment was defined by performance: (a) at least 1.5 SD below the mean for age on at least one of TWF Accuracy Score, Rosner raw score, CELF-R Receptive Language Score, or CELF-R Expressive Language Score; or (b) at least 1 SD below the mean for age on two or more of these scores" (Oram et al., 1999, p. 74). As a result of the testing, the 53 children with ADHD were divided into two groups: those with ADHD only (25 children) and those with ADHD and language impairment (28 children). This particular study was actually part of a larger study conducted by Tannock and colleagues (1998) in which children referred for medical treatment of ADHD (but not referred due to concerns about language) were given several standardized language tests in addition to assessment of auditory processing, conversational and narrative language, cognitive functioning, and academic skills. Oram and colleagues further hypothesized as to which tasks would be most problematic for the children with ADHD. These included tasks "requiring high levels of sustained attention, inhibition, working memory, or planning/organization" (p. 73). A list of the tasks and their nonlinguistic demands is found in Table 13–4.

Results were as follows:

- On most subtests, the ADHD-only and control groups did not differ in their performance, with both groups doing significantly better than the group of children with ADHD and LI.

- On the CELF-R subtests, the ADHD-only children and the controls performed within normal limits, but the children with ADHD and LI scored more than 1 SD below the mean on two subtests and borderline for two other subtests.

- On the three CELF-R expressive language subtests, the controls and ADHD-only children did better than the ADHD-LI group.

- On the three CELF-R expressive language subtests, those children with ADHD only did significantly worse than the controls on the Formulated Sentences, Word Structure, and Sentence Assembly subtests.

TABLE 13–4   Nonlinguistic demands of standardized language tasks on systems impaired in ADHD

Nonlinguistic Demand	Subtest	Description
Sustained attention	CELF-R Listening to Paragraphs	Listen to narrative paragraphs
	TWF Description Naming	Listen to three-part word definitions
	CELF-R Oral Directions	Listen to multipart directions
Inhibition	CELF-R Oral Directions	Do not point until examiner says "Go"
Working memory	CELF-R Oral Directions	Remember all parts of direction while executing each step
	CELF-R Word Classes	Remember four words while selecting two related in meaning
	CELF-R Formulated Sentences	Remember target word while formulating a sentence using it
	Rosner Level VII	Remember target syllable to delete while segmenting multisyllabic word
Planning/ Organization	CELF-R Sentence Assembly	Avoid making same arrangements of word groups that already were unsuccessful

Source: From "Assessing the language of children with attention deficit hyperactivity disorder," by J. Oram, J. Fine, C. Okamoto, and R. Tannock. In *American Journal of Speech-Language Pathology* 8 (1). Copyright February 1999 by American Speech-Language-Hearing Association.

- On the Sentence Assembly subtest, "only the mean score for the group with ADHD+LI approached clinical levels" (p. 76).

- Mean scores for all three groups were within the normal range on the Word Structure subtest.

- The differences in performance by the ADHD-only and control groups on the Word Structure and Sentence Assembly subtests were not clinically relevant.

- Both ADHD groups scored at least within the borderline range on the Formulated Sentences subtest, making this subtest "more challenging in children with ADHD relative to their unaffected peers, even in the absence of LI" (p. 77).

On the Formulated Sentences subtest, there were three patterns of errors by the children with ADHD only: no response, missing clause, and responses with the target at the beginning. Because these three responses occurred more frequently in the ADHD-only group than in the controls, it is possible that they were a factor in the lower scores achieved by the ADHD-only group. The ADHD-LI group scored even lower than the ADHD-only group, indicating that their language weaknesses also contributed to poor performance on the Formulated Sentences subtest. Another factor that may have contributed to the lower performance on the Formulated Sentences subtest is pragmatics. All the children with ADHD exhibited pragmatic deficits such as displaying poor turn-taking skills, providing insufficient and ambiguous information, talking excessively and inappropriately, and having difficulty initiating and maintaining a topic. All of these findings have implications for the assessment of language disorders in children with ADHD.

MULTICULTURAL ISSUES IN ASSESSMENT OF SCHOOL-AGE CHILDREN

Demographic Issues

The United States conducts a census every 10 years, and just completed the 2010 Census. Based on information from the U.S. Census of 2000 (see Tables 13–5 and 13–6), it is estimated that approximately 36 million people in the United States (13%) speak English as a second language.

This data shows that the number of children in the United States who speak English as a second language has a significant impact on the caseloads of speech-language pathologists, particularly those in schools located in large urban areas. As a profession, we have taken great strides over the last 20 years in distinguishing language differences from language delays and disorders; we have not kept pace with the demographic changes in terms of assessment materials available that are appropriate for this population, nor has our curriculum in a majority of graduate schools kept pace. All graduate programs must show evidence of addressing multicultural issues in their curriculum, but I suspect that a majority of speech-language pathologists do not feel prepared to work with this population. In 1995, Owens reported that over 33 percent of ASHA-certified speech-language pathologists had at least one bilingual client in their caseload, yet over 80 percent of those clinicians did not feel confident in their abilities to treat bilingual clients.

think about it

How, as a profession, can we better prepare today's speech-language pathologists and audiologists to provide adequate and appropriate services to those who speak English as a second language?

TABLE 13–5 Breakdown of population by origin in U.S. Census, 2000

National Origin/Race	Number	Percent of Population
White alone	211,460,626	75.1%
Black or African American alone	34,658,190	12.3%
Hispanic or Latino alone	14,891,303	5.3%
Asian alone	10,242,998	3.6%
American Indian or Alaskan Native alone	2,475,956	0.9%
Native Hawaiian or other Pacific Islander alone	398,835	0.1%
Other or Combination Race/Origin	7,491,562	0.28%
TOTAL for U.S., 2002	281,421,906	100%

Source: Compiled from U.S. Census, 2000. www.census.gov/prod/2001pubs.

TABLE 13–6 Breakdown of population by race in U.S. Census, 2000

Race/Origin	Number	Percent of Population
White	211,460,626	75.1
Other than White	69,961,280	24.9
Other than White and Black/African American	35,500,654	13%

Source: Compiled from U.S. Census, 2000. www.census.gov/prod/2001pubs.

Special Considerations

If the clinician conducting an evaluation is not fluent in the child's language, it is necessary to find a colleague who is. If another clinician cannot be located, it is acceptable to use an interpreter. Taking the time to train the translator in test administration, paying particular attention to the use of inadvertent nonlinguistic cues, is critical. It is strongly recommended that one interpreter be used consistently with a client (ASHA, 1989). It is also important to remember that a word-for-word translation of English into any other language is not possible. Thus, the validity and reliability of any test that is translated by an interpreter is affected.

Interpreters can also be of benefit when analyzing language samples when the clinician and client speak different languages or dialects of the same language. The clinician should collect language samples in several different contexts to check for code switching and dialect use. Monologue and dialogue settings should be analyzed, as well as static tasks such as describing objects, dynamic tasks such as narration, and abstract tasks such as expressing opinions (Owens, 1995).

In cases in which a dialectal difference occurs but not English as a second language, it is important to compare the presence of dialectal variations in oral language and written language. In any vernacular, differences occur in the functional and structural properties of language used for writing and spoken language (Rubin, 1987). Rubin also pointed out that research shows that African Americans show fewer instances of Black English vernacular in their written language than in their spoken language.

Linguistic and Cultural Differences

Difficulty with English is the primary reason for referral for determination of eligibility for special education placement. Minority children also are known to have a greater dropout rate, frequently are less successful in school, and are, in fact, overrepresented in special education classes and underrepresented in classes for gifted students (Polakow, 1993). Until 1983, ASHA recognized several minority groups based on physical, mental, or hearing handicaps. At that time, it adopted the federal government's designation of minority groups as consisting of Blacks, Hispanics, Asians, and Native American Indians (including Native Alaskans). One of the complicating issues is that what constitutes a difference or a disorder in one culture may not be one in another setting. For example, Native American children are taught that it is disrespectful to establish eye contact with their elders. This lack of eye contact could be interpreted as a pragmatic deficit by a clinician who is not familiar with the culture of the Native Americans. Unfortunately, very few data exist, particularly from Third World countries, to define a communication disorder. According to a sociocultural perspective, the clinician must keep in mind that a difference or disorder exists on a continuum related to culturally based norms for that speech community. Nonetheless, clinicians must be prepared to assess and treat individuals from different cultural and linguistic backgrounds. In fact, not only is it logical and ethical, but also it is federally mandated that the assessment and remediation of communication disorders in minority language speakers require specific skills and background knowledge. These skills are discussed more thoroughly in Chapter 14.

When one is assessing children who are linguistically and culturally different, there are many factors that require attention from the speech-language pathologist. Some of these considerations are diagrammed in Figure 13-1. As depicted in the model, the first thing that should be done is to screen language of standard American English (SAE)-speaking students. If the child fails, he or she should then be screened using a test standardized on the child's linguistic-cultural group, if available. Based on the child's

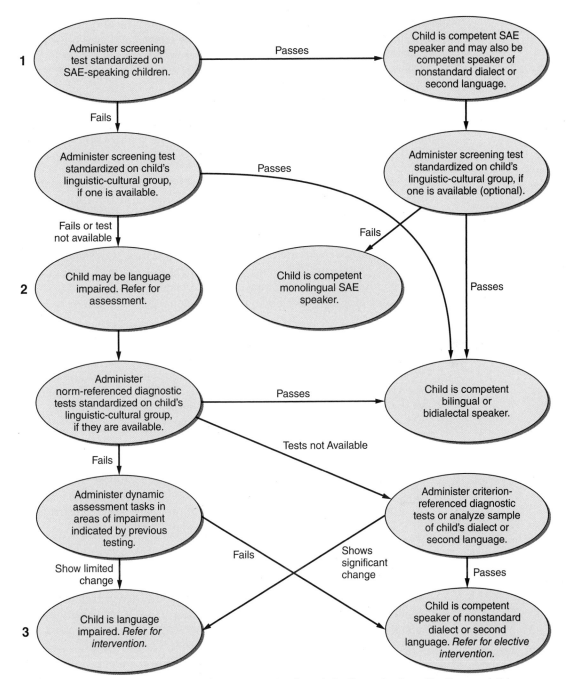

FIGURE 13–1   Model of differential diagnosis for linguistically and culturally diverse children. (*Source:* Language and linguistically-culturally diverse children, by S. Long. In *An introduction to children with language disorders,* (3rd ed.), edited by V. A. Reed, Figure 9.1, p. 326. Copyright Pearson Education, Inc., 2005.)

performance, he or she then continues for further testing and intervention or is determined to be competent in his or her native language. It is important to remember that children may demonstrate a language deficit in English but be competent in their native language.

Legal Mandates Related to Multicultural Issues

Several federal and case laws address the assessment and treatment of individuals from multicultural backgrounds.

- *P.L. 95-561 (The Bilingual Education Act of 1978; Title VII of the Elementary and Secondary Education Act of 1968).* Reauthorized in 1978, P.L. 95-561 provided federal assistance for programs to aid children speaking limited English.

- *Equal Education Opportunity Act (EEOA) of 1974.* The EEOA stated that education opportunities could not be denied to an individual because of the failure by an educational agency to take appropriate action to overcome language barriers that impede equal participation by its students.

- *Diana v. Board of Education (1970).* This case addressed the over-identification of children of Mexican migrant workers for placement in special education classes. Upon investigation, it was ascertained that the children were being tested in English, even though, for the majority of the children, Spanish was their first language and their English was extremely limited. The ruling in this case mandated that children should be tested in their native language.

- *Lau v. Nichols (1974).* "No equality of treatment" was the issue in San Francisco, where more than half of the students of Chinese descent received no instruction to overcome English-language deficiencies. A Supreme Court decision led to a resolution to give special instruction to teach English to the students of Chinese descent.

- *Martin Luther King, Jr., Elementary School v. Ann Arbor School District Board (1979).* This is a case that addressed the legitimacy of Black English. The parents of several African American children believed that the academic progress of their children was being hindered and impeded, particularly in language-based classes such as reading and spelling, by a lack of understanding and appreciation of Black English. Speech-language pathologists were designated by the courts to take an active role in assisting teachers to be sensitive to cultural dialects while providing instruction in standard English. This case is often referred to as the case that found the Black English dialect to be a legitimate and distinct dialect with cultural origins that deserved recognition and acceptance.

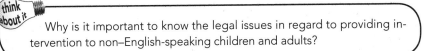

think about it — Why is it important to know the legal issues in regard to providing intervention to non–English-speaking children and adults?

SUMMARY

P.L. 94-142, P.L. 99-457, and IDEA have all played a key role in determining the importance of adequate evaluations of school-age children. IDEA mandates increased services in the areas of assessment and intervention and serves to heighten health care professionals' awareness of the importance of early intervention. The final determination of a child's disorder and eligibility for therapy should be a synthesis of the clinician's knowledge of norms, adequate testing procedures and techniques, test results, observations, effective and empathetic relationships, and creative intuition.

CASE STUDY

History

Mary is an 11-year-old girl in the fifth grade at Clark Elementary School. Her developmental history and Mrs. Wagner's pregnancy with Mary are unremarkable. Mr. Wagner has reported that he struggled with reading and was a "slightly below average student" when he was in school, but he was never tested or diagnosed with a reading problem. Mary's learning problems were first apparent toward the end of second grade. Mary is repeating fifth grade and continues to struggle academically. She was initially evaluated by a school psychologist 2.5 years ago when she was in third grade and was found to have low-average intellectual functioning with a full-scale IQ of 85. She was further tested by the school's speech-language pathologist, who determined that Mary has a moderate to severe language disorder with apparent deficits in auditory processing. After more than 2 years of group therapy at Clark, Mary has demonstrated little progress. Mary's parents have brought her to the Communicative Disorders Diagnostic Clinic (CDDC) at Memorial Hospital for further assessment.

Evaluation

On September 9, 2010, Mary was tested for language-based learning disabilities at the CDDC at Memorial Hospital. Tests administered included the Token Test—Revised, the Woodcock-Johnson Psychoeducational Battery, the Test of Language Development—Intermediate (TOLD-I), and the Word Test. Additional nonstandardized diagnostic procedures were also done.

(continues)

CASE STUDY (continued)

On the Token Test—Revised, Mary's overall age standard score of 496 and overall grade standard score of 495 were within the average performance range. On each subtest of the TOLD-I, she scored more than 1 standard deviation below the mean. A summation of her scores on the TOLD-I is as follows.

Subtest	Raw Score	Percentile	Standard Score
Sentence Combining	11	9	6
Characteristics	38	37	9
Word Ordering	9	5	5
Generals	7	2	4
Grammatic Comprehension	6	9	6

On the Word Test, Mary achieved a raw score of 21 with an age equivalent of 7:9. Results of the Woodcock-Johnson Psychoeducational Battery Tests of Cognitive Ability are as follows.

Cluster	Grade Score	Age Score	Percentile
Verbal Ability	5:6	10:8	50
Reasoning	1:0	3:10	<1
Perceptual Speed	2:8	8:4	9
Memory	2:8	8:0	17

On the Broad Cognitive Ability Scale, Mary achieved an age score of 7:4 and a grade score of 1:8. This is equivalent to a moderately deficient functioning level. On the Tests of Achievement, Mary performed as follows.

Cluster	Grade Score	Age Score	Functioning Level
Reading	2:3	7:6	Severely deficient
Mathematics	1:7	6:11	Severely deficient
Written	1:8	7:4	Severely deficient
Knowledge	4:7	10:0	Average

On the Calculation subtest, Mary added all problems including the subtraction and multiplication problems, only completing 4 of 13 correctly. Mary's strongest performance was on the Blending subtest, and her lowest performances were on the Analysis and Synthesis subtest and the Concept Formation subtest. She was also weak on the Dictation subtest.

Mary was asked to write a brief narrative about her best friend. In this narrative, which consisted of six sentences, Mary wrote two incomplete sentences (e.g., "Go to school twogather"), and used simple sentence structure for the remaining four sentences (e.g., "April is nice. she is my friend sins preskool"). She used two adjectives and used capital letters inconsistently.

Mary was able to complete two-step commands in order (10 of 10), but completed only 6 of 10 three-step commands in the proper sequence.

Behavioral Observations

Mary is a pleasant young lady who put forth excellent effort during the testing session. She occasionally would get frustrated on the tasks presented and frequently inquired as to how she was doing on the tests. Mary professed that she does not like school and wishes her mother would arrange for home schooling.

Summary

This evaluation found that Mary has difficulties in math, reading, spelling, and verbal expression skills in addition to the previously determined deficits in auditory processing.

Recommendations

Recommendations given to the parents and sent to the school include the following:

- It would be beneficial for Mary to be tested by a reading specialist to determine her level of phonemic awareness and phonological memory prior to initiating a therapy program that targets reading and spelling skills. Participation in a multisensory, phonetics-based reading therapy program such as the Barton program, the LiPS program, or the Orton-Gillingham method is recommended.

- Address auditory discrimination, auditory memory, and visual memory skills. Mary possibly may benefit from the use of an FM system in her classroom.

- Incorporate problem-solving activities into the academic and therapy settings.

- Minimize visual and auditory distractions in the school room and home study area.

- The clinician shared Mary's thoughts about attending school and suggested that the parents consider an alternative school setting. There is a Montessori school in town that goes from kindergarten to eighth grade, and all children who attend the school have reading, spelling, and other language-based academic difficulties. There is a full-time speech-language pathologist on staff who works collaboratively with the teachers to facilitate development of language skills that impact on academic ability. Mary expressed an interest in visiting this school, and the parents were given the principal's name and phone number. Perhaps this would be a happy compromise between mainstreamed public school and home schooling.

REVIEW QUESTIONS

1. Language screening identifies a child's strengths and weaknesses in language tasks and results in a specific diagnosis.
   a. True
   b. False

2. When comparing the assessment of preschoolers and school-age children, typically more cognitive assessment is included in the testing of preschoolers than in the testing of school-age children.
   a. True
   b. False

3. Factors that result in the onset of a language or communication problem or both, are _____ factors.

   a. Precipitating

   b. Perpetuating

   c. Predisposing

4. A set of auditory skills that integrates what is heard with language at the cortical level is

   a. Auditory perception

   b. Auditory acuity

   c. Auditory processing

5. The speech-language pathologist should analyze a student's fictional and personal narrative to determine the student's level of semantic and syntactic complexity and maturity.

   a. True

   b. False

6. Assessment batteries for language-based learning disabilities should include

   a. Modality-specific testing

   b. Tests of language and cognition

   c. Comparison of verbal and nonverbal skills

   d. All of the above

7. Which of the following can be tested through the analysis of a spontaneous language sample?

   a. Mean length of utterance

   b. Use of morphosyntactic structures

   c. Lexicon

   d. Pragmatics

   e. All of the above

   f. a, c, and d

   g. a, b, and d

   h. a, b, and c

8. Which of the following cases address over-identification of minority children as having speech and/or language deficits?

   a. *Diana v. Board of Education*

   b. *Lau v. Nichols*

   c. The Bilingual Education Act

   d. *Martin Luther King, Jr. Elementary School v. Ann Arbor School District*

    e. All of the above

    f. a, c, and d

    g. a, b, and c

    h. a, b, and d

9. Some schools use discrepancy testing as a means of justifying educational assistance for a child.

    a. True

    b. False

10. Auditory perception and auditory processing can be used interchangeably.

    a. True

    b. False

REFERENCES

American Speech-Language-Hearing Association (ASHA) (1983). Social dialects. *Asha, 25,* 23–27.

American Speech-Language-Hearing Association (ASHA). (1989). Clinical management of communicatively handicapped minority language populations. *ASHA Desk Reference, 4,* IV-2–IV-6.

American Speech-Language-Hearing Association (ASHA) (1996). Central auditory processing: Current status of research and implications for clinical practice: Technical report. http://www.asha.org/docs/html/TR1996-00241.html

American Speech-Language-Hearing Association (ASHA) (2005). (Central) Auditory Processing Disorders [technical report]. Available from www.asha.org/policy.

Aram, D., Ekelman, B., & Nation, J. (1984). Preschoolers with language disorders: Ten years later. *Journal of Speech and Hearing Research, 27,* 232–244.

Baran, J., Musiek, F., Gollegly, K., et al. (1987, November 15). Auditory duration pattern sequences in the assessment of CANS pathology. Paper presented at the American Speech-Language-Hearing Association annual meeting, New Orleans.

Barkley, R. A. (2000). *Taking charge of ADHD: The complete authoritative guide for parents.* New York: Guildford Press.

Bates, E. (1976). *Language in context.* New York: Academic Press.

Berk, R. A. (1984). *Screening and diagnosis of children with learning disabilities.* Springfield, IL: Thomas.

Bliss, L. S. (2002). *Discourse impairments: Assessment and intervention applications.* Boston: Allyn and Bacon.

Bloom, L. (1973). *One word at a time: The use of single-word utterances before syntax.* The Hague, The Netherlands: Mouton.

Brinton, B., & Fujiki, M. (1989). *Conversational management with language-impaired children: Pragmatic assessment and intervention.* Rockville, MD: Aspen Publishers.

Brown, R. (1973). *A first language.* Cambridge, MA: Harvard University Press.

Brown, A. (1978). Knowing when, where, and how to remember: A problem in meta-cognition. In R. Glaser (ed.), *Advances in instructional psychology*. Hillsdale, NJ: Lawrence Erlbaum.

Carrow-Woolfolk, E. (1999). Comprehensive assessment of spoken language. Circle Pines, MN: American Guidance Service, Inc.

Catts, H. (1991). Early identification of dyslexia: Evidence from a follow-up study of speech-language impaired children. *Annals of Dyslexia, 41,* 163–177.

Catts, H. (1993). The relationship between speech-language impairments and reading disabilities. *Journal of Speech and Hearing Research, 36,* 948–958.

Chapman, R. (1978). Comprehension strategies in young children. In J. Kavanaugh and W. Strange (eds.), *Speech and language in the laboratory, school, and clinic* (pp. 308–327). Cambridge, MA: MIT Press.

Chapman, S. (1997). Cognitive-communication abilities in children with closed head injury. *American Journal of Speech-Language Pathology, 6,* 50–58.

Chapman, S., Levin, H., & Culhane, K. (1995). Language impairment in closed head injury. In H. Kirschner (ed.), *Handbook of neurological speech and language disorders* (pp. 387–414). New York: Marcel-Dekker.

Chapman, S. B., Ulatowska, H. K., Franklin, L. R., Shobe, J. L., Thompson, J. L., & McIntire, D. D. (1997). Proverb interpretation in fluent aphasia and Alzheimer's disease: Implications beyond abstract thinking. *Aphasiology, 11,* 337–350.

Coggins, T., & Carpenter, R. (1981). The communicative intention inventory: A system for coding children's early intentional communication. *Applied Psycholinguistics, 2,* 235–251.

Damico, J. (1985). Clinical discourse analysis: A functional approach to language assessment. In C. S. Simon (ed.). *Communication skills and classroom success:* Assessment of language-learning disabled students. San Diego, CA: College-Hill Press.

Damico, J. (1991). Clinical discourse analysis: A functional approach to language assessment. In C. Simon (ed.), *Communication skills and classroom success: Assessment and therapy methodologies for language and learning disabled students* (pp. 165–206). Eau Claire, WI: Thinking Publications.

Damico J. (1993). Language assessment in adolescents: Addressing critical issues. *Language, Speech, and Hearing Services in Schools, 24,* 29–35.

DeBonis, D. A., & Moncrieff, D. (2008, February). Auditory processing disorders: An update for speech-language pathologists. *American Journal of Speech Language Pathology, 17*(1), 4–18.

Dore, J. (1974). A pragmatic description of early language development. *Journal of Psycholinguistic Research, 4,* 343–350.

Emerick, L. L., & Haynes, W. O. (1986). *Diagnosis and evaluation in speech pathology.* Englewood Cliffs, NJ: Prentice Hall.

Evans, J. L., and Craig, H. (1992) Language sampling collection and analysis: Interview compared to freeplay assessment contexts. *Journal of Speech and Hearing Research, 35,* 343–353.

Fey, M. C. (1986). *Language intervention with young children.* Needham Heights, MA: Allyn and Bacon.

Flavell, J. H. (1977). *Cognitive development.* Englewood Cliffs, NJ: Prentice Hall.

Flavell, J. H., & Wellman, H. (1977). Metamemory. In R. Kail and J. Hagen (eds.), *Perspectives on the development of memory and cognition*. Hillsdale, NJ: Lawrence Erlbaum.

Friel-Patti, S. (1999, October). Clinical decision-making in assessment and intervention of central auditory processing disorders. *Language, Speech, and Hearing Services in the Schools, 30*(4), 345–352.

Gardner, M. F. (1996). Test of auditory perceptual skills–revised. Hydesville, CA: Psychological and Educational Publishers, Inc.

German, D. J. (1986). *Test of word finding*. Allen, TX: DLM Teaching Resources.

Goffman, L., & Leonard, J. (2000). Growth of language skills in preschool children with specific language impairment: Implications for assessment and intervention. *American Journal of Speech-Language Pathology, 9*, 151–161.

Greenhalgh, K. S., & Strong, C. J. (2001). Literate language features in spoken narratives of children with typical language and children with language impairments. *Language, Speech, and Hearing Services in the Schools, 32*, 114–125.

Grela, B. G., & Leonard, L. B. (2000). The influence of argument-structure complexity on the use of auxiliary verbs by children with SLI. *Journal of Speech, Language, and Hearing Research, 43*, 1115–1125.

Hammill, D. D. (1998). *Detroit test of learning aptitude—4*. Austin, TX: Pro-Ed.

Hegde, M. N. (1996). *Pocket guide to assessment in speech-language pathology*. Clifton Park, NY: Delmar, Cengage Learning.

Holston, J. T. (1992, February). *Assessment and management of auditory processing problems in children*. Paper presented at the Winter Conference of the Florida Speech-Language-Hearing Association, Gainesville, FL.

Hughes, D., McGillvray, L., & Schmidek, M. (1997). *Guide to narrative language: Procedures for assessment*. Eau Claire, WI: Thinking Publications.

Jerger, J., & Jerger, S. (1974). Auditory findings in brainstem disorders. *Archives of Otolaryngology, 99*, 342–349.

Katz, J. (1962). The use of staggered spondaic words for assessing the integrity of the central auditory system. *Journal of Audiology Research, 2*, 327–337.

Keith, R. W. (1986). *SCAN: A screening test for auditory processing disorders*. San Antonio, TX: Psychological Corporation.

Keith, R. W. (1988). Central auditory tests. In N. J. Lass, L. V. McReynolds, J. L. Northern, and D. E. Yoder (eds.), *Speech, language, and hearing. Vol. 3: Hearing disorders* (pp. 1215–1236). Philadelphia: W. B. Saunders.

Keith, R. W. (1999). Clinical issues in central auditory processing disorders. *Language, Speech, and Hearing Services in the Schools 30*(4), 339–344.

Keith, R. W. (2000). *Random gap detection test*. St. Louis, MO: Auditec.

Larson, V. L., & McKinley, N. (1995). *Language disorders in older students: Preadolescents and adolescents*. Eau Claire, WI: Thinking Publications.

Lee, L. (1974). *Developmental sentence analysis*. Evanston, IL: Northwestern University Press.

Lindamood, P. C., & Lindamood, C. (1979). Lindamood auditory conceptualization test. Boston, MA: Pearson.

Mandler, J., & Johnson, N. (1977). Remembrance of things passed: Story structure and recall. *Cognitive Psychology, 9*, 111–151.

McCabe, A., Bliss, L., Barra, G., & Bennett, M. (2008, May). Comparison of personal versus fictional narratives of children with language impairment. *American Journal of Speech-Language Pathology, 17,* 194–206.

McCauley, R. J. (2001). *Assessment of language disorders in children.* Mahwah, NJ: Lawrence Erlbaum Associates Publishers.

Miller, J. (1981). *Assessing language production in children: Experimental procedures.* Baltimore, MD: University Park Press.

Musiek, F. (1983). Assessment of central auditory dysfunction: The dichotic digits test revisited. *Ear and Hearing, 4,* 79–83.

Nelson, K. (1973). Structure and strategy in learning to talk. *Monographs of the Society for Research in Child Development, 38*(1–2, Serial No. 149).

Nelson, N. W. (1998). *Childhood language disorders in context: Infancy through adolescence* (2nd ed.). Boston: Allyn and Bacon.

Nicholas, L., & Brookshire, R. (1993). A system for quantifying the informativeness and efficiency of the connected speech of adults with aphasia. *Journal of Speech and Hearing Research, 36,* 338–350.

Nippold, M. (1998). *Later language development: The school-age and adolescent years* (2nd ed.). Austin, TX: Pro-Ed.

Northern, J. L., & Downs, M. P. (1991). *Hearing in children* (4th ed.). Baltimore, MD: Williams & Wilkins.

Oram, J., Fine, J., Okamoto, C., & Tannock, R. (1999). Assessing the language of children with hyperactivity disorder. *Journal of Speech-Language Pathology, 8*(1), 72–80.

Owens, R. (1995). *Language disorders: A functional approach to assessment and intervention* (2nd ed.). Boston: Allyn and Bacon.

Owens, R. (1996). *Language development: An introduction* (4th ed.). Boston: Allyn and Bacon.

Paul, R. (2001). *Childhood language disorders in context: Infancy through adolescence* (2nd ed.). Boston: Allyn and Bacon.

Pinheiro, M. (1977). Test of central auditory function in children with learning disabilities. In R. Keith (ed.). *Central auditory dysfunction.* New York: Grune & Stratton.

Polakow, V. (1993). *Lives on the edge: Single mothers and their children in the other America.* Chicago: University of Chicago Press.

Proctor, A. (1989). Stages of normal noncry vocal development in infancy: A protocol for assessment. *Topics in Language Disorders, 10*(1), 43–56.

Retherford, K. (1993). *Guide to analysis of language transcripts* (2nd ed.). Eau Claire, WI: Thinking Publications.

Richard, G. J., & Hanner, M. A. (1995). Language processing test–3. Los Angeles, CA: Western Psychological Services.

Rosner, J., & Simon, D. P. (1971). The auditory analysis test: An initial report. *Journal of Learning Disabilities, 4,* 384–392.

Rossetti, L. (1990). *Infant-toddler assessment: An interdisciplinary approach.* Boston: Little, Brown & Co.

Roth, F., & Spekman, N. (1986). Narrative discourse: Spontaneously generated stories of learning disabled and normally achieving students. *Journal of Speech and Hearing Disorders, 51,* 8–23.

Rubin, D. L. (1987). Divergence and convergence between oral and written communication. *Topics in Language Disorders, 7*(4), 1–18.

Rumelhart, D. (1975). Notes on a schema for stories. In D. Bobrow and A. Collins (eds.), *Representation and understanding: Studies in cognitive science* (pp. 211–236). New York: Academic Press.

Sattler, J. M. (1988). *Assessment of children.* San Diego, CA: Author.

Schow, R. L., & Nerbonne, M. A. (1996). *Introduction to audiologic rehabilitation.* Needham Heights, MA: Simon & Schuster Company.

Scott, C. (1988). Spoken and written syntax. In M. Nippold (ed.), *Later language development: Ages nine through nineteen* (pp. 49–55). Austin, TX: Pro-Ed.

Semel, E., Wiig, E. H., & Secord, W. (1987). *Clinical evaluation of language fundamentals—revised.* New York: The Psychological Corporation, Harcourt Brace Jovanovich.

Shaywitz, K., & Cherry-Wilkinson, L. (1982). Age-related differences in metalinguistic awareness. In S. Kaczaj (ed.), *Language development. Vol. 2: Language, thought, and culture.* Hillsdale, NJ: Lawrence Erlbaum.

Stark, R. E., Bernstein, L., Condino, R., Bender, M., Tallal, P., & Catts, H. (1984). Four-year follow-up study of language impaired children. *Annals of Dyslexia, 34,* 49–68.

Stein, N., & Glenn, C. (1979). An analysis of story comprehension in elementary school children. In R. Freedle (ed.), *New directions in discourse processing, 2* (pp. 53–120). Norwood, NJ: Ablex.

Swain, D. & Long, N. (2004). Auditory processing abilities test. Novato, CA: Academic Therapy Publications.

Tannock, R., Fine, J., & Ickowicz, A. (1998). Language abilities of children with attention deficit hyperactivity disorder. *Journal of Child Psychology, 21,* 103–117.

Templin, M. C. (1957). Certain language skills in children, their development, and interrelationships. *Institute of Child Welfare Monograph Series, No. 26.* Minneapolis, MN: University of Minnesota Press.

Thorndyke, P. (1977). Cognitive structures in comprehension and memory of narrative discourse. *Cognitive Psychology, 9,* 77–110.

Ulatowska, H., Chapman, S., Highley, A., & Prince, J. (1998). Discourse in healthy old-elderly adults: A longitudinal study. *Aphasiology, 12,* 619–633.

United States Census Bureau. (2000). *U.S. Census 2000.* Retreived June 1, 2010 from www.census.gov/prod/2001pubs.

van Kleeck, A. (1984). Metalinguistic skills: Cutting across spoken and written language and problem solving abilities. In G. Wallach and K. Butler (eds.), *Language learning disabilities in school-age children* (pp. 53–89). Baltimore, MD: Williams & Wilkins.

Wagner, R. K., Torgesen, J. K., & Rashotte, C. A. (1999). Comprehensive test of phonological processing. Austin, TX: Pro-Ed.

Wallach, G. P., & Butler, K. G. (1994). *Language learning disabilities in school-age children and adolescents: Some principles and applications.* New York: Macmillan.

Weiss, A., & Johnson, C. (1993). Relationships between narrative and syntactic competencies in school-age hearing-impaired children. *Applied Psycholinguistics, 14,* 35–59.

Weiss, A. L., Tomlin, J. B., & Robins, D. A. (2000). Language disorders. In J. B. Tomlin, H. L. Morris, & D. C. Spriesterbach (Eds.), *Diagnosis in Speech-Language Pathology* (2nd ed.). Clifton Park, NY: Delmar, Cengage Learning.

Westby, C. (1994). The effects of culture on genre, structure, and style of oral and written texts. In G. Wallach and K. Butler (eds.), *Language learning disabilities in school-age children and adolescents* (pp. 180–218). New York: Merrill-Macmillan College Publishing Company.

Wetherby, A., & Prizant, B. (2002). *Communication and symbolic behavior scales— developmental profile (CSBS-DP).* Baltimore, MD: Brookes Publishing.

Woodcock, R. W., & Johnson, M. B. (1977). *Woodcock-Johnson psycho-educational battery.* Allen, TX: DLM Teaching Resource.

Woodcock, R. W., McGrew, K. S., & Mather, N. (2001a). *Woodcock-Johnson III tests of achievement.* Itasca, IL: Riverside.

Woodcock, R. W., McGrew, K. S., & Mather, N. (2001b). *Woodcock-Johnson III tests of cognition.* Itasca, IL: Riverside.

Young, M. (1985). Central auditory processing through the looking glass: A critical look at diagnosis and management. *Journal of Childhood Communication Disorder, 9,* 31–42.

Zachman, L., Huisingh, R., & Barrett, M. (1992). *The listening test.* East Moline, IL: LinguiSystems.

Chapter 14

Treatment in the School-Age Population

LEARNING OBJECTIVES

After completion of this chapter, the reader will be able to:

1. Discuss some factors that could negatively impact the accomplishment of therapy goals for school-age children.

2. Discuss some special issues that need to be considered when planning and implementing language therapy for adolescents.

3. Compare and contrast the three primary models of intervention in the schools.

4. Discuss the four steps of Merritt and Culatta's view of collaboration in the problem-solving process.

5. Discuss the steps involved in planning and implementing the therapy process.

6. Discuss some of the academic changes and demands that occur beginning in third grade.

7. Discuss the importance of developing metalinguistic skills and their impact on academic success.

8. Discuss the focus of language therapy for adolescents, including critical thinking, listening, and writing.

9. Differentiate between and discuss the three philosophies regarding provision of therapy services to individuals from minority cultural groups.

INTRODUCTION

Language-impaired children are students who are unable to use language to fulfill the academic and social demands of school (Naremore, Densmore, & Harman, 1995). One of the first steps in the therapeutic process is to set the goals, objectives, and procedures that will guide the therapy for the school-age child. According to Van Hattum (1985), three questions should guide the determination of goals, objectives, and procedures for therapy. The first question is, "What does the child need to communicate successfully in his or her environment?" This question is particularly important to address in terms of the several environments (e.g., home, school, social settings) in which school-age children function. A second question that should be addressed is, "What skills is the child currently demonstrating?" Using the four-box system (see Chapter 6), this question should be answered in terms of the communicative and noncommunicative strengths that the child exhibits in the different environments. The third question has its impact after the new skills have been learned in the therapy setting. At that time, the major question facing the clinician is, "How do I facilitate the child's use of the newly learned skills in his or her natural environment?" It is also important to be sure that the goals and objectives are appropriate for the child's age and overall cognitive abilities. Table 14–1 delineates six questions that can be used as guidelines for determining the appropriateness of the goals and objectives that the clinician has developed for therapy.

With regard to question 1 in Table 14–1, the environments of a school-age child are greatly expanded in comparison to those of a preschool child. Therefore, the issue of environmental demands is much more critical when setting goals and objectives for school-age children. The usefulness and relevance of the goals, as expressed in question 2, can be determined only in light of the different environments in which the child functions on a daily basis. The use of the skills in the child's daily environment leads to the issue expressed in questions 3 and 4 in Table 14–1 with regard to the maintenance and generalization of the skills. The fifth question brings forth a critical concern. Perhaps one of the hardest jobs in determining goals and objectives is to be sure that the steps are appropriate in their demands. If steps are too big, the student does not make efficient progress and may become discouraged. If the steps are too small, critical therapy time is wasted on reviewing what is already known. This ties in with question 6 in that it is important that the objectives be achievable. Many times emotional, physical, or mental capacity problems may exist that affect the achievability of the goals and objectives. Given the potential for emotional distress due to unmet goals, particularly in older elementary and middle school–age children, the answers to questions 5 and 6 are critical for success with school-age children in speech-language therapy.

When planning therapy for adolescents, it is first important to look at the educational commitment of the student. Does this student value education, or does he or she resent being in school (Larson & McKinley, 1995)?

TABLE 14–1   Deciding if goals and objectives are appropriate

1. Do the goals and objectives take the student's environmental demands into consideration?

2. Are the goals and objectives useful and relevant?

3. Can the goals and objectives be transferred and maintained?

4. Do the goals and objectives provide a foundation for response generalization?

5. Can the objectives be broken down into smaller steps?

6. Are the goals achievable?

Source: Delmar/Cengage Learning

Does the child complete homework assignments? Is he or she motivated to achieve? What are his or her educational aspirations? A student who does not value the education he or she is receiving is likely to be negative about most attempts at therapy. Therefore, extra time needs to be spent developing a rapport with the student and making him or her understand the importance of achieving the therapy goals that have been set. Children with language-based learning disabilities often have a negative attitude toward school because of a feeling of failure that is based on poor academic performance due to the learning disability. In these cases, it is important to gain the trust of the student and help him or her see the educational relevance of the objectives in speech-language therapy (Larson & McKinley, 1995). A high school student recently started therapy for dyslexia at a local clinic. After several sessions, the clinician asked her whether she thought the therapy was helping. The student replied that she understood her history lessons for the first time and had even volunteered to read aloud in class. Clearly, this student made the connection between what was happening in therapy and the changes it could create in the classroom.

Second, tied in with the student's educational commitment are his or her values. Does the student value the educational process? Does the student care about the feelings of other people? Does the student value helping other people? The student should be asked these questions as part of the history-gathering process so that the values can be taken into account when developing the goals and objectives for therapy (Larson & McKinley, 1995).

Third, a special issue with adolescents is social competence, which taps into issues related to self-esteem, assertiveness, decision-making skills, friend-making abilities, planning skills, and the student's personal view of his or her own future. As seen in Chapter 9, self-esteem and depression are major concerns when working with adolescents with language-based learning disabilities.

Providing therapy for students with language-based learning disabilities is a multi-dimensional issue. Careful consideration needs to be given to establishing rapport with the student, particularly students beyond the elementary school years. For the therapy to be successful, the student must see the value of the therapy and have a sense of trust in the clinician.

ELIGIBILITY FOR THERAPY

Children who are considered language impaired as preschoolers may have their condition variously labeled as a reading disability or a learning disability in elementary schools (Bashir et al., 1983; Snyder, 1984; Wallach & Liebergott, 1984). Thus, it is important to understand the school environment, the curriculum, the child's language abilities, interactive learning styles, and the child's language problems when planning intervention for school-age children with language-based learning disabilities.

When determining eligibility for therapy, the clinician can look toward exclusionary criteria, discrepancy criteria, or both (Naremore, Densmore, & Harman, 1995). Using exclusionary criteria, the therapist diagnoses the language-based learning disability based on the fact that the child has language or learning problems that are not related to mental handicaps, sensory impairments, or physical conditions. If the clinician uses discrepancy criteria, he or she is typically referring to a gap between the child's expected level of language achievement based on his or her overall intellectual functioning and sociocultural opportunities and his or her language abilities. The discrepancy can be in any or all of the components of language and can affect both receptive and expressive language (Naremore, Densmore, & Harman, 1995).

ASHA published a paper in 1989 in which the association took issue with using discrepancy definitions to determine eligibility for therapy. Specifically, one of the concerns was the possible use of a single aspect of language to validate the presence of a discrepancy. The association also was concerned about poor availability of age-appropriate and psychometrically valid testing instruments for the school-age population. This is not as much of a problem today as it was in 1989, but that concern is still valid if a clinician applies labels using inadequate standardized testing. Related to the lack of age-appropriate and valid testing instruments is the fact that tests are developed on the basis of different theoretical constructs and standardized on different populations. Thus, it can be psychometrically incorrect to compare test scores from different tests. Many tests also fail to provide important qualitative information regarding the nature of the learning or language deficits (ASHA, 1989). These are certainly critical concerns when determining a label for a child's disorder that may be needed to qualify for services in the schools. In fact, ASHA went so far as to say that "the exclusive use of a discrepancy formula as a required procedure for determining eligibility for language intervention should be viewed with extreme caution and avoided whenever possible" (ASHA, 1989, p. 115).

> **think about it**
> Find out the criteria in your local school district and/or state for the placement of school-age children in language therapy. Do you think the criteria are reasonable and appropriate? Why or why not?

MODELS OF INTERVENTION

Historically, school-based clinicians primarily have employed the pull-out method for therapy. Using this model, students were assigned to specific times for therapy, and the clinician would take the children to the speech-language therapy room, where he or she would provide therapy before taking the child back to the classroom. The pull-out model places an extra demand on the classroom teacher because the clinician relies on the teacher to provide feedback as to how well the child is generalizing his or her therapy skills into the classroom.

The collaborative model of intervention, as illustrated in Figure 14–1, is a partnership between the teacher and the speech-language pathologist and is becoming increasingly popular among school-based speech-language pathologists. In the collaborative model, each professional has a view of the "whole child," not myriad professional viewpoints (Naremore, Densmore, & Harman, 1995). The collaborative model, also known as classroom-based intervention or curriculum-based intervention, focuses on learning strategies and using them in materials related to the curriculum. The underlying philosophy of the collaborative model is that "language learning is intrinsic to literary development" (Naremore, Densmore, & Harman, 1995).

In 1991, ASHA supported the collaborative model as the most efficient and effective model of intervention for students with language-based learning disabilities in public schools (ASHA, 1991). Merritt and Culatta (1998) viewed collaboration as a problem-solving process consisting of four steps: identification of the problem, planning of intervention, implementation, and evaluation. During the identification phase, the teachers and clinicians work together to write behavioral objectives consisting of a description of the behavior that needs to be changed, the conditions under which the behavior will occur, and the criteria for measuring progress. Examples of behavioral objectives for speech-language pathology are shown in Table 14–2.

Collaborative model. Classroom-based or curriculum-based intervention that focuses on learning strategies and using them in materials related to the curriculum.

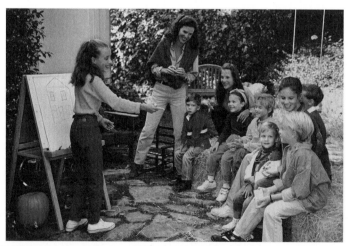

FIGURE 14–1 In the collaborative model, the speech-language pathologist and teacher work together in the classroom to facilitate generalization of skills in the academic setting. (*Source: Delmar/Cengage Learning.*)

TABLE 14–2 Samples of behavioral objectives

Andrew will independently match the phonemes /b/, /p/, /s/, and /t/ with the corresponding grapheme with 90 percent accuracy on 20 trials.

With no more than two verbal prompts from the clinician, Nicole will place five story strips in the proper sequence for three different stories.

Sam will list one synonym for each of the 10 words on a vocabulary list with 80 percent accuracy.

Source: Delmar/Cengage Learning

During the identification stage, the clinician also presents any baseline data against which progress will be measured and identifies the most problematic behaviors to determine the priority in which multiple goals will be addressed.

During the stage in which the intervention is planned, the involved personnel brainstorm ideas and do the equivalent of a feasibility study to develop a realistic action plan and timeline. The implementation stage consists of putting the plan into action, following the timeline, and collecting the data. In the final stage—evaluation of the program—the teachers and clinicians compare the pre- and postintervention data and make a decision as to whether to continue with the intervention, revise the goals, or terminate the intervention (Merritt & Culatta, 1998).

In spite of ASHA's strong support of the collaborative model, there has been some hesitancy on the part of educators to adopt this service delivery model. General educators have been found to be less favorable toward within-class services (the foundation of the collaborative model) but do agree that it is less detrimental academically, as the children remain in the classroom. Furthermore, both regular and special education teachers have questioned the teacher's need to be in class when the speech-language pathologist is present (Sanger, Hux, & Griess, 1995). Clinicians adopting the collaborative model must stress that it is based on *collaboration* between the classroom teacher and the clinician. It is not intended that the speech-language pathologist be a temporary substitute for the teacher. Rather, both professionals should work as a team in coordinating language therapy goals, objectives, and procedures with curricular demands in the classroom.

In the consultative model, the speech-language pathologist provides indirect therapy through workshops and individualized input to classroom teachers on appropriate methods for encouraging effective speech and language skills. In this model, the clinician provides preventive and direct intervention information. Other indirect methods of therapy include counseling, tutoring, and adapting education materials to intermingle communication and language into the standard classroom curriculum. A comparison of all three models is in Table 14–3.

Consultative model. A service delivery model in which the speech-language pathologist provides indirect therapy through in-service and input to classroom teachers on appropriate methods for encouraging effective speech and language skills.

TABLE 14–3 Direct service and consultation models

Model Type	Options	Description
Direct service	Pull-out	The SLP* provides services in individual or small group sessions in a setting separate from the regular education classroom; goals and objectives typically are unrelated to curricular demands; teacher may or may not reinforce approaches.
	Pull-in (parallel instruction)	The SLP conducts individual or small group sessions in the classroom and incorporates specific speech and language objectives within a curricular focus; teacher assists in generalizing skills.
Consultation	Instructional consultation	The SLP is a consultant to the classroom teacher, assisting in interpreting formal and informal assessment data, developing intervention approaches, and monitoring progress.
	Monitoring	The SLP observes the student in the classroom context and collects data relative to established language goals and objectives.
	Prereferral assistance teacher	The SLP participates in a problem-solving team that attempts to meet the educational needs of children in the classroom by varying instructional approaches and strategies.

*SLP: Speech-language pathologist
Source: From "Collaborative partnerships and decision-making," by J. DiMeo, D. D. Merritt, and B. Culatta. In *Language intervention in the classroom*, edited by D. D. Merritt and B. Culatta, p. 74. Clifton Park, NY: Delmar, Cengage Learning, 1998.

Individualized education plan (IEP). Required by IDEA, the academic plan required for all students who are in special education or related services in the public schools.

INDIVIDUALIZED EDUCATION PLANS (IEPs)

Individualized education plans (IEPs) are supposed to address four domains: curriculum and learning environment, independent functioning, social and personal concerns, and communication. The curriculum and learning environment incorporate the academic subjects, including reading, writing, listening, speaking, mathematics, and problem solving. With the passage of IDEA, *transition* became a major focus of the IEP to encourage educators to consider what skills a student needs to make the transition from school to work. Thus, the curriculum portion of the IEP includes job preparation, use of tools and technology, and employability skills.

Independent functioning includes personal care (daily living skills) and self-management, which addresses personal planning, decision making, and appropriate conduct in daily living and work roles. The social and personal domains concentrate on working with others, focusing on group and interpersonal relationships. With regard to communication, the IEP needs to address the student's ability to participate effectively in communication exchanges.

The IEP should also specify the level of functioning the child is expected to achieve. At the *independent* level of functioning, the student is capable of working and living independently, even though occasional assistance may be needed. For the student to achieve independent functioning, his or her IEP needs to address functional academics and functional daily living and working skills. The *supported* level of functioning means that the student is expected to be capable of living and working in a supported setting. This student needs skills that address daily living tasks and activities and skills that can maximize independence and personal effectiveness. Finally, a level of functioning may be specified as *participatory*. This means that the student is capable of participating in major life activities but requires extensive support systems. The student needs opportunities for participation in tasks and activities of daily living. Regardless of the level of expected functioning, it is critical that the curriculum focuses on functional goals and objectives. In other words, subjects need to provide real-life applications to facilitate the generalization of the academic preparation to the work place. "A Case for Teaching Functional Skills" (Lewis, 1987) is provided in the case study in Chapter 8. It is an eloquent story that highlights the importance of providing therapy that is based on functional goals for school-age children with language delays and disorders.

TREATMENT SEQUENCE

Regardless of the student's age and the type of language-based learning disability, a general sequence of events is part of planning and implementing the therapy process. The first step is to select the target behavior. This ties in very closely with the evaluative-planning process because an appropriate assessment protocol that is properly administered can provide the necessary baseline data from which to select the language skills to be targeted in therapy.

A second step is to plan the sequence in which the targets will be addressed in therapy. Most children who have a language-based learning disability have difficulty with a number of aspects of language. Thus, it is the job of the clinician to prioritize the objectives. The ability to task analyze a goal is absolutely critical at the planning stage of therapy. Task analysis is important because many of the language and communication objectives people use incorporate a chained sequence of behaviors. The clinician must know the components of the skill in order to plan effective and efficient therapy. Objectives and procedures need to be small enough to be readily achievable, yet not so small that the student does not progress at a satisfactory rate in therapy. Using the four-box system, a clinician can ascertain the strengths and weaknesses that were identified in the assessment process to help prioritize the skills to be addressed in therapy. The information and data gathered from the assessment process also are critical in the documentation of baselines. Baselines reflect the student's level of performance prior to intervention. Baselines help document the need for therapy, serve as a basis for documenting improvement, and establish the clinician's accountability (Hegde, 1996).

The third step involves writing the therapy plan. This includes the selection of stimulus materials and the determination of which procedures will be used. At this point, the clinician defines the expected cause-and-effect considerations by selecting stimuli to facilitate the accuracy and rate of responses from the student. Materials should be age appropriate and in accordance with the child's level of functioning. For example, when teaching reading to a child in middle school, it is important to use literature that is not significantly beyond the child's level of ability yet is appropriate for the student in terms of the content and interest level. Complexity of the responses should be graded on a continuum from words, to phrases, then to simple shorter sentences. As the child progresses, longer and more complex sentences should be used, followed by establishing maintenance of the skills from each level (Hegde, 1996).

Maintenance. The independent use of therapy skills in a person's natural settings.

Generalization. The addition of new stimuli or environmental factors to elicit the same response obtained in a controlled setting.

Another consideration when writing the therapy plan is the development of a maintenance and generalization plan. It does not do any good for a child to be able to develop and use new language skills in a controlled setting if there is no plan to incorporate the skills into the child's daily settings and activities.

The fourth step in the therapy process is putting the plans for therapy, maintenance, and generalization into action. The goal is to establish the new skills in a controlled setting, then to practice the skills to ensure that they are generalized and maintained when stimuli and reinforcement schedules are changed. The clinician should always be moving toward effective communication. Strategies to facilitate the movement toward conversation include the ability to initiate and maintain a topic. Turn taking and eye contact should also be addressed. The child should also be taught conversational repair strategies, such as requesting verification when a message is not understood (Hegde, 1996). Once the child can maintain a skill in a controlled setting, the emphasis shifts to the generalization of the skills into the child's daily environments and routines.

The final step in the treatment process is reviewing the data and making any needed modifications. This evaluative process leads to a decision on whether to modify current goals, objectives, or procedures and whether to continue or dismiss the child from therapy.

INTERVENTION WITH ELEMENTARY SCHOOL–AGE CHILDREN

During the elementary school years, the development of literacy skills predominates in the academic curriculum. As mentioned previously, the transition in third grade from "learning to read" to "reading to learn" (Roth & Worthington, 2001, p. 146) represents a major milestone in the academic world. Other academic demands include increasingly complex written and oral language and the use of narratives as part of the instructional protocol for teaching more advanced language forms. It is assumed that, by the time the child enters third grade, he or she has mastered skills needed to succeed academically and socially. Some of these skills are the development of good work habits, the ability to work independently, self-organization skills, and "rapid and automatic application of knowledge" (Roth & Worthington, 2001, p. 146). Children with a history of language and/or phonological deficits may experience difficulty with these aspects of their schooling.

Development of Metalinguistic Skills

Metalinguistic skills are needed for a child to be able to analyze his or her language and its functions. They are critical in order for the child to manipulate the components of language so that he or she can appreciate humor, understand idioms, provide definitions of words, and use phonemic awareness tasks including segmentation of words and blending of sounds to create words (Roth & Worthington, 2001). The development of metalinguistic skills gives the child a basis from which he or she can analyze his or her language. This is a critical foundational skill for the development of phonological and morphological awareness skills, which are the focus of improving literacy.

Improving Literacy

Various approaches can be utilized to facilitate literacy growth in school-age children. Specific intervention programs for children diagnosed with reading disabilities are discussed in Chapter 10. The focus in this chapter is on children with language disabilities who are struggling academically.

Speech-language pathologists providing therapy for school-aged children, particularly those in third grade and up, should provide "curriculum-relevant and strategic-based language intervention" (Wallach, Charlton, & Christie, 2009, p. 201). A student's success in the classroom is affected by internal and external factors. The internal factors are the inherent skills and knowledge the student brings to the classroom; the external factors include the content and structure of the classroom materials, the teaching style used in the classroom, and the task demands. Our job is to teach students strategies that enable them to comprehend the classroom curriculum and facilitate meeting the various task demands. The curricular content that has been covered in the classroom should serve as the context for our interventions; we should not be teaching new curricular content in therapy. Again, our focus should be teaching the students strategies for learning (Wallach, Charlton, & Christie, 2009).

Integration of Metacognitive and Metalinguistic Skills in Intervention

When planning intervention with school-age children, the clinician should implement strategies that provide the students with tools that can be used to interpret the content of his or her textbooks. Wallach, Charlton, and Christie (2009) discussed derived literacies and fundamental literacies. Derived literacies are the style and form specific to a subject area. For example, the style of writing and the lexicon of a math book are dramatically different for the style of writing and lexicon of a history book. Students need fundamental literacies ("being fluent in a language, understanding the different discourses of that language, and reading and writing that language") (p. 204) in order to read and comprehend derived literacies (treating history as a language that is different from math language). The implication of this is that students need to develop comprehension strategies that are specific to the various content areas of the academic curriculum.

> **Derived literacies.** Literacy style and form specific to a subject area.
>
> **Fundamental literacies.** Having fluency in a language, understanding that language's discourses, and being able to read and write that language.

Specific skills that should be addressed include:

- Making syntactic transformations while keeping the same meaning of the sentence (e.g., active and passive forms of the same sentence)

- Understanding different types of expository text (descriptive, persuasive, compare and contrast, and problem–solution)

- Understanding the meaning and use of "*similar to, different from, was caused by, is the result of, prior to, after*" (Wallach, Charlton, & Christie, 2009, p. 203)

- Knowing how to decipher the meaning of a sentence by breaking it down into smaller linguistic units (i.e., its semantic and syntactic components)

- Identifying the main idea and the supportive information in a sentence or paragraph

- Using graphic organizers such as maps and diagrams to analyze the content of a sentence

- Focusing on "content and structure knowledge" (Wallach, Charlton, & Christie, 2009, p. 205)

Morphological Awareness and Phonological Awareness

Wallach, Charlton, and Christie (2009) focused on semantic and syntactic analysis of content to facilitate comprehension. Kirk and Gillon (2009) focused on morphological awareness as a key component of improving literacy. Morphological awareness involves breaking down words into the distinct morphemes that comprise each word. Kirk and Gillon studied the impact of increased understanding of morphology on spelling performance of children aged 8:7 to 11:1 years who had specific spelling difficulties. They particularly focused on "orthographic rules that apply when suffixes are added to the base word" (Kirk & Gillon, 2009, p. 341).

Kirk and Gillon (2009) found that intervention that integrates morphological awareness with orthographic and phonological awareness positively impacts reading and spelling development in school-age children. Teaching skills such as adding prefixes and suffixes to base words, segmenting words into their component morphemes, and teaching "semantic relationships between morphologically complex words" (p. 342) resulted in growth in phonological decoding, reading, and spelling. Butyniec-Thomas and Woloshyn (1997) demonstrated the advantages of teaching morphological awareness in content as opposed to drill for the best results, and Kirk and Gillon (2009) stressed the need to learn orthographic patterns as opposed to memorization of word lists.

Phonological awareness (breaking down words into syllables and phonemes) and morphological awareness play significant roles in the development of reading and spelling in school-age children. Siegel (2008) found that morphological awareness was a bigger contributor to the development of reading and spelling skills than were phonological awareness and oral-language skills. This is in contrast to the work of Carlisle (1995) and others who have found that phonological awareness is the key component to reading success. However, Siegel (2008) and Kirk and Gillon (2009) both based their studies on older children than did Carlisle. Carlisle's subjects were in kindergarten through second grade; Siegel's subjects were 12 years old, and Kirk and Gillon's subjects were 8:7 to 11:1. It could be that phonological awareness is more important in the early stages of learning to read (when words are less complex), and morphological awareness is more important in the later stages of reading.

Thus, the inclusion of morphological awareness, particularly when combined with orthographic awareness activities, is critical in intervention with school-age children with language learning disabilities, including reading and spelling disabilities.

Narratives

Speech-language pathologists often use narratives as a means of assessing children's and adolescents' growth in the use of form and content. As discussed in Chapter 13, different types of narratives yield results that are at variance with each other. For example, children with language learning disabilities do better on personal narratives than they do on fictional narratives. This may be due to the fact that they engage in personal narratives more frequently than fictional narratives. The importance of this observation is that we tend to teach narratives using these types of fictional narratives; that is, we give the student a topic or a wordless picture book and ask him or her to create a story about that topic or book. We typically focus on improving narrative ability using fictional narratives. However, evidence shows that improvement in the ability to produce fictional narratives does not translate into improved personal narratives, particularly during the elementary school years. There appears to be only a marginal correlation between fictional and personal narratives (McCabe, Bliss, Barra, & Bennett, 2008). Based on a review of the literature, McCabe and colleagues recommended that therapists and teachers focus on the development of personal narratives with elementary school children, then focus on fictional narratives in middle school. Therapists should monitor the types of grammatical structures the child uses in his or her narratives, the lexical variety, and the integration of story elements into the narratives as part of an over-all program designed to improve language and communication in school-aged children and adolescents (Greenhalgh & Strong, 2001).

Narrative-based therapy should focus on developing oral narratives and literate (written) narratives. When engaging a school-age child or adolescent in an oral narrative, the speech-language pathologist should encourage conversation focusing on one topic. She or he should ask *wh-* questions to encourage the student to provide more information, and offer nonspecific prompts such as "uh-huh" and "tell me more" to encourage adding more information in the continuation of the narrative (McCabe, Bliss, Barra, & Bennett, 2008). Therapy should include teaching story structure and sequencing of events through the use of temporal words such as *first*, *next*, and *last*. Gradually, elaborations such as "descriptors, causal factors, emotions, and dialogue" can be incorporated into the narratives (McCabe, Bliss, Barra, & Bennett, 2008, p. 201).

Three Language Teaching Methods

Olswang and Bain (1991) described three intervention methods based on the amount of structure used in the therapy process. The first one, *milieu teaching*, involves providing therapy in the child's natural environments. Goals and activities are based on the interests and attention of the child, and natural reinforcements in the environment promote language growth. Procedures include incidental teaching, mand-model teaching, and delay (Warren & Yoder, 1994). In incidental teaching the therapist, teacher, and caregivers build language into the child's daily activities and routines. A variety of techniques can be used, and the teaching is highly dependent on the interests of the child. Mand-model intervention is the more typical therapy approach in that it is adult-directed, with the adult presenting a stimulus, asking for a particular response, and, if necessary, providing a prompt to elicit the response. If the child responds correctly, he or she is reinforced by the clinician. If the child responds incorrectly, the clinician uses a variety of techniques to elicit the desired response. Using delay as a teaching technique must be done carefully in order not to frustrate the child. In using delay, the adult looks expectantly at the child for about 15 seconds while waiting for an appropriate request for an action or object. Lack of response from the child can be met with modeling the desired behavior, then waiting again (Reed, 2005).

The second model is *joint action routines*, or script therapy, as it is sometimes called. In joint action routines, the adult sets up "interactive, systematic repetitions of events in which each partner has predictable language and behavioral patterns to complete" (Reed, 2005, p. 476). The routines set up the need to communicate in a contrived social situation. As the child's involvement in the routines increases, language demands become more complex. It is hoped that the child will generalize the routines to his or her natural environment, but this is sometimes problematic.

The most structured teaching method, *inductive teaching*, is the third model proposed by Olwsang and Bain (1991). The child looks for patterns in communicative exchanges that are developed and manipulated by the adult. This procedure assumes that the induction process is an innate process, and that if the communicative exchanges are arranged correctly, the child will hypothesize, or induct, the rule governing the pattern of the exchanges.

Most therapists use a combination of the three models, with the child's abilities and interests guiding which one is implemented at any given time.

GROUP THERAPY

It is common in school-based therapy to see children in groups (see Figure 14–2). This can be quite intimidating to a clinician, particularly in the neophyte years. A critical determinant of the success of group therapy is putting together the "right" group.

In some settings, block scheduling is used. In block scheduling, clinicians have no control over when the children come to therapy. The entire school is scheduled in blocks, with children going to "specials" as a class. In this type of scheduling, all children from one or more classrooms are blocked into a speech-language therapy time based on the class schedule, not on the basis of the child's abilities or disabilities. This can result in a group in which the children have little more in common than being eligible for therapy.

In these circumstances, it is necessary to divide the group into subgroups based on commonality of objectives or based on diagnosis. This author

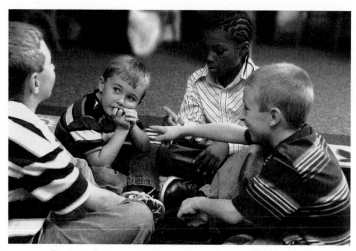

FIGURE 14–2 Group therapy allows children to interact with and support each other to facilitate improvement in their language and communication skills. (*Source: Delmar/Cengage Learning.*)

prefers to base the subgroups on commonality of objectives or symptomology, not diagnosis. As seen throughout this book, children with the same diagnostic label can be vastly different, so it does not make sense to group children on basis of diagnosis.

Once the children are divided into subgroups, a schedule can be made for each subgroup. For example, the author worked in a school for children with special needs that utilized block scheduling. At the middle school level, there were four classrooms. Two of the classes were scheduled to send their eligible students to therapy on Mondays and Wednesdays, and the other two classes came on Tuesday and Thursdays. One group had 10 students; the other group had 12 students. Fortunately, she had an aide. She would work intensively with a group of four while the aide worked with the others. One at a time, students would rotate out of the aide's group and go work on an assignment independently behind a partition. Two job-skill deficits adolescents with cognitive disabilities typically have are (1) not asking for help or clarification when needed, and (2) not announcing that they are finished with a task and need more work. Thus, the independent work station was set up to facilitate these skills. The student had to call for help if he or she could not complete the task, or announce that he or she had finished the task. When that was done, he or she could go to the reward corner and choose a reward task to work on for 10 minutes. The reward tasks included things like looking at books or working on an educational computer game. After those 10 minutes, he or she would rejoin the aide's group. Thus, each child spent 10 minutes in each of the four stations within each 45-minute block.

Another consideration in working with groups is whether to use matched groups or stair-step groups. Matched groups consist of students who are all working on similar goals and objectives and are at approximately the same functioning level. Stair-step groups consist of a variety of students at different levels. In stair-step groups, the clinician can set up a situation in which student A can serve as a model for student B, student B can serve as a model for student C, and so on. The clinician serves as the model for student A. Stair-step groups are more difficult to organize initially but are more effective in the long run. If you do not have the luxury of an aide and/or being able to divide the group into subgroups as discussed in the previous paragraph, the stair-step group can be quite efficient.

Whether one uses matched groups or stair-step groups, the clinician can keep all the students engaged by asking them to critique another student's response. For example, the clinician can turn to student B and ask him or her what student A said, or (when student A is correct), ask student B if student A was correct. This keeps them listening to each other and engaged in the group instead of losing attention when they are not being directly addressed by the clinician.

Data collection in a group can be a challenge. One method used that worked well was to give each student in the group a paper cup in which to put tokens when they were disbursed by the clinician. A green token meant the response was correct, a yellow token meant the response was an approximation of the desired response, a red token signified an incorrect response, and a blue token meant no response. Choose a goal on which to take data on that day for each child. At the end of the day you could take each child's cup, count the tokens, and record the data. Through this system, take data on all the children in the group at the same time and never have to break eye contact or the classroom rhythm to record data.

think about it

Why is most therapy in schools group therapy? In your opinion, is it an effective means of providing intervention?

INTERVENTION WITH ADOLESCENTS

Roth and Worthington (2001) delineated three main stages of adolescence, as explained in Table 14–4. The development of metalinguistic skills continues in this age period, with increased ability to use and appreciate humor, proverbs, metaphors, and idioms. The use of figurative language enhances oral and written language as the child learns to "go beyond the conventional meaning of language for correct interpretation or use" (Roth &

TABLE 14–4 Stages of adolescence and corresponding therapeutic emphasis

Stage	Age	Therapeutic Emphasis Area
Early	10–14	Developing communication skills for academic and personal-social purposes
Middle	14–16	Facilitation of communication skills for academic, personal-social, and vocational goals
Late	16–20	Developing communication skills for personal-social and vocational purposes

Source: Adapted from *Treatment resource manual for speech-language pathology* (2nd ed.), by F. P. Roth and C. K. Worthington. Copyright 2001 by Delmar, Cengage Learning.

Worthington, 2001, p. 158). Other advances in language include increased mean length of utterance and increased complexity of sentences, the use of linguistic cohesion devices, expository writing, and continued development of lexicon and word knowledge. Metalinguistic skills are a major target of intervention with adolescents with language-based learning disabilities. They play a role in both oral and written language, and they facilitate the acquisition and use of independent problem-solving strategies (van Kleeck, 1994).

Within the confines of the different disorders, one can generally say that therapy for adolescents should focus on critical thinking strategies, listening skills (particularly important because most high school teaching models revolve around lectures), and written and oral language comprehension and production. In other words, it is particularly important that children in this age group be taught *how* to learn as opposed to *what* to learn. McKinley and Larson (1985) reported that when therapy focuses on teaching learning strategies, the child is more likely to "generalize basic skills across situations, settings, and curricula" (p. 4).

As presented in Chapter 13, it is critical to involve the adolescent in the stages of therapy by explaining the diagnostic and therapeutic processes and addressing the adolescent regarding the results of the assessment and development of therapy goals. The goals must be ones that are meaningful to the adolescent if he or she is expected to willingly participate in the therapeutic process. In addition, it is critical for the speech-language pathologist to stress the impact of achieving the set goals on future schooling and employment.

think about it
Most adolescents balk at coming to therapy in the public school setting. How can you convince the reluctant student to participate in therapy? What can you do to minimize the stigma associated with receiving special education services in middle and high school?

ADDRESSING WRITTEN LANGUAGE PROBLEMS IN CHILDREN WITH LANGUAGE-BASED LEARNING DISABILITIES

Written language poses a different set of problems than does oral language. Wong and colleagues (1991) identified problems these children have with written language as including "lower-order cognitive problems in spelling, punctuation, and grammar, and higher-order cognitive and metacognitive problems in planning, writing fluency, revising, and awareness of audience" (p. 117). They proposed an interactive teaching model to assist children with written language assignments. In an interactive model, the clinician engages the older elementary children or adolescents in oral discourse to help them clarify the theme of their writing and to help them identify any ambiguous statements in their written narratives. Therapy for written language is best implemented in a collaborative approach involving the academic teachers and the speech-language pathologist.

TREATMENT OF AUDITORY PROCESSING DISORDERS

Given the impact an auditory processing disorder can have on an individual's social, educational, and academic success, early identification and intervention are critical. Early intervention enables the clinician to take advantage of the plasticity and cortical reorganization abilities of the brain. In most cases, treatment includes environmental analysis and modification through the use of devices such as personal FM systems and classroom, workplace, or home amplification. Environmental manipulation is critical in the treatment of APD because the language deficit most affected by APD is the comprehension of spoken language (ASHA, 1996).

In addition, treatment should include training in the interhemispheric transfer of information activities such as "using interaural temporal offsets and intensity differences, as well as other unimodal (e.g., linking prosodic and linguistic acoustic features) and multimodal (e.g., writing to dictation, verbally describing a picture while drawing) interhemispheric transfer exercises" (ASHA, 2005, p. 11).

Keith (1999) wrote that management of APD should consist of modification of the environment, perceptual training, compensatory training, and cognitive training. Modification of the environment includes the use of assistive listening devices as well as classroom amplification. Other environmental changes can include improving the acoustics of the classroom, providing preferential seating, and assigning a "listening buddy" to assist the child with APD.

Auditory training, including "procedures targeting intensity, frequency, and duration discrimination; phoneme discrimination and phoneme-to-grapheme skills; temporal gap discrimination; temporal ordering or sequencing; pattern recognition; localization/lateralization; and recognition of auditory information presented within a background of noise or competition" should be incorporated into any treatment plan for an individual with APD (ASHA, 2005, p. 11). Compensatory strategies can be used to develop auditory skills that can improve the academic skills and perceptual processes. These include training in auditory figure-ground, auditory memory, phonemic synthesis, speech sound discrimination, auditory analysis, and prosody.

Cognitive therapy should focus on monitoring and self-regulating skills needed for message comprehension and problem solving. Included in cognitive therapy are activities that address language training, organizational skills, and development of the lexicon. These also incorporate the following skills: following directions, using written notes, listening and anticipating what will be said, asking relevant questions, and answering questions (Keith, 1999).

MULTICULTURAL ISSUES IN LANGUAGE THERAPY

One of the first questions the clinician should ask when faced with serving a student whose first language is not English is, "Am I prepared to assess and work with students of other cultures who have various language-learning difficulties?" Providing treatment for multicultural students goes beyond knowing the child's native language. Clinicians must understand the child's native culture as well. Thus, it is important for clinicians to update their knowledge and skills with regard to cultural diversity. Another major question is, "How do I encourage positive interaction between myself and the client?" The answer to this question takes on extra meaning when reviewing the culturally accepted practices that affect pragmatics and interactions in non–English-speaking students. For example, in some cultures, it is considered a major transgression to touch someone's head. This could certainly have an impact on a clinician who is putting ear phones on a student or performing an oral-facial examination. Clinicians must be aware of verbal and nonverbal rules used by the student who speaks a minority language to avoid inadvertent insults, thus damaging the client–clinician relationship.

The ultimate goal in providing therapy to students from non–English-speaking backgrounds is equity. That is, it is important to give all students what they need to perform equally well in their academic and social pursuits. Addressing both verbal and nonverbal pragmatics is necessary when teaching multicultural students.

Impact of Theories of Language Development

Skinner espoused the behaviorist theory of language development. This viewpoint emphasizes the form of language, not necessarily the cognitive processes that underlie language and abstract thinking. Using behaviorist theory, language is taught in a stimulus-response paradigm. Although this type of theoretical approach to language therapy has a role in some therapies, it can be disastrous for students who have limited English proficiency (LEP) because it ignores many of the pragmatic issues that form a foundation for communication.

The nativist viewpoint of language development states that children have innate structures that enable language to develop when stimulated by the environment. Chomsky was the major proponent of the nativist theory, but as with the behaviorist approach, the emphasis is on form, and, in this case, syntax in particular.

Proponents of the interactionist theory of language development believe that language development interacts with cognition. In this theory, having a great variety of experiences means that there are greater opportunities to learn language. The interactionist approach is the most effective one to use with individuals who are learning English as a second language. The ability to address form, content, and use through a pragmatic approach to learning a second language should not be underestimated. However, the clinician should keep in mind that narrative performances "among various cultural, ethnic, and linguistic groups may differ greatly" (Owens, 1995, p. 62). Standard English relies primarily on word order to convey meaning, whereas many other languages tend to use more inflectional morphemes to convey meaning (Nelson, 1993). Also, speakers in other cultures tend to use more paralinguistic devices than does most of the American culture (Owens, 1995).

A Continuum of Proficiency in English

ASHA (1985) outlined a continuum of proficiency in English:

1. Bilingual English proficient

2. Limited English proficient

3. Limited in English and the minority language

The association also developed clinical competencies needed to serve each of these three groups. Clients who are bilingual English proficient are equally or more fluent in English than in their native language. If the communication disorder is in English, the speech-language pathologist does not have to be proficient in the minority language. However, the clinician must have enough base knowledge to distinguish between dialectal differences influenced by the minority language and the communication disorder. This includes knowing the rules that govern the use of the minority language and knowledge of contrastive phonological, grammatical, semantic, and pragmatic features of the minority language. The clinician must also be knowledgeable about nondiscriminatory testing procedures (ASHA, 1985).

The second group on the continuum includes persons who are considered to be limited English proficient. These are the students who are proficient in their native language but have limited mastery of the English language. In these cases, assessment and treatment must be conducted in the native language. Thus, the clinician must have native or near-native fluency in the minority language and English. He or she must also know normative processes for speech and language acquisition in the minority language, both oral and written. The clinician must be able to administer and interpret formal and informal assessment procedures to distinguish between a language difference and a language disorder. Again, the clinician should be sensitive to cultural factors affecting communication and its remediation (ASHA, 1985).

Students who are limited in both English and their minority language constitute the third group on the continuum. In these cases, the clinician must be fluent in English and the child's native language. It is important to assess the child in both languages to determine if one is dominant over the other. The same competencies required for working with students who have limited English proficiency apply to this segment of the continuum. Which language is used for intervention depends on the assessment results (ASHA, 1985).

Language Education

School-based clinicians may provide services in the instruction of English as a second language or in teaching a nonstandard dialect. For most of these students, therapy is considered an elective service, stemming from a desire to acquire more standard English production. Therefore, unless a disorder is present in the native language, the child does not qualify for services in the schools under Section 504 of the Rehabilitation Act or under IDEA. However, funding from other sources within the district may be used to cover the costs of providing therapy.

To provide these therapeutic services, the clinician must be competent and knowledgeable in at least three areas. First, the clinician must be familiar with linguistic features of the child's dialect. Second, he or she must understand linguistic contrastive analysis. Third, the clinician must have an appreciation of the effects of attitudes toward dialects.

Therapy must emphasize language structure, language use, and language as a facilitator of cognition. The practical use of the language in a variety of settings also must be emphasized (Taylor, 1992). As with almost all language instruction, a multimodality, multifunctional approach is most beneficial. It is also important to remember that proficiency in English at the elementary ages does not guarantee successful use of English in middle school and high school because of the differences in the language demands and use at the different age levels (Nelson, 1993).

There are three philosophies regarding whether or not to provide dialect intervention to children in the schools. The *no intervention* view states that community dialects are culturally adequate. Therefore, the stance should be to forgo intervention and permit the children to use the language of their home speech community. Proponents of the *bidialectal* view believe that it is important to respect and preserve the students' native dialects, but that it is also important to teach them to master the prevalent dialect so they can use it when expected or required to do so. The third philosophy is the *eradication* view. In this viewpoint, community dialects have no value and should not be preserved. The children should be taught the prevalent dialect and instructed to use it in all settings at all times. The school-based clinician must be aware of these philosophies and know if one philosophy takes precedence over another within his or her own school setting.

Knapp, Turnbull, and Shields (1990) addressed the issue of how children from impoverished homes succeed in school. They found that these children can rise to the challenges presented in the academic setting when the following occur:

1. Teachers respect the students' cultural and linguistic backgrounds and communicate this appreciation to them in a personal way.

2. The academic program encourages students to draw and build on the experiences they have at the same time that it exposes them to unfamiliar experiences and ways of thinking.

3. The assumptions, expectations, and ways of doing things in school—in short, its culture—are made explicit to these students by teachers who explain and model these dimensions of academic learning (p. 5).

When these conditions are met, not only do children from poverty benefit, but so do those from any minority culture.

NELB and LEP

NELB and *LEP* are acronyms used to identify children as being of non–English language background or as limited English proficient. Typically, these terms are used to refer to speakers of English as a second language. However, it is important to remember that a child could be of a non–English language background but still be proficient in English. Likewise, it is possible to be limited English proficient without being of a non–English language background. Although these thoughts may seem trivial, they emphasize that clinicians and educators should not make hasty assumptions about a child based on his or her dialect or knowledge of the English language when English is a second language.

The Pygmalion effect states that individuals live up to expectations placed on them. Thus, if our expectations are lowered for children with dialects or language differences, it is probable that these children will show, in accordance with the expectations, limited progress in their academic and social skills. In a lecture to students at the University of Florida, Bernardo Garcia, director of the Office of Multicultural Student Language Education in the Florida Department of Education, proposed that we rename the acronym *LEP* to represent a more positive perspective. For example, he proposed that *LEP* could stand for "language-enhanced pupils" because many educators equate *LEP* with "lower expectation pupil" (Garcia, 1994). It is certainly something to consider. The real issue is "How meaningfully does this individual communicate?" not how well his or her language represents the standard dialect.

> *think about it*
>
> A student from France has enrolled in the school where you are a speech-language pathologist. She is in the United States for one year while her father is on sabbatical at the local university. Her English is limited. What is your role in this child's education (if you have one), and what can you do to help ensure she has a meaningful educational experience during that year?

SUMMARY

Individuals with language-based learning disabilities, especially those that affect reading, spelling, and writing, often face an uphill battle to overcome these deficits. When structuring the treatment for these students, clinicians must avoid fostering a sense of failure and helplessness. Learned helplessness can be decreased by rewarding completed work with positive reinforcement and meaningful feedback. Promoting active involvement in the learning process and scheduling breaks to avoid mental fatigue also help to improve the student's abilities to sustain his or her attention on the task at hand. Teaching children to self-check their own work is likewise critical in decreasing learned helplessness because the children learn to rely on themselves for positive feedback instead of relying on others. Similarly, teaching about the learning disability is of critical importance (Goldsworthy, 1996). The speech-language pathologist should teach the student and his or her classmates what it means to have a learning disability and how it affects reading, spelling, writing, and communication. The more a student understands his or her disability, the more he or she can learn about strategies to overcome it.

Knowledge and personal understanding of the nature of the learning disability can help to prevent the depression and feelings of frustration that often become overriding factors. This is critical to understand because there are times when depression and frustration can overwhelm the child and interfere with remediation of the problems. An effective, comprehensive program focuses on the strategies needed for effective reading, spelling, and writing but is not limited to the mechanics of these skills. It is just as important to teach the children to concentrate, listen, and control their attention so that they can persist with a task until it is completed successfully.

In conclusion, there are a variety of techniques that can be used for intervention, but they all have a common set of goals. Specifically,

> critical steps of all of these curriculum-based language intervention strategies are to (1) identify zones of significance (contextually based needs); (2) analyze the communicative demands of the event or situation; (3) observe the individual's current attempts to meet those demands; (4) provide intervention to assist the individual to acquire new knowledge, skills, and strategies: (5) mediate the contextual demands to make them more accessible; and (6) keep in mind the desired outcome of independent functioning in the real world. (Nelson, 1998, p. 433)

CASE STUDY

History

David is a 9-year-old male who was diagnosed at the Dyslexia Center as having developmental dyslexia. His diagnosis was based on a discrepancy between test scores of oral language and test scores of reading, spelling, and phonological awareness. He has been in dyslexia therapy for one semester. He was scheduled for 22 sessions between January and April and attended all sessions. Therapy was based on the Lindamood Phoneme Sequencing Programs (LiPS).

David is in the fourth grade at Pine Hills Elementary School. He is an average student, getting mostly Bs and Cs on his report card. He is quite social and has several friends. He plays baseball in the local youth league, and also plays soccer.

Behavioral Observations During Therapy

David cooperated and worked diligently in all therapy sessions. He was very motivated to succeed. He responded well to verbal reinforcement. His mother observed each session and practiced his therapy goals at home between therapy sessions. She requested a set of LiPS cards to use at home to practice the LiPS labels, mouth movements, and corresponding sounds and symbols.

Long-Term Goals

- David will complete all levels of the LiPS program. This includes (1) all voiced and unvoiced consonants, (2) all vowels, (3) tracking, spelling, and reading one-syllable

(continues)

CASE STUDY *(continued)*

words, and (4) tracking, reading, and spelling multisyllabic words.

- David will improve his scores on the Lindamood Auditory Conceptualization Test (LACT).
- David will improve his scores on the Test of Phonological Awareness (TOPA).

Short-Term Goals

The LiPS program is a multisensory, multifaceted program of phonemic awareness training, based on a phonological foundation and rooted in the motor-articulatory feedback theory. This program facilitates perception of contrasts between speech sounds and the order of sounds in syllables in words, a critical skill needed for reading and spelling. A distinctive feature of the program is that the student is taught to self-correct, rather than being given the right answers.

- Lip Poppers: David will say the sound, label, and write the symbols for the sounds /p/ and /b/ with 85 percent accuracy.
- Tongue Tappers: David will say the sound, label, and write the symbols for the sounds /t/ and /d/ with 85 percent accuracy.
- Tongue Scrapers: David will say the sound, label, and write the symbols for the sounds /k/ and /g/ with 85 percent accuracy.
- Lip Coolers: David will say the sound, label, and write the symbols for the sounds /f/ and /v/ with 85 percent accuracy.
- Skinny Air Sounds: David will say the sound, label, and write the symbols for the sounds /s/ and /z/ with 85 percent accuracy.

- Tongue Coolers: David will say the sound, label, and write the symbols for the sounds /th/ (voiceless) and /th/ (voiced) with 85 percent accuracy.
- Fat Air Sounds: David will say the sound, label, and write the symbols for the sounds /sh/ and /zh/ with 85 percent accuracy.
- Fat Pushed Air Sounds: David will say the sound, label, and write the symbols for the sounds /ch/ and /j/ with 85 percent accuracy.
- Nose Sounds: David will say the sound, label, and write the symbols for the sounds /m/, /n/, and /ng/ with 85 percent accuracy.
- Wind Sounds: David will say the sound, label, and write the symbols for the sounds /w/, /h/, and /wh/ with 85 percent accuracy.
- Lifters: David will say the sound, label, and write the symbols for the sounds /l/ and /r/ with 85 percent accuracy.
- Round Vowel Sounds: David will say the sound, label, and write the symbols for the sounds /oo/ (as in the words *book* and *look*) and /oe/ with 85 percent accuracy.
- Open Vowel Sounds: David will say the sound, label, and write the symbols for the sounds /o/ and /au-aw/ with 85 percent accuracy.
- Smile Vowel Sounds: David will say the sound, label, and write the symbols for the sounds /ee/, /I/, /e/, /ae/, /a/, and /u/ with 85 percent accuracy.
- Slider Vowel Sounds: David will say the sound, label, and write the symbols for the sounds /ie/, /ue/, /ou-ow/, and /oi-oy/ with 85 percent accuracy.

Results

Goals	Accuracy	Goal Met (+)/Not Met (−)
Lip Poppers		
Say	100%	+
Label	100%	+
Write	100%	+
Tongue Tappers		
Say	100%	+
Label	100%	+
Write	100%	+
Tongue Scrapers		
Say	100%	+
Label	100%	+
Write	100%	+
Lip Coolers		
Say	100%	+
Label	100%	+
Write	100%	+
Skinny Air Sounds		
Say	100%	+
Label	100%	+
Write	100%	+
Tongue Coolers		
Say	100%	+
Label	100%	+
Write	100%	+
Fat Air Sounds		
Say	92%	+
Label	100%	+
Write	100%	+

(continues)

CASE STUDY *(continued)*

Fat Pushed Air Sounds		
Say	100%	+
Label	100%	+
Write	100%	+
Nose Sounds		
Say	100%	+
Label	100%	+
Write	100%	+
Wind Sounds		
Say	100%	+
Label	100%	+
Write	100%	+
Lifters		
Say	100%	+
Label	100%	+
Write	100%	+
Round Vowel Sounds		
Say	95%	+
Label	100%	+
Write	100%	+
Open Vowel Sounds		
Say	100%	+
Label	100%	+
Write	100%	+
Smile Vowel Sounds		
Say	100%	+
Label	100%	+
Write	100%	+
Slider Vowel Sounds		
Say	92%	+
Label	100%	+
Write	100%	+

Procedures

David labeled, described, and categorized sounds and the symbols associated with the sounds. He also tracked one-syllable words with colored blocks. David played games during the second half of each therapy session to enforce the sounds, symbols, and labels that he was learning. The following is a list of the games David played in therapy:

- David played "Memory" using the sounds he was currently learning in therapy. The symbols that he was learning in therapy were written on individual pieces of colored construction paper. Then these pieces of paper were turned face down on the table. David took turns with the clinician turning over two pieces of paper at a time to try and find a match. Every time David turned a card over he was asked to produce the sound that the symbol represents and to label what group it was in.

- David played "Go Fish" using the sounds he was currently learning in therapy. The symbols that David was learning in therapy were written on individual pieces of colored construction paper. These pieces of paper were then distributed to David and the clinician. The object was to get matches by asking the other player for certain sounds. For example, David might ask the clinician if she had an /l/. For every match made by either player, David was asked to produce the sound that corresponded to the symbol and to label what group it was in.

- Pictures of different objects were presented to David who was then asked to name the object or picture, produce the initial sound in the word in isolation, and label the sound. He was given three different symbols to choose from.

- David played a game in which he jumped to letter symbols on the floor after the clinician produced a sound. All the sounds were previously learned in therapy, so this was a review game.

- David played "Guess Who" in which he answered a question about something he was working on in therapy in order to get a turn.

- David played "Bingo" using the sounds he learned in therapy.

Summary of Results of Short-Term Goals

David met all of his short-term goals for this semester. He has now mastered all the consonant sounds and vowel sounds. David loved playing games, so incorporating games into his therapy sessions proved to be a valuable method to reinforce what he had learned. It was quite apparent that he practiced at home with his mother, and this was a major factor in his rapid progress.

Recommendations

It was recommended that David attend intensive individual summer therapy to complete the LiPS program for reading and spelling. It is also recommended that David's mother continue to practice at home with him to reinforce what is learned in therapy.

(continues)

CASE STUDY *(continued)*

Therapy goals for next semester should include the following:

- Review the vowels: round sounds, open sounds, smile sounds, and sliders.
- Introduce the Crazy Rs.
- Practice auditory recognition and discrimination for the initial sounds in words. One way to do this is to present David with an object or picture, then ask him to name it, produce the initial sound of the word in isolation, and label the sound. For example, when shown a picture of a cat, David will respond, "That's a cat; it starts with /k/, which is a tongue scraper."
- Practice counting the number of syllables in words by clapping or pounding each syllable beat on the table as he says the word aloud.

REVIEW QUESTIONS

1. Which of the following is a form of direct therapy?
   a. Consultation
   b. Pull-out model
   c. Collaborative model
   d. Both a and c
   e. Both b and c
   f. Both a and b

2. When does the emphasis in traditional reading instruction shift from basic skills to content acquisition?
   a. Grade 3
   b. Grade 4
   c. Grade 5
   d. Grade 6

3. Which of the following represent the domains that must be addressed on a child's education plan at school?
   a. Curriculum
   b. Independent functioning
   c. Social and personal
   d. Communication
   e. All of the above
   f. a, b, and d
   g. a, c, and d

4. An _____ must be written annually for school-age children receiving speech-language services in the schools.

   a. Individualized Family Service Plan (IFSP)

   b. Interventional Plan of Education (IPE)

   c. Individualized Education Plan (IEP)

   d. Progress report such as a SOAP note

5. Generalization is the gradual withdrawal of prompts and guidance to allow the stimulus to elicit the response.

   a. True

   b. False

6. The interactionist approach is the most effective one to use with individuals who are learning English as a second language.

   a. True

   b. False

7. The measured level of ability prior to intervention is

   a. Documentation of soft signs

   b. Sensory Integration

   c. Task analysis

   d. Baseline

8. Exclusional criteria for determining placement in therapy is based on

   a. The gap between the child's expected level of achievement and his or her intellectual and social achievement levels compared to his or her language abilities

   b. The presence of a documented language and/or learning problem in the absence of cognitive, sensory, or physical handicaps

9. Which of the following theories on dialect intervention in the schools is most ethical?

   a. The no intervention view

   b. The bidialectal view

   c. The eradication view

10. Of the three models of language intervention described by Olswang and Bain, the _____ model is the most structured.

    a. Milieu teaching

    b. Joint action routines

    c. Inductive teaching

REFERENCES

American Speech-Language-Hearing Association (ASHA). (1985). Clinical management of communicatively handicapped minority language populations. *ASHA Desk Reference, 4,* IV-2–IV-6.

American Speech-Language-Hearing Association. (1989, March). Issues in determining eligibility for language intervention. *ASHA, 31,* 113–118.

American Speech-Language-Hearing Association. (1991). A model for collaborative service delivery for students with language-learning disorders in public schools. *ASHA, 33*(Suppl. 5), 44–50.

American Speech-Language-Hearing Association Task Force on Central Auditory Processing Consensus Development. (1996, July). Central auditory processing: Current status of research and implications for clinical practice. *American Journal of Audiology, 5*(2), 41–54.

American Speech-Language-Hearing Association. Working Group on Auditory Processing Disorders. (2005, February). (Central) auditory processing disorders. *ASHA Technical Report.*

Bashir, A., Kuban, K., Kleinman, S., & Scavuzzo, S. (1983). Issues in language disorders: Considerations of cause, maintenance, and change. In J. Miller, D. Yoder, and R. Schiefelbush (eds.), *ASHA Reports,* 92–106.

Butyniec-Thomas, J., & Woloshyn, V. E. (1997). The effects of explicit-strategy and whole language instruction on students' spelling ability. *Journal of Experimental Education, 65,* 293–302.

Carlisle, J. E. (1995). Morphological awareness and early reading achievement. In L. B. Feldman (ed.), *Morphological aspects of language processing* (pp. 189–209). Hillsdale, NJ: Erlbaum.

Garcia, B. (1994). Personal communication.

Goldsworthy, C. L. (1996). Developmental reading disabilities: A language-based treatment approach. Clifton Park, NY: Delmar, Cengage Learning.

Greenhalgh, K. S., & Strong, C. J. (2001). Literate language features in spoken narratives of children with typical language and children with language impairments. *Language, Speech, and Hearing Services in the Schools, 32,* 114–125.

Hegde, M. N. (1996). *A coursebook on language disorders in children.* Clifton Park, NY: Delmar, Cengage Learning.

Keith, R. W. (1999). Clinical issues in central auditory processing disorders. *Language, Speech, and Hearing Services in the Schools, 30*(4), 339–344.

Kirk, C., & Gillon, G. T. (2009, July). Integrated morphological awareness intervention as a tool for improving literacy. *Language, Speech, and Hearing Services in the Schools, 40,* 341–351.

Knapp, M. S., Turnbull, B. J., & Shields, P. M. (1990). New directions for educating the children of poverty. *Educational Leadership, 48*(1), 4–8.

Larson, V. L., & McKinley, N. (1995). *Language disorders in older students: Preadolescents and adolescents.* Eau Claire, WI: Thinking Publications.

Lewis, P. (1987, December). A case for teaching functional skills. *TASH Newsletter* (The Association for Persons with Severe Handicaps).

McCabe, A., Bliss, L., Barra, G., & Bennett, M. (2008, May). Comparison of personal versus fictional narratives of children with language impairments. *American Journal of Speech-Language Pathology, 17,* 194–206.

Merritt, D. D., & Culatta, B. (1998). *Language intervention in the classroom.* San Diego, CA: Singular Publishing Group.

Naremore, R. C., Densmore, A. E., & Harman, D. R. (1995). *Language intervention with school-age children: Conversation, narrative, and text.* San Diego, CA: Singular Publishing Group.

Nelson, N. W. (1993). *Childhood language disorders in context: Infancy through adolescence.* New York: Macmillan Publishing Company.

Nelson, N. W. (1998). *Childhood language disorders in context: Infancy through adolescence* (2nd ed.). New York: Macmillan Publishing Group.

Olswang, L., & Bain, B. (1991). Intervention issues for toddlers with specific language impairments. *Topics in Language Disorders, 11,* 69–86.

Owens, Robert E. (1995). *Language disorders: A functional approach to assessment and intervention.* Boston: Allyn & Bacon.

Reed, V. A. (2005). *An introduction to children with language disorders* (3rd ed.). Boston: Allyn & Bacon.

Roth, F. P., & Worthington, C. K. (2001). *Treatment resource manual for speech-language pathology* (2nd ed.). Clifton Park, NY: Delmar, Cengage Learning.

Sanger, D. D., Hux, K., & Griess, K. (1995). Educators' opinions about speech-language pathology services in the schools. *Language-Speech-Hearing Services in the Schools, 26*(1), 75–86.

Siegel, L. (2008). Morphological awareness skills of English language learners and children with dyslexia. *Topics in Language Disorders, 28*(1), 15–27.

Snyder, L. (1984). Developmental language disorders: Elementary school age. In A. Holland (ed.), *Language disorders in children: Recent advances* (pp. 129–158). San Diego, CA: College-Hill Press.

Taylor, J. S. (1992). *Speech-language pathology services in the schools* (2nd ed.). Boston: Allyn & Bacon.

Van Hattum, R. (1985). *Organization of speech-language services in schools: A manual.* San Diego, CA: College-Hill Press.

van Kleeck, A. (1994). Metalinguistic development, In G. P. Wallach and K. G. Butler (eds.), *Language learning disabilities in school-age children and adolescents: Some principles and applications* (2nd ed., pp. 53–98). Boston: Allyn & Bacon.

Wallach, G. P., Charlton, S., & Christie, J. (2009, April). Making a broader case for the narrow view: Where to begin? *Language, Speech, and Hearing Services in the Schools, 40,* 201–211.

Wallach, G. P., & Liebergott, J. W. (1984). Who shall be called "learning disabled?" Some new directions. In G. P. Wallach and K. C. Butler (eds.), *Language learning disabilities in school-age children.* Baltimore: Williams & Wilkins.

Warren, S. F., & Yoder, P. J. (1994). Communication and language intervention: Why a constructivist approach is insufficient. *Journal of Special Education, 28,* 248–258.

Wong, B. Y., Wong, R., Darlington, D., & Jones, W. (1991). Interactive teaching: An effective way to teach revision skills to adolescents with learning disabilities. *Learning Disabilities Research & Practice, 6,* 117–127.

Appendix A

Suggested Reading List on Language Abnormalities in Preschool Children

(Note: Some of the books on this list cover language delays, disorders, and differences from infancy through adolescence. Thus, some of the books on this list would also be appropriate on the school-aged list.)

Accardo, P. J. (2008). *Capute & Accardo's neurodevelopmental disabilities in infancy and childhood. Volume I: Neurodevelopmental diagnosis and treatment* (3rd ed.). Baltimore, MD: Paul H. Brookes Publishing Company.

Accardo, P. J. (2008). *Capute & Accardo's neurodevelopmental disabilities in infancy and childhood. Volume II: The spectrum of neurodevelopmental disabilities* (3rd ed.). Baltimore, MD: Paul H. Brookes Publishing Company.

Alvares, R. L., & Downing, S. F. (1998). A survey of expressive communication skills in children with Angelman syndrome. *American Journal of Speech-Language Pathology, 7*, 1–24.

American Speech-Language-Hearing Association. (1987). *Learning disabilities and the preschool child* [position statement]. Available from www.asha.org/policy.

American Speech-Language-Hearing Association, Committee on Augmentative Communication. (1989). Competencies for speech-language pathologists providing services in augmentative communication. *ASHA, 31*, 107–110.

American Speech-Language-Hearing Association, Committee on Language Learning Disorders. (1989). Issues in determining eligibility for language intervention. *ASHA, 31*, 113–118.

American Speech-Language-Hearing Association, Committee on Mental Retardation and Developmental Disabilities. (1989). Mental retardation and developmental disabilities curriculum guide for SLPs and audiologists. *ASHA, 31*, 94–96.

American Speech-Language-Hearing Association. (1990). The roles of SLPs in service delivery to infants, toddlers, and their families. *ASHA, 32*(Suppl. 2), 4.

American Speech-Language-Hearing Association. (1991). Position statement: Augmentative and alternative communication. *ASHA, 33*(Suppl. 5), 8.

American Speech-Language-Hearing Association. (1991). Report: Augmentative and alternative communication. *ASHA, 33*(Suppl. 5), 9–12.

American Speech-Language-Hearing Association. (1992). Guidelines for meeting the communication needs of persons with severe disabilities. *ASHA, 34*(Suppl. 7), 1–8.

American Speech-Language-Hearing Association. (1993). *Definitions of communication disorders and variations* [relevant paper]. Available from www.asha.org/policy.

American Speech-Language-Hearing Association. (2002). *Knowledge and skills needed by speech-language pathologists with respect to reading and writing in children and adolescents* [knowledge and skills]. Available from www.asha.org/policy.

American Speech-Language-Hearing Association, Working Group on Auditory Processing Disorders. (2005, February). (Central) auditory processing disorders. *ASHA Technical Report.*

Baker, D. (2008, July). Illiteracy in America. Available from trivani.wordpress.com/2008/07/13/illiteracy-in-america.

Batshaw, M. L., Pelligrino, L., & Roizen, N, J. (eds.). (2007). *Children with disabilities* (6th ed.), Baltimore, MD: Paul H. Brookes Publishing Company.

Berk, L. (2004). *Development through the lifespan.* Boston: Allyn & Bacon.

Bernstein, D. K., & Levey, S. (2009). Language development: A review. In D. K. Bernstein and E. Tiegerman-Morris (eds.), *Language and communication disorders in children* (pp. 28–100). Boston: Allyn & Bacon.

Bernstein, D. K., & Tiegerman-Farber, E. (2002). *Language and communication disorders in children* (4th ed.). Boston: Allyn & Bacon.

Billeaud, F. P. (1998). *Communication disorders in infants and toddlers: Assessment and intervention* (2nd ed.). Boston: Butterworth-Heinemann.

Bishop, D. V. M., & Adams, C. (1990). A prospective study of the relation between specific language impairment, phonological disorder, and reading retardation. *Journal of Child Psychology and Psychiatry, 31,* 1027–1050.

Bishop, D. V. M., & Edmundson, A. (1987). Specific language impairment as a maturational lag: Evidence from longitudinal data on language and motor development. *Developmental Medicine and Child Neurology, 29,* 442–459.

Blackman, J. A. (2000). Attention-deficit/hyperactivity disorder in preschoolers. *Pediatric Clinics of North America, 46,* 1011–1025.

Bloom, L., & Lahey, M. (1978). *Language development and language disorders.* New York: John Wiley & Sons.

Blosser, J. L., & DePompei, R. (1994). *Pediatric traumatic brain injury: Proactive intervention.* San Diego, CA: Singular Publishing Group.

Bregman, J. D. (2005). Definitions and characteristics of the spectrum. In D. Zager (ed.). *Autism spectrum disorders: Identification, education, and treatment* (pp. 3–46). Mahwah, NJ: Lawrence Ehrlbaum.

Brinton, B., Fujiki, M., & Higbee, L. (1998). Participation in cooperative learning activities by children with specific language impairment. *Journal of Speech, Language, and Hearing Research, 41,* 1193–1206.

Brinton, B., Fujiki, M., Montague, E. C., & Hanton, J. L. (2000). Children with language impairment in cooperative work groups: A pilot study. *Language, Speech, and Hearing Services in Schools, 31,* 252–264.

Britt, R. R. (2009). 14 percent of United States adults can't read. *Live Science.* Available from www.livescience.com/culture/090110-illiterateadults.html.

Brock, S. E., & Slone, M. (n.d.). Autism spectrum disorders (Part 1): Case finding and screening. In-service at Irvine Unified School District.

Brown, I., & Percy, M. (eds.). (2007). *A comprehensive guide to intellectual and developmental disabilities.* Baltimore, MD: Paul H. Brookes Publishing Company.

Brown, R. A. (1973). *A first language: The early stages.* Cambridge, MA: Harvard University Press.

Buckendorf, G. R. (2008). *Autism: A guide for educators, clinicians, and parents.* Greenville, SC: Thinking Publications.

Chomsky, N. (1982). *Some concepts and consequences of the theory of government and binding.* Cambridge, MA: The MIT Press.

Coleman, T. J., & McCabe-Smith, L. (2000). Key terms and concepts. In T. J. Coleman (ed.), *Clinical management of communication disorders in culturally diverse children* (pp. 3–12). Boston: Allyn & Bacon.

Condouris, K., Meyer, E., & Tager-Flusberg, H. (2003, August). The relationship between standardized measures of language and measures of spontaneous speech in children with autism. *American Journal of Speech-Language Pathology, 12*(3), 349–358.

Crystal, D. & Varley, R. (1993). *Introduction to language pathology* (3rd ed.). San Diego, CA: Singular Publishing Group.

Curenton, S. M. (2011). Multicultural issues. In J. N. Kaderavek (ed.), *Language disorders in children: Fundamental concepts of assessment and intervention* (pp. 383–412). Boston: Allyn & Bacon.

Elman, J. L., Bates, E. A., Johnson, M. H., Karmiloff-Smith, A., Parisi, D., & Plunkett, K. (1996). *Rethinking innateness: A connectionist perspective on development.* Cambridge, MA: The MIT Press.

Fletcher, P., & MacWhinney, B. (eds.). (1995). *The handbook of child language.* Oxford, England: Blackwell.

Fujiki, M., & Brinton, B. (1995). The performance of younger and older adults with retardation on a series of language tasks. *American Journal of Speech-Language Pathology, 4,* 77–86.

Fujiki, M., Brinton, B., & Clarke, D. (April, 2002). Emotional regulation in children with specific language impairment. *Language, Speech, and Hearing Services in Schools, 33,* 102–111.

Gerber, S. E. (1998). *Etiology and prevention of communicative disorders* (2nd ed.). San Diego, CA: Singular Publishing Group.

Gertner, B. L., Rice, M. L., & Hadley, P. A. (1994). Influence of communicative competence on peer preferences in a preschool classroom. *Journal of Speech and Hearing Research, 37,* 913–923.

Girolametto, L., Weitzman, E., & Greenberg, J. (2003, August). Training day care staff to facilitate children's language. *American Journal of Speech-Language Pathology, 12*(3), 299–311.

Gleason, J. B. (2005). *The development of language* (6th ed.). Boston: Allyn & Bacon.

Goffman, L., & Leonard, J. (2000, May). Growth of language skills in preschool children with specific language impairment: Implications for assessment and intervention. *American Journal of Speech-Language Pathology, 9*(2), 151–161.

Grandin, T. (1997). A personal perspective on autism. In D. Cohen and F. Volkmar (eds.). *Handbook of autism and pervasive developmental disorders* (2nd ed.) (pp. 1032–1042). New York: John Wiley & Sons.

Hagberg, B. S., Miniscalco, C., Gillberg, C. (2010). Clinic attendees with autism or attention deficit/hyperactivity disorder: Cognitive profile at school age and its relationship to preschool indicators. *Research in Developmental Disabilities: A Multidisciplinary Journal, 31*(1), 1–8.

Hall, L. J. (2009). *Autism spectrum disorders: From theory to practice.* Upper Saddle River, NJ: Pearson.

Halle, J., Brady, N. C., & Drasgow, E. (2004, February). Enhancing socially adaptive communicative repairs of beginning communicators with disabilities. *American Journal of Speech-Language Pathology, 13*(1), 43–54.

Hart, B., & Risley, T. (1995). *Meaningful differences in the everyday experience of young American children.* Baltimore, MD: Paul H. Brookes Publishing Company.

Hegde, M. N., & Maul, C. A. (2006). *Language disorders in children: An evidence-based approach to assessment and treatment.* Boston: Allyn & Bacon.

Hegde, M. N., & Pomaville, F. (2008). *Assessment of communication disorders in children: Resources and protocols.* San Diego, CA: Plural Publishing, Inc.

Hulit, L. M., & Howard, M. R. (2002). *Born to talk: An introduction to speech and language development.* Boston: Allyn & Bacon.

Johnson, B. A. (1995). *Language disorders in children: An introductory clinical perspective.* Clifton Park, NY: Delmar, Cengage Learning.

Johnson, C. J., Beitchman, J. H., Young, A., Escobar, M., Atkinson, L., Wilson, B., et al. (1999). Fourteen year follow up of children with and without speech/language impairments: Speech/language stability and outcomes. *Journal of Speech, Language, and Hearing Research, 42*(3), 744–760.

Justice, L. M., Chow, S., Capellini, C., Flanigan, K., & Colton, S. (2003, August). Emergent literacy intervention for vulnerable preschoolers: Relative effects of two approaches. *American Journal of Speech-Language Pathology, 12*(3), 320–332.

Justice, L. M., & Ezell, H. K. (2002, February). Use of storybook reading to increase print awareness in at-risk children. *American Journal of Speech-Language Pathology, 11*(1), 17–29.

Justice, L. M., Skibbe, L., & Ezell, H. (2006). Using print referencing to promote written language awareness. In T. A. Ukrainetz (ed.), *Contextualized language intervention: Scaffolding preK–12 literacy achievement* (pp. 389–428). Eau Claire, WI: Thinking Publications.

Kaderavek, J. N. (2011). *Language disorders in children: Fundamental concepts of assessment and intervention.* Boston: Allyn & Bacon.

Kaufman, N. J., & Larson, V. L. (2007). *Asperger syndrome: Strategies for solving the social puzzle.* Greenville, SC: Thinking Publications University.

Kumin, L. (2003). *Early communication skills for children with Down syndrome: A guide for parents and professionals.* Bethesda, MD: Woodbine House.

La Paro, K. M., Justice, L., Skibbe, L. E., & Pianta, R. C. (2004, November). Relations among maternal, child, and demographic factors and the persistence of preschool language impairment. *American Journal of Speech-Language Pathology, 13*(4), 291–303.

Layton, T, Crais, E., & Watson, L. (eds.). (1999). *Handbook of early language impairment in children: Nature.* Clifton Park, NY: Delmar, Cengage Learning.

Lizardi, L. O. (2000). *A connectionist approach to language acquisition.* ERIC #ED39434.

McCauley, R. J. (2001). *Assessment of language disorders in children.* Mahwah, NJ: Lawrence Erlbaum Associates.

McGreer, M. M. (2009). House passes burden of health care costs to the illiterate, and poor. Available from *www.*associatedcontent.com/.../house_passes_burden_of_ health_care.html.

McLaughlin, S. (2006). *Introduction to language development* (2nd ed.). Clifton Park, NY: Delmar, Cengage Learning.

Mentis, M., & Lundgren, K. (1995). Effects of prenatal exposure to cocaine and associated risk factors on language development. *Journal of Speech and Hearing Research, 8*(6), 1303–1318.

Monten, M. (2007, March). More than one-third of Washington, D.C. residents are functionally illiterate. *State of Adult Literacy 2006.* Available from www.proliterach.org.

National Center for Education Statistics. (2006). A first look at the literacy of America's adults in the 21st century. Available from nces.ed.gov/NAAL/PDF/2006470.pdf.

National Center for Education Statistics. (2007). Literacy in everyday life: Results from the 2003 National Assessment of Adult Literacy. *NCES 2007-480.* Washington, D.C.: United States Department of Education. Available from www.nces. ed.gov/Pubs2007/2007480.pdf.

National Early Intervention Longitudinal Study (NEILS). (2007, January). *Early intervention for infants and toddlers with disabilities and their families: Participants, services, and outcomes.*

National Institute for Literacy. (n.d.). Literacy in the United States. Available from www.policyalmanac.org/education/archives/literacy.shtml.

National Joint Committee on Learning Disabilities. (2007, October). *Learning disabilities and young children: Identification and intervention* [technical report]. Available from www.asha.org/policy.

Nelson, N. W. (2010). *Language and literacy disorders: Infancy through adolescence.* Boston: Allyn & Bacon.

Neuman, S. B. (2008). *Educating the other America: Top experts tackle poverty, literacy, and achievement in our schools.* Baltimore, MD: Paul H. Brookes Publishing Company.

Nippold, M. A, Mansfield, T. C., Billow, J. L., & Tomblin, J. B. (2009, August). Syntactic development in adolescents with a history of language impairments: A follow-up investigation. *American Journal of Speech-Language Pathology, 18*(3), 241–251.

Nippold, M. A., & Schwarz, I. E. (1996). Children with slow expressive language development: What is the forecast for school achievement? *American Journal of Speech-Language Pathology, 5,* 22–25.

Oller, J. W., & Oller, S. D. (2010). Autism: The diagnosis, treatment, and etiology of the undeniable epidemic. Sudbury, MA: Jones and Bartlett.

Owens, R. E., Jr. (2004). *Language disorders: A functional approach to assessment and intervention* (4th ed.). Boston: Allyn & Bacon.

Parker, F., & Riley, K. (1994). *Linguistics for non-linguists: A primer with exercises* (2nd ed.). Boston: Allyn & Bacon.

Paul, R. (2001). *Language disorders from infancy through adolescence* (2nd ed.). St. Louis, MO: Mosby.

Payne, K. T., & Taylor, I. L. (2010). Multicultural differences in human communication and disorders. In N. Anderson and G. H. Shames (eds.). *Human communication disorders: An introduction* (8th ed.). Boston: Pearson Education, Inc.

Pinker, S. (1999). *Words and rules: The ingredients of language.* New York: Basic Books.

Plante, E., & Vance, R. (1995). Diagnostic accuracy of two tests of preschool language. *American Journal of Speech-Language Pathology, 4,* 70–76.

Polakow, V. (1993). *Lives on the edge: Single mothers and their children in the other America.* Chicago: University of Chicago Press.

Prelock, P. A. (2006). *Autism spectrum disorders: Issues in assessment and intervention.* Austin, TX: Pro-Ed.

Reichle, J., Beukelman, D., & Light, J. (eds.). (2002). *Exemplary practices for beginning communicators: Implications for AAC.* Baltimore, MD: Paul H. Brookes.

Rescorla, L. (2009, February). Age 17 language and reading outcomes in late talking toddlers: Support for a dimensional perspective on language delay. *Journal of Speech, Language, and Hearing Research, 52*(1), 16–30.

Roberts, J. E., Mirrett, P., Anderson, K., Burchinal, M., & Neebe, E. (2002, August). Early communication, symbolic behavior, and social profiles of young males with fragile X syndrome. *American Journal of Speech-Language Pathology, 11(3),* 295–304.

Roberts, J. E., Prizant, B., & McWilliam, R. A. (1995, May). Out-of-class versus in-class service delivery in language intervention: Effects on communication interactions with young children. *American Journal of Speech-Language Pathology, 4,* 87–94.

Rossetti, L. M. (1986). *High risk infants: Identification, assessment, and intervention.* San Diego: College-Hill Press.

Rossetti, L. M. (1996). *Communication intervention: Birth to three.* Clifton Park, NY: Delmar, Cengage Learning.

Rumelhart, D. E., & McClelland, J. L. (1986). On learning past tenses of English verbs. In J. L. McClelland, D. E. Rumelhart, and The PDP Research Group, *Parallel distributed processing: Explorations in the microstructure of cognition. Vol. 1: Foundations.* Cambridge, MA: Bradford Books/MIT Press.

Rvachew, S., Nowak, M., & Cloutier, G. (2004, August). Effect of phonemic perception training on the speech production and phonological awareness skills of children with expressive phonological delay. *American Journal of Speech-Language Pathology, 13*(3), 250–263.

Rvachew, S., Ohberg, A., Grawburg, M., & Heyding, J. (2003, November). Phonological awareness and phonemic perception in 4-year-old children with delayed expressive phonology skills. *American Journal of Speech-Language Pathology, 12*(4), 463–471.

Shipley, K. G., & McAfee, J. G. (2009). *Assessment in speech-language pathology: A resource manual* (4th ed.). Clifton Park, NY: Delmar, Cengage Learning.

Shprintzen, R. J. (1997*). Genetics, syndromes, and communication disorders.* San Diego, CA: Singular Publishing Group, Inc.

Shprintzen, R. J. (2000). *Syndrome identification for speech-language pathology: An illustrated pocket guide.* Clifton Park, NY: Delmar, Cengage Learning.

Shulman, B. B., & Capone, N. C. (2010). *Language development: Foundations, processes, and clinical applications.* Sudbury, MA: Jones and Bartlett.

Sicile-Kira, C. (2004). *Autism spectrum disorders.* New York: Perigee.

Sigman, M., & Capps, L. (1997). *Children with autism: A developmental perspective.* Cambridge, MA: Harvard University Press.

Snowling, M. J., Adams, C., Bishop, D. V. M., & Stothard, S. E. (2001). Educational attainments of school leavers with a preschool history of speech-language impairment. *International Journal of Language and Communication Disorders, 36,* 173–183.

Snowling, M. J., Bishop, D. V., & Stothard, S. E. (2006, August). Psychosocial outcomes at 15 years of children with a preschool history of speech-language impairment. *Journal of Child Psychology and Psychiatry and Allied Discipline, 47,* 759–765.

Snyder, L. E., & Scherer, N. (2004, February). The development of symbolic play and language in toddlers with cleft palate. *American Journal of Speech-Language Pathology, 13*(1), 66–80.

Tattershall, S. (2002). *Adolescents with language and learning needs: A shoulder to shoulder collaboration.* Clifton Park, NY: Delmar, Cengage Learning.

Thal, D. J., Bates, E., Goodman, J., & Jahn-Samilo, J. (1997). Continuity of language abilities: An exploratory study of late- and early-talking toddlers. *Developmental Neuropsychology, 13,* 239–274.

Thal, D. J., & Tobias, S. (1992). Communicative gestures in children with delayed onset of oral expressive vocabulary. *Journal of Speech and Hearing Research, 35,* 1281–1289.

Tiegerman-Farber, E. (1995). *Language and communication intervention in preschool children.* Boston: Allyn & Bacon.

Tomblin, J. B., Hardy, J. C., & Hein, H. A. (1991, October). Predicting poor-communication status in preschool children using risk factors present at birth. *Journal of Speech and Hearing Research, 34,* 1096–1105.

Ukrainetz, T. A. (2006). *Contextualized language intervention: Scaffolding preK–12 literacy achievement.* Eau Claire, WI: Thinking Publications University.

Van Keulen, J. E., Weddington, G. T., & DeBose, C. E. (1998). *Speech, language, learning, and the African American child.* Boston: Allyn & Bacon.

Volkmar, F., Paul, R., Klin, A., & Cohen, D. (eds.). (2005). *Handbook of autism and pervasive developmental disorders.* New York: John Wiley & Sons.

Wetherby, A. M., & Prizant, B. M. (2002). *Communication and symbolic behavior scales developmental profile.* Baltimore, MD: Paul B. Brookes Publishing Company.

Wolfe, V., Presley, C., & Mesaris, J. (2003, August). The importance of sound identification training in phonological intervention. *American Journal of Speech-Language Pathology, 12*(3), 282–288.

Woods, J. J., & Wetherby, A. M. (2003, July). Early identification of and intervention for infants and toddlers who are at risk for autism spectrum disorder. *Language, Speech, Hearing Services in the Schools, 34,* 180–193.

Zager, D. (ed.). (2005). *Autism spectrum disorders: Identification, education, and treatment* (3rd ed.). Mahwah, NJ: Lawrence Erlbaum Associates.

Appendix B

Suggested Reading List on Language Abnormalities in School-Age Children

American Speech-Language-Hearing Association, Committee on Augmentative Communication. (1991, March). Report: Augmentative and alternative communication. *ASHA, 33*(Suppl. 5), 9–12.

American Speech-Language-Hearing Association, Task Force on Central Auditory Processing Consensus Development. (1996, July). Central auditory processing: Current status of research and implications for clinical practice. *American Journal of Audiology, 5*(2), 41–54.

American Speech-Language-Hearing Association. (2001). Role and responsibilities of speech-language pathologists with respect to reading and writing in children and adolescents [position statement]. Available from www.asha.org/policy.

American Speech-Language-Hearing Association. (2001). Role and responsibilities of speech-language pathologists with respect to reading and writing in children and adolescents [guidelines]. Available from www.asha.org/policy.

American Speech-Language-Hearing Association, Working Group on Auditory Processing Disorders. (2005, February). (Central) auditory processing disorders. *ASHA Technical Report.*

Barkley, R. A. (2000). Taking charge of ADHD: The complete, authoritative guide for parents (rev. ed.). New York: The Guilford Press.

Berk, L. E. (2004). *Development through the lifespan* (3rd ed.). Boston: Allyn & Bacon.

Bernard-Opitz, V. (1982, February). Pragmatic analysis of the communicative behavior of an autistic child. *Journal of Speech and Hearing Disorders, 47,* 99–110.

Bliss, L. S. (2002). *Discourse impairments: Assessment and intervention applications.* Boston: Allyn & Bacon.

Blosser, J. L., & DePompei, R. (2003). *Pediatric traumatic brain injury: Proactive intervention* (2nd ed.). Clifton Park, NY: Delmar, Cengage Learning.

Bogaert-Martinez, E. (2007). Assessment and treatment of traumatic brain injury within the ECHCS polytrauma system of care. Available from www.dol.gov/vets/grants/07conference/TB.

Bopp, K. D., Brown, K. E., & Mirenda, P. (2004, February). Speech-language pathologists' roles in the delivery of positive behavior support for individuals with developmental disabilities. *American Journal of Speech-Language Pathology, 13*(1), 5–19.

Bourassa, D. C., & Treiman, R. (2001, July). Spelling development and disability: The importance of linguistic factors. *Language, Speech, and Hearing Services in the Schools, 32*(3), 172–181.

Brinton, B., & Fujiki, M. (1993, October). Language, social skills, and socio-emotional behavior. *Language, Speech, and Hearing Services in the Schools, 24,* 194–198.

Carlisle, J. E. (1995). Morphological awareness and early reading achievement. In L. B. Feldman (ed.), *Morphological aspects of language processing* (pp. 189–209). Hillsdale, NJ: Erlbaum.

Carroll, J. M., Snowling, M. J, Hulme, C., & Stevenson, J. (2003). The development of phonological awareness in preschool children. *Developmental Psychology, 39,* 913–923.

Catts, H. W., Fey, M. D., Zhang, X., & Tomblin, J. B. (2001). Eliminating the risk of future reading difficulties in kindergarten children: A research-based model and its clinical implemenation. *Language, Speech, and Hearing Services in the Schools, 32,* 38–50.

Centers for Disease Control. (2007). *Attention deficit hyperactivity disorder (ADHD).* Available from www.cdc.gov/nchs/fastats/adhd.htm.

Condouris, K., Meyer, E., & Tager-Flusberg, H. (2003, August). The relationship between standardized measures of language and measures of spontaneous speech in children with autism. *American Journal of Speech-Language Pathology, 12*(3), 349–358.

Connor, D. F. (2002). Preschool attention deficit hyperactivity disorder: A review of prevalence, diagnosis, neurobiology, and stimulant treatment. *Journal of Developmental and Behavioral Pediatrics, 23,* 51–59.

DeBonis, D. A., & Moncrief, D. (2008, February). Auditory processing disorders: An update for speech-language pathologists. *American Journal of Speech Language Pathology, 17*(1), 4–18.

Ebert, K. A., & Prelock, P. A. (1994, October). Teachers' perceptions of their students with communication disorders. *Language, Speech, and Hearing Services in the Schools, 25,* 211–214.

Ellis, L., Schlaudecker, C., & Regimbal, C., (1995, January). Effectiveness of a collaborative consultation approach to basic concept instruction with kindergarten children. *Language, Speech, and Hearing Services in the Schools, 26,* 69–74.

Fey, M. E., Long, S. H., & Finestack, L. H. (2003, February). Ten principles of grammar facilitation for children with specific language impairments. *American Journal of Speech-Language Pathology, 12*(1), 3–15.

Finkelstein, E., Corso, P., Miller, T., et al. (2006). *The incidence and economic burden of injuries in the United States.* New York: Oxford University Press.

Fujiki, M., Brinton, B., & Clarke, D. (April, 2002). Emotional regulation in children with specific language impairment. *Language, Speech, and Hearing Services in Schools, 33,* 102–111.

Gallagher, T. (1993, October). Language skill and the development of social competence in school-age children. *Language, Speech, and Hearing Services in the Schools, 24,* 199–205.

Gillon, G. T. (2000). The efficacy of phonological awareness intervention for children with spoken language impairment. *Language, Speech, and Hearing Services in the Schools, 31,* 126–141.

Greenhalgh, K. S., & Strong, C. J. (2001). Literate language features in spoken narratives of children with typical language and children with language impairments. *Language, Speech, and Hearing Services in the Schools, 32,* 114–125.

Hart, B., & Risley, T. R. (1995). *Meaningful differences in the everyday experience of young American children.* Baltimore, MD: Paul H. Brookes Publishing Company.

Hart, B., & Risley, T. R. (1999). *The social world of children learning to talk.* Baltimore, MD: Paul H. Brookes Publishing Company.

Haynes, W. O., Moran, M. J., & Pindzola, R. H. (1999). *Communication disorders in the classroom: An introduction for professionals in school settings.* Dubuque, IA: Kendall/Hunt.

Hummel, L., & Prizant, B. (1993, October). A socioemotional perspective for understanding social difficulties of school-age children with language disorders. *Language, Speech, and Hearing Services in the Schoosl, 24,* 216–224.

Johnson, C. J., Beitchman, J. H., Young, A., Escobar, M., Atkinson, L., Wilson, B., et al. (1999). Fourteen-year follow-up of children with and without speech/language impairments: Speech/language stability and outcomes. *Journal of Speech, Language, and Hearing Research, 42*(3), 744–760.

Kamhi, A. G., & Catts, H. W. (1989). *Reading disabilities: A development language perspective.* Boston: College-Hill Press.

Kaufmann, S. S., Prelock, P. A., Weiler, E. M., Creaghead, N. A., & Donnelly, C. A. (1994, July). Metapragmatic awareness of explanation adequacy: Developing skills for academic success from a collaborative communication skills unit. *Language, Speech, and Hearing Services in the Schools, 25,* 174–180.

Keith, R. W. (1999). Clinical issues in central auditory processing disorders. *Language, Speech, and Hearing Services in the Schools, 30*(4), 339–344.

Kirk, C., & Gillon, G. T. (2009, July). Integrated morphological awareness intervention as a tool for improving literacy. *Language, Speech, and Hearing Services in the Schools, 40,* 341–351.

Koppenhaver, D. A., Coleman, P. P., Kalman, S. L., & Yoder, D. E. (1991, September). The implications of emergent literacy research for children with developmental disabilities. *American Journal of Speech-Language Pathology, 1,* 38–44.

Kuder, S. J. (2003). *Teaching students with language and communication disabilities* (2nd ed.). Boston: Allyn & Bacon.

Langolis, J. A., Kegler, S. R., Butler, J. A., et al. (2003). Traumatic brain injury-related hospital discharges: Results from a fourteen state surveillance system, 1997. *Morbidity and Mortality Weekly Reports, 52*(55-04), 1–18.

Langolis, J. A., Rutland-Brown, W., & Thomas, K. E. (2004). *Traumatic brain injury in the United States: Emergency department visits, hospitalizations, and deaths.* Atlanta, GA: Centers for Disease Control and Prevention, National Center for Injury Prevention and Control.

Larivee, L. S., & Catts, H. W. (1999). Early reading achievement in children with expressive phonological disorders. *American Journal of Speech-Language Pathology, 8,* 118–128.

Larson, V. L., & McKinley, N. (1995). *Language disorders in older students: Preadolescents and adolescents.* Eau Claire, WI: Thinking Publications.

Lyon, G. R., Fletcher, J. M., Shaywitz, S. E., Shaywitz, B. A., Torgesen, J. K., Wood, F., et al. (2001). Rethinking learning disabilities. In C. E. Finn Jr., A. J. Rotherham, and C. R. Hokanson Jr. (eds.), *Rethinking special education for a new century* (pp. 259–287). Washington, DC: Thomas B. Fordham Foundation.

McCabe, A., Bliss, L., Barra, G., & Bennett, M. (2008, May). Comparison of personal versus fictional narratives of children with language impairment. *American Journal of Speech-Language Pathology, 17,* 194–206.

McCauley, R. J. (2001). *Assessment of language disorders in children.* Mahwah, NJ: Lawrence Erlbaum Associates.

Merritt, D. D., & Culatta, B. (1998). *Language intervention in the classroom.* San Diego, CA: Singular Publishing Group.

Nathan, L., Stackhouse, J., Goulandris, N., & Snowling, M. J. (2004). The development of early literacy skills among children with speech difficulties: A test of the "critical age" hypothesis. *Journal of Speech, Language, Hearing Research, 47,* 377–391.

National Center for Education Statistics. (2007). Literacy in everyday life: Results from the 2003 National Assessment of Adult Literacy. *NCES 2007-480.* Washington, D.C.: United States Department of Education. Available from www.nces.ed.gov/Pubs2007/2007480.pdf.

National Institute for Literacy (n.d.). Literacy in the United States. Available from www.policyalmanac.org/education/archives/literacy.shtml.

National Institute of Neurological Disorders and Stroke. (2002, February). *Traumatic brain injury: Hope through research.* NIH Publ. #902-158. Bethesda, MD: National Institutes of Health.

Nelson, N. W. (1994, September). Speech-language pathology: Moving toward the 21st century: Traumatic brain injury. *American Journal of Speech-Language Pathology, 3,* 39–41.

Nelson, N. W. (1994, September). School-aged language: Bumpy road or super-expressway to the next millennium? *American Journal of Speech-Language Pathology, 3,* 29–31.

Nelson, N. W. (2010). *Language and literacy disorders: Infancy through adolescence.* Boston: Allyn & Bacon.

Neuman, S. B. (2008). *Educating the other America: Top experts tackle poverty, literacy, and achievement in our schools.* Baltimore, MD: Paul H. Brookes Publishing Company.

Norris, J. A. (1992, September). Some questions and answers about whole language. *American Journal of Speech-Language Pathology, 1,* 11–14.

Pastor, P. N., & Reuben, C. A. (2008, July). Diagnosed attention deficit hyperactivity disorder and learning disability: United States 2004–2006. National Center for Health Statistics. *Vital Health Statistics, 10*(237). Available from www.cdc.gov/nchs/data/series/sr_10/Sr10-237.pdf.

Paul, R. (2001). *Language disorders from infancy through adolescence* (2nd ed.). St. Louis, MO: Mosby.

Philofsky, A., Fidler, D. J., & Hepburn, S. (2007, November). Pragmatic language profiles of school-age children with autism spectrum disorder and Williams syndrome. *American Journal of Speech Language Pathology, 16*, 368–380.

Pinborough-Zimmerman, J., Satterfield, R., Miller, J., Bilder, D., Hossain, S., & McMahon, W. (2007, November). Communication disorders: Prevalence and comorbid intellectual disability, autism, and emotional/behavioral disorders. *American Journal of Speech-Language Pathology, 16*(4), 359–367.

Polakow, V. (1993). *Lives on the edge: Single mothers and their children in the other America.* Chicago: University of Chicago Press.

Raitano, M. A., Pennington, B. F., Tunick, B. F., Boada, R., & Shriberg, L. D. (2004). Pre-literacy skills of subgroups of children with speech sound disorders. *Journal of Child Psychology and Psychiatry, 45*, 821–835.

Ratner, V., & Harris, L. (1994). *Understanding language disorders.* Eau Claire, WI: Thinking Publications.

Records, N. L., Tomblin, J. B., & Freese, P. P. (1992, January). The quality of life of young adults with histories of specific language impairment. *American Journal of Speech-Language Pathology, 1*, 44–53.

Reed, V. A. (2005). *An introduction to children with language disorders* (3rd ed.). Boston: Allyn & Bacon.

Reif, S. F. *How to reach and teach ADD/ADHD children.* Eau Claire, WI: Thinking Publications.

Russell, N. K. (1993, April). Educational considerations in traumatic brain injury: The role of the SLP. *Language, Speech, and Hearing Services in the Schools, 24*, 67–75.

Rvachew, S. (2006, May). Longitudinal predictors of implicit phonological awareness skills. *American Journal of Speech Language Pathology, 15*, 165–176.

Rvachew, S., Ohberg, A., Grawburg, M., & Heyding, J. (2003). Phonological awareness and phonemic perception in 4-year-old children with delayed expressive phonology skills. *American Journal of Speech Language Pathology, 12*, 463–471.

Sanger, D. D., Hux, K., & Belau, D. (1997, February). Oral language skills of female juvenile delinquents. *American Journal of Speech-Language Pathology, 6*, 70–76.

Sanger, D., Hux, K., & Griess, K. (1995, January). Educators' opinions about speech-language pathology services in schools. *Language, Speech, and Hearing Services in the Schools, 26*, 75–86.

Semrud-Clikeman, M. (2001). *Traumatic brain injury in children and adolescents: Assessment and intervention.* New York: The Guilford Press.

Sicile-Kira, C. (2004). *Autism spectrum disorders: The complete guide to understanding autism, Asperger's syndrome, pervasive developmental disorder, and other ASDs.* New York: Perigree.

Siegel, L. (2008). Morphological awareness skills of English language learners and children with dyslexia. *Topics in Language Disorders, 28*(1), 15–27.

Simon, C. S. (1991). *Communication skills and classroom success.* Eau Claire, WI: Thinking Publications.

Snowling, M. J., Bishop, D. V. M., & Stothard, S. E. (2000). Is preschool language impairment a risk factor for dyslexia in adolescence? *Journal of Child Psychology and Psychiatry, 41,* 587–600.

Stanovich. K. E. (2000). *Progress in understanding reading: Scientific foundations and new frontiers.* New York: Guilford Press.

Storch, S. A., & Whitehurst, G. J. (2002). Oral language and code-related precursors for reading: Evidence from a longitudinal structural model. *Developmental Psychology, 38,* 934–947.

Stothard, S. E., Snowling, M. J., Bishop, D. V. M., Chipchase, B. B., & Kaplan, C. A. (1998, April). Language-impaired preschoolers: A follow-up into adolescence. *Journal of Speech, Language, and Hearing Research, 41,* 407–418.

Tattershall, S. (2002). *Adolescents with language and learning needs: A shoulder to shoulder collaboration.* Clifton Park, NY: Delmar, Cengage Learning.

Thurman, D., Alverson, C., Dunn, K., Guerero, J., & Sniezek, J. (1999). Traumatic brain injury in the United States: A public health perspective. *Journal of Head Trauma and Rehabilitation, 14*(6), 602–615.

Towne, R. L., & Entwisle, L. M. (1993, April). Metaphoric comprehension in adolescents with traumatic brain injury and in adolescents with language learning disability. *Language, Speech, and Hearing Services in the Schools, 24,* 100–107.

United States Military Defense. (March, 2009). The U.S. military's brain injury program. Available from www.defenseindustrydaily.com/173m-for-us-militarys-brain-injury-program-03511/.

Wagovich, S. A., & Newhoff, M. (2004, November). The single exposure: Partial word knowledge growth through reading. *American Journal of Speech-Language Pathology, 13*(4), 316–328.

Wallach, G. P., & Butler, K. B. (1994). *Language learning disabilities in school-age children and adolescents.* New York: Merrill Publishers.

Wiig, E., & Wilson, C. C. (1994, October). Is a question a question? Passage understanding by preadolescents with learning disabilities. *Language, Speech, and Hearing Services in the Schools, 25,* 241–250.

Wilcox, M. J., Kouri, T. A., & Caswell, S. B. (1991, September). Early language intervention: A comparison of classroom and individual treatment. *American Journal of Speech-Language Pathology, 1,* 49–62.

Appendix C

Suggested Reading List on Multicultural Aspects of Language Disorders

American Speech-Language-Hearing Association, Committee on the Status of Racial Minorities. (1983). ASHA position paper on social dialects. *ASHA, 25,* 23–24.

American Speech-Language-Hearing Association. (1989). ASHA definition: Bilingual speech-language pathologists and audiologists. *ASHA, 31,* 93.

American Speech-Language-Hearing Association. (1993). Definitions of communication disorders and variations. *ASHA, 35*(Suppl. 10), 33–39.

American Speech-Language-Hearing Association. (1993). Guidelines for gender equity in language use. *ASHA, 35*(Suppl. 10), 42–46.

Brice, A. E. (2002). *The Hispanic child: Speech, language, culture and education.* Boston: Allyn & Bacon.

Britt, R. R. (2009). 14 percent of United States adults can't read. *Live Science.* Available from www.livescience.com/culture.

Cole, L. (1993, September). Implications of the position on social dialects. *ASHA, 25,* 25–27.

Coleman, T. J. (2000). *Clinical management of communication disorders in culturally diverse children.* Boston, MA: Allyn & Bacon.

Craig, H. K., & Washington, J. A. (1995, January). African-American English and linguistic complexity in preschool discourse: A second look. *Language, Speech, and Hearing Services in the Schools, 26,* 87–93.

Craig, H. K., & Washington, J. A. (2002, February). Oral language expectations for African American preschoolers and kindergartners. *American Journal of Speech-Language Pathology, 11*(1), 59–70.

663

Hart, B., & Risley, T. (1995). *Meaningful differences in the everyday experience of young American children.* Baltimore, MD: Paul H. Brookes Publishing Company.

Justice, L. M., Chow, S., Capellini, C., Flanigan, K., & Colton, S. (2003, August). Emergent literacy intervention for vulnerable preschoolers: Relative effects of two approaches. *American Journal of Speech-Language Pathology, 12*(3), 320–332.

Justice, L. M., & Ezell, H. K. (2002, February). Use of storybook reading to increase print awareness in at-risk children. *American Journal of Speech-Language Pathology, 11*(1), 17–29.

Langdon, H. W., & Cheng, L. L. (1992). *Hispanic children and adults with communication disorders: Assessment and intervention.* Gaithersburg, MD: Aspen Publishers.

La Paro, K. M., Justice, L., Skibbe, L. E., & Pianta, R. C. (2004, November). Relations among maternal, child, and demographic factors and the persistence of preschool language impairment. *American Journal of Speech-Language Pathology, 13*(4), 291–303.

McGreer, M. M. (2009). House passes burden of health care costs to the illiterate, and poor. Available from www.associatedcontent.com/.../house_passes_burden_of_health_care.html.

Molrine, C. J., & Pierce, R. S. (2002, May). Black and white adults' expressive language performance on three tests of aphasia. *American Journal of Speech-Language Pathology, 11*(2), 139–150.

Monten, M. (2007, March). More than one-third of Washington, D.C. residents are functionally illiterate. *State of Adult Literacy 2006.* www.proliterach.org.

National Assessment of Adult Literacy. (2003). Key concepts and features of the 2003 National Assessment of Adult Literacy. Available from nces.ed.gov/NAAL/PDF/2006471_1.pdf.

National Center for Education Statistics. (2006). A first look at the literacy of America's adults in the 21st century. Available from nces.ed.gov/NAAL/PDF/2006470.pdf.

National Center for Education Statistics. (2007). Literacy in everyday life: Results from the 2003 National Assessment of Adult Literacy. *NCES 2007-480.* Washington, D.C.: U.S. Department of Education. Available from www.nces.ed.gov/Pubs2007/2007480.pdf.

National Institute for Literacy. (n.d.). Literacy in the United States. Available from www.policyalmanac.org/education/archives/literacy.shtml.

Neuman, S. B. (2008). *Educating the other America: Top experts tackle poverty, literacy, and achievement in our schools.* Baltimore, MD: Paul H. Brookes Publishing Company.

Payne, K. T., & Taylor, I. L. (2010) Multicultural differences in human communication and disorders. In N. Anderson and G. H. Shames (eds.), *Human communication disorders: An introduction* (8th ed.). Boston: Pearson Education, Inc.

Rodriguez, B. L., & Olswang, L. B. (2003, November). Mexican-American and Anglo-American mothers' beliefs and values about child-rearing, education, and language impairment. *American Journal of Speech-Language Pathology, 12*(4), 452–462.

Terrell, B. Y. (1993, November). Multicultural perspectives: Are the issues and questions different? *ASHA, 35,* 51–52.

Thomas-Tate, S., Washington, J., & Edwards, J. (2004, May). Standardized assessment of phonological awareness skills in low-income African-American first graders. *American Journal of Speech-Language Pathology, 13*(2), 182–190.

van Keulen, J. E., Weddington, G. T., & DeBose, C. E. (1998). *Speech, language, learning, and the African-American child.* Boston: Allyn & Bacon.

Vaughn-Cooke, F. B. (1993, September). Improving language assessment in minority children. *ASHA, 25,* 29–34.

Appendix D

Memoirs, Biographies, and Autobiographies Related to Communication Disabilities

Books About Preschool Children

Title	Author	Topic
A Real Boy: A True Story of Autism, Early Intervention, and Recovery	C. Adams	Autism
A Child Called Noah	J. Greenfield	Autism
A Place for Noah	J. Greenfield	Autism
Let Me Hear Your Voice: A Family's Triumph over Autism	C. Maurice	Autism
George and Sam	C. Moore	Autism
10 Things Ever Child with Autism Wishes You Knew	E. Notbohm	Autism
The Siege: The First 8 Years of an Autistic Child	C. Park	Autism
Making Peace with Autism: One Family's Story of Struggle, Discovery, and Unexpected Gifts	S. Senator	Autism
Unraveling the Mystery of Autism and Pervasive Developmental Disorder: A Mother's Story of Research and Recovery	K. Seroussi and B. Rimland	Autism
The Boy Who Loved Windows	P. Stacey	Autism
A Real Boy: Autism Shattered Our Lives and Made a Family from the Pieces	C. Stevens and N. Stevens	Autism
Born on a Blue Day	D. Tammett	Autism

Title	Author	Topic
Nobody Nowhere: The Remarkable Autobiography of an Autistic Girl	D. Williams	Autism
Blue Sky July	N. Wyn	Autism
Knowing Jesse	M. Leone	Cerebral Palsy
Expecting Adam	M. Berg	Down syndrome
Life As We Know It	M. Berube	Down syndrome
Road Map to Holland	J. G. Groneberg	Down syndrome
Broken Cord	M. Dorris	Fetal alcohol syndrome
Changed by a Child	B. Gill	Developmental disabilities

Books About School-Age Children

Title	Author	Topic
Autism? Asperger's? ADHD? ADD?	D. Burns	Autism
The Game of My Life	J. McElwain with D. Paisner	Autism
How Can I Talk If My Lips Don't Move?	T. Mukhopadhyay	Autism
Emergence: Labeled Autistic	M. Scariano	Autism
10 Things Your Student with Autism Wishes You Knew	V. Zysk	Autism
A Different Life: Growing Up Learning Disabled and Other Adventures	Q. Bradlee	Learning disabilities
A Special Education: One Family's Journey Through the Maze of Learning Disabilities	D. Buchman	Learning disabilities
Coping with a Learning Disability	L. Clayton and J. Morrison	Learning disabilities
The Short Bus: A Journey Beyond Normal	J. Mooney	Learning disabilities
Smart but Stuck	M. Orenstein	Learning disabilities
That Went Well: Adventures in Caring for My Sister	T. Dougan	Intellectual disabilities
The Secret Life of the Dyslexic Child	R. Frank and K. Livingston	Dyslexia
Reading Davie: A Mother's Journey Through the Labyrinth of Dyslexia	L. Weinstein	Dyslexia
The Out-of-Sync Chid: Recognizing and Coping with Sensory Processing Disorder	C. Kranowitz and L. Miller	Sensory Processing Disorder
Driven to Distraction	E. Hallowell and J. Ratey	ADHD
Delivered from Distraction	E. Hallowell and J. Ratey	ADHD

(continued)

Books About Adults with Communication Disorders

Title	Author	Topic
Thinking in Pictures	T. Grandin	Autism
The Real Rain Man: Kim Peek	F. Peek	Autism
The Life and Message of the Real Rain Man: Journey of a Mega Savant	F. Peek and L. Hanson	Autism
Look Me in the Eye: My Life with Asperger's	J. Robinson	Asperger's syndrome
Riding the Bus with My Sister: A True Life Journey	R. Simon	Intellectual disabilities
Facing Learning Disabilities in the Adult Years	J. Shapiro	Learning disabilities
Hanging by a Twig: Adults with Learning Disabilities	C. Wenn	Learning disabilities
You Mean I'm Not Crazy?: The Classic Self-Help Book for Adults with ADD	K. Kelly	ADHD
The Day Donny Herbert Woke Up	R. Blake	Prolonged coma
I Raise My Eyes to Say Yes	R. Sienkiewicz-Meyer and S. Kaplan	Cerebral palsy
The Diving Bell and the Butterfly	J-D. Bauby	Locked-in syndrome
Love is Ageless	J. Bryan	Alzheimer's disease
Death in Slow Motion: A Memoir of a Daughter, Her Mother, and a Beast Called Alzheimer's	E. Cooney	Alzheimer's disease
When it Gets Dark: An Enlightened Reflection of Life	T. DeBaggio	Alzheimer's disease
Losing My Mind: An Intimate Look at Life with Alzheimer's	T. DeBaggio	Alzheimer's diseas
Stolen Mind: The Slow Disappearance of Ray Doernberg	M. Doernberg	Alzheimer's disease
Dancing with Rose	L. Kessler	Alzheimer's disease
Finding Life in the Land of Alzheimer's: One Daughter's Hopeful Story	L. Kessler	Alzheimer's disease
The 36 Hour Day	N. Mace and P. Robins	Alzheimer's disease
Mom, Are You There? Finding a Path to Peace Through Alzheimer's	K. Negri	Alzheimer's disease
Caring for Mother: A Daughter's Long Goodbye	V. Owens	Alzheimer's disease
Another Name for Madness	M. Roach	Alzheimer's disease
Alzheimer's from the Inside Out	R. Taylor	Alzheimer's disease
My Stroke of Insight	J. T. Bolte	Aphasia
The Man Who Lost His Language: A Case of Aphasia	S. Hale	Aphasia

Title	Author	Topic
After Stroke	D. Hinds	Aphasia
Striking Back at Stroke	C. Hutton and L. Caplan	Aphasia
My Year Off: Recovering Life After Stroke	R. McCrum	Aphasia
A Mind of My Own: A Memoir of Recovery from Aphasia	H. Mills	Aphasia
The Man Who Mistook His Wife for a Hat	O. Sachs	Aphasia
Aphasia, My World Alone	H. Wulf	Aphasia
Where Is the Mango Princess? A Journey Back from TBI	C. Crimmins	TBI
TBI Hell: A Traumatic Brain Injury Really Sucks	G. Gosling	TBI
Smile and Jump High	D. Lloyd, S. Kehoe, and D. Lloyd	TBI
Head Cases: Stories of Being Injured and Its Aftermath	M. Mason	TBI
Over My Head: A Doctor's Own Story of Head Injury from the Inside Out	C. Osborn	TBI
I'll Carry the Fork!	K. Swanson	TBI
In an Instant	L. Woodruff and B. Woodruff	TBI
Awakenings	O. Sacks	Pseudo-Parkinson's disease
Lucky Man: A Memoir	M. Fox	Parkinson's disease

Books About People with Hearing Impairment

Title	Author	Topic
Talk with Me: Giving the Gift of Language and Emotional Health to a Hearing Impaired Child	E. Altman	Hearing impairment
Rebuilt: My Journey Back to the Hearing World	M. Chorost	Hearing impairment
Train Go Sorry: Inside a Deaf World	L. Hager	Hearing impairment
Odyssey of Hearing Loss: Tales of Triumph	M. Harvey	Hearing impairment
The Story of My Life	H. Keller	Hearing impairment
A Journey into the Deaf World	H. Lane, R. Hoffmeister, and B. Behan	Hearing impairment
Listening	H. Merker	Hearing impairment
A Quiet World: Living with Hearing Loss	D. Myers	Hearing impairment

(continued)

Title	Author	Topic
Deaf Culture	C. Paden and T. Humphries	Hearing impairment
Inside Deaf Culture	C. Paden and T. Humphries	Hearing impairment
In Silence: Growing Up Hearing in a Deaf World	R. Sidransky	Hearing impairment
Missed Connections: Hard of Hearing in a Hearing World	B. Stenross	Hearing impairment
The Unheard: A Memoir of Deafness and Africa	J. Swiller	Hearing impairment
Hands of My Father: A Hearing Boy, His Deaf Parents, and the Language of Love	M. Uhlberg	Hearing impairment
Loss for Words	L. A. Walker	

General Books on Disabilities

Title	Author	Topic
The Elephant in the Playroom	D. Brodey	Developmental disabilities
You Will Dream New Dreams: Inspiring Personal Stories by Parents...	S. Klein and K. Schive	Developmental disabilities
Special Children, Challenged Parents: The Struggles and Rewards of Raising a Child with a Disability	R. Naseef	Autism
Through the Glass Wall	H. Buten	Autism
No Pity: People with Disabilities Forging a New Civil Rights Movement	J. Shapiro	General disabilities
Social Perceptions of People with Disabilities in History	H. Covey	General disabilities
A Different Kind of Perfect: Writings by Parents on Raising a Child with Special Needs	C. Dowling	Disabilities in children
Shut Up About Your Perfect Kid	G. Gallagher and P. Konjoian	Disabilities in children
Reflections from a Different Journey: What Adults with Disabilities Wish All Parents Knew	S. Klein and J. Kemp	Disabilities in children
What About Me: Growing Up with a Developmentally Disabled Sibling	B. Siegel	Disabilities in children
Thinking About Dementia: Culture, Loss, and the Anthropology of Senility	A. Leibing and L. Cohen	Dementia
Inside Alzheimer's: How to Hear and Honor Connections with a Person Who Has Dementia	N. Pearce	Alzheimer's disease

Answers to Review Questions

Chapter 1

1. A
2. D
3. C
4. A
5. B
6. A
7. B
8. B
9. B
10. A

Chapter 2

1. E
2. B
3. D
4. B
5. A
6. B

7. A
8. B
9. B
10. B

Chapter 3

1. C
2. C
3. B
4. B
5. A
6. C
7. A
8. D
9. D
10. A

Chapter 4

1. B
2. A

3. A
4. E
5. D
6. B
7. B
8. D
9. C
10. A

Chapter 5

1. B
2. A
3. D
4. D
5. A
6. B
7. A
8. A
9. B
10. B

Chapter 6

1. C
2. B
3. D
4. B
5. A
6. B
7. B
8. B
9. A
10. B

Chapter 7

1. A
2. B
3. A
4. A
5. C
6. A
7. C
8. C
9. B
10. D

Chapter 8

1. A
2. A
3. B
4. C
5. A
6. B
7. A
8. B
9. A
10. B

Chapter 9

1. B
2. A
3. D
4. D
5. D
6. B
7. A
8. B
9. A
10. A

Chapter 10

1. B
2. C
3. A
4. D
5. B
6. A
7. B
8. A
9. B
10. A

Chapter 11

1. D
2. B
3. B
4. B
5. C
6. D
7. A
8. C
9. B
10. A

Chapter 12

1. B
2. B
3. A
4. B
5. B
6. C
7. B
8. A
9. E
10. B

Chapter 13

1. B
2. B
3. A
4. C
5. A
6. D
7. E
8. H
9. A
10. B

Chapter 14

1. E
2. A
3. E
4. C
5. B
6. A
7. D
8. B
9. B
10. C

Glossary

A

Abstract thought processes Thinking beyond the limits of a fact and developing opinions and expansion on a given piece of information.

Acting-out tasks Tasks in which the clinician offers a set of instructions on what the child must complete; the clinician needs to ascertain that the child is truly responding to the examiner's questions and not performing tasks that he or she knows due to real-world familiarity with the item.

Adaptability The ability to adjust to new or changing circumstances.

Affective control Inappropriate affect and expression of emotions.

Alphabetic principle The dictum governing how specific sounds in a language are represented by specific spelling patterns.

Alternate-form reliability Evaluating the reliability of a test by having the child take two different forms of the same test, then comparing the performance on each form.

Alternating attention The ability to shift attention between tasks that have different cognitive demands.

Anomia Lack of the ability to recall names of people, common objects, and places.

Aphasia Impairment of the abilities to comprehend and express language resulting from acquired neurological damage.

Appetite control The ability to delay gratification, which is typically problematic for children with ADHD.

Apraxia A neurological deficit in the cortex that hinders one's ability to make voluntary motor movements even when the muscles function normally.

Aprosodia The inability to either produce or comprehend the affective components of speech or gesture.

Assessment process The process of interviewing, observing, and testing an individual to determine the nature, extent, and severity of his or her language disorder, delay, or difference.

Associative control Control that enables a person to maintain a conversation by stating issues that are relevant to the conversation.

Association A pattern of malformations occurring at an unusual rate with no known etiology.

Attention deficit disorder The presence of behavior that typically includes inattention, hyperactivity, and impulsivity exceeding that expected by children at a given age.

Auditory acuity The sharpness and clarity with which sound is perceived by the ear.

Auditory discrimination The ability to identify specific sounds by their source and/or acoustical properties.

Auditory perception The ability to hear specific environmental and speech sounds.

Auditory processing A set of skills, including auditory discrimination, auditory analysis, auditory attention, and auditory memory, that integrate what is heard with language.

Auditory processing disorder Difficulties with functions of language based on input to and feedback from the auditory system, including problems with auditory discrimination, lateralization, recognizing auditory patterns, and localizing sound.

Auditory sequential memory The ability to remember sounds, words, phrases, and sentences in a specified sequence.

B

Backward chaining A series of sequenced behaviors in which the last steps of the sequence are taught first, working backward to the beginning of the chain; frequently used to teach self-help skills.

Baseline The preintervention measurement of a patient's skills.

Behavior control Impulsive behavior due to a poorly organized central nervous system.

Behaviorism Like empiricism, the belief that a child's language is not innate but develops when verbalizations are positively reinforced.

Behavior modification The implementation of an intervention plan to change, modify, or correct an individual's behavior.

Brachycephaly Head shape characterized by tallness of the head and flatness of the back of the head due to premature fusion of the coronal sutures.

C

Causality The reactivation of a spectacle or event by bodily movement (e.g., turning the key to have a toy car reactivate).

Central deafness Damage to the eighth nerve in the brain stem or to the cortex.

Cephalometric measures Measurements of the size of the head.

Chromosomal disorder A disorder in the structure or number of chromosomes or both.

Circumlocution The use of an indirect manner of expression to describe an object or event when the name cannot be recalled; e.g., saying "That thing you use to unlock the door" instead of "key."

Clinical assumptions What clinicians judge to be true, although they may not observe or measure attributes related to these events directly.

Clinical facts Statements made about events that actually took place and were directly observed or measured by the clinician.

Closed-head injury A nonpenetrating brain injury in which the skull may be intact or fractured, but the meninges are intact.

Code switching The ability of an individual to switch dialects or languages depending on the communicative situation.

Cognitive determinism The belief that cognition relies on language for a child to understand his or her experiences; the child's knowledge of the world is expressed through his or her language, with meaning preceding form.

Collaborative activities Those activities that involve the joint participation and cooperation of the members of a group.

Collaborative model Classroom-based or curriculum-based intervention that focuses on learning strategies and using them in materials related to the curriculum.

Co-morbidity The coexistence of one or more disorders.

Conductive hearing loss A breakdown in the ability of the middle ear to receive acoustic signals from the environment and then to transmit the acoustical information to the inner ear.

Confrontational naming The naming of items as the child is confronted with the item by the clinician.

Construct validity The degree to which a test measures a theoretical construct or trait.

Consultative model A service delivery model in which the speech-language pathologist provides indirect therapy through in-service and input to classroom teachers on appropriate methods for encouraging effective speech and language skills.

Content bias The effect of a dialectal or cultural difference on the responses of an individual to a test item.

Content validity A systematic examination of the relevance of the responses given to test items in order to ascertain how well the test covers a representative sample of the skills to be assessed.

Contrecoup injury A brain injury occurring opposite from the impact as the brain bounces from the point of impact to the opposite side of the skull.

Correlation coefficient A number that represents the degree of relationship between two sets of scores.

Coup injury Injury at the point of impact, occurring when a blow to the head results in the brain moving and slamming against the point of impact.

Craniosynostosis Premature fusion of the bones of the cranium.

Criterion-referenced test A nonstandardized probe used to study a language construct in more depth than is normally associated with standardized tests.

Criterion-related validity How effectively a test predicts an individual's behavior, abilities, or both in specific situations.

Cryptorchidism Undescended testicles.

Culture The philosophies, ideas, arts, and customs of a group of people that are passed from one generation to the next.

D

Delayed gratification The ability to continue providing the correct and expected behaviors even when a delay exists between the response and the provision of reinforcement.

Diadochokinetic tasks Tasks requiring rapid repetitive movements of the articulators; frequently elicited by having the child repeat p^t^k^ as quickly as possible.

Dialect Systematic, patterned, rule-governed variations in a language.

Diffuse lesion A lesion in which the damage is spread throughout a large area of the brain or several small areas, resulting in comprehensive deficits.

Discrepancy criterion The measurable difference between a child's achievement and his or her expected achievement based on IQ.

Divided attention Determining how much attention to give to each activity.

Dysarthria A motor speech disorder resulting from generalized weakness of the oral musculature.

Dysgraphia Impaired ability to write, usually due to brain damage.

Dyslexia Difficulty learning to read, often due to neurological deficit.

Dysnomia Loss of ability to name people, places, or things; may also be referred to as anomia.

Dysplasia Underdevelopment of tissue.

E

Echolalia The unmodified involuntary or voluntary repetition of what is said to the child.

Embedded sentences Compound sentences in which a minimum of two independent clauses are combined to form one sentence.

Emotional regulation The ability to control one's emotions and express them appropriately based on the myriad components of a setting.

Empiricism The belief that a child's language is not innate but develops as a result of experiences.

Epicanthal fold A fold of skin, sometimes crescent-shaped, on the inner and sometimes outer corners of the eyes.

Ethnography The study of language use for communicative purposes, considering social and cultural factors.

Etiology Causative factors that lead to a delay or disorder.

Executive tasks Activities such as setting goals, initiating tasks, self-monitoring, self-evaluating, keeping schedules, and managing time well.

Exorbitism Bulging of the eyes beyond the socket of the orbit.

Expressive language The ability to convey a message through conventional means using words and symbols; the content of what is expressed.

Extrinsic causes Factors in the environment of the child that interfere with development.

F

Face validity How well test items represent what they claim to test.

Fading The gradual withdrawal of prompts used to facilitate a response.

Fissure A deep furrow in the brain; also known as a sulcus.

Fluent aphasia Aphasia in which the initiation and production of speech are intact, but deficits occur in semantics and comprehension.

Focal control The ability to select what is important and attend to that over all other distractions and information.

Focal lesion A lesion in which the impact is concentrated in one small area of the brain.

Focused attention The requirement that a child complete an activity, usually under a time constraint.

Forward chaining A series of sequenced behaviors in which the first steps of the sequence are taught first; the typical chaining approach used in teaching academic skills.

Functional magnetic resonance imaging (fMRI) An MRI of the brain done while the patient performs specific tasks so the radiologist can visualize the mechanisms of the brain activated with each tasks.

Functional Memory Memory needed to recall previously learned information, to learn new information, to remember situational details, and to function independently.

Functional outcome Environmentally based results of therapy that can be generalized to the patient's natural settings; expected results of therapy that can readily be integrated into the patient's natural environment.

G

Generalization The addition of new stimuli or environmental factors to elicit the same response obtained in a controlled setting.

Genetic Specific characteristics or traits passed from one generation to the next in the genes.

Glossoptosis Displacement of the tongue into a downward and/or posterior position.

Graduated prompting In diagnostic therapy, the co-occurrence of assessment and treatment, with the child being tested for stimulability on a language construct.

Grammatic closure The ability to determine the missing elements in a sentence.

Gyrus A rounded elevation in the cerebral hemispheres.

H

Hydrocephalus Abnormal accumulation of fluid within the cranium, placing undue pressure on the brain tissues.

Hypercalcemia Abnormally elevated calcium levels in the blood.

Hyperkinetic Having persistent and exaggerated motor movements.

Hyperlexic. Recognizing and reading words exceeding one's cognitive and language levels, yet having little or no comprehension of what is said or read.

Hyperphagia Compulsive eating for an extended period of time.

Hyperreflexia. Abnormally high reactions when reflexes are stimulated.

Hypertonia. Abnormally high muscle tone; sometimes referred to as spasticity.

Hypogonadism Underdevelopment and decreased function of sex organs.

Hyporeflexia Abnormally low responses when the reflexes are stimulated.

Hypotonia Abnormally low muscle tone; sometimes referred to as athetosis.

Hypoxia A decrease in the amount of oxygen delivered to or utilized by a body organ, or both

Hypsistaphylia A high, narrow palate.

I

Identification tasks Tasks in which the child is asked to identify a picture or object that is named by the clinician.

Illocutionary force The intention of a speech act.

Illocutionary stage The social stage of communication development in which the child is interactive and communication efforts are intentional, although some of the communication may still be nonverbal.

Impulsivity Acting without premeditation, thought, or concern about consequences.

Incidental learning Learning that results from routine interactions with the environment.

Individualized Education Plan (IEP) Required by EAHCA and IDEA, the academic plan required for all students who are in special education or related services in public schools.

Intrinsic causes Factors within the child, such as neurological damage, that interfere with development.

J

Jargon Correctly articulated utterances with appropriate prosody; typical of children aged 10–14 months; decreases as words emerge.

Joint attention The sharing of visual and auditory attention to the same stimulus.

Judgment tasks Tasks that require the child to make a determination of the accuracy or reasonableness of a statement made by the clinician.

K

Kinesthetic Relating to the sensation of movement of joints, muscles, and tendons.

L

Language acquisition device (LAD) Not a specific structure, but rather a conglomeration of innate capacities of language that governs the input and output of language form.

Language-based learning disability A single disorder that manifests itself in different ways at various points in development as communicative contexts and learning tasks change.

Language delay The acquisition of normal language competencies at a slower rate than would be expected given the child's chronological age and the level of functioning.

Language difference Language behaviors and skills that are not in concert with those of the person's primary speech community or native language.

Language disorder A disruption in the learning of language skills and behaviors; typically includes language behaviors that are not considered part of normally developing linguistic skills.

Language parameters Aspects of language that form the basis of linguistic functioning.

Learned helplessness A state of inaction that a child learns because his or her needs are constantly anticipated by his or her caregivers so that there is little or no need for the child to communicate or initiate communication.

Learning disability Any one of a heterogeneous set of learning problems that affect the acquisition and use of listening, speaking, writing, reading, mathematical, and reasoning skills.

Lexicon A composite list of the words and signs that comprise an individual's vocabulary.

Linguistic competence The language user's underlying knowledge about the system of rules of the language he or she is using to communicate.

Linguistic performance The use of a person's linguistic knowledge in daily communication.

Linguistic universals The shared principles that underlie the variety of languages and form the foundation for a relatively universal structure of language.

Linguistic verbs Verbs that refer to acts of speaking, such as *said* or *told*.

Locutionary stage The social stage of communication development during which the child develops intentional, linguistic communication and speech consists primarily of nouns and labels.

M

Maintenance The independent use of therapy skills in a person's natural settings.

Mean length of utterance (MLU) Average length of a sample of utterances spoken by an individual; can be measured in terms of number of words, or number of morphemes

Means-end A language parameter in which the child has the ability to use foresight in simple problem solving (e.g., using a dowel to obtain an object that is out of reach).

Meningitis An inflammation of the meninges lining the brain and/or spinal column.

Mental effort control Work at concentrating, resulting in mental fatigue when excess energy is expended on focal control.

Mental verbs Verbs that refer to different acts of thinking, such as *decided* or *thought*.

Mentalism Often associated with nativism, the mentalist philosophy posits that one's knowledge is derived from innate mental processes.

Metacognition The ability to develop alternative ways to solve a problem or resolve a situation, the ability to form hypotheses and task analyze them in a constructive manner, and the capacity to make personal decisions.

Metacognitive skills Those skills that enable a child to solve problems, form hypotheses, analyze his or her thoughts, and make a decision.

Metalinguistic devices The ability to think about and analyze language in a critical manner, including the ability to understand humor, multiple meanings, inferences, and figurative language.

Metalinguistic skills Skills that allow an individual to think about language in a critical manner and to make judgments with regard to the accuracy and appropriate use of language skills and functions; form the basis for effective ability to think about language, thus allowing the interpretation of language.

Metanarrative skills The ability to analyze stories, extract appropriate details from a story, and comprehend a story.

Metapragmatic skills Conscious and intentional awareness of ways in which to use language effectively in different contexts.

Metathesis The reversal of the position of two sounds in a word (e.g., "aks" for "ask").

Microcephaly Head size smaller than the age- and gender-appropriate size.

Micrognathia A very small lower jaw that is frequently paired with a recessed chin.

Modality According to Fillmore, one of two components of sentences, which looks at the influence of semantics on grammar, particularly as applied to verb tense, the question form, and negation.

Modeling The demonstration of a desired behavior to elicit an imitative response.

Morphology Units of meaning that make up the grammar of language by modifying meaning at the word level.

Multimodality approach An approach to therapy that incorporates information from all sensory systems to teach a conceptual element.

Mutism Not speaking; may be selective, meaning a child does not talk in certain settings, or elective, meaning there is no organic or physical disability that prevents the child from talking.

N

Nativism The idea that the capacity to develop language is innate, with language knowledge coming to fruition as the child matures biologically.

Nonfluent aphasia Slow, labored speech, word retrieval deficits, and motor planning deficits due to a lesion or lesions in the anterior language area and left premotor cortex (Broca's area).

Nonliteral language Language that is abstract and symbolic.

Nystagmus Uncontrollable rapid eye movements.

O

Otitis media Inflammation of the middle ear.

Otitis media with effusion Inflammation of the middle ear accompanied by the accumulation of infected fluid.

P

Paraphasia The unintentional substitution of an incorrect word for an intended word.

Penetrating head injury An open head injury resulting in a fracturing or perforation of the skull, with the meninges becoming torn or lacerated.

Percentile scores The percentage of individuals in the standardization sample for an age level who scored below a predetermined raw score.

Perceptual-cognitive skills The integration of thinking and organizing sensory input.

Peripheral hearing loss Conductive hearing losses and losses related to malfunction of the inner ear.

Perlocutionary stage The social stage of communication development during which the child is interactive but uses nonverbal and unintentional communication.

Perpetuating factors Factors that result in the persistence of a language and/or communication deficit.

Perseveration Unintentional repetitive movements or vocalizations.

Phoneme–grapheme correspondence The association of a printed letter with the sound it makes.

Phonemic awareness Recognizing that words are made up of sounds and understanding the differences between phonemes.

Phonemic segmentation The act of breaking down a word into sounds.

Phonemic synthesis The act of combining sounds presented in isolation into a single word.

Phonological processing Understanding of the sound system of a language.

Phonology The distribution and sequencing or organization of phonemes within a language.

Placebo effect An inactive treatment that has a suggestive effect on the individual's symptomology.

Polydrug exposure The use of multiple drugs, including alcohol, by a pregnant mother.

Postlingual hearing loss The acquisition of a hearing loss after the development of speech and language.

Pragmatics The social use and functions of language for communication.

Precipitating factors Factors that result in the onset of the language and/or communication problem.

Predisposing factors Factors that dispose or incline an individual toward an impairment related to his or her language and communication skills.

Prelingual hearing loss The acquisition of a hearing loss prior to the development of speech and language.

Preoperational skills Skills needed to emerge into conceptual thinking and leading to prelogical thought.

Presymbolic level The stage of communication that precedes the use of gestures, words, and actions to denote specific language concepts or words.

Principles Summary statements of experimental evidence that provide the rules from which treatment procedures are developed.

Procedures Concrete, measurable, and objective clinical activities based on the experimental evidence that form the foundation for therapy outlined in principles.

Processing How the child handles information that is presented to him or her visually and aurally.

Prognathism Abnormal facial construction in which the upper and/or lower jaws project forward.

Prompt A supplementary antecedent that is added to the original stimulus to increase the probability of a correct response.

Proposition According to Fillmore, the second component of a sentence, which regulates the relationship between nouns and verbs.

Propositional force The literal meaning of a sentence.

Proptosis Bulging of the eyes.

Prosody The use of tone and accent to embellish spoken language.

Prospective Memory memory involved in remembering to do daily activities at the appropriate time

Psycholinguistics The study of language structures and processes that undergird the ability to speak and understand language.

Psychostimulants Medications that have antidepressant effects and stimulate the production of dopamine, which acts on the frontal lobe to improve executive functions.

Q

Quality control A person's ability to provide an explanation for his or her own actions.

R

Rapport A harmonious connection between two individuals based on mutual respect and a level of trust.

Reliability The consistency of a test in measuring what it claims to measure in the same individual on reexamination.

Retrograde amnesia A common sequela of traumatic brain injury that creates difficulty in remembering the events that led up to the accident.

S

Scaffolding system A "stair-step" approach to problem solving in a group consisting of students at varying levels of ability, in which a high-functioning child provides a model for a lower-functioning child.

Screening The administration of short tests to determine if a child's language is within normal limits or if he or she needs to be referred for a complete diagnostic procedure.

Scripts Scenarios designed to facilitate language development and the application of language skills to reading.

Segmentation The breaking down of sentences into words, words into syllables, and syllables into phonemes.

Selective attention The attention needed to focus on what is important among myriad stimuli.

Semantics The knowledge and ideas a person has about the objects and events in his or her world; the content of language.

Sensorimotor skills Skills involving the integration of sensory feedback and motor behaviors.

Sensorimotor stages Stages of development that precede early symbolic communication, characterized by the development and integration of the sensory and motor systems of the child.

Sensorineural hearing loss Hearing loss due to malfunctioning of the inner ear or damage to the acoustic nerve.

Sensory integration The organization and interpretation of input from various sensory systems of the body.

Sequence A disorder in which many of the anomalies are actually secondary disorders caused by a single anomaly, which sets off a chain reaction of changes in the developing embryo that result in other anomalies.

Shaping The differential reinforcement of successive approximations to a specified target to create a new behavior.

Skill A sequence of responses that are learned through the coordination of various motor and sensory systems and are eventually organized into complex response chains.

Sociolinguistics The study of social and cultural influences on language structures.

Soft signs Possible early indicators that, taken as a group, could be warning signs for a possible language-based learning disability.

Speech acts In a communicative exchange, expressions verbalized by the speaker, such as receiving information, giving information, or acknowledging an individual (greeting and departing words).

Speech community A group of people who routinely and frequently use a shared language to interact with each other.

Standard deviation A statistical measurement used to document the disparity between an individual's test score and the mean.

Standard score A score obtained by converting the raw score to a weighted raw score that takes into account the average score and the variability of scores of children of that age.

Standardized test A test that has been evaluated using a sample of individuals that represents a broad cross-section of cultural groups. Standardized tests offer norms that allow a comparison of a child's performance on a test with those in the standardization sample.

Stereotypical phrases Fixed, unvarying utterances that are often heard produced by others and are used in excess by children with social interaction deficits.

Stereotypic speech The unintentional use of a real or invented word or phrase that has little meaning.

Stimulability The degree to which a child can imitate a language construct presented by the clinician; the less intervention is needed, the more the child is stimulable.

Strabismus The deviation of the eye(s) from center when looking forward.

Subcortical pathways Interconnections in the brain that lie below the cerebral cortex.

Survival language Knowing the lingo associated with peer language and knowing how to be part of a peer group through appropriate actions and communication styles.

Sustained attention The ability to remain on task, but without the time constraints of focused attention.

Symbolic level Communication in which the individual understands the relationships between words and objects and events (i.e., that the words represent the objects and events).

Syndrome The presence of multiple anomalies in the same individual, with all of those anomalies having a single cause.

Syntax Appropriate, rule-based ordering of words in connected discourse.

T

Tactile defensiveness A pronounced dislike of being touched, usually accompanied by a negative emotional reaction.

Task analysis The breaking down of a task into small steps that must be accomplished individually before the whole task can be completed.

Test-retest reliability Evaluating the reliability of a test by having the child take the same test on two separate occasions (usually within a 6-month period) and comparing the child's performance on each test.

Therapy The process of establishing and habituating new skills, then generalizing the skills to the client's natural environment.

Topic-associated narrative A series of narratives linked to a topic, with no particular theme or point to the narrative.

Topic-centered narrative A tightly structured discourse on a single topic or a series of closely related topics and events.

Total-task presentation A series of sequenced behaviors, all of which must be done completely and in sequence in order to master the skills and be reinforced.

Transformational generative grammar (TGG) A theory of rules, or transformations, that govern how syntactic components of our speech are combined to express language.

V

Validity The degree to which a test measures what it is designed to measure, and how well it does so.

Vigilance The attention skills needed to develop and use a memory bank.

Index

Phonlogical processing, 457
Phonological awareness, 629
  instruction in, 465–466
  training program, outline of, 180
Phonological coding in working memory, 402
Phonological deficits, 405–406
Phonological processing, 417–423
Phonology deficits, 20
Physical assistance, 285
Physical symptoms, of TBI, 542
Piagetian sensorimotor stage, 288
PICO, 320–321
Pictographic writing systems, 183
Picture Exchange Communication System (PECS), 144–146
Pierre Robin sequence. *See* Robin sequence/Stickler syndrome
Pierre Robin syndrome. *See* Robin sequence/Stickler syndrome
Pivotal response training (PRT), 137
Placebo effect, 509
Play-Doh, 121
Polydrug-exposed infants, 86–88
Post assessment conference, 220–221
Post head injury, 563–565
Postlingual hearing loss, 76
Posttraumatic amnesia (PTA), 531
Poverty, modification of environmental factors of, 283
Prader-Willi syndrome, 64–68
  information source for, 68
  language characteristics of children with, 66–67
  physical characteristics associated with, 64–65
  speech characteristics of children with, 66–67
Pragmatic deficits, 410–412
Pragmatic domain, 22–24
Pragmatics, 22
Precipitating factors, 579
Predictive validity, 203
Predisposing factors, 579
Predominantly hyperactive-impulsivity, 491
Predominantly inattention, 491
Prelingual hearing impairment, 76
Prematuriy/high-risk infancy, language disorders associated with, 80–82
  cytomegalovirus (CMV) infection, 81–82
  failure to thrive (FTT), and premature babies, 80
Prenatal exposure to drugs, interventions for infants, 290–291. *See also* alcohol/drugs, prenatal exposure to
Preoperational skills, 443
Preponderance of evidence, 319
Pre-reading, 402–403
Preschool children
  emergent literacy, development of, 294–295
  intellectual disabilities, therapy approaches, 287–289
  language assessments of, 252–255
  language deficits in, 191–223
  language delays in, 257–296
  language development in, 163–171, 362–364
  language disorders in, 167, 257–296
  language impairments in, 362–364
  literacy/linguistic success in, 161–186
  speech impairments in, 362–364
  treatment of, 257–296

Preschool Language Assessment Instrument, 2nd ed., 254
Preschool Language Scale, 4th ed., 254
Preschool Language Scale—3 (PLS-3), 556
Presidents Commission on Excellence in Special Education (PCESE), 321
Presymbolic level, 213
Primitive narratives, 184–185
Principles. *See also* therapeutic principles
  alphabetic, 466
  defined, 272
  language development, 9
  special education law, 305
  therapeutic, 269–271
Priori criteria, 324
Problem, defining, 197–199
Procedures, defined, 273
Processes/processing, 506
  abstract thought, 365
  assessment, 194
  attention demanding control, 395
  auditory, 591
  central auditory, 591
  evaluative-planning, 280–283
  phonological, 417–423, 457
  scientific model to diagnostic, 197–222
  test-teach-retest, 216
Processing-dependent tasks, 462
Professional interaction, 276
Professional wisdom, 318
Proficiency stage. *See* fixation stage of development
Profound intellectual disabilities, 93–94
Prognathism, 40
Project Read, 466–467
Promoting Alternative Thinking Strategies (PATHS), 294
Prompting, graduated, 462
Prompting hierarchy, 284
Prompting with verbal assistance, 286
Proposition, 12
Propositional force, 13
Proptosis, 61
Prose literacy, 370
Protoimperatives, 266
Psychiatric disorders, 47
Psychoeducational Battery, 214
Psychoeducational Profile (PEP), 133
Psycholinguistic theory of language development, 11
Psychosocial examination, 556
Psychosocial impairment, 549
Psychostimulants, 508
Pygmalion effect, 639–640

Q

Qualitative literacy, 370
Quality control, 497
Queensland University Inventory of Literacy (QUIL), 556
Questions
  evidence-based practice/education, posing, 320–321
  interview, 198–199
  preceding test selection, 202–204